Introduction to Audiology Today

James W. Hall, III

Nova Southeastern University

University of Florida

Salus University

University of Pretoria South Africa

PEARSON

Boston   Columbus   Indianapolis   New York   San Francisco   Upper Saddle River
Amsterdam   Cape Town   Dubai   London   Madrid   Milan   Munich   Paris   Montréal   Toronto
Delhi   Mexico City   São Paulo   Sydney   Hong Kong   Seoul   Singapore   Taipei   Tokyo

Executive Editor & Publisher: Stephen D. Dragin
Editorial Assistant: Michelle Hochberg
Marketing Manager: Joanna Sabella
Development Editor: Jenny Gessner
Production Editor: Karen Mason
Production Coordination: Walsh & Associates, Inc.

Electronic Composition: Jouve
Text Design and Illustrations: Jouve
Cover Designer: Laura Gardner
Cover Photo Credits: Kstudija/Shutterstock and
3Art/Shutterstock

Text Photo Credits: Jerry Northern, pp. 6, 129; James W. Hall, III, pp. 55, 91, 97, 98, 100, 105, 114, 159, 218, 274, 303, 365, 387, 388, 404, 479, 484; Peter Dallos, p. 70; Frank Musiek, p. 79; Diane Guercio, pp. 95, 218; Robin Hamill-Ruth, p. 96; Vickie Ledon, pp. 104, 108, 192, 193; Elizabeth Aiken, pp. 107, 275; Herb Weitman/WUSTL Photos, p. 166; Susan Jerger, p. 177; Etymotic Research, Inc., p. 195; James Jerger, p. 215; David Kemp, p. 236; Deborah Hayes, p. 254; Jack Katz, p. 256; Robert Keith, p. 256; Don Jewett, p. 273; Nina Kraus, p. 281; Bruce Taylor, p. 290; Richard Gans, p. 312; Kathleen Campbell, p. 342; Sharon Kujawa, p. 348; Linda Hood, p. 370; Teri James Bellis, p. 378; Ruth Bentler, p. 399; Harvey Dillon, p. 403; Carol Flexer, p. 417; Kristine English, p. 424; David Luterman, p. 429; Patricia Kricos, p. 435; Rich Tyler, p. 457; David Baguley, p. 466; Christie Yoshinago-Itano, p. 478; Cheryl deConde Johnson, p. 481. All other photo credits appear on the page with the image.

Copyright © 2014 by Pearson Education, Inc. All rights reserved. Manufactured in the United States of America. This publication is protected by Copyright, and permission should be obtained from the publisher prior to any prohibited reproduction, storage in a retrieval system, or transmission in any form or by any means, electronic, mechanical, photocopying, recording, or likewise. To obtain permission(s) to use material from this work, please submit a written request to Pearson Education, Inc., Permissions Department, One Lake Street, Upper Saddle River, New Jersey 07458, or you may fax your request to 201-236-3290.

Many of the designations by manufacturers and sellers to distinguish their products are claimed as trademarks. Where those designations appear in this book, and the publisher was aware of a trademark claim, the designations have been printed in initial caps or all caps.

Between the time website information is gathered and then published, it is not unusual for some sites to have closed. Also, the transcription of URLs can result in typographical errors. The publisher would appreciate notification where these errors occur so that they may be corrected in subsequent editions.

Library of Congress Cataloging-in-Publication Data

Hall, James W. (James Wilbur)
  Introduction to audiology today / James W. Hall III.
    p. ; cm.
  Includes bibliographical references and index.
  ISBN-13: 978-0-205-56923-6
  ISBN-10: 0-205-56923-4
  I. Title.
  [DNLM: 1. Audiometry—methods.   2. Audiology.   3. Ear Diseases—diagnosis.
4. Ear Diseases—rehabilitation.   5. Hearing—physiology. WV 272]
  RF294
  617.8'075—dc23
                                                              2013015368

3   16

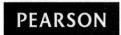

ISBN-10: 0-205-56923-4
ISBN-13: 978-0-205-56923-6

In memory of my first mentor
James W. Hall, Jr., O.D.
(1922–2012)

With deep gratitude to my audiology father
James Jerger, PhD

With love to my wife and best friend
Missy Hall

Brief Contents

Contents

PART II   Audiology Procedures and Protocols   87

Chapter 4   Preparing for Hearing Assessment   87

PART III   Patient Populations   315

Preface

The importance of the sense of hearing cannot be overemphasized. Within months after birth and even before an infant utters one word, the sense of hearing is shaping brain development. The sense of hearing plays a critical role in a child's acquisition of speech, language, and communication in general. As a child enters school, hearing influences a child's reading skills and academic performance.

Hearing loss and related disorders like balance problems are often early signs of a wide variety of diseases affecting children or adults. Results of hearing testing contribute to earlier identification and more effective treatment for many diseases. Hearing loss is very common in older adults but often not recognized by physicians and family members. Most people don't realize that adults with untreated hearing loss experience reduced quality of life and loss of income each year due to their communication difficulties. And problems with hearing and listening are not uncommon in persons with disorders involving the nervous system like traumatic brain injury and dementia. In fact, recent research in elderly populations confirms a clear connection between hearing loss and decline in mental functions.

It's important for teachers, speech pathologists, and health professionals to have an understanding of hearing and hearing loss. *Introduction to Audiology Today* was written for students in communicative sciences and disorders and related areas of study. In reading the book you will learn about how we hear. You'll gain an appreciation for the profession of audiology and the ways audiologists detect, diagnose, and treat hearing loss. You'll discover in this book that audiologists greatly improve the quality of life of children and adults with hearing and related disorders.

Organization

Parts

This book is organized into four parts. Part I: Profession and Principles of Audiology introduces the reader to the profession of audiology, to sound, and to the ear. Chapters in Part II, Audiology Procedures and Protocols, review the test procedures and protocols used to evaluate hearing from the ear to the brain including techniques for hearing testing of infants and young children. Part III, Patient Populations, is a review of diseases that cause hearing loss and other explanations for hearing loss such as exposure to excessive noise and advancing age. The final part, Audiologic Management Technology, Techniques, and Rehabilitation, is devoted to a summary of modern technologies and evidence-based techniques for effective management of hearing loss and related disorders including balance disturbances.

Features

Each chapter in *Introduction to Audiology Today* includes features to facilitate learning.

- Learning Objectives, a Chapter Focus, and Key Terms at the beginning of each chapter orient the reader to important content and new vocabulary that will follow. Three additional features appear in each chapter to enhance reader interest in the content and to facilitate learning.

- Clinical Connections are brief notations that relate information in the chapter to audiology practice, specifically the diagnosis and management of hearing loss and related disorders.

- WebWatch features direct readers to Internet resources on topics covered in the chapter including video clips illustrating clinical techniques and procedures.

- The Leaders and Luminaries feature includes a brief biographical sketch and a photograph of some of the persons who've made especially important contributions to audiology or hearing science. The Leaders and Luminaries feature is intended to bring the subject matter to life. The feature also reminds readers that the growth of audiology is due to the tireless efforts of individual audiologists and hearing scientists.

- Each chapter concludes with two features: one is called Pulling It All Together, which summarizes succinctly the topics covered in the chapter, and the second is a list of relevant Readings for students who seek additional information.

- A detailed Glossary at the end of the book provides easy access to definitions of new terms that are important in understanding hearing and hearing loss.

- Following the Glossary is a compilation of all References cited within the book to guide students to primary sources of information plus an author index and a comprehensive subject index.

Overview

Introduction to Audiology Today is a new textbook offering students a fresh overview of the broad scope of a dynamic profession. An introduction to hearing and hearing disorders is likely to be of benefit to all students who are thinking about a career in speech pathology, audiology, education, or any aspect of healthcare.

- After a review of the profession of audiology in Chapter 1, the reader is introduced to two areas of basic knowledge that audiologists apply every day in their clinical practice: the principles of sound and functional anatomy of the auditory system from the ear to the brain. The review includes current research findings that have improved our understanding of hearing and how persons with hearing loss can be helped.

- Clinically oriented chapters on test techniques and procedures incorporate case studies to illustrate the practical application of newly learned information. For example, chapters that review pure tone and speech audiometry are followed with cases demonstrating how test findings are recorded on an audiogram and analyzed in the description of degree, configuration, and type of hearing loss.

- Chapter 4 focuses on preparation for hearing assessment with discussion of timely and clinically important topics not included in other textbooks, including patient privacy and security and prevention of medical errors in audiology. Chapter 7 is devoted to the challenging topic of masking principles and procedures.

- Diseases involving the peripheral or central auditory system are reviewed in Chapters 11 and 12. The review includes a number of diagrams and photographs to increase the reader's appreciation of how selected diseases affect the auditory system. The chapters emphasize the impact of peripheral and central disorders on hearing function and also the audiologist's role in the diagnosis and medical referral of such patients. The practice of audiology goes far beyond hearing testing. The final section of the book is devoted to a discussion of modern rehabilitation technologies and techniques. Chapter 13 focuses on technology, including devices like hearing aids, cochlear implants, and FM systems. Chapter 14 emphasizes the critical role of aural rehabilitation and counseling in management of children and adults with hearing loss. Chapter 15 is set aside for a review of false or exaggerated hearing loss, tinnitus, and hyperacusis. These three clinical entities are commonly encountered in audiology practice, but they aren't accurately described or categorized as diseases.

- The final chapter, 16, highlights how audiologists provide effective management of a handful of remarkably different types of patients.

Supplements

- The Instructor Manual for the book is provided to enhance the learning experience. It includes dozens of case reports highlighting test findings for children and adults with different types of hearing loss. The case reports correspond to material covered in different chapters such as pure tone audiometry, speech, audiometry, masking, and then the clinical application of objective tests like acoustic immittance measures, otoacoustic emissions, and other diagnostic test procedures. The case reports introduce students to how test results are plotted on an audiogram and how findings are analyzed and interpreted in the diagnosis of hearing loss. The presentation of case reports progresses from a discussion of rather basic testing of patients with common auditory disorders to more challenging diagnostic hearing assessments.
- The **Instructor Manual and Test Bank** also contain additional pedagogical features. Measure Your Learning is a series of multiple-choice, fill-in-the-blank, or true/false questions for each chapter that assess the readers' grasp of important factual information.
- **PowerPoint Slides** include key concept summarizations, diagrams, and other graphic aids to enhance learning. They are designed to help students understand, organize, and remember core concepts and theories.

Acknowledgments

No one writes a book alone and in isolation. This book is a product of 40 years of audiological inspiration, education, and experience. I'm indebted to instructors at Northwestern University in the years 1971–1973 who introduced me to audiology while I was a master's degree student in Speech Pathology, particularly Earl Harford, Tom Tillman, and Noel Matkin. Occasional hallway greetings from Raymond Carhart may have subconsciously influenced my career.

In my first position at Methodist Hospital and Baylor College of Medicine in Houston Texas, James Jerger was the perfect mentor for a young and motivated speech pathologist who was interested in converting to audiology. Since then hundreds of audiology colleagues and several very supportive otologists have contributed directly to my career development and indirectly to the writing of this book. And, along the way, I benefited immeasurably from clinical interactions with thousands of patients.

The following persons provided consistently valuable reviews of the manuscript for this book: Judith T. Blumsack, Auburn University; Gerald Church, Central Michigan University; Gary Cottrell, University of Wisconsin, River Falls; Colleen A. McAleer, Clarion University; James McCartney, California State University, Sacramento; Larry Medwetsky, Rochester Hearing and Speech Center; Colleen M. O'Rourke, Georgia State University; Joseph Smaldino, Illinois State University; Jennifer Smart, Towson University; Suzanne Thompson, Iona College; Denise Tucker, The University of North Carolina at Greensboro; Laura Ann Wilber, Northwestern University; and Christopher K. Zalewski, University of Maryland. I look forward to personally thanking each reviewer for his or her good advice.

Last but certainly not least, I thank Steve Dragin and Karen Mason at Pearson and a production team including Kathy Whittier, John Shannon, Michael Walsh, and Jenny Gessner for their efforts and patience in guiding my manuscript on its long and sometimes tedious journey to publication.

About the Author

James W. Hall III received a bachelor's degree in biology from American International College, a master's degree in speech pathology from Northwestern University, and his PhD in audiology from Baylor College of Medicine under the direction of James Jerger. Since then he has held clinical and academic audiology positions at major medical centers throughout the United States. Throughout his career Dr. Hall has also maintained a clinical practice, participated in funded research, and served as a clinical instructor and mentor to Doctor of Audiology students. He now holds appointments as Extraordinary Professor in the Department of Communication Pathology at the University of Pretoria in South Africa and Adjunct Professor in the Department of Audiology at Nova Southeastern University. He also manages James W. Hall III Audiology Consulting LLC.

Dr. Hall is one of the thirty-four founders of the American Academy of Audiology (AAA). Since then he's served the AAA as convention program chair and also on numerous boards, committees, and task forces. In 2012 he received the Distinguished Achievement Award from the Academy.

Dr. Hall's major clinical and research interests are electrophysiology, auditory processing disorders, tinnitus/hyperacusis, and audiology applications of tele-health. He regularly lectures throughout the United States and internationally on these and other audiology and hearing-related topics. Dr. Hall is the author of over 170 peer-reviewed journal articles, monographs, or book chapters. He's also authored or co-authored seven textbooks, including the *Handbook of Auditory Evoked Responses, The Handbook of Otoacoustic Emissions,* the *New Handbook of Auditory Evoked Responses, Audiologists' Desk Reference (Volumes I and II), Objective Assessment of Hearing,* and *Otoacoustic Emissions: Principles, Procedures & Protocols.*

More information about Dr. Hall including access to many of his presentations and publications is available on his website: www.audiologyworld.net.

1 Audiology Yesterday and Today

LEARNING OBJECTIVES

In this chapter, you will learn:

- What an audiologist is and what an audiologist does
- About the profession of audiology
- How the relatively new profession of audiology began
- About the education of audiologists and the Doctor of Audiology degree
- The different work settings where audiologists are employed
- About a variety of career options in audiology
- The kinds of hearing healthcare services that audiologists provide
- That audiology is growing around the world
- The credentials an audiologist needs for clinical practice
- Why audiology is highly ranked as a career choice

KEY TERMS

Audiology
Audiometers
Board certification
Clinical scholar
Cochlear implants
Code of ethics
Doctor of Audiology degree
Educational audiologist
Hearing aids
Hearing science
Industrial audiology
Licensure
Otolaryngology
Otology
Pediatric audiology
Prevalence
Scope of practice

CHAPTER FOCUS

Audiology is a relatively young profession. In this chapter you'll learn about the profession and the kinds of services audiologists provide to people with hearing loss and related disorders. You'll read about some of the remarkable scientists whose work laid the foundation for a profession devoted to diagnosis and treatment of hearing loss. Then you'll discover that the profession of audiology emerged from a need during World War II to provide nonmedical help to soldiers who suffered hearing loss during their military service. You will be introduced in the chapter to Raymond Carhart who is widely recognized as the "Father of Audiology." Carhart essentially founded the new profession and contributed in many ways to audiology throughout his productive career.

Audiology is a highly dynamic profession. For over sixty years audiology has undergone constant change and development. We'll highlight in the chapter some of the major developments and advances in the scope of audiology and the services that audiologists provide. This will naturally lead into a discussion of the education of audiologists, including a description of the Doctor of Audiology (AuD) degree. You'll gain awareness of the many career options available to audiologists today. The chapter concludes with a dozen reasons to consider audiology as a career.

To help you learn the new vocabulary, terms first listed in this chapter are identified by **bold font**, listed among **Key Terms**, and defined in a Glossary at the end of the book.

What Is Audiology?

Audiology is the health profession responsible for caring for persons with hearing loss and related problems. "Audiologists are the primary healthcare professionals who evaluate, diagnose, treat, and manage hearing loss and balance disorders in adults and children" (American Academy of Audiology, 2010). Table 1.1 lists some of the various responsibilities and activities of audiologists. An audiologist usually specializes in one or more of the types of clinical services shown in this table. Some audiologists provide services only to children whereas other audiologists limit their practice to adult patients.

Audiologists evaluate and treat persons with hearing loss across the age spectrum, from newborn infants to elderly adults. Hearing loss is a common condition and healthcare problem. Estimates of the **prevalence** of hearing loss are quite impressive. The term *prevalence* refers to the number of cases of a specific disease or disorder like hearing loss in a given population of people at a specific time. For example, an estimate of prevalence of hearing loss can be made for children or adults living in the United States in the year 2013.

Hearing loss is the third most prevalent chronic health condition among elderly adults who are eligible for Medicare. Approximately one-third of adults between the ages of 65 and 74 have a significant hearing loss that interferes with communication, and the proportion with hearing loss increases to almost one-half for adults over the age of 75 (National Institute on Deafness and Other Communication Disorders, 2010). Although the prevalence of hearing loss in children is lower than it is for adults, the consequences for children are often much more serious. Up to six of every 1000 children are born with some degree of hearing impairment, and the proportion of children with hearing loss increases considerably in the preschool years (JCIH, 2007; Fortnum et al., 2001). Also, about three out of four children in the United States will have an ear infection before they are 3 years old (National Institute on Deafness and Other Communication Disorders, 2010). Ear infections are a common cause for hearing loss in children.

Audiologists are nonphysician healthcare professionals who treat hearing loss using techniques other than medicine or surgery. The majority of patients with hearing loss do not have an underlying disease or disorder that can be treated with drugs or surgery. Over three-fourths

TABLE 1.1

Professional responsibilities and clinical services that audiologists provide. Most audiologists specialize in selected clinical areas on the list.

- Evaluate and diagnose hearing loss and vestibular (balance) disorders
- Prescribe, fit, and dispense hearing aids and other amplification and hearing assistance technologies
- Provide auditory rehabilitation and training to improve listening skills and communication in persons with hearing loss
- Design and implement programs for hearing conservation and protection in persons at risk for hearing loss due to excessive noise exposure
- Design and implement newborn hearing screening programs
- Assess and treat children and adults with hearing problems involving the brain, known as central auditory processing disorders
- Evaluate candidacy of persons with severe hearing loss for management with cochlear implants; program cochlear implants for specific patient needs; provide habilitation or rehabilitation of children and adults with cochlear implants.
- Assess and treat persons with bothersome tinnitus (noise in the ears like ringing or buzzing)
- Perform monitoring of auditory and facial nerve function during surgical procedures to prevent disorders and improve outcome

Source: Adapted from the American Academy of Audiology.

of persons seeking help for hearing loss require the services of audiologists rather than physi-cians (Hall, Freeman, & Bratt, 1994; Zapala et al., 2010).

Audiologists work closely with physicians in the evaluation and management of persons with hearing loss, balance problems, and related disorders. In fact, a sizable proportion of audiologists work in medical settings with physicians who are ear specialists. **Otolaryngology** is the medical specialty that includes treatment of ear disease. Otolaryngologists are surgi-cal physicians with advanced education and training related to the ear, nose, and throat. **Otology** is a subspecialty of otolaryngology. Otologists have expertise in the medical and surgical management of ear diseases. These physician specialists make important contributions to the diagnosis and treatment of some patients with hearing prob-lems. However, audiologists are the healthcare professionals with pri-mary responsibility for caring for persons with hearing loss and related disorders. Later in the chapter you'll learn more about different settings where audiologists work and the types of clinical services audiologists provide.

 WebWatch

You can learn more about audiology and the work of audiologists at the How's Your Hearing? Ask an Audiologist website.

Audiology Yesterday

Scientific Foundation

The scientific underpinnings of audiology can be traced to the late 1800s. Talented physicists, biologists, experimental psychologists, and physicians in Europe and particularly Germany made important discoveries that were necessary for an understanding of the ear and hearing (Feldmann, 1970). Research produced fundamental information about the nature of sound, the structure and function of the ear, and how the brain responds to sound.

The first generation of formally trained hearing scientists was born at the end of the 1800s. **Hearing science** is the branch of scientific study that investigates the auditory system and how it responds to sound. Some areas of study within hearing science include anatomy, physi-ology, psychoacoustics, and auditory neuroscience. There are researchers who conduct inves-tigations only on animals, whereas other researchers focus on human auditory functioning. Hearing scientists in the first half of the twentieth century discovered a number of principles concerned with sound and the auditory system.

One of the first and most famous hearing research centers in the United States was the Psychoacoustic Laboratory (PAL) at Harvard University in Cambridge, Massachusetts. An impressive collection of scientists at the PAL conducted research that formed the foundation of our understanding of how the auditory system functions. These researchers also developed some of the equipment and techniques used in hearing assessment today. Four of the "big names" in hearing science who conducted research at the PAL were Hallowell Davis, Robert Galambos, Ira Hirsh, and Georg von Békésy. Georg von Békésy was a Hungarian-born bio-physicist who in 1961 won the Nobel Prize in Physiology or Medicine for his work on how the ear functions. Later in the book you'll learn more about these remarkable hearing scien-tists and their important contributions to audiology.

The Bell Labs in New York and later New Jersey were another hotbed of hearing research in the early 1900s. Motivated by a commitment to greatly improve communication with tele-phone technology, the Bell Labs hired innovative scientists who in turn developed some of the first devices for hearing testing and also conducted critical research on speech perception. Harvey Fletcher is the most famous of the early hearing scientists at Bell Labs. The pioneer-ing contributions of Fletcher are highlighted in Leaders and Luminaries in Chapter 2. A recent popular book entitled *The Idea Factory: Bell Labs and the Great Age of American Innovation* chronicles this exciting era of discovery (Gertner, 2012).

In the 1920s and 1930s several prominent otolaryngologists in the United States began to use what came to be known as **audiometers** in clinical hearing assessment. An audiometer is a device specifically designed for hearing testing. The operator of an audiometer selects different types of sounds and, using earphones or loudspeakers, presents them to the person being tested at precise volume levels.

A nonphysician named Cordia C. Bunch played a prominent role in pioneering attempts to systematically evaluate hearing. He summarized his research findings and years of patient experiences in a classic book entitled simply *Clinical Audiometry* (Bunch, 1943). When he died unexpectedly at the age of 57, C. C. Bunch was on the faculty at Northwestern University in Evanston, Illinois. In the years just before his death he mentored a young student named Raymond Carhart.

Birth of Audiology

The profession of audiology in the United States was conceived during World War II. Large numbers of soldiers, sailors, airmen, and marines suffered from hearing loss caused by exposure to high-intensity sounds during military service. Physicians were unable to treat the noise-induced hearing problems with medicine or surgery. A handful of officers in the military were assigned the task of developing and providing a rehabilitative program for these servicemen. There were no formally educated or trained audiologists at the time. Indeed, there is considerable discussion and debate about the exact origin of the term *audiology* and when persons in the new profession were first called audiologists (Newby, 1979; Jerger, 2009). Most of the officers in charge of hearing rehabilitation had a pre-war background in speech or some other aspect of communication.

An important component of the military rehabilitation effort for hearing loss was amplification. **Hearing aids** were used to amplify the volume of sound in hopes of facilitating communication in hearing-impaired soldiers. Figure 1.1 depicts a World War II soldier undergoing an evaluation for hearing aid fitting in a military hearing clinic. Hearing aids at the time were cumbersome and quite simple in comparison to the sophisticated hearing instruments available today. Even now amplification is the most common approach to rehabilitation of persons with hearing loss. You'll learn in Chapter 13 about modern hearing aid technology.

Raymond Carhart was prominent among those who did their best to provide care to hearing-impaired servicemen at selected military hospitals in the United States (Jerger, 2009). He is featured as a Leader and Luminary here in recognition of his remarkable contributions to audiology. In 1945, immediately after the war, Carhart returned to a faculty position as speech pathologist at Northwestern University. Recognizing the need for nonmedical healthcare providers who were specifically trained to provide services to persons with hearing impairment, Carhart was instrumental in creating one of the first formal educational programs for audiologists. Raymond Carhart is known as the "Father of Audiology" in recognition of his important role in the development of the profession as well as his many contributions to clinical audiology.

Over a dozen other audiology educational programs were developed in the late 1940s and early 1950s, mostly in the midwestern part of the United States. Some of the new audiology programs began through the efforts of those who had provided hearing services in the military during World War II.

FIGURE 1.1

A soldier undergoing hearing testing in the World War II era. The patient is in a fabricated sound-treated room. He has a hearing-aid earphone in his ear connected with a cable to a hearing aid about the size of a cell phone above his head. The soldier is undergoing testing to determine how well he hears with the hearing aid. Looking through the window in the sound room you'll see a technician or tester in the adjacent room. Photo with appreciation to Jerry Northern, PhD.

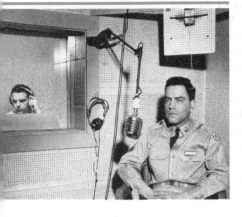

LEADERS AND LUMINARIES

Raymond Carhart (1912–1975)

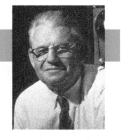

Dr. Carhart earned his bachelor's degree in speech and psychology at Dakota Wesleyan University and a master's degree in speech pathology, experimental phonetics, and psychology at Northwestern University, where he also received his PhD in 1936. Except for 1944 to 1946, when he served in the U.S. Army Medical Corps as Director of the Acoustic Clinic at Deshon General Hospital in Pennsylvania, Carhart remained at Northwestern University throughout his career. There, in 1947, Carhart established the first the academic program in audiology.

Carhart exerted significant influence on the development of the new profession of audiology. His leadership was evidenced by his long tenure as head of the department and hearing clinics at Northwestern University as well as his service to professional organizations and the National Institutes of Health (NIH), by whom he was awarded a Research Career Award in 1963. Throughout his productive career Carhart conducted basic hearing research and highly varied clinical studies, leading to major advances in the quality of audiology practice and patient services. Widely appreciated as a highly effective teacher, he successfully led 45 of his students to completion of doctoral degrees or postdoctoral studies. Dr. Carhart is known as the "Father of Audiology" in well-deserved recognition of his incomparable contributions to the field.

Audiology Grows Up

The first generation of formally educated audiologists entered the profession in the 1950s. A substantial proportion of them graduated with a PhD and went on to pursue an academic career in teaching and research. These early academic audiologists contributed to the creation of additional educational programs at universities around the United States. As a result, the profession of audiology underwent rapid growth and expansion during this period. Among the newly minted audiologists, there is no question that James Jerger was the "most likely to succeed."

With Raymond Carhart as his mentor at Northwestern University, Jerger quickly made a name for himself in the new profession. He is universally known for conducting innovative clinical research and disseminating the findings in a steady stream of scientific publications. Among his many accomplishments, Jerger is particularly well known for his development of new and valuable clinical tests for more accurate diagnosis of hearing loss. You'll encounter the name James Jerger often in subsequent chapters as his important contributions to audiology are cited in discussions of various clinical procedures. He is featured in Leaders and Luminaries in Chapter 8.

Major Developments in the New Profession

Audiology grew steadily during the 1960s and even more so in the 1970s as the initial wave of baby boomers entered college and then graduate programs. Many audiologists found employment in hospitals and other medical facilities, working closely with otolaryngologists and other physicians in the diagnosis of hearing loss. Other audiologists provided clinical services in freestanding speech and hearing centers, took positions as classroom or clinical instructors in universities, or cared for children with hearing impairment in public schools.

Strategies and techniques for diagnosis of hearing loss developed rapidly during this era. One key motivation for the expansion of diagnostic hearing testing was early identification of potentially life-threatening tumors affecting the auditory nerve that runs from the ear to the brain. Back then brain-imaging technology was not yet available for clinical diagnosis. Hearing tests offered the best option for detection of tumors involving the auditory system.

In the late 1970s a modest number of enterprising audiologists left the security of institutional employment to open private practices. These audiologists were among the first to provide rehabilitative services that included the fitting and dispensing of amplifying devices for persons with hearing loss. At the time hearing aid dispensing and sales was not commonplace or accepted practice. Indeed, the professional organization then representing audiologists declared that it was unethical for audiologists to be involved in hearing aid dispensing. The movement toward independent clinical practice of audiology and the inclusion of hearing aid dispensing as a clinical service was a turning point in the evolution of audiology as an autonomous profession.

Audiology scope of practice continued to expand throughout the 1980s and 1990s. The advent of computer technology and scientific advances like digital signal processing led to more sophisticated hearing tests and more effective options for treating patients with hearing loss. Audiologists increasingly provided diverse clinical services that went beyond diagnosis of hearing loss and management with hearing aids. Some of the new services were provided outside the confines of the audiology clinic.

Audiologists took on a wide assortment of new clinical duties such as assessment and management of persons with vestibular disorders, monitoring hearing function of patients undergoing surgery that could damage the auditory system, hearing screening of newborn infants in the intensive care nursery setting (see Leaders and Luminaries feature on Marion Downs), and the evaluation and rehabilitation of patients with severe hearing loss who were candidates for surgical implantation of electrical hearing devices.

L E A D E R S   A N D   L U M I N A R I E S

Marion Downs

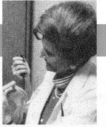

Marion Downs earned her bachelor's degree in political science and English from the University of Minnesota and in 1951 her master's degree in audiology from the University of Denver. She's also received an honorary Doctor of Science from the University of Colorado and an honorary Doctor of Human Services from the University of Northern Colorado. Early in her career Dr. Downs was involved in providing audiology and speech pathology services in a Veteran's Administration facility in Denver. In the early 1960s she worked in an otolaryngology clinic at the University of Colorado School of Medicine where she initiated the revolutionary practice of fitting hearing aids on infants by the age of 6 months. Dr. Downs recognized that early intervention for hearing loss was critical, even though the typical age of hearing aid fitting at the time was 2 to 3 years.

She has remained committed to promoting newborn hearing screening, early intervention for hearing loss, and pediatric audiology in general. In 1969 Dr. Downs played an essential role in the development of the Joint Committee on Infant Hearing and then in the 1990s in the implementation of universal newborn hearing screening in the United States and elsewhere in the world. Dr. Downs has published over 100 articles and several books, including a highly popular textbook co-authored with colleague Jerry Northern entitled *Hearing in Children*. The book has undergone many editions and been translated in multiple foreign languages.

Approaching the age of 100 years, Marion Downs is an inspirational and beloved leader and luminary in audiology. She's has certainly earned the honorary title "Mother of Pediatric Audiology." A search of Marion Downs on the Internet, for example, the Silver Planet website, should provide some interesting information.

Education of Audiologists
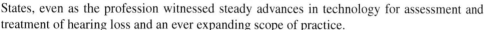

 ClinicalConnection

Audiologists now have unprecedented access to a variety of techniques for diagnosis of hearing in persons of all ages, from infants only a few hours old to elderly adults. In later chapters of the book, you'll learn about these techniques and how they are applied in hearing testing and diagnosis of hearing loss.

Historical Perspective

In the early years, most audiologists entered the profession with a bachelor's degree. A relatively small number went on to pursue a PhD degree, in preparation for an academic career in teaching and/or research. As the profession developed in the 1960s, educational requirements for the practice of audiology expanded to include a clinically oriented two-year master's degree program. The master's-level educational model persisted for the next thirty years in the United States, even as the profession witnessed steady advances in technology for assessment and treatment of hearing loss and an ever expanding scope of practice.

Early in the 1990s, farsighted leaders in the profession recognized the need for clinically oriented doctoral level education in audiology. Audiology needed an educational model resembling other health professions, such as optometry and dentistry. It was simply not possible for a two-year program to provide the coursework and clinical experience necessary to adequately prepare students for a career in audiology.

The transition from a master's to a doctoral level of graduate education was a major challenge for the profession of audiology. The change was not enthusiastically endorsed or even accepted by some audiologists in academic and clinical settings. Fortunately for the profession, in the late 1990s, visionaries at a handful of well-respected universities pushed forward with the development of coursework and curricula leading to a four-year **Doctor of Audiology degree** (or AuD). The movement gathered momentum and within a relatively short time period the AuD became the entry level degree for the practice of audiology.

The Doctor of Audiology (AuD) Degree

A bachelor's degree is necessary for entry into Doctor of Audiology programs. Some students applying to Doctor of Audiology programs have an undergraduate background in communicative disorders. Other applicants enter audiology graduate study with degrees in a variety of other areas, such as psychology, biology, English, or music. Some undergraduate coursework in mathematics and the sciences is strongly recommended, particularly courses in biology, chemistry, and physics.

Doctor of Audiology or AuD programs generally include three years of coursework and supervised clinical experience plus a fourth-year clinical externship. Table 1.2 shows a sample curriculum leading to an AuD, including didactic courses and clinical practicum requirements.

Review of this table shows that the first two years include classroom and didactic courses, covering introductory and basic information pertaining to audiology. As the program progresses there is a greater emphasis on clinical courses and rotations through different clinical services.

Each semester, Doctor of Audiology students participate in closely supervised clinical practicum experiences in addition to receiving classroom instruction. Students in the first year of the AuD program are allotted time for observation of different clinical activities. For example, a student might go to a hospital speech and hearing center every Tuesday morning to watch audiologists as they test patients for hearing loss using different devices and techniques. Or a student might observe newborn infants undergoing hearing screening in the nursery of a local hospital.

As the students complete more advanced clinical coursework in the AuD curriculum they also spend a designated amount of time each week in specific clinical settings. Students at

T A B L E   1 . 2   Sample curriculum for courses in a four-year Doctor of Audiology program. Courses are listed for fall, spring, and summer semesters of the first three years.

YEAR 1

Fall

Basic Auditory Sciences (3): Nature of sound, structure, and function of auditory system, frequency selectivity, auditory filtering, and psychoacoustics of pure tones and complex sounds.

Amplification I (2): Theoretical and applied understanding of current technology in amplification systems for hearing impaired.

Hearing Aid Analysis Lab (1): Advanced analysis and description of electroacoustic properties of hearing aids.

Principles of Audiological Evaluation (3): Advanced procedures in speech audiometry, masking, and audiogram interpretation.

Anatomy and Physiology of the Auditory System (2): In-depth coverage of anatomy and physiology of auditory system to support understanding of auditory function in persons with healthy auditory mechanisms and those with specific disorders.

Anatomy and Physiology of Balance (1): The anatomy and physiology of balance and the nature of balance disorders.

Initial Clinical Experience in Audiology (1): For beginning graduate students in audiology. Opportunity to engage in various phases of audiology practice under supervision.

Spring

Clinical Clerkship (1): Beginning level audiology practicum.

Clinical Auditory Electrophysiology (3): Auditory electrophysiological measures used in clinical assessment, including auditory brainstem response (ABR) and otoacoustic emissions (OAEs).

Pediatric Audiology (3): Seminar in pediatric issues in audiology.

Deaf Culture (1): Issues in deafness.

Audiological Rehabilitation – Adults (2): Exploration of theoretical and clinical literature. Description of assessment and management strategies.

Occupational & Environmental Hearing Conservation (3): Seminar in hearing conservation and noise control.

Summer

Clinical Clerkship (1): Beginning level audiology practicum.

Peripheral and Central Auditory Disorders (Clinical Decision Making) (2): Clinical decision making: case-based exercises in problem solving in clinical audiology.

Medical Audiology (2): Differential diagnosis of hearing impairment.

Functional Human Neuroanatomy (4): Intensive readings, lectures, and labs in specialized fields of neuroscience and allied disciplines.

YEAR 2

Fall

Clinical Practice in Hearing Assessment (2): Audiology internship rotations.

Audiological Rehabilitation – Children (2): Exploration of theoretical and clinical literature. Assessment and therapy techniques for children.

Amplification II (2): Digital and programmable technology in hearing aids.

Auditory Processing Disorders (3): Anatomy and physiology of central auditory nervous system and disorders of auditory processing that occur in humans. Focus on evaluation and treatment of auditory processing disorders.

Statistical Methods in Social Research I (3): Descriptive statistics, estimation, significance tests, two-sample comparisons, methods for nominal and ordinal data, regression and correlation, introduction to multiple-regression measures and their use in clinical practice.

Spring

Clinical Practice in Hearing Assessment (2): Audiology internship rotations.

Communication in Aging (3): Characteristics of and management approaches for communication disorders found with some frequency in elderly. Communication enhancement stressed.

Introduction to Graduate Research (3): Critical evaluation of research design and analysis for graduate students in audiology.

Amplification III (3): Theoretical and applied understanding of current and future technology in amplification systems in (a) recent advances in programmable and digital hearing aids, (b) hearing aid selection procedures for special populations, (c) assistive learning devices, and (d) classroom amplification systems.

Cochlear Implants I (3): Principles and procedures for implant management from pre-candidacy evaluations through postoperative therapies.

Summer

Clinical Practice in Hearing Assessment (4): Audiology internship rotations.

Professional Issues in Hearing Care Delivery (3): Federal and state regulations, audiological jurisprudence, audiological management, and interfacing with other professionals.

Auditory Pharmacology (2): Introduction to pharmacology, with particular attention to auditory-vestibular system effects.

YEAR 3

Fall

Graduate Practicum (5): Clinical practicum for AuD students.

Psychosocial Aspects of Hearing Loss (2): Psychological implications of hearing impairment. Specifically psychoeducational, psychosocial, and counseling strategies and rehabilitation procedures for patient and family management.

Advanced Auditory Electrophysiology (3): Advanced seminar in auditory electrophysiological measures and their use in clinical practice, including electrocochleography (ECochG), cortical auditory evoked responses, nonauditory evoked responses, electroneuronography (ENoG), and neurophysiological monitoring.

Audiology Research Project (3): Completion of the audiology research project required for the AuD degree.

Spring

Graduate Practicum (4): Clinical practicum for AuD students.

Cochlear Implants II (3): Advanced techniques in implant management.

Vestibular Disorders (2): Mechanics and physiology of disorders of balance, and approaches to diagnostic assessment and rehabilitation.

Counseling Skills for Non-Counselors (3): Counseling skills in didactic communication and in small groups.

YEAR 4: EXTERNSHIP YEAR

Source: Adapted from the University of Florida.

FIGURE 1.2

A Doctor of Audiology student preparing to conduct hearing testing of an adult patient. The elderly patient is sitting in a sound-treated room. When testing begins, the student will sit in front of an audiometer in the adjacent control room. Courtesy of GN Otometrics.

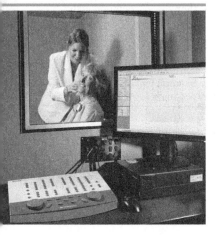

this point have a general knowledge and understanding of hearing, hearing testing, and hearing loss. In fact, students have actually spent time practicing hearing testing either on a computer device or with fellow students. Figure 1.2 shows a Doctor of Audiology student in a clinic performing a common hearing test with an older adult patient.

Over the course of the four-year graduate program, students progress from assisting in the provision of various clinical services to actually testing and treating patients under the supervision of a preceptor who is an instructor in the AuD program. For the most part, the students' clinical experiences parallel the topics covered in the courses listed in Table 1.2. Later in the book you'll learn all about the different tests that audiologists use in hearing assessment of children and adults. You'll also be introduced to a variety of techniques and technologies that audiologists apply in the management of persons with hearing and related disorders.

Admission Requirements. Students applying to a Doctor of Audiology program with a bachelor's degree are typically required to submit an official transcript for undergraduate work and letters of recommendation. Doctor of Audiology programs at most universities also require applicants to take the Graduate Record Examination (GRE).

The timeframe for application to Doctor of Audiology programs varies from one university to the next but the deadline is usually in January or February of the year the student will begin graduate studies. Almost all students begin their Doctor of Audiology program in late summer or early fall of the academic year because there is little flexibility in the class schedule for the programs. The majority of Doctor of Audiology programs require four years for completion, including a fourth-year externship experience. However, several universities with concentrated curriculum formats offer three-year programs.

WebWatch

AuD programs offered at different universities are listed in the student program page of the American Academy of Audiology's (AAA) website. University links will take you to websites for specific Doctor of Audiology programs where you can learn more about the faculty, the curriculum, clinical learning opportunities, admission requirements, and financial information.

Distance Learning Doctor of Audiology Programs. During the transition in audiology education from the master's to the doctoral level, four major universities developed programs that allow practicing audiologists to pursue the AuD degree while still working. In a distance learning program faculty members at a university and sometimes guest faculty from other universities or work settings teach courses online, utilizing special computer programs. Students also learn by reading articles and books and by viewing DVD videos of lectures and clinical procedures. Distance learning technology and programs have become commonplace in many academic areas.

A distance learning educational option for earning the new AuD was essential for the relatively smooth and rapid conversion of audiology from a master's to a doctoral level. When the first AuD programs were developed most practicing audiologists held a master's degree. From the late 1990s onward, thousands of practicing audiologists took the opportunity to pursue their AuD via distance learning. Figure 1.3 shows that the majority of audiologists now hold a doctoral degree. Two universities continue to offer a distance learning option for a Doctor of Audiology degree to audiologists with a master's degree.

Wanted ... PhD Audiologists!

The demand for audiologists with research skills, interests, and experience is considerable, and it is steadily increasing. Audiologists usually complete a PhD program in preparation for an academic career that focuses on teaching and research. Faculty members with PhDs are

needed in university graduate programs to educate future generations of audiologists. There is also a demand for PhD-level audiologists who have the skills to conduct original research on hearing
and related topics. Research is the foundation upon which clinical
audiology rests.

PhD-level audiologists are in high demand to a large extent
because the number of new graduates entering academic institutions is less than the number of audiology faculty members who
are retiring at the end of their careers. There is another factor
contributing to the shortage of PhD audiologists in academic settings. Newly graduated PhD-level audiologists now sometimes opt
for a career in an industrial setting where they are well compensated financially. **Industrial audiology** might involve conducting
research in the laboratories of a manufacturer of hearing aids, or of
other devices or equipment.

The Clinical Scholar

A select number of universities offer the opportunity for highly
motivated students to complete a combined Doctor of Audiology
degree and PhD program. Universities offering both the AuD and
PhD degrees are included among those listed on the website of
the American Academy of Audiology. The usual sequence of a combined-degree program
is to first fulfill requirements for the AuD, including intensive clinical experience during
the fourth-year externship. Students then continue on with individualized coursework in a
highly focused area, in addition to "research tools" courses such as statistics and experimental
design. The combined program includes research projects and dissertation research under the
guidance of a mentor and a doctoral committee.

A combined AuD/PhD program is an efficient route that leads to the credentials required
for a **clinical scholar**. A clinical scholar is a professional who has expertise in providing
patient services combined with research education and experience.
Some of the courses required in the AuD curriculum also apply toward
the PhD degree. Audiologists who complete an AuD/PhD program are
well prepared to conduct clinical research and to assume a leadership
role in academic audiology for years to come. Most graduates who
earn both AuD and PhD degrees are employed in major university
environments where their work combines the three traditional areas
of an academic career ... research, teaching, and professional service.

The Profession of Audiology Today

Current Clinical Services

Students in Doctor of Audiology programs complete coursework in all
aspects of clinical audiology. As they progress through an AuD program, students also acquire, under supervision, clinical experience
with diverse test procedures required for assessment of hearing loss in
patients of all ages. In addition, AuD students gain experience with strategies and techniques
for nonmedical treatment of hearing loss. Students often discover in their classroom or clinical
studies a particular interest in certain aspects of audiology or in providing services to patients
with a particular type of problem. Sometimes the clinical preference is simply to work only
with pediatric or only with adult patients.

F I G U R E   1 . 3

The proportion of audiologists with different academic
degrees. Most audiologists now hold a doctoral-
level degree. Courtesy of the American Academy of
Audiology.

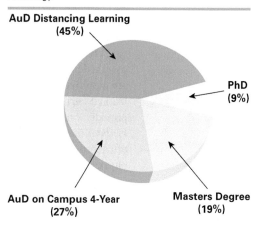

AuD Distancing Learning (45%)

PhD (9%)

AuD on Campus 4-Year (27%)

Masters Degree (19%)

WebWatch

"The Student Academy of Audiology (SAA) is the
national student organization of the American
Academy of Audiology that serves as a collective
voice for students and advocates for the rights,
interests, and welfare of students pursuing
careers in audiology. The SAA introduces
students to lifelong involvement in activities that
promote and advance the profession of audiology
and provides services, information, education,
representation, and advocacy for the profession
and the public we serve." You'll find plenty of
interesting information about audiology as a
career at the SAA website.

Students' interests strongly influence their decision on what kind of fourth-year clinical externship position they will seek. For example, a student with an interest in adults may choose to complete a fourth-year externship in a Veterans Administration (VA) Medical Center, whereas a student with an interest in pediatric audiology might seek a fourth-year position in a children's hospital. The desire to focus on certain types of patients or clinical services also guides decisions on employment following graduation. Different professional activities, responsibilities, and clinical services of audiologists were summarized earlier in Table 1.1.

A word about terminology is appropriate here. The term *medical audiologist* is sometimes used in describing one of the specialties in the profession. A sizable proportion of audiologists are employed in medical settings but there is no formal medical audiologist specialty. You learned earlier in the chapter that audiologists are not physicians and also that audiologists provide nonmedical treatment to persons with hearing impairment. For these reasons the term *medical audiologist* is not accurate. Furthermore, audiologists employed in medical settings often provide a wide range of clinical services independently, without collaboration with physicians.

You'll now learn about some of the different types of clinical services and career specialties available to audiologists. This is just a brief introduction to the varied facets of the profession. Each chapter of the book includes more discussion about the information audiologists apply in their practice and about what an audiologist does each day to help people with hearing loss and related disorders. You may wish to review the table of contents to get a glimpse of some of the topics covered later in the book. If you find yourself curious about a particular type of patient, a specific clinical service, or one of the work settings reviewed in this chapter, it's okay to look ahead and read more about the topic.

Adult Audiology. One practical and real-world way to categorize audiology specialization or focus is to consider the age of the patients served. Some audiologists provide services mostly or entirely to adult patients. For example, an audiologist working in a VA Hospital or VA Medical Center sees only adult patients. Audiologists who care for adult patients see a variety of different types of hearing problems. Audiologists in a VA medical setting also need to be skilled in the administration of a number of different tests for diagnosis of hearing loss and very familiar with hearing aids and other devices for management of patients. In other words, there are clear subcategories of services within the rather broad category of adult audiology. As an example, audiologists who limit their practice to an adult patient population may further specialize in the assessment and treatment of persons with a certain type of problem such as those who are dizzy or who have vestibular or balance disorders. Audiologists who see only pediatric patients will also find specialization opportunities.

Pediatric Audiology. **Pediatric audiology** is a true specialty. Pediatric audiology specialty certification is one of only two areas of specialty certification available through the American Board of Audiology (ABA). Audiologists provide services to children in a variety of different work settings, ranging from private practice clinics to public schools to children's hospitals. An audiologist in any given pediatric work setting may offer a wide assortment of different services.

WebWatch

The website for the Academy of Doctors of Audiology or ADA is a good source for information on private practice options in audiology. The mission of the ADA is " . . . the advancement of practitioner excellence, high ethical standards, professional autonomy and sound business practices in the provision of quality audiologic care."

ClinicalConnection

Children are not just little adults. Special techniques and clinical skills are required to consistently obtain accurate hearing test results from young children and to implement an effective plan for treating their hearing loss. You'll read about many test and treatment techniques throughout the book.

There are many different pediatric audiology services. Some audiologists focus mostly on newborn hearing screening and diagnosis of hearing loss in infants using test procedures often performed while the child is sleeping. Other audiologists in the same clinic coordinate treatment and management of children after hearing loss is confirmed. And **educational audiologists** who work closely with speech pathologists in a public school setting provide various services to children aged 5 to 18 years.

Teachers, Preceptors, and Mentors. Three groups of audiologists function as vital links in helping students to make the transition from entry into a Doctor of Audiology program to emergence four years later as competent audiologists. Teachers in the Doctor of Audiology program are the first link. Most instructors of AuD students are audiologists themselves. A faculty member typically teaches certain courses or "specializes" in selected subject areas. You might say that these university faculty members themselves form a specialty in audiology.

Clinical preceptors play a second and very important part in the AuD educational process. Most Doctor of Audiology programs have an on-campus clinic and also partner with multiple local clinical sites where students can gain practical experience. Most university medical center and off-campus clinics would provide services to patients even if there were no AuD program. Audiologists working in these clinics have two sets of responsibilities. First and foremost, the preceptor is responsible for providing high-quality hearing care to the patient.

The preceptor's other responsibility is to supervise and instruct students who are assigned to the clinic during their AuD program. Audiologists working "in the trenches" and supervising students are the glue that holds a Doctor of Audiology program together and assures its success.

Finally, successful education of Doctor of Audiology students depends on clinical audiologists working in settings that serve as sites for the fourth-year externship experience. Some AuD students complete an externship on their university campus, but most apply to and are accepted at an off-campus clinical site. It's not uncommon for students to complete the fourth-year externship in a hospital clinical facility or audiology practice far away from the university, in another part of the country. The externship is like a job in that the student has daily clinical duties within a typical work week. However, the student is always under the supervision of one or more clinical audiologists who serve as on-the-job instructors and mentors.

A Diversity of Work Settings

Audiologists perform their work in a variety of settings. Table 1.3 shows the percentage of audiologists in the United States employed in a particular work setting based on information from a 2011 survey. Average annual salary is also shown for each of the different settings. In discussing audiologist work settings we'll return a few times to the information in this table. Some full-time audiologists work in more than one of the settings in the list. For example, there are audiologists who maintain a private practice or work within a physician practice and also teach as an adjunct instructor at a local university Doctor of Audiology program.

WebWatch

The American Academy of Audiology has developed clinical education guidelines for audiology externships that" . . . define and outline the competencies of the preceptor, and the roles and responsibilities of both the preceptor and the university for the externship year." You can read more about externships and responsibilities of preceptors at its website.

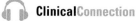
ClinicalConnection

Audiology is a clinical profession. Much of the teaching in a Doctor of Audiology program is practical and conducted in a clinical setting rather than during didactic lectures in a classroom. In other words, students learn from clinical supervisors and patients as well as from books and PowerPoint presentations. During their AuD education, students must acquire skills in performing tests and analyzing test results. Students must also develop confidence and competency in interacting positively with patients of various ages, with different hearing and related disorders.

TABLE 1.3
Proportion of audiologists employed full time (12 months), ranked according to work setting. Average annual compensation is also shown for each work setting.

Setting	Percent Employed	Total (Full-Time) Compensation
Otolaryngology Practice	23	$75,863
Private Practice-Owner/Partner	14	$128,408
University/Teaching Hospital	12	$75,286
Hospital	11	$75,606
Private Practice-Employee	9	$73,829
Private Clinic (non-profit)	6	$73,532
Private Clinic (for -profit)	3	$99,317
University	3	$90,276
Veterans Administration Hospital	5	$82,713
Manufacturer	5	$103,100
Non-Otolaryngology Practice	3	$74,566
Other	3	$73,403
Federal Government	2	$87,943
Public School	2	$82,458
Corporate Audiology Group Practice	1	$88,341

Source: American Academy of Audiology 2011 Compensation and Benefits Report (July 12, 2012).

General and Teaching Hospitals. Audiologists are healthcare professionals. Table 1.3 confirms that common work settings for audiologists include hospitals, physician practices, and other medical facilities where patients receive healthcare. The majority of audiologists are employed in medical settings. These include different types of hospitals (e.g., teaching, VA, children's) and practices that also include such health professionals as physicians, psychologists, speech pathologists, and therapists.

Audiologists work more closely with otolaryngologists (ENT specialists) than other groups of physicians. Collaboration of audiologists and otologists (ear subspecialists in otolaryngology) is particularly common. The two professions often provide services to the same patients with ear or hearing complaints. There are numerous parallels in the daily activities of professional audiologists and otolaryngologists in a teaching hospital. A teaching hospital is affiliated with a university that includes a school of medicine and often other colleges or schools for health-related professions. Services in the hospital are provided by physicians, nurses, and other health professionals, with the assistance of students or residents in training for a health profession. Audiologists and otologists in teaching hospitals and medical centers share involvement in the three academic missions of teaching, clinical services, and research.

Children's Hospitals. Children's hospitals are special places for healthcare. Most major cities in the United States have children's hospitals that enjoy a reputation for expertise and excellence in pediatric healthcare. Audiologists are employed in all children's hospitals. Clinical and research collaboration between audiologists and otolaryngologists is commonly found in children's hospitals. Audiologists functioning as a team in a children's hospital provide comprehensive services, ranging from assessment of hearing loss in infants and young children, to diagnosis of hearing loss in children who have rare medical conditions, to treatment of hearing loss with the latest technology and techniques.

In short, audiologists in children's hospitals are often best suited for evaluation and nonmedical treatment of children with complex forms of hearing disorder. It is important to note that audiologists in other settings also provide diagnostic and rehabilitative services to infants and young children, including audiologists working in teaching hospitals and private clinics.

Veterans Administration (VA) Hospitals. Many hundreds of audiologists employed in VA Hospitals and Medical Centers throughout the United States and in Puerto Rico provide valuable services to men and women who have served in the US Armed Forces. Patients range from elderly veterans of World War II, to those nearing retirement age who served during the Vietnam era, to young veterans of the wars in Iraq and Afghanistan. Employment in a VA audiology service is rewarding professionally. Also, as shown in Table 1.3, VA audiologists are well compensated for their work.

Over the past sixty years thousands of practicing audiologists have benefited from clinical training at a VA Medical Center during their graduate studies. The positive impact of the VA system on the education of audiologists and, conversely, the influence of the profession of audiology on the hearing healthcare of VA patients cannot be overstated.

Military Audiology. You learned earlier in the chapter that audiology in the United States was a direct outgrowth of efforts during World War II to help servicemen with hearing impairment. Audiologists continue to fulfill this important mission. Indeed, the role audiologists play in the U.S. Army, Navy, and Air Force has expanded considerably over the years.

Around the world hundreds of audiologists serve as officers in the U.S. military. These audiologists are involved in various professional activities, including diagnosis of hearing loss and vestibular disorders, hearing conservation to prevent noise- and combat-induced hearing loss, and critical administrative tasks to assure standard of care is provided to all servicemen and servicewomen. Audiologists fulfill their duties at major military installations in the United States and in other countries, as well as unlikely venues like ships and medical facilities within combat zones. The U.S. military also offers fourth-year externship opportunities for students enrolled in a Doctor of Audiology program.

Universities and Research Laboratories. High-quality state-of-the-art clinical services for patients with hearing and related problems rest on a foundation of basic and clinical research. Basic hearing research usually focuses on the anatomy and physiology of the auditory system and on the principles and mechanisms underlying hearing. Studies are often carried out in laboratories with animals as subjects and funded with research grant money from the National Institutes of Health or some other

 ClinicalConnection

In Chapters 4 through 10, you'll learn about various devices and techniques available to audiologists for the assessment of hearing loss. Diseases and disorders associated with hearing loss are reviewed in Chapters 11 and 12. The remainder of the book is devoted to a discussion of modern options for management of hearing loss.

 WebWatch

Audiology has a strong tradition of clinical service in Veterans Administration (VA) Hospitals and Medical Centers. A substantial number of audiologists are employed in VA facilities across the United States and in Puerto Rico. Large states with a high proportion of elderly citizens like Florida often have more than a dozen VA facilities. For more information review the website of the Association of VA Audiologists.

 WebWatch

Hearing research is a high priority in the VA healthcare system and has been from the earliest years of audiology. One of the premier sites for hearing research is the Veterans Administration National Center for Rehabilitative Auditory Research, or NCRAR, in Portland, Oregon. The NCRAR website (www.ncrar.research.va.gov) is filled with information about ongoing and past research projects and conferences, as well as mentoring and training opportunities.

 WebWatch

You can learn more about opportunities for audiologists in the U.S. Army, Air Force, and Navy at the website for the Military Audiology Association (http://militaryaudiology.org) or websites for the U.S. Army and Army Medical Research, U.S. Navy, and U.S. Air Force.

funding agency. Laboratory studies might, for example, be designed to answer a research question about how exposure to excessive noise damages the ear and whether certain drugs minimize the damage. Basic research does not directly affect patient care, although this is often a long-term goal.

In contrast, clinical research is conducted with human subjects, often in a medical center or university facility where patient services are provided. As a rule the results of clinical research are applied almost immediately. Research results contribute to more accurate identification or diagnosis of hearing loss or to more effective treatments for hearing loss in children or adults.

An example of clinical research is a study to determine whether a new automated device designed to better detect hearing loss in newborn infants actually meets that objective. Or a research study might be set up to determine whether a new technical hearing aid feature actually improves a person's ability to understand speech in noisy listening conditions.

Audiologists and other scientists with research training and experience conduct experiments in laboratory settings or studies in a clinical setting. Research audiologists usually hold a PhD degree or a combined AuD/PhD degree. Figure 1.4 shows an audiologist with an AuD/PhD at a major research center who conducts basic and clinical hearing studies. The importance of research to clinical practice has been appreciated since Raymond Carhart and others conducted auditory studies back in the 1950s. The quality of clinical services and the future of audiology as a profession are still dependent on a solid research foundation.

Industry and Manufacturers. In recent years an increasing number of audiologists have elected to take positions with hearing-related companies. Some of the companies manufacture equipment used to test hearing and others manufacture devices used in the management of persons with hearing loss. The latter include companies that design, build, and market hearing aids and also complex electrical devices like **cochlear implants**.

You'll learn all about cochlear implants in Chapters 13, 14, and 16. Briefly, a cochlear implant is a device for converting sound energy from speech into an electrical signal that stimulates the auditory nerve running from the ear to the brain. Audiologists and speech pathologists have the main responsibility for rehabilitation and training of patients with cochlear implants. Persons with severe damage to the ear and very severe hearing loss are usually able to communicate effectively following cochlear implantation and appropriate rehabilitation.

Manufacturers of hearing aids, cochlear implants, and other hearing-related devices employ audiologists in various capacities, including laboratory research, customer (audiologist) education and training, and also sales. The industry or manufacturing career option appeals to audiologists for a variety of reasons. Review of the data on financial compensation in Table 1.3 highlights another factor in the growing popularity of industry as a work setting.

Global Audiology

The Internet has contributed importantly to the communication of audiologists in countries around the world. Improved communication has also led to increased collaboration in clinical and education activities among audiologists in the United States and their colleagues in other countries.

Most audiologists are located in the United States and other developed countries. Over 90% of persons with hearing loss, however, live in countries with little or no access to audiologists. One reason for the

FIGURE 1.4

An audiologist with an AuD degree and a PhD degree conducting basic hearing research in a laboratory setting. Courtesy of Christopher Spankovich, MPH, AuD, PhD.

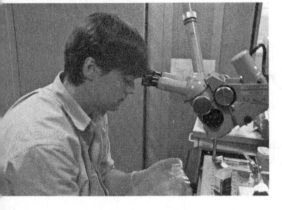

growing interest and efforts in global audiology is recognition of the need to "export" hearing-related clinical services and educational opportunities to the underserved regions of the world (Swanepoel & Hall, 2010; Swanepoel et al., 2010).

Different Educational Models. There are considerable differences in the education and training of audiologists from one country to the next. The Doctor of Audiology approach described earlier is rather unique to the United States. In some European countries like Sweden and Italy audiologists are physicians who have elected to specialize in providing services to persons with hearing loss, including nonsurgical management. In other countries such as the United Kingdom, Canada, Australia, and New Zealand audiologists practice with a master's level degree. And, in many regions of the world where there are formal educational programs, audiologists are qualified to practice in collaboration with physicians and other healthcare professionals after completion of a bachelor's degree.

Tele-Audiology. *Tele-audiology* is a term coined for audiology applications of tele-health or tele-medicine. Research has proven that the quality of hearing services is comparable, whether an audiologist is in the same location as the patient or in another part of the world. Test equipment with Internet capability can be used to perform hearing assessments of children and adults in remote locations where there is no access to audiologists. Technology also permits treatment of hearing loss via tele-audiology (Swanepoel & Hall, 2010; Swanepoel et al., 2010). Tele-audiology applications worldwide will continue to grow rapidly due to advances in instrumentation and the large unmet demand for audiology services in many parts of the world.

 ClinicalConnection

Tele-audiology is a term coined for audiology applications of telehealth or telemedicine. As a result of advances in technology, including broadband Internet connectivity, it is now possible to screen for hearing loss, test hearing, and treat hearing loss with an audiologist in one location and the patient somewhere else, even in another country. Remote provision of clinical audiology services is now becoming a reality.

 WebWatch

The Internet has greatly increased interest in global audiology as well as communication and collaboration among audiologists from different countries throughout the world. Some of the many websites devoted to global audiology issues are Audiology Resources (worldaudiology); the International Society of Audiology (ISA); Audiology World (www.audiologyworld.net), and American Academy of Audiology.

Professional Issues and Organizations

Credentials and Codes

Licensure. Each state in the United States requires that audiologists hold a license to practice. The purpose of state regulation of audiologists and other health professionals is to protect citizens of the state who are consumers of healthcare services. **Licensure** requirements now include completion of a Doctor of Audiology degree, a minimum number of hours of supervised clinical experience, and a passing score on a national examination in audiology. Audiologists with a master's degree who were practicing in a state before the relatively recent requirement for an AuD are "grandfathered" under the new regulations. They are permitted to maintain their state license and continuing practicing. Some states also have regulations pertaining to personnel who provide support to audiologists, including audiologist assistants. Support personnel work under direct supervision of a licensed audiologist (American Academy of Audiology, 2010).

Certification. Although not required as part of the regulation for state licensure, many audiologists hold some type of certification in audiology. One example is certification available from the American Board of Audiology (ABA). The ABA is "an autonomous organization ... dedicated to enhancing audiologic services to the public by promulgating universally recognized standards in professional practice. The ABA encourages audiologists to exceed these prescribed standards, thereby promoting a high level of professional development and ethical practice." Audiologists must apply for **Board certification**.

Completion of regular and well-defined continuing education is required to maintain certification. Continuing education (CE) activities include participation in professional conferences, self-paced readings, and other forms of audiology instruction. The ABA also offers specialty certification in cochlear implants and in pediatric audiology for audiologists who qualify. Audiologists are awarded specialty certification only after demonstrating a sufficient amount of clinical experience plus a passing score on a rigorous written examination.

(i) **Web**Watch

The American Board of Audiology or ABA is one of the major entities for credentialing audiologists for clinical service. It is "an autonomous organization dedicated to enhancing audiologic services to the public by promulgating universally recognized standards in professional practice." The ABA offers students in Doctor of Audiology programs an option for provisional Board certification.

Scope of Practice and Code of Ethics. Audiologists must practice within a scope of activities defined according to professional organizations. The rather broad scope of practice encompasses the diverse assessment and treatment procedures and techniques described throughout this book. Published statements detailing the **scope of practice** of audiology are accessible on the websites of the American Academy of Audiology and the American Speech-Language-Hearing Association. These documents outline activities that are within the expertise of members of the profession.

Documents defining the **code of ethics** guiding audiologists in their clinical practice and other professional activities are also available on the websites of the American Academy of Audiology (AAA) and the American Speech-Language-Hearing Association (ASHA). According to the AAA the two-part Code of Ethics ". . . specifies professional standards that allow for the proper discharge of audiologists' responsibilities to those served, and that protect the integrity of the profession." Alleged violations of ethical conduct are taken very seriously.

Organizations

For approximately forty years audiologists were members in and were represented professionally by the American Speech-Language-Hearing Association (ASHA). In addition to professional representation at the national level, benefits of membership included several scientific journals and the option of annual attendance at a national convention for continuing education and interaction with colleagues. ASHA is a large organization with over 150,000 members. The majority of members are speech pathologists, with audiologists accounting for a less than 5% of total membership.

In 1988 a group of thirty-four audiologists gathered in Houston, Texas, at the invitation of Dr. James Jerger to discuss the need for a professional home "of, by, and for audiologists." The meeting led directly to the formation of the American Academy of Audiology (AAA). The founders created an organizational structure including a president, a board of directors, and other necessary committees for representation of the profession. The new organization immediately developed a bimonthly communication known as *Audiology Today* and in 1990 began publishing a scientific journal called the *Journal of the American Academy of Audiology.*

The AAA since its modest beginning has rapidly grown to membership exceeding 10,000 audiologists from the United States and many other countries. For each year since 1989 the AAA has held an annual professional convention. Currently called AudiologyNow!, the convention takes place each spring in a major U.S. city. It is the largest gathering of audiologists in the world. You are encouraged to review the AAA website. It contains a wide assortment of information about the profession and hearing-related topics.

Students in Doctor of Audiology programs have their own organization called the Student Academy of Audiology, or SAA. The group meets annually at the AudiologyNow! convention, where it organizes a variety of events for student education, interaction, and pre-professional development. At most universities with Doctor of Audiology programs students have organized local SAA chapters. One mission of the SAA groups is to introduce undergraduate students to the profession of audiology.

There are now also a number of state academies of audiology in the United States where audiologists can conveniently meet once or twice a year for continuing education and social interaction. You'll quickly find the academy of audiology for your state with an Internet search using the key words "audiology" and the name of the state.

In addition, several smaller research-oriented organizations hold annual meetings for the education of audiologists and hearing scientists and for dissemination of research findings. The American Auditory Society (AAS) annual meeting is one of the more popular research gatherings.

A Highly Ranked Profession

Audiology is a well-recognized and highly ranked profession. *US News & World Report* listed audiology as one of the best careers in 2006, 2007, 2008, and 2009. The Buzzle website placed audiology in the list of up-and-coming careers in 2012. And CareerCast ranked audiologist at number 6 on a listing of 200 jobs. For comparison purposes, dentist was 33, nurse was 38, physician was right behind at 40, and attorney was 87.

A Dozen Reasons to Consider a Career in Audiology

- Audiologists Are in Demand. The supply of audiologists available to provide hearing care in the United States is inadequate to meet the demand for services. The shortage of audiologists is far more serious elsewhere in the world.

- Audiology Is Highly Ranked as a Health Profession. You'll find ample evidence for this statement among national surveys and rankings of jobs in general and health careers in particular.

- Variety of Work Settings. You've learned already that audiologists have the choice of a wide variety of work environments and venues, ranging from medical facilities to private practice offices and public schools.

- Children, Adults, or Both ... It's Your Decision. Unlike some health professionals, audiologists provide services to patients of all ages, from newborn infants to elderly adults. Some audiologists are very interested in limiting their practice to patients in a specific age category, whereas other audiologists enjoy the challenge and daily diversity associated with patients of all ages.

- Many Specialties to Choose From. Related to the variety of work settings and the age spectrum is the option for developing a high level of expertise and primary clinical focus in a single specialty, or in several related areas. We've highlighted some audiology specialties in this chapter. You'll learn more about them and other specialties throughout the book.

- Audiology Is a Dynamic and Growing Profession. The profession of audiology is not static. Since its beginning over sixty years ago audiology has consistently expanded in scope and complexity. Audiologists twenty or even ten years ago would never have envisioned the profession as it is today. In another ten years we will probably be able to make the same statement about the constantly changing nature of audiology.

- Reasonable Hours and Comfortable Work Environment. Audiologists typically work in safe and comfortable settings. Clinical or teaching duties are almost always completed within daytime working hours. Unlike some health professionals, audiologists are not required to be "on call" or perform clinical work on weekends.

- Less Stress. The group CareerCast in 2011 ranked audiology at number 1 as the least stressful job. In its words: "An Audiologist diagnoses and treats hearing problems by attempting to discover the range, nature, and degree of hearing function. The job is not

(i) **Web**Watch

Audiology and speech pathology are ranked highly among health professions and among jobs in general. You can find details about rankings of audiology and speech pathology on several websites, such as:

- American Academy of Audiology
- Occupational Outlook Handbook, Department of Labor (www.bls.gov/ooh/healthcare /audiologists.htm)
- CareerCast
- Buzzle: search for audiologists, what is an audiologist, clinical audiologist-salary, audiologist education requirements

typically physically demanding or stressful, but it does require a keen attention to detail and focused concentration."

- **Professional Satisfaction, Respect, and Rewards.** You'll gain further appreciation of this positive aspect of the profession as you read the book. You'll learn about the many important ways audiologists can help children and adults. Audiologists are rewarded daily with the knowledge that their patients have improved quality of life. As awareness of audiology has grown, the profession has earned respect from healthcare colleagues and from the public.

- **Competitive Compensation.** Table 1.3 provided some information about average financial compensation for audiologists in different work settings. Hardworking audiologists can earn a very good living while still taking satisfaction in helping people.

- **Service as an Officer in the U.S. Military.** For some this is a good reason to consider a career in audiology. Audiologists enter the U.S. Army, Navy, or Air Force at an officer rank. During their professionally rewarding military service, audiologists can earn a competitive salary while also fully developing their audiology skills. Upon discharge or "retirement" from service at a relatively young age, an audiologist can pursue other career options while receiving a government pension.

- **Become an Audiologist and See the World.** Audiologists can often "write their ticket" when it comes to choosing a location to practice their craft. Audiologist openings are available in most parts of the United States and in many other locations in the world. Audiologists who develop an international reputation through their research or with publications like journal articles and books are often in high demand as lecturers and speakers at professional conferences and workshops in the United States and elsewhere in the world.

PULLING IT ALL TOGETHER

Audiologists are the only nonphysician healthcare professionals who assess, diagnose, and manage hearing loss, balance problems, and related disorders in adults and children. In this chapter you were introduced to the many clinical services audiologists now provide to persons across the age span. Diagnostic services range from hearing screening of newborn infants to diagnosis of hearing loss and related disorders caused by a diverse assortment of diseases. Rehabilitative or treatment services include management of patients with hearing loss using technology such as hearing aids and cochlear implants. You also learned in this chapter that audiologists work in many different settings, including hospitals, physician clinics, schools, private practice offices, and even military installations. Education in four-year Doctor of Audiology programs prepares students for the challenges of practicing as licensed audiologists. Finally, you are now aware of the many reasons audiology today is a highly ranked as career option.

READING

Jerger, J. (2009). *Audiology in the USA*. San Diego: Plural Publishing.

2 Sound, Acoustics, and Psychoacoustics

LEARNING OBJECTIVES

In this chapter, you will learn:

- What is meant by the terms *vibration, displacement, inertia,* and *elasticity*
- About the properties of sound, including frequency, intensity, and duration
- The meaning of words used to describe sound, including phase and wavelength
- About decibels and how they are used to describe sound intensity and pressure
- How sound levels are specified and verified with a sound level meter
- What is meant by the term *psychoacoustics*
- Psychoacoustic principles, like loudness and pitch
- How to describe the sounds used in hearing testing, pure tones, speech, and noise
- Why an understanding of sound is important in hearing testing

CHAPTER FOCUS

A discussion of sound involves many new concepts and technical terms. Some of the terminology may be unfamiliar to you. To help you learn the new vocabulary, terms first introduced in this chapter are identified by **bold font**, listed among **Key Terms**, and defined in a Glossary at the end of the book. An introduction to audiology and an understanding of hearing requires a review of the major properties of sound and types of sounds. In their daily practice, audiologists regularly apply the concepts of sound and use the terminology you are about to learn. An introduction to any profession or discipline, such as medicine, law, teaching, speech pathology, or audiology, requires the mastery of a new language and, really, a new way of thinking. In reading this chapter you'll be exposed to concepts and terms that are essential for an understanding of the profession and practice of audiology.

KEY TERMS

Amplitude
Condensation
Cycle
Damping
decaPascal (daPa)
Decibel (dB)
Displacement
Elasticity
Forced vibration
Frequency
Inertia
Instantaneous displacement
Intensity
Inverse square law
Loudness
Oscillate
Period
Phase
Pitch
Psychoacoustics
Pure tones
Rarefaction
Reference equivalent threshold sound pressure levels (RETSPLs)
Resonance frequency
Simple harmonic motion
Sound level meter
Sound pressure level (SPL)
Temporal integration
Tuning fork
Vibration
Wavelength

INTRODUCTION

Every day, audiologists work with various types of sound. You might say that sound is one of the tools of the audiology trade. Thus, an understanding of sound is necessary for the practice of audiology. The audiologist identifies, quantifies, describes, precisely defines, and manipulates sound when accurately evaluating hearing function. Audiologists use sound as a signal or a stimulus to assess hearing.

Let's consider just a few ways audiologists incorporate different sounds in testing the hearing of children and adults. The simplest and most common of hearing tests involves tones at specific frequencies. An audiologist presents the tones through earphones to a patient beginning at a comfortable listening level. The tones are then systematically decreased in volume until the patient can no longer hear them. The goal of this test is to determine hearing threshold, that is, the softest level of the tone that the patient can detect.

The basic hearing evaluation often includes one or more tests that measure how well the patient recognizes different speech sounds. The patient might be asked to repeat two-syllable words, like "hot dog" or "baseball," while the volume of the words is decreased until they can no longer be heard and repeated accurately. Or, the patient might repeat single-syllable words such as "yes or "burn" at a comfortable listening level while the audiologist tallies the number of words the patient repeats correctly.

Sometimes testing estimates problems that a hearing-impaired person experiences in the real world, such as struggling to understand what people are saying in a noisy setting. During routine hearing testing of one ear, audiologists often present noise sounds to the other ear. It is important for an audiologist to assure that a patient's response to sound isn't coming from the non-test ear.

This is only a small sampling of the types of sounds used in hearing testing. Later in the book you'll read about other types of sounds that are used in various hearing tests.

We'll now discuss three fundamental physical properties of sound and their psychological counterparts. The discussion proceeds from simple sounds to more complex sounds, including speech sounds and musical sounds.

Properties of Sound

Vibrations

The story about sound must begin with a discussion of *vibrations*. Sound is **vibration** of air particles produced by the vibration of an object or objects. It's quite easy to think of daily experiences with vibrating objects that produce sound. Your day might start when the alarm on your smartphone rudely announces that it's time for you to get up. Vibrations of a small loudspeaker somewhere in the smartphone produces the sounds you selected for the alarm. Or you may have awoken during the night to the annoying loud sound produced by vibration of the soft tissues at the back of someone's throat. That's right, someone was snoring. Perhaps you had trouble falling asleep because you heard a rhythmic low-pitch thumping sound from an expensive sound system in an adjacent dorm room or apartment.

While taking a shower soon after waking you might hear the pleasant background sound produced by the turbulence of water rapidly shooting out of the showerhead and cascading down to strike the floor. Before even leaving for school you may be exposed to many and various other sounds produced by vibrations associated with assorted fluids such as coffee dripping or a toilet flushing, vibrating vocal folds generating a human voice, or the clanging and clattering sounds produced by hard objects like dishes striking each other. You might listen to voices or music produced by the vibrations of the large speaker in your entertainment center or the miniature but high-quality speakers in the earplugs of your MP3 player. Vibrations and the sounds associated with them occur 24/7 everywhere in our environment. We'll first discuss two properties necessary for vibrations.

Inertia and Elasticity. The properties of *inertia* and *elasticity* are necessary for an object to vibrate. An object will remain motionless or inert, in a resting state, unless some force acts upon it. **Inertia** of an object is the tendency of the object to remain at rest or inactive unless disturbed by an external force. Take, for example, the strings on a guitar. The guitar may sit for days on a stand in a room with the guitar strings completely motionless. The guitar is certainly capable of producing sound, but first some external force like your fingers must move the guitar strings. Most objects also have the property of **elasticity**, or springiness. Just as a stretched band will immediately return toward its original motionless position if released, an object that is changed or moved from its original inert state will return to its original position.

An object may move back and forth one time to produce a single vibration. More commonly, however, the object moves back and forth in *simple harmonic motion* or *oscillation*. **Simple harmonic motion** is the simplest form of vibratory motion. The word **oscillate** is derived from the Latin word meaning "to swing." Pluck a guitar string once and the string will return to and then pass through its original position, moving to and fro multiple times before coming to rest.

The vibrations of an object and the sounds produced by the vibrations are affected by the properties of the object, including length, stiffness, and mass. Let's take a moment to describe each of these terms. *Length* is a familiar quantity, defined in terms of units that are small, such as millimeters (mm), to meters, to even larger units like kilometers (km). *Stiffness* is a property related to the springiness and elasticity of an object. An object with more stiffness requires more force to compress it. The opposite of stiffness is compliance. Objects that are more compliant are less stiff and vice versa. *Mass* is a property of all matter that is defined with units such as milligrams (mg), grams, and kilograms (kg). It's important to keep in mind that mass is not equivalent to weight. Weight is determined by measuring the effect of gravity on mass. Objects in space and outside the influence of earth's gravity may be weightless but they still have mass.

The concepts of inertia and elasticity in vibration can be illustrated with various physical objects. One object designed specifically to vibrate is a *tuning fork*. Figure 2.1 shows a tuning fork. The metal **tuning fork** consists of a stem that's held in the user's hand and two prongs (tines) that form a U shape. A tuning fork is set into vibration when the tines of the tuning fork are struck against the palm of the user's other hand. When set into motion the tines of the tuning fork oscillate inward and outward.

Condensation and Rarefaction. The vibration of an object temporarily increases the air pressure and the density of air molecules on one side of the object. The increase in pressure of air molecules near the object spreads to nearby air molecules and continues to spread or propagate through a medium, such as air, in the form of a sound wave. Regions of increased pressure are known as **condensation**. The root word in the word *condensation* is *condense*, which means "more compact." Right behind this wave of increased air pressure is a region of reduced air pressure, known as **rarefaction**. *Rarify* is the root word in the word *rarefaction*. It means "less dense or compact."

FIGURE 2.1

A tuning fork. Image © Unkreativ/Shutterstock.

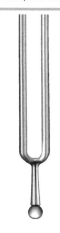

ClinicalConnection

Very few people utter the terms *rarefaction* and *condensation* in everyday conversations. However, audiologists who perform specialized hearing tests involving the measurement of brain responses to sound use the terms on a regular basis. Brain responses are activated when rarefaction and condensation pressure sounds are delivered to the ears. In Chapter 9, you'll learn how different auditory brain responses elicited with rarefaction or condensation sounds can be used to evaluate auditory function in children and adults.

Let's return to the tuning fork as an example of a vibrating object, as illustrated in Figure 2.2A. Regions of rarefaction and condensation of air molecules correspond respectively to the inward and outward movement of the tuning fork tines. Figure 2.2B illustrates this concept. The different shades represent the different types of gas within typical air. Increased density of air molecules and condensation is shown by a darker appearance. The lighter regions represent decreased density of air molecules and rarefaction. The changes in air pressure corresponding to sound occur many times each second, at the frequency of the sound wave.

Displacement. **Displacement** occurs when an object is displaced from one point to another point. Displacement of tuning fork tines away from the resting or starting position corresponds to a point on a simple harmonic waveform. The simple harmonic waveform is usually plotted over a time period of one or more cycles. A **cycle** is movement away from one point and return movement to the same point in the same direction. The word *cycle* is derived from the Greek word for "circle." The time required for completion of one complete cycle of movement is called the **period** of the waveform. The period of a waveform from the beginning to the end of a cycle is on the order of milliseconds, or even a fraction of a millisecond.

The waveform in Figure 2.2C illustrates a simple harmonic waveform and the concepts of cycle and period. The waveform is directly related to the displacement of the tuning fork shown

FIGURE 2.2

A vibrating tuning fork is depicted in the top portion of the figure (labeled **A**). Just below is an illustration of rarefaction and compression (condensation) waves in sound produced by vibration of the tuning fork (labeled **B**). Pressure waves from vibration of a tuning fork are shown as a sine wave in the lower portion of the figure (labeled **C**) and, to the right, the complete cycle of a tuning fork vibration is shown as a circle, with degrees corresponding to different portions of the cycle (labeled **D**).

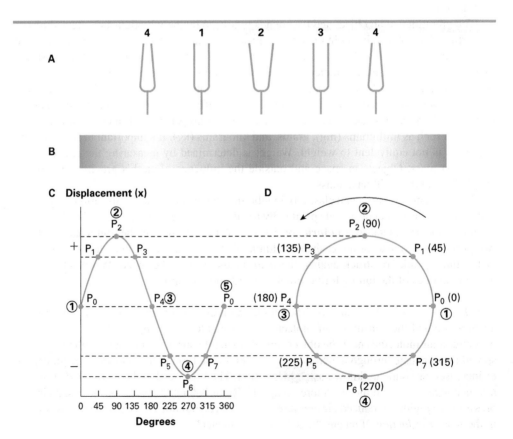

in the top portion of the figure (Figure 2.2A). Due to elasticity, the object returns to and then through its resting position, reaching another point of displacement at a maximum distance from the starting point before returning back to the starting point. A cycle is a complete trip from the starting point outward to the positive and negative extremes and then back to the starting point.

Now look closely at Figure 2.2D. You'll see that simple harmonic vibrations of the tuning fork can be plotted with a circular diagram. Outward movement away from the resting point is plotted as a positive value, whereas inward movement is plotted as negative value. The wave-form crosses zero displacement as the object passes momentarily through the starting position some time after movement began.

The displacement of a vibrating object must be described in relation to time. Displacement is constantly changing over time. At any given time or any instant the location of the vibrating object is described as **instantaneous displacement**, abbreviated **d(t)**, for displacement (d) at a specific time (t). For example, the displacement of the guitar string will be different at any specific time.

Displacement in a waveform is referred to as **amplitude**. Amplitude of a simple harmonic waveform can be expressed in different ways. Figure 2.3 illustrates how amplitude can be calculated from baseline to the peak. The baseline is the midpoint or the starting point in a typical waveform. Amplitude is measured from the baseline to the positive or the negative amplitude extreme for the waveform. The second approach is to calculate the difference in displacement between a positive and a negative peak. Figure 2.3A shows how amplitude is measured from the positive amplitude extreme to the negative amplitude extreme.

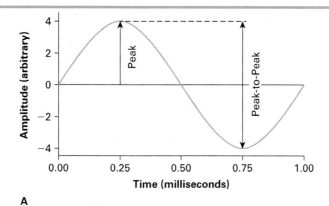

A

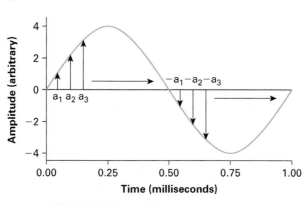

$$RMS = \sqrt{[a_1^2 + a_2^2 + a_3^2 + ... + (-a_1^2) + (-a_1^2) + (-a_1^2) + ...] / \#a\text{'s}}$$

B

FIGURE 2.3

Calculation of amplitude for a sine wave using three approaches: Peak amplitude (labeled **A**), peak-to-peak amplitude (labeled **A**) and, below, root mean square (RMS) amplitude (labeled **B**). One cycle of the wave is complete in a time period of 1 ms. *Source: From Audiology: Science to Practice.* (p. 48), by Steven Kramer. Copyright © 2008 Plural Publishing, Inc. All rights reserved. Modified and reproduced with permission.

Root-mean-square (RMS) amplitude. Root-mean-square amplitude is a third way of expressing amplitude of a waveform. Figure 2.3B shows how amplitude values for many points on the waveform are squared and totaled. The root mean square of the sum is then calculated.

A brief explanation of the rationale for RMS method of determining amplitude of a waveform is needed here. A simple waveform has equal positive and the negative amplitudes corresponding to upward and downward points on the waveform. Simply averaging amplitudes at all of the positive and negative points along the waveform would yield a sum of zero. Zero amplitude would be an inaccurate description of amplitude for the waveform. RMS amplitude is obtained by first squaring all of the instantaneous amplitudes on the waveform, thus eliminating negative values. All of the squared values are averaged and the square root of the average is calculated.

The RMS technique is often used to accurately quantify amplitude of sounds in hearing research. You'll encounter the term *RMS amplitude* in reading articles and books about sound, hearing, and music. Although the RMS approach appears to require complicated calculations, it's quickly performed with laboratory instrumentation.

Damping. If vibrations were to take place in an environment free from any resistance, then the maximum displacement would remain constant and the vibration would continue on indefinitely. However, some resistance to vibration is always present here on earth, including friction encountered in an air medium. Decrease of a vibration due to resistance is referred to as **damping**. As a result of damping the amplitudes in a waveform decay or fade away over time. Damping of the waveform begins almost immediately, and the amplitude of the displacement gradually decreases. A few seconds after a tuning fork is struck or a guitar string is plucked one time, vibrations at the natural frequency of the object decrease and sound gradually becomes inaudible. That is, amplitude values diminish to a value of 0. The tuning fork or guitar string returns to a motionless state.

Vibration will be maintained as long as a constant force is applied to the object to keep it in motion. This is referred to as **forced vibration**. During forced vibration the continuous supply of energy offsets damping due to friction. In the case of forced vibration produced by an external force, the consistent regular repetition of the displacement back and forth is maintained. There are many possible examples of ongoing forced vibration. One example would be a trumpet player holding a note while continuing to blow air evenly into the mouthpiece.

Media for Sound Production. A *medium* is a necessary ingredient for the production of sound. Media, the plural of medium, include air, water, and solid substances. Energy from vibration of an object travels away from an object through a medium. Without a medium, vibrations are not transmitted away from an object. The typical medium for sound is air. Air consists of molecules representing a mixture of different gases. Oxygen is the heaviest gas in air, and hydrogen is the lightest. The gas that accounts for the greatest volume in air is nitrogen.

At sea level there are about 2.7×10^{19} molecules in a cubic centimeter. Air molecules are always moving about randomly and bumping into nearby molecules or any object that is within the space occupied by the air. The technical term for the constant movement of air molecules is *Brownian motion*, a term that honors Robert Brown (see Table 2.1). Because the amount of Brownian motion is directly related to the temperature of air, it is also sometimes referred to as *thermal motion*. The constant collisions of very large numbers of air molecules create static pressure, the pressure that is measured by a barometer.

Although air is the medium for most of the sound we hear, sound can also transmitted through liquid and solid. An example of the former is hearing the sound of a distant boat

TABLE 2.1   Brief biographies of persons contributing to our understanding of sound and vibration

Robert Brown (1773–1858): Brown was a British botanist. Although earlier scientists described Brownian movement, Brown is given credit for discovering the random movement of particles in a medium (e.g., air). According to reports, Brown was using a microscope to study particles of pollen on the surface of water when he noticed rapid and random movement of very small particles within each pollen grain. The theory behind Brownian motion has since been applied in the explanation of a variety of phenomena, including, believe it or not, activity of the stock market!

Heinrich Hertz (1857–1894): Heinrich Rudolph Hertz was a German physicist. Born in Hamburg and educated at the University of Berlin, Hertz studied under Hermann von Helmholtz, a famous scientist who made important contributions to knowledge of the function of the ear. Hertz expanded upon the electromagnetic theories of British physicist James Clark Maxwell by showing that electricity can be transmitted via electromagnetic waves. His work laid the foundation for development of the wireless telegraph and telephone. Remarkably, Hertz's invaluable contributions to science occurred while he was still a young man. He died just before his 37th birthday.

Blaise Pascal (1623–1662): Blaise Pascal was a brilliant and highly talented French philosopher, theologian, writer, inventor, physicist, and mathematician. While still a teenager Pascal invented a mechanical calculation machine, and soon after he made major new contributions to mathematics, including geometry and calculus. Pascal began his scientific career with studies of fluids, hydrodynamics, vacuums, and pressure, the topic of greatest relevance to our interest in sound. In addition to having his name given to a unit of pressure, a computer programming language was named in his honor. Plagued by poor health all of his life, Blaise Pascal died several months after his 39th birthday.

Alexander Graham Bell (1847–1922): A. G. Bell was born in Edinburgh, Scotland. His father and his grandfather were very interested in speech and communication. In addition, Bell's mother began to lose her hearing when he was a child, and his wife was deaf. As a teenager he began to study acoustics and to develop more effective ways of communicating with his mother. A. G. Bell's interest and research on electricity, sound, speech, and methods for electrically transmitting speech (e.g., the telephone) were initially Influenced by the writings of Helmholtz. Bell played an important role in the early development of telecommunications devices, such as the telephone, and also made contributions in the field of the education of persons who are deaf or hearing impaired. A brief biography cannot do credit his varied and substantial scientific contributions and inventions. Giving the name "decibel" to a unit of sound developed at Bell Laboratories is just one way Bell has been honored. Detailed information on his long and highly productive life can be found in more than a dozen book-size biographies.

engine while underwater in a lake or the ocean. Sound can also be transmitted through a combination of two media, like air and a solid.

Frequency

Introduction. Frequency of sound is a fundamental and very practical concept in clinical audiology. Almost every hearing evaluation involves the manipulation of sound frequency. The concept of frequency and related parameters of sound are explained and illustrated in multiple ways in this section of the chapter. You've already been introduced to the concept of frequency.

Remember the example of the guitar string? The vibrations or oscillations of the guitar strings determined the *frequency* of the sound produced by the guitar. **Frequency** is influenced by properties of a vibrating object. When a guitar string is plucked, frequency of vibration increases as *length* of the vibrating portion of the string is shortened and, conversely, frequency decreases as the vibrating portion of the string is lengthened. *Stiffness* (or its reciprocal, compliance) of an object is also a factor affecting vibration. The frequency of vibrations increases directly as stiffness of the object is increased and vice versa. For example, a more taut guitar string produces a higher frequency of vibration. If tension on the guitar string is decreased, vibration frequency decreases. Finally, the *mass* of an object also affects the frequency of vibrations. Thicker guitar strings produce lower-frequency vibrations, whereas thinner guitar strings produce higher-frequency vibrations.

Now we'll explore further the essential topic of sound frequency, beginning with the simplest of sounds.

Sine Waves and Pure Tones. A sine wave or sinusoid represents a single frequency. The word *sinusoid* means "like a sine." The time course of simple harmonic motion can be described by the sine function of trigonometry. Interestingly, the word sine is derived from the medieval Latin word for "fold in a garment." Indeed, the regular undulating appearance of the sine wave does resemble a fold in a piece of clothing. Sine waves are commonly referred to as **pure tones**.

WebWatch

You'll find an abundance of information about sound on the Internet. A good example is the Physics Classroom website. Click on the Multimedia Studies link and scroll down to the Waves, Sound, and Light category. There you'll have access to additional descriptions of sound, along with simulations of different sound-related concepts like the sound waves produced by a tuning fork or a guitar string.

You've already been introduced to two other terms, cycle and period, that are used to describe sine waves. The frequency of a sound is described as the number of cycles per unit of time, usually in seconds. The term *cycle* was illustrated in Figure 2.2. A vibration cycle is, very simply, defined as one completion vibration. A cycle may be described with a starting point anywhere on a waveform. The *period* of a waveform is the time required for completion of one cycle of vibration, from the starting point through the wave to the same point moving in the same direction. A period is usually described in subdivisions of seconds, like milliseconds (ms).

Figure 2.4 shows waveforms for three different frequencies. Frequency of the pure tones increases from top to bottom in the figure. Frequency of each sound is determined by the number of cycles of the sound occurring in 1 second (1000 ms). For example, for the top waveform the frequency is 5 cycles per second or 5 *Hz*. Hz is the abbreviation for *Hertz*, a term named after scientist Heinrich Hertz. Table 2.1 includes biographical sketches of Hertz and other persons whose names are attached to important hearing terms. In audiology the abbreviation *Hz* is typically used to refer to cycles per second (cps).

ClinicalConnection

Sinusoidal sounds of different frequencies are commonly used to evaluate hearing. Audiologists typically refer to sinusoids as pure tone sounds or simply pure tones. Hearing ability is usually tested for pure tones at specific frequencies like 250 Hz, 500 Hz, 1000 Hz, 2000 Hz, 4000 Hz, and 8000 Hz. You'll learn in Chapter 5 about the different clinical tests involving pure tone sounds.

A waveform of 20 Hz is shown at the bottom of Figure 2.4. There are 20 cycles in the 1-second time frame. The frequencies illustrated in the figure are quite low in comparison to those used to test hearing. A frequency of 1000 Hz is one of the test tone frequencies commonly employed in hearing testing. A sound with a frequency of 1000 Hz or 1000 cycles in 1 second has one cycle per millisecond. Frequencies of sounds may also be described in units of kilohertz. A frequency of 1000 Hz is 1 KHz.

Next we'll summarize the relation of the terms *frequency* and *period* using a few simple equations and a figure. The relation of the frequency and the period of a sound is described by the equations:

$$\text{frequency} = 1/\text{period} \qquad \text{period} = 1/\text{frequency}$$

In these equations, frequency (f) of the sound is in Hertz (Hz) and the period of the sound is in either seconds or milliseconds (ms).

As the equations reveal, there is a reciprocal or inverse relation between the frequency and the period of a sound. That is, as one property of sound increases, the other decreases. The longer the period, or the time required for completion of one cycle of a sound, the lower the frequency, and vice versa. Higher frequency sounds have shorter periods and lower frequency sounds have longer periods.

This principle will now be illustrated with solutions of the equations for three common audiometric test frequencies, 500 Hz, 1000 Hz, and 2000 Hz, with the period expressed in seconds (sec). Keep in mind that 1 second is 1000 milliseconds (ms):

500 Hz

frequency = 500 Hz

period = 0.002 sec or 2 ms

frequency in Hz = 1/period in sec

500 Hz = 1/0.002 sec

period = 1/frequency in Hz

0.002 sec = 1/500 Hz

1000 Hz

frequency = 1000 Hz

period in sec = 0.001 sec or 1 ms

frequency in Hz = 1/period in sec

1000 Hz = 1/0.001 sec

period = 1/frequency

0.001 sec = 1/1000 Hz

2000 Hz

frequency = 2000 Hz

period = 0.0005 sec or 0.5 ms

frequency in Hz = 1/period in sec

2000 Hz = 1/0.0005 sec

period = 1/frequency

0.0005 sec = 1/2000 Hz

FIGURE 2.4

Pure tones of different frequencies plotted on the same time scale (1 second). Frequency of each sound can be calculated by dividing the number of cycles of the sound (labeled with numbers) into the time period of 1 second (1000 ms). For example, frequency = 1000/5 = 200 Hz.

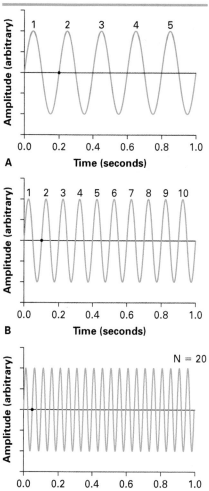

Let's return for moment to Figure 2.4. It shows waveforms that illustrate the relation between the frequency and period of a sine wave. If you again examine the waveforms for each frequency, you'll see a dark dot marking the end of one cycle. The period or time that's required to complete one cycle of a waveform is shorter for high frequency tones and progressively longer for lower frequency tones.

Phase. Two other properties of a simple pure tone or sine wave will now be introduced: *phase* and *wavelength*. The **phase** of a sine wave or pure tone is the point at which the wave begins. Any sine wave must begin at some point. Phase is described in degrees (°) or degrees of angle. The simplest way to understand this concept is to again consider a circle divided into degrees from 0° to 360°. This concept was illustrated earlier in Figure 2.2D. A resting or starting point for a sine wave of 0 degrees, or zero phase, is usually depicted on a horizontal line.

The concept of phase might be more easily understood by considering the childhood game jumping rope. Let's say that you and a friend decide to spend some time jumping rope. Since a third friend is not available to join in the game, you cleverly tie one end of a 10-foot rope to a nearby tree. You grasp the other end of the rope in your right hand while your trusting friend stands midway along the length of the rope. You then begin to rotate your right arm in a clockwise direction in order to swing the rope in a big regular circular movement.

Where was your hand when you began to swing the rope? There are a variety of possible starting points. Let's assume your hand was initially at waist height and your forearm was extended horizontally forward. You first moved the rope by rotating your hand upward and to the left. You continued to rotate your hand to a high point and then downward through a position waist high. Your hand continued to move downward to a low point, to the right, and then back up to the starting point.

Of course, you repeated these motions faster and maybe with more force to create a large and smooth arc in the rope around your friend. In this example, the starting phase for the movement of your arm was 0 degrees, with the rope horizontal. You then moved your hand through the rest of a circle (90, 180, 270, to 360 degrees). However, you could also have started the rotary movement of your hand at any other point, perhaps at the high point of 90 degrees in the circle or at the low point, 270 degrees in our example. In any event, once the rope was swinging around and around in a large arc, and your friend jumped over the rope every time it brushed past the ground, the movement was the same regardless of the starting point.

The Greek letter theta (θ) is often used as a symbol for starting phase. The term *phase* is used to describe any starting point for a sine wave. Displacement of a waveform at the starting point is zero. Over the course of one complete cycle of the sine wave, there are points representing different locations from 0 to 360 degrees.

Figure 2.5 illustrates how a sine wave could begin at any of these points. Each of the sine waves labeled Figure 2.5A begins at 0 degrees. A starting point of 0 degrees for a waveform is considered *standard phase*. Sine waves that start at the same point are *in phase*. Now, look closely at the waveforms labeled Figure 2.5B. The top sine wave begins at 0 degrees. The lower waveform begins at 90 degrees, or a starting point one quarter of a period later than standard phase. Waveforms with different starting points, like those in Figure 2.5B, are *out of phase*. Now inspect the lowest set of waveforms in Figure 2.5C. One begins at 90 degrees and the other at 270 degrees, a difference of 180 degrees. The term *opposite phase* is used to describe waveforms that are 180 degrees out of phase.

Wavelength. The **wavelength** of a sine wave is the distance from some point on a sine wave to a second point 360 degrees after the beginning or the point at which the next cycle begins. Wavelength is described in feet, inches, meters, or centimeters. Sometimes wavelength is determined from the beginning to the end of a cycle of the wave. Or wavelength can be calculated as the distance from one region of condensation to the next region of condensation or one region of rarefaction to the next region of rarefaction. The Greek letter lambda (λ) is used as a symbol for wavelength. The period and wavelength of a waveform are similar concepts: period is measured in time whereas wavelength is measured in distance. We'll focus here on wavelength.

The wavelength of a sound is related to its frequency. Speed of sound is a factor in the relationship between wavelength and frequency. Speed of sound is described in meters per second (m/sec) or in feet per second (ft/sec). Recall that the speed of sound is 1100 ft/sec or 345 m/sec. The relationship of wavelength, frequency, and speed of sound is defined with the equation:

$$\lambda = v/f$$

FIGURE 2.5

Phase relation is shown for three sets of sinusoidal waveforms of the same frequency. Waveforms labeled **A** are **in phase**. Each waveform begins at a phase of 0 degrees. Waveforms labeled **B** are **out of phase** (one begins at 0 degrees, or standard phase, and the other at 90 degrees). Waveforms labeled **C** are of **opposite phase,** or 180 degrees out of. *Source:* Mullin, William J.; Gerace, William J.; Mestre, Jose P.; Velleman, Shelley L., *FUNDAMENTALS OF SOUND WITH APPLICATIONS TO SPEECH AND HEARING, 1st Ed.,* © (2003). Reprinted and Electronically reproduced by permission of Pearson Education, Inc., Upper Saddle River, New Jersey.

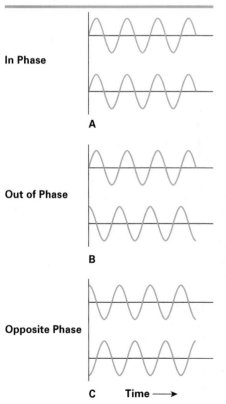

In Phase

A

Out of Phase

B

Opposite Phase

C   Time ⟶

where wavelength is designated by the Greek symbol lambda (λ), speed of sound is indicated with "v" for velocity, and frequency of sound is represented by "f."

If we insert some real values for the frequency of sound in this equation, the relationship of wavelength to frequency is readily apparent. Let's solve the equation for wavelength using three different frequencies: 220 Hz, 1000 Hz, and 4000 Hz. Wavelength will be calculated for speed of sound described in feet/second (1100) and also in meters/second (345).

λ = v/f or λ = 1100/220 Hz or λ = 5.0 feet
λ = v/f or λ = 345/220 Hz or λ = 1.57 meters

λ = v/f or λ = 1100/1000 Hz or λ = 1.1 feet
λ = v/f or λ = 345/1000 Hz or λ = 0.34 meter

λ = v/f or λ = 1100/4000 Hz or λ = 0.28 feet
λ = v/f or λ = 345/4000 Hz or λ = 0.09 meter

The equation defines an inverse relationship between wavelength and frequency of a sound wave. From these examples, it's clear that lower frequency sine waves have longer wavelengths, and vice versa. Figure 2.6 illustrates graphically this relation between frequency of a tone and its wavelength.

Resonance. All vibrating objects have a natural or **resonance frequency**. That is, with the application of force an object vibrates or oscillates more readily and more efficiently and with less loss of energy at one frequency than any other frequency. Resonance frequency (f_r) is also known as the natural vibration frequency of the object.

You'll recall our earlier discussion about the effect of certain properties of an object on the frequency of its vibrations, specifically its length, stiffness, and mass. Resonance frequency is also dependent on the physical characteristics of the object, like size and shape, as well as the volume of air enclosed within the object.

Tuning forks offer a clear example of resonance. You may wish to examine again the tuning fork shown in Figure 2.1. The size or mass of the tuning fork determines the resonance frequency. Smaller size is associated with higher frequencies and larger size with lower frequencies. Each tuning fork is constructed to produce a specific frequency when set into vibration, such as 256 Hz or 512 Hz. A tuning fork always produces its designated resonance frequency, whether a skilled health professional or a novice like a college student strikes it. In contrast, many objects in nature when set into vibration produce multiple frequencies and a complex pattern of resonance rather than a single frequency.

Resonance frequency is perhaps best appreciated with examples involving music. The frequency of sound varies greatly when a drummer strikes a big bass drum instead of a smaller snare drum, or a tall and thin bongo drum rather than a short and squat bongo drum, or a drum instead of a cymbal. Let's also consider stringed musical instruments. The different sounds produced with a violin, a viola, a cello, or a bass are determined by the length, stiffness, and

🎧 Clinical Connection

The resonance frequency of an object is largely determined by the properties of mass and stiffness. In Chapter 8, you'll again encounter these terms and we'll discuss their application in the evaluation of how the ear functions. Mass and stiffness are measured in a common clinical test procedure that measures movement of the eardrum and the middle ear structures. Abnormalities of the two properties cause various patterns of hearing loss.

FIGURE 2.6

The relationship between frequency and wavelength is shown for tones of 4000 Hz, 1000 Hz, 500 Hz, and 220 Hz.

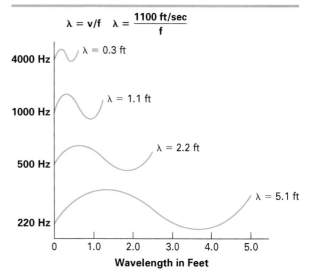

mass of the strings in combination with the resonance frequency of the volume contained by the specific size and shape of the wooden instrument.

Each resonating object or resonator vibrates at its own resonance frequency rather than at the frequency of the driving force. For example, different drums produce different frequencies even when a drummer strikes them the same way. Another common musical example of resonance frequency is the delicate wine or champagne glass that dramatically shatters when an opera singer holds a single pitch that is at the resonance frequency for the glass. The resonance of a cylinder, tube, or pipe filled with air depends on its length, its width, its volume, and whether it's open at one end.

Intensity

Intensity of a sound is related to the maximum displacement or the amplitude of a waveform. To illustrate the concept of intensity and amplitude, we'll return again to the example of sound produced by a guitar string. How far the guitar string is initially displaced and how far the string moves back and forth determines the amplitude of vibration and the resulting intensity of the sound. Intensity is a term like frequency that audiologists use dozens of times each day. Audiologists repeatedly manipulate the intensity of sounds in hearing testing. Rare is the procedure performed by an audiologist in the clinic that doesn't involve increasing and decreasing sound intensity or at least checking the intensity of a stimulus sound. A clear understanding of sound intensity is required for the practice of audiology.

Clinical Connection

Almost all hearing tests involve the presentation of sounds of different intensity levels. Intensity levels are carefully selected and often manipulated in tests that screen the hearing of newborn infants, rather simple hearing tests that measure how well a person can detect faint sounds, and more complex procedures that assess a patient's response to speech sounds.

Force and Pressure. The concept of sound intensity is directly related to the displacement or amplitude of air molecules and to sound pressure. We reviewed displacement of air molecules earlier in the chapter. Oscillating movements of air molecules produced by a vibrating object produce sound pressure.

Let's take a moment to review the concept of pressure. Pressure is a force exerted on an area. The amount of force and of sound pressure is directly related to the amount of vibration of an object, its displacement, and the velocity of the vibration. Pressure increases or decreases with changes in the strength and speed of the vibration. And, pressure is inversely related to the area it is distributed over. If a given pressure is spread over a greater area, then the pressure for any small portion of the area is lower. Conversely, pressure increases if it is applied to a smaller area.

A simple experiment will illustrate this point. Take a pencil or a pen and press the point of the pencil or pen firmly against your arm. Notice carefully the pressure sensation and maybe even discomfort that you feel. Now, turn the pencil or pen around and with the same firm pressure push the eraser or blunt end against your arm. You applied about the same amount of force in both conditions, but you felt considerably greater pressure when the force was exerted over the small area under the point of the writing instrument than over the larger area of the other end.

The oscillating movement of air molecules produced by a vibrating object and transmitted through the air as regions of condensation and rarefaction create increased pressure on the tympanic membrane. Movement of the tympanic membrane is one of the early steps in the hearing process.

Units of Force and Pressure. Some consistent units for force and area are needed to meaningfully describe and define sound pressure. We need units that are capable of quantifying the small amounts of force that set the tympanic membrane in motion. The *dyne* is a unit of force commonly used in audiology and hearing science. A dyne is the amount of force required to accelerate 1 gram 1 cm/$\sec^2$. Dyne is from the Greek word *dunamis*, meaning "power." It's no coincidence that the word dyne is imbedded within the word "dynamite."

A common unit of pressure is the micro-Pascal, abbreviated μPa. The μPa is a tiny fraction (a millionth) of a *Pascal.* The **decaPascal**, abbreviated **daPa**, is a larger unit of pressure. The term *Pascal* honors Blaise Pascal, a French scientist who is highlighted with a brief biography in Table 2.1. The forces and pressures used in describing human hearing are necessarily small because the ear is highly sensitive to sound. The minimum amount of force that is detected by a healthy young ear is approximately 0.0002 dyne/cm^2 corresponding to a pressure of 20 μPa.

Power and Intensity. Power is another measure of the strength or magnitude of sound. Sound power is the total amount of acoustical energy exerted over a unit of time. The Watt is a unit of energy that is used in describing sound power. A small unit of power called an **erg** is used to describe hearing. A Watt is equivalent to 1 million ergs/sec. Sound intensity is defined as sound power exerted over a unit of area. Typical units of sound power are watts/cm^2. Sound intensity is expressed with the formula:

$$\text{Intensity (watts/cm}^2) = \frac{\text{Power (watts)}}{4\pi \times \text{radius(cm)}}$$

Defining the Decibel (dB). Audiologists regularly apply the concept of the *decibel (dB)* in manipulating sound and using sound meaningfully in a clinical setting. As described below, four concepts are important for understanding the decibel as used in audiology and hearing science. The **decibel** is a:

- Logarithmic unit
- Ratio of one sound power to another specified reference sound power or one sound pressure to another specified reference sound pressure
- Relative measure, not an absolute measure
- Unit for sound power and also for sound pressure

A decibel (dB) is one-tenth of a bel (B). The "B" in the abbreviation dB is always capitalized. Scientists employed at the Bell Telephone Laboratories in the 1920s coined the term *bel* to honor Alexander Graham Bell. Table 2.1 includes a brief biography of this talented person. Another comment about the term *decibel* is appropriate here. The word *decibels* is used when referring to more than 1 decibel. However, the abbreviation dB is used to indicate one or many decibels. For example, we would say "the sound increased from 1 decibel to 20 decibels," but "the sound increased from 1 dB to 20 dB."

 ClinicalConnection

Manipulation of sound intensity level expressed in dB is an essential component of audiology. Hearing loss is described in decibels. It is therefore important for students enrolled in audiology courses and for practicing audiologists to understand the concept of the decibel.

We'll now consider why the decibel is used to describe levels of sound pressure. The human ear is capable of responding to an incredible range of sound pressures. Sound pressures involved in hearing range from tiny amounts of pressure on the order 20 μPa, which barely moves the thin and delicate eardrum (tympanic membrane), all the way up to magnitudes of pressure on the order of 200,000,000 μPa that are 100,000,000,000,000 times more intense. The lowest sound pressures, at 20 μPa, are just detectable to a person with normal hearing. These levels represent the threshold for hearing, whereas at the other extreme the highest sound pressures represent a level that produces the sensation of pain. Take a moment to count all those zeros! The ratio of the maximum pressure of sound that can be perceived by the human ear before the perception of pain to the minimum amount of sound that the ear can just detect is well over a million. Believe it or not, the ratio of power from the maximum sound to auditory threshold is well over a trillion.

The decibel is a logarithmic unit. The word *logarithm* is derived from two Greek words: *logos*, meaning "ratio," and *arithmos*, which means "number." A logarithm, abbreviated "log," is a number (the base) that is multiplied a specific number of times, such as 2, 3, 4, and so forth. The number of times the number is multiplied is referred to as an *exponent*. For the decibel, the logarithm base is 10. A logarithmic unit like the dB is needed to describe the vast range of sound pressures involved in hearing.

Sound Pressure and Sound Intensity. A few equations are used to define and describe the decibel and make calculations involving sound intensities and sound pressures. Each of the equations includes the ratio of one intensity or pressure value (I_2 or P_2) to a reference intensity (I_R) or pressure (P_R).

Sound Intensity (Intensity Level or IL):

$$Bel(IL) = \log (I_2/I_R)$$

and

$$decibel \text{ or } dB \text{ (IL)} = 10 \times \log (I_2/I_R)$$

Sound pressure (Sound Pressure Level or SPL):

$$dB \text{ (SPL)} = 10 \times \log (P_2^2/P_R^2)$$

or

$$dB \text{ (SPL)} = 10 \times 2 \times \log (P_2/P_R)$$

or

$$dB \text{ (SPL)} = 20 \times \log (P_2/P_R)$$

To put these equations into words, the decibel is 10 times the log of the ratio of a sound intensity to the reference intensity, and 20 times the log of the ratio of a sound pressure to the reference sound pressure. Notice that the square of the ratios of the two pressures (P_2^2/P_R^2) is equivalent to two times the pressure ratios (P_2/P_R). That is, squaring the argument of a logarithm is equal to doubling the logarithm. Therefore, $10 \log P_2^2/P_R^2$ is the same as $20 \log P_2/P_R$. Sound intensity is equivalent to the square of sound pressure. Table 2.2 summarizes the relations of ratios of sound pressure to actual intensity levels and sound pressure levels for some common sounds.

Calculation of Sound Intensities and Sound Pressures. Keeping the above equation for sound intensity level in mind, the calculation of sound intensity levels in dB is quite straightforward once the ratio is known. For example, when two sounds are different by 3, 4, or 5 orders of magnitude, such as $\log_{10} 10^3$, or $\log_{10} 10^4$, or $\log_{10} 10^5$, they are different by 30, 40, or 50 dB. Remember, in describing and calculating decibels the ratio of sound powers is multiplied $\times$ 10 and the ratio of sound pressures is multiplied $\times$ 20.

Let's consider for a moment two sounds that differ by 40 dB. The two sound powers differ by a ratio of 10,000:1. There are 4 zeros in 10,000. The number 10 is multiplied by itself 4 times (10^4) to produce the number 10,000, $10 \times \log 10,000$ is the same as 10 x 4, and $10 \times 4 = 40$. When making the same calculations for two sounds with pressure rather than power, the acoustic pressures of the two sounds differ by a ratio of 100:1. There are 2 zeros in 100. The number 10 is multiplied by itself 2 times to produce the number 100. And $20 \times \log 100$ is the same as 20×2, and $20 \times 2 = 40$.

Summing two sound powers in dB results in an additional 3 dB. For example, if sound from one loudspeaker is 50 dB and then a sound of 50 dB is also presented from a second loudspeaker, the increase in intensity is 3 dB or a total of 53 dB IL. To calculate the addition

TABLE 2.2 The relations of ratios of sound intensity and sound pressure to actual intensity levels and sound pressure levels for some common sounds

Intensity in dB SPL	Ratio of Sound Pressure to Reference Level	SPL (dynes/cm²)	Sounds
0	1:1	.0002	Absolute human hearing threshold for a 3000-Hz pure tone
20	10:1	.002	A whispered voice at 4 feet
40	100:1	.02	A quiet room
50	316:1		A typical office
60	1,000:1	.2	Average level of soft conversation 5 feet from the speaker
70	3,160:1		Moderately intense conversational level
80	10,000:1	2.0	Average level of shouting at a distance of about 5 feet, or the sound of heavy traffic
90	31,600:1		Elevated train, or pneumatic drill at 10 feet
100	100,000:1	20.0	Symphony orchestra, or rivet gun at 35 feet
120	1,000,000:1	200.0	Sound of a jet airplane engine, or MP3 player at high volume
140	10,000,000:1	2000.0	Loud sound causing pain

Source: Adapted from Mueller, H. G., III, & Hall, J. W., III. (1998). *Audiologists' desk reference, vol. II,* p. 683. San Diego: Singular Publishing Group.

of two sound intensities, it's necessary to memorize that the log of the number 2 or $\log_{10} 2$ is 0.3. As an illustration, let's say that one loud speaker in a room or in your car produces sound at 70 dB IL. You then activate a second speaker at the same sound intensity level. Fortunately for anyone near the speakers, the combined sound produced by the two speakers is not 140 dB IL. That very high sound level is at the threshold of pain, or the level of sound that just produces a sensation of pain. Combining the output of the two speakers doubles the sound power. Sound power is increased by an order of 2. Inserting the number 2 into the equation above:

$$dB\ (IL) = 10 \times \log\ (I_2/I_R)$$

or

$$dB\ (IL) = 10 \times \log\ 2$$

or

$$dB\ (IL) = 10 \times 0.3 = 3\ dB$$

Similarly, adding together two sound pressures in dB doesn't double the amount of decibels. Instead, combining the sound pressure levels adds 6 dB. The same general calculation is made, but with the equation for sound pressure levels. That is:

$$dB \ (SPL) = 20 \times \log \ (P_2/P_R)$$

or

$$dB \ (SPL) = 20 \times \log \ 2$$

or

$$dB \ (SPL) = 20 \times 0.3 = 6 \ dB$$

The sound pressure level is equal to the reference value when the ratio of P_2/P_R is 1:1. The $\log_{10}$ (logarithm to the base 10) is 10^0 and the value is zero (0). In audiology, this would represent a hearing threshold of 0 dB. Sound would be first detected at a sound pressure level of 0 dB. This corresponds to normal hearing. When the ratio of the two pressure levels (P_2/P_R) is 100:1, then the logarithm is 2 because $10^2 = 100$. So, inserting the logarithm of 2 into the equation above), we have:

$$dB \ (SPL) = 20 \times \log \ 1 = 20 \ dB$$

Once the ratio is known and the above equations are memorized, the calculation of sound intensity levels for even multiples of the number 10 is essentially done with a tally of the number of zeroes in the sound level. For example, a ratio of 10,000:1 involves 4 zeros or 10^4. The log is 4 and inserting 4 into the equation (dB (IL) = 10×4) yields 40 dB IL.

i **Web**Watch

The Internet offers a wide assortment of instructional aids, tutorials, and reviews to help you better understand the decibel. There are even dB demonstrations on YouTube. Perform an Internet search with the key words "understanding the decibel" to begin your search for these instructional resources.

Measurement of Sound. Before continuing on with the review of intensity of sound and the decibel, we'll take a moment to discuss sound level measurement. Sound level is measured and quantified with a *sound level meter*. A sound level meter plays an important role in verifying the accuracy of the levels of sounds used in hearing testing. A **sound level meter** is a device that always consists of several components, including a microphone for detecting sound and converting acoustic energy to an electrical signal that can then be quantified in decibels and a meter like a needle or an digital display representing the measured sound levels. Figure 2.7 shows a sound level meter.

Sounds measured with the sound level meter are in reference to 20 μPa or 0.0002 dyne/cm^2. Prior to any measurements, a sound level meter is calibrated according to well-established standards such as those developed by the American National Standards Institute (ANSI). Calibration standards are the same for all sound level meters. However, the devices vary considerably in terms of features, flexibility, and price. In fact, a variety of sound level measurement applications can now be downloaded to many smartphones.

Sound level meters used in audiology clinics are sophisticated devices capable of multiple sound level measurements including processing of sound data like maximum, minimum, and average sound levels and spectral characteristics. They are also capable of long-term storage of sound data. Sound measurement data on a sophisticated device can be uploaded to a computer with special software for further analysis and printing. Verification and calibration of sounds used as stimuli in hearing testing are done with this type of sound level meter.

FIGURE 2.7

A sound level meter for documenting sound intensity in dB SPL. Courtesy of 3M Detection Solutions.

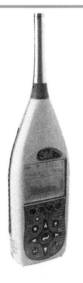

Calibration. The accuracy of hearing research and clinical hearing test results depend on precise calibration of equipment. The purpose of calibration is to document the precise

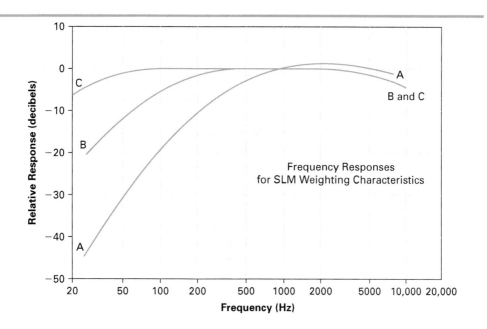

Frequency Responses
for SLM Weighting Characteristics

FIGURE 2.8

Sound level meter weighting networks. The dBA weighting is used most often for sound measurements in audiology. *Source: Martin, Frederick N.; Clark, John Greer, INTRODUCTION TO AUDIOLOGY, 11th Ed.,* © 2012. Reprinted and Electronically reproduced by permission of Pearson Education, Inc., Upper Saddle River, New Jersey.

level of sounds and to verify that the equipment including earphones and loudspeakers are performing properly. Sounds are calibrated with a sound level meter using a physical reference for decibels (dB) called **sound pressure level (SPL)**.

Sound level meters feature different weighting scales that alter the response of the device to sound within the low-frequency region. Figure 2.8 shows the most common weighting scales. The term *weighting* means that sound energy within a specific frequency region is given more or less emphasis. The A weighting curve, known as the *dBA scale*, has considerably less weight for low-frequency sound. When we discuss loudness of sound a little later in the chapter, you'll see how the dBA curve resembles the response of the human ear to low-frequency sounds.

 ClinicalConnection

Regular calibration of hearing test equipment in an audiology clinic is very important both to verify the level of stimulus sounds and to assure accuracy of test results. You'll learn more about equipment calibration with sound level meters in Chapter 4.

Different References for Decibels. Decibels without any further description are only numbers lacking any dimension or meaning. The dimension or specific reference used in the ratio of sounds must be defined whenever decibels are cited in the description of sound. A reference or comparison point for sound pressure is needed to describe sound pressure levels in a meaningful way. The sound pressure that we are interested in must be compared to a standard.

The common reference sound pressure level used in audiology and hearing science is 0.0002 dyne/cm^2. The term *dyne* was mentioned earlier, when the concept of force was introduced. A **dyne** is the force required to move a single gram (1 gr) with an acceleration of 1 cm/sec^2. You will immediately conclude that 0.0002 dyne/cm^2 is a very small amount of force. Think about how little effort you would expend pushing a tiny object that weighs only 1 gram a distance of only one cm (about ½ inch). However, 0.0002 dyne/cm^2 is the common reference for sound because it represents the smallest amount of pressure striking the tympanic membrane that is detectable.

As you've learned, sound pressure and sound intensity are not the same. However, the term *intensity* is commonly used in clinical audiology to refer to the volume or level of sound.

The intensity of sounds is always described in decibels (dB). Audiologists regularly use at least three different descriptors for decibels. Each description has a different reference for sound.

Sound is sometimes described in *dB SPL (sound pressure level)* in an audiology clinic. For example, dB SPL is used in calibrating with a sound level meter the sounds produced by test equipment. Audiologists also document sound level in dB SPL when verifying the function of hearing aids and other devices designed for people with hearing loss. And, the level of sound used in some special hearing test procedures is measured in dB SPL.

Sound intensity is described in *dB HL (hearing level)* for most hearing test procedures performed in an audiology clinic. Hearing test results and hearing losses are not reported in dB SPL. The reference point for dB HL is 0 dB HL or "audiometric zero." By definition, 0 dB HL is the faintest sound detected by the average young person with normal hearing. The intensity of various sounds used in hearing testing is always described in dB HL.

The term dB sensation level or *dB SL* is a third descriptor for intensity level. The reference for a sound in dB SL is a specific patient's hearing level. In other words, the sounds are presented at an intensity level that is a certain number of decibels above the faintest level of sound that the person can detect. The term *threshold* is used to describe the faintest level of sound a person can detect. Hearing thresholds in an audiology clinic are often measured for different type of sounds, like tones and speech sounds. You'll learn about other descriptors for sound intensity level later in the book.

To reiterate an important point, the reference for sound intensity should be stated whenever decibels are mentioned. Statements such as "The intensity of the car horn was 50 dB" or "The patient could just hear a sound level of 40 dB" are not very meaningful because the decibel description is incomplete. On the other hand, the meaning is very clear when the reference for decibels is specified. For example, "The motorcycle noise was measured at 90 dBA SPL at a distance of 30 feet." The abbreviation dBA SPL indicates that sound pressure level was measured with a sound level meter using the A scale. Or, "Ms. Johnson's hearing threshold for 1000 Hz was 40 dB HL" is quite meaningful because it refers to sound intensity with a precisely defined unit for dB that is used in clinical hearing measurement.

Duration

Time plays an important role in sound production and sound perception. The phrase "**temporal** properties of sound" describes the various features of sound that involve time. One temporal property of sound is its **duration**. Duration is the length of time from the beginning to the end of a sound. Some very brief sounds are only fractions of a second in duration and are described in milliseconds. Other sounds may last for seconds or even longer.

Dimensions of Duration. Figure 2.9 illustrates terms used to describe duration of a sound: the *onset*, the *rise time*, the *plateau*, the *fall time*, and the *offset*. The onset is the initial portion of the sound. It is defined as the time from the beginning of the sound at the baseline to the point where maximum amplitude is first reached. The plateau is the segment of sound during which amplitude is consistent or unchanging. Not all sounds have a plateau component of duration. The offset is the final portion of the sound. It consists of the time required for the sound to decrease in amplitude from the maximum point to zero amplitude or back to the baseline. All sounds have an onset and an offset, although very brief or transient sounds are almost instantly on and off.

There is a well-appreciated relation or trade-off between duration and frequency or spectrum of sound. The term *spectrum* refers to the frequency content of a sound. Figure 2.10 shows the relation between duration and frequency in a simple diagram. The duration of the tone is shown on the left side of Figure 2.10, whereas the spectrum is shown to the right.

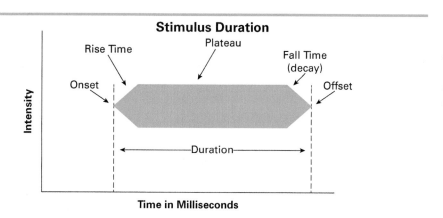

FIGURE 2.9

Illustration of the duration of a stimulus, including stimulus onset, plateau, and offset.

A pure tone or sinusoidal sound has a comparatively long duration. Duration of a pure tone sound may be on the order of seconds, as shown in the top portion of the figure. The spectrum of a pure tone is a single pure tone frequency. Spectrum of a 1000-Hz tone is shown on the right side of Figure 2.10.

A tone with a short duration of 4 ms is depicted in the middle portion of Figure 2.10. A time of 4 ms is only 1/250th of a second. Very brief tonal sounds are referred to as *tone bursts*. Although most of the energy of the tone burst in Figure 2.10 is at 1000 Hz, you'll notice in the right portion of the figure that the spectrum extends somewhat above and below 1000 Hz.

An extremely brief *click* sound is shown in the lower portion of Figure 2.10. The term *click* is used for a sound duration of only 100 microseconds or one-tenth of a millisecond (0.1 ms). One millisecond is 1/1000 of a second. The broad spectrum of the click extends from low to high frequencies, as shown to the right. You'll discover in Chapter 9 that very brief sounds like clicks and tone bursts are used to perform special hearing testing of infants and young children.

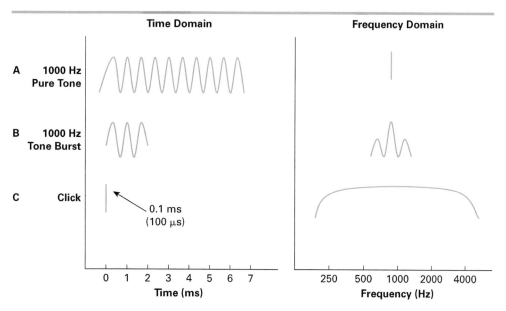

FIGURE 2.10

Illustration of the relation between the duration in the time domain and the spectrum or frequency content for three sounds including a pure tone **(A)**, a tone burst **(B)**, and a click **(C)**.

ClinicalConnection

The unavoidable trade-off between the duration of sound and its spectrum influences the selection of stimuli used in certain clinical test procedures. Some brain responses used in hearing testing of infants and young children are activated only with stimuli of very brief duration. In Chapter 9, you'll learn how audiologists select sounds for auditory response measurement.

The examples of sounds shown in Figure 2.10 summarize the inevitable trade-off between duration and frequency of sound. Very brief transient sounds always consist of a broad range of frequencies, whereas sounds of relatively long duration like pure tones have a spectrum limited to a single frequency.

Psychoacoustics

Up to this point in the chapter, we've focused on the physical properties of sounds. Acoustics is the study of physical properties of sounds. **Psychoacoustics** describes human perception of these physical properties of sound. Psychoacoustics is the study of the psychological or sensory response to the acoustical features of sound. We'll now review psychoacoustical sensations associated with frequency, intensity, and duration of sounds.

Pitch

Pitch is the subjective perception or the psychological attribute of the frequency of a sound. Frequency of a sound can be precisely measured with electronic instruments and described unequivocally in Hz (cycles per second). Low-frequency sounds correspond to low pitches, whereas sounds with high frequencies are perceived as high in pitch. The correspondence between frequency and pitch is quite obvious. However, there isn't a 1:1 relationship between the physical measure of frequency and the psychological perception of pitch. You'll recall from the earlier discussion of logarithms and the decibel that the human auditory system operates over a very wide range of sound intensities. Similarly, the auditory system compresses a broad range of frequencies into a smaller range of perception. For example, a twofold increase in frequency doesn't result in two-fold change in pitch.

In psychoacoustics, pitch is described with the *mel* unit. The term *mel* is derived from the word *melody*. When listening to the melody of a song, we're constantly comparing sounds of different pitches. Pitch can be measured on scale first described by psychoacoustics researchers back in the 1930s (Stevens, Volkman, & Newman, 1937). Figure 2.11 illustrates the *mel scale*. It is a perceptual scale of pitches judged by listeners to be equal distances from each other. On the mel scale, 1000 mels is the pitch of a 1000-Hz tone at an intensity level 40 dB above a listener's threshold for the sound, or 40 dB SL. When pitch perception is measured in mels, sounds are manipulated so that the listener describes them as half the pitch of the reference tone, twice or three times the pitch of the reference tone, and so forth. The mel and the mel scale are important for studying and describing the relationship between frequency and pitch. However, the terms are not regularly used in clinical audiology.

FIGURE 2.11

The mel scale, depicting the relation between pitch (in mels) and frequency (in Hz). *Source:* Martin, Frederick N.; Clark, John Greer, *INTRODUCTION TO AUDIOLOGY, 11th Ed.,* © 2012. Reprinted and Electronically reproduced by permission of Pearson Education, Inc., Upper Saddle River, New Jersey.

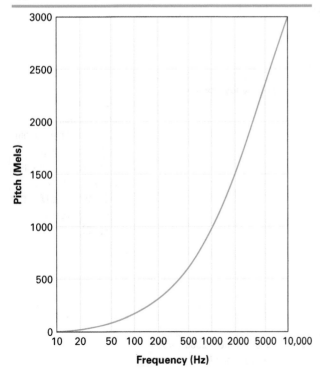

Just Noticeable Difference (JND). Discrimination (detection of a difference) between two sounds is a fundamental auditory skill. One psychoacoustical measurement strategy requires the listener (the subject) in an experiment to match the pitch of a sound to another reference or standard sound. A unit of measurement for the discrimination between two sounds is called the *just noticeable difference*, or *JND*. It's sometimes indicated by the Greek character or symbol "△." The symbol △ is a shorthand way to express "delta," meaning a difference or change. For example, the JND for frequency (f) is sometimes abbreviated as △f.

Other phrases sometimes used to describe this concept include *just noticeable change, difference threshold*, and *difference limen*. The word "limen" is derived from the Latin word for threshold. In measuring JND, the researcher determines whether a listener can detect a very small difference between two sounds. The difference is systematically made smaller or larger until the researcher finds the smallest difference between two sounds that the listener can distinguish most of the time.

Frequency discrimination is the ability to distinguish a difference between two frequencies. It is a psychoacoustic task involving pitch perception. The frequencies are often spaced very close together. Measurement of frequency discrimination is quite time consuming. As a result, it's typically made with subjects in an experimental setting but not with patients in a clinical setting. Figure 2.12 shows the general relationship of the frequency of a 40-dB sound to the JND for frequency, the △f. Recall that the difference threshold or JND for frequency is the smallest difference between two different frequencies that can be detected by a listener. You can see in Figure 2.12 that the difference threshold (△f) is smallest for low frequencies, below 500 Hz. Then the △f increases for frequencies above about 2000 Hz.

Loudness

You'll recall from our earlier discussion that the word *frequency* describes a physical property of sound, whereas the term *pitch* is used to describe human perception of frequency. Similarly, the term *intensity* refers to a physical property of sound pressure. The subjective or

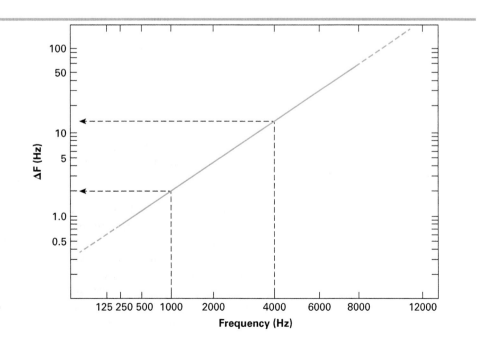

FIGURE 2.12

The relationship between the absolute frequency of sound (on the X-axis) and the ability to discriminate just noticeable differences in frequencies of two sounds (on the Y-axis). *Source:* Durrant, John D.; Feth, Lawrence L., *HEARING SCIENCES: A FOUNDATIONAL APPROACH, 1st Ed.,* © 2012, p. 13. Reprinted and Electronically reproduced by permission of Pearson Education, Inc., Upper Saddle River, New Jersey.

L E A D E R S   A N D   L U M I N A R I E S

Harvey Fletcher (1884–1981)

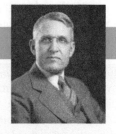

Harvey Fletcher earned his bachelor's of science degree from Brigham Young University in 1907. Fletcher and his new wife moved to Chicago from Utah in hopes that he would be accepted to the University of Chicago. He was required to repeat four years of undergraduate study before earning the first PhD summa cum laude ever awarded there. Dr. Fletcher's doctoral work was completed under the direction of Robert Millikan, an experimental physicist and Nobel laureate who is best known for his discoveries on the charge of electrons and his work on the photoelectric effect.

Returning to Utah, Dr. Fletcher was the first faculty member with a PhD to teach at BYU, and he soon became chair of the Physics Department.

Within a few years, Dr. Fletcher accepted a position at Western Electric in New York City. Soon after he was appointed Director of Physical Research at Bell Telephone Laboratories, where he began an illustrious and highly productive career. Dr. Fletcher with colleagues completed many fundamental studies of sound and psychoacoustics and published germinal articles and books. He is recognized for making many contributions to hearing science and audiology. Dr. Fletcher is also known as the "Father of Stereophonic Sound."

Even a cursory search of the Internet reveals many excellent sources of information about Harvey Fletcher.

psychological term for intensity is **loudness**. Greater amounts of sound pressure and higher intensity levels are perceived as louder. Loudness decreases as sound intensity decreases.

The terms *loudness* and *loud* should not be used interchangeably with the term *intensity*. Intensity is a physical property of sound, whereas loudness is a psychological attribute corresponding to the perception of intensity. Sometimes intensity and loudness are mistakenly equated. You might hear a statement such as: "The band last night was really loud. Using the sound level meter app on my smartphone, I measured the loudness in the back of the club at 90 dB!" In this case, the listener perceived the music as loud but the sound level meter feature on the smart phone measured the sound pressure level of the music, not the loudness.

Loudness level has its own special unit, called the *phon*. It's important to be mindful that the decibel is a unit of intensity rather than loudness. The perception of loudness varies for different frequencies. Loudness levels in phons can be plotted across the range of frequencies heard by normal-hearing persons. The lines extend from low to high frequencies. Representations of loudness levels in phons are known as *equal loudness contours*, or sometimes *Fletcher Munson curves*. Among the classic psychoacoustical papers written during the 1930s was a detailed description of loudness by Harvey Fletcher and a colleague named Wilden Munson (Fletcher & Munson, 1933). Fletcher is featured in Leaders and Luminaries a little earlier in this chapter.

Figure 2.13 is a graph of equal loudness contours. The lowest line in the figure, representing 0 phons, is the level at which sound is first detected (or the hearing threshold) for each frequency. The graph clearly shows that the human ear is less sensitive to lower frequencies. You'll recall that the dBA weighting curve for sound level measurements shown previously in Figure 2.8 also showed decreased response for lower-frequency sounds.

Returning to Figure 2.13, let's focus for a moment on one of the higher equal loudness contours, for example, a loudness level of 90 phons. Except for the very high-frequency region, the equal loudness contour is almost a flat line at an intensity level of 100 dB. Compare the

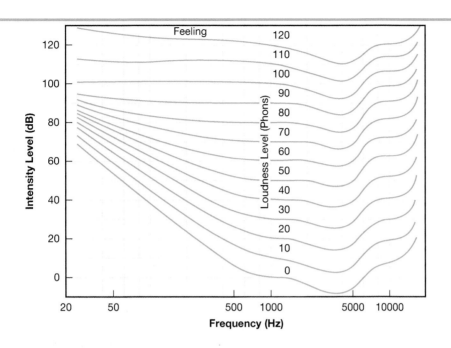

FIGURE 2.13

Equal loudness contours showing the relation between loudness (in phons) and intensity (in dB) as a function of frequency. *Source:* Martin, Frederick N.; Clark, John Greer, *INTRODUCTION TO AUDIOLOGY, 11th Ed.,* © 2012. Reprinted and Electronically reproduced by permission of Pearson Education, Inc., Upper Saddle River, New Jersey.

difference between the 90-phon line and the 0-phon line for a very low-frequency sound, versus a 1000 Hz tone. Loudness grows much more quickly from threshold to the 90-phon level for the low-frequency tones than for tones in the mid- to higher frequency region.

Just Noticeable Difference for Intensity. The concepts reviewed in the discussion of frequency discrimination and the just noticeable difference (JND) for frequency also apply to intensity discrimination. The smallest difference in intensity that can be detected is indicated by the expression $\triangle I$. The smallest difference in intensity ($\triangle I$) detected by a normal hearer decreases modestly as intensity of the sound increases. This trend in JND or $\triangle I$ for intensity of sounds is relatively consistent across the range of frequencies that we use for communication.

WebWatch

Animations and tutorials on psychoacoustical concepts, such as pitch, loudness, and JNDs, are available on a variety of websites. You'll be taken directly to them with an Internet search using key words like "understanding loudness" or "understanding pitch."

Duration

Temporal Integration. Detection of a sound is influenced by duration of the sound. The technical term **temporal integration** is used to describe the relationship between duration of sound and its detection by the auditory system of the listener.

The concept of threshold for sound was discussed in the section on sound intensity. Duration has no effect on the threshold for a sound for sounds lasting longer than one second (1000 ms). However, progressively poorer detection is associated with sound durations of less than one second and especially for sounds shorter than 300 ms.

Figure 2.14 shows the increased threshold for short duration sounds. You'll see that the line representing the threshold for sound begins to curve upward when the duration of sound decreases below about 300 ms. Greater intensity levels are required for detection of very brief sounds. The threshold for detection of sound in dB increases as the duration of the sound decreases.

Just Noticeable Difference for Duration. The concept of JND or difference limen applies also to the duration of sound. Measurement of the JND for duration is not an easy task. You'll

FIGURE 2.14

Illustration of the relation between the duration of sound and the threshold for detection of the sound. The relation is known as temporal integration. *Source:* Adapted from Durrant, John D.; Feth, Lawrence L., *HEARING SCIENCES: A FOUNDATIONAL APPROACH, 1st Ed.*, © 2012, p. 8. Reprinted and Electronically reproduced by permission of Pearson Education, Inc., Upper Saddle River, New Jersey.

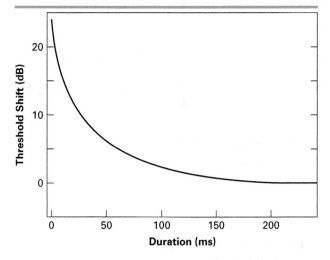

ClinicalConnection

Measurement of temporal auditory abilities using gap detection techniques has long been a part of experimental hearing studies. As reviewed in Chapter 9, gap detection tests are now also available for clinical assessment of certain types of hearing problems in children and adults.

recall from our discussion of frequency/pitch and intensity/loudness that one property of sound may interact with another. In the area of hearing research called psychoacoustics, inevitable interactions among frequency, intensity, and duration of sound are sometimes referred to as "confounding variables." Interactions among the properties of sounds make measurements quite complicated and sometimes confusing. For example, there's an influence of intensity on frequency and an influence of duration on detection and threshold of sound. It's almost impossible to measure one property of sound without considering and accounting for other properties of sound.

Gap Detection. Although not directly related to the actual duration of sound, another temporal aspect of sound is the time interval or the gap between two or more sounds. Sounds are rarely heard in isolation. This statement is particularly true for speech sounds. In hearing assessment, the length of time between sounds is referred to as the *inter-stimulus interval*. The expression $\triangle T$ is often used to indicate the smallest detectable difference in duration between different sounds.

Relatively large time gaps between sounds, such as 50 or 100 ms, are easily detected. At the other extreme, even a person with normal auditory function will not detect a very small gap or silent period between two sounds. For example, two sounds with a gap between them of 1 ms are heard as a single sound. A listener will begin to hear two distinct sounds as the silent gap between sounds is increased to a certain number of milliseconds. The minimal gap in time that is required to perceive two sounds rather than one sound is influenced by many factors, including the type of the stimulus (e.g., noise versus tone), the intensity of the stimulus, the age of the listener (especially young children and elderly adults), and whether the listener's auditory function is normal or disordered.

Audibility of Sound

Now that we've reviewed the main properties of sound . . . frequency, intensity, and duration . . . and the interaction among these properties, you have the background information required to grasp the concept of the *threshold of audibility*. Audibility of a sound occurs at the faintest intensity level of the sound that can be detected. Audibility of sound varies greatly, depending on the properties of sound reviewed earlier in the chapter, including frequency, phase, duration, and intensity. Detection of sound is a basic and simple auditory process. Formal and careful experiments of auditory thresholds for pure tone signals were initially conducted in the 1930s (e.g., Fletcher & Munson, 1933; Stevens, 1935). Measurement of auditory sensitivity for simple pure tone sounds remains an important and very common goal in clinical hearing testing.

Minimal Auditory Field (MAF) and Minimal Auditory Pressure (MAP)

Two general approaches for measuring the threshold of audibility are known as *minimal auditory field (MAF)* and *minimal auditory pressure (MAP)*. Minimal auditory field (MAF) thresholds are auditory thresholds measured with the listener sitting in a sound-treated room facing a loudspeaker at a distance of 1 meter. The listener is not wearing earphones. In this measurement condition, the listener hears in a *binaural* condition (using both ears). Intensity levels for signals used to measure thresholds are verified precisely with a calibration process before MAF measurements are carried out. Intensity is verified by placing the microphone of a sound level meter in the same location in the sound-treated room that will be occupied by the listener's head. Then, a listener's auditory thresholds are determined.

Minimal auditory pressure (MAP) is the other general approach for measuring threshold of audibility. MAP measurement is performed with pure tone signals presented to the listener via earphones. Each ear is tested separately, in a *monaural* listening condition. Again, intensity levels for the sounds are first carefully verified with a sound level meter.

Reference Equivalent Threshold Sound Pressure Levels (RETSPLs)

The rather lengthy term **reference equivalent threshold sound pressure levels** and the odd abbreviation **RETSPLs** refer to the values that are determined from calibrating sounds with a sound level meter connected to a device with a cavity of a specific size. The device, called a coupler, is designed for connecting the microphone of a sound level meter to some type of earphone. You were introduced to sound level meters earlier in the chapter.

Table 2.3 shows sound measurement values for a collection of frequencies.

| Frequency (Hz) | Free Field | Earphone | |
	MAF	TDH[a]	Insert[b]
125	22	45	26
250	11	27	14
500	4	13.5	5.5
750	2	9.0	2
1000	2	7.5	0
1500	0.5	7.5	2
2000	−1.5	9.0	3
3000	−6	11.5	3.5
4000	−6.5	12.0	5.5
6000	2.5	16.0	2
8000	11.5	15.5	0
Speech	-----	20.0	12.5

TABLE 2.3
Reference equivalent threshold sound pressure levels (RETSPLS) for different clinical transducers (earphones).

a: TDH 49/50 BS9A earphone

b: ANSI S3.6 reference thresholds measured with HA-2 (2 cc coupler) with rigid tube

The RETSPLs were measured according standards of the American National Standards Institute (ANSI, 2004). Hearing researchers and clinical audiologists around the world adhere closely to these or other standards. A brief explanation is needed for the data displayed in Table 2.3. Thresholds are shown for a *sound field* condition in which sounds were presented to the listener with a loudspeaker. In an audiology clinic, sound field measurements are made in a sound-treated room. Similar measurements in a *free field* are made by auditory scientists in a laboratory using a special type of sound-treated room known as an anechoic room. Thresholds are also displayed for measurements with two types of earphones commonly used in clinical audiology.

Differences in threshold among the pure tone frequencies are readily apparent. You'll also notice in Table 2.3 that threshold levels vary depending on how sounds are delivered to a listener. Thresholds are different for loudspeakers than for earphones that fit over the ear, and again different for earphones that are inserted into the ear canal.

 ClinicalConnection

It would be reasonable to question whether reference equivalent threshold sound pressure levels or RETSPLs are really relevant to hearing testing. The answer is definitely "yes." The accuracy of hearing testing is dependent on knowing the exact intensity level of sounds presented with test equipment to a patient. Careful documentation of RETSPLs with a sound level meter connected to a device representing an ear is an important step in insuring that estimations of hearing status and hearing loss are accurate.

Propagation of Sound

Speed of Sound

As noted earlier in the chapter, sound travels or is propagated through a medium that is solid, liquid, or air. Speed of sound is defined by the distance the sound wave travels during a unit of time, such as a second. Sound travels faster in denser media like solids and liquids than in air. The average speed of sound traveling in air from point A to point B is 1100 feet per second or 345 meters per second. Three major factors influence the speed of sound through air, including (1) temperature, (2) moisture or humidity, and (3) barometric pressure. The speed of sound increases as temperature increases, humidity increases, and/or pressure increases.

Inverse Square Law

The intensity of sound decreases as sound waves travel farther from the source of the sound. The explanation for this statement is that displacement of air molecules produced by a vibrating object decreases as the distance from the object increases. Sound propagates or radiates outward in all directions from the vibrating object.

In the optimal acoustical environment, there are no objects or other irregularities within the space to interfere with sound and no reflections of the sound.

The decrease in intensity of sound associated with the increased distance from the source of the sound is described quite precisely. The intensity of any sound is inversely proportional to the squared distance that the sound has traveled. This principle is known as the **inverse square law**. The relation of the decrease in sound intensity to the distance traveled is described by the following equation:

$$I \propto K (P/4\pi r^2)$$

In this equation, I = intensity of a sound, K = a constant that accounts for the density of the medium (e.g., air) and the speed of sound, $\propto$ is the symbol for proportionality, P = the power of sound at the source of the sound, π = pi, and r = the distance from the source of the sound to the point where sound is measured, or the ear of the listener.

Sound power decreases 6 dB and sound pressure also decreases 6 dB as the distance from the source is doubled. Also according to the inverse square law, when the distance between the source of a sound and its measurement location (or between the source of the sound and the listener) decreases, the sound power or pressure increases by 6 dB.

Examining the equation again, you'll see that increases or decreases in the value of "r" (the symbol for distance from the source of sound) produce these predictable effects on sound intensity.

Interference with Propagation of Sound

Sound waves can interact or interfere with each other in different ways. Two general categories of sound wave interactions or interference are *reinforcement* and *cancellation*. Reinforcement is also referred to as *constructive interference,* whereas cancellation is also known as *destructive interference.*

Figure 2.15 illustrates a simple interaction of two or more waves. Constructive interference is illustrated with the waves labeled A on the left side of Figure 2.15. Imagine that the waves are traveling in the direction indicated by the arrows in the figure. The pressures for each wave eventually add to or *reinforce* each other, creating a greater pressure when the instantaneous displacement or pressure of two sound waves that interact is in the same direction. You'll recall that displacement of a vibrating object and resulting sound pressures are constantly changing over time. Instantaneous displacement is the displacement at a specific time.

Cancellation of waves is shown as B in the right part of Figure 2.15. Close examination of the different waveforms reveals two or more waves of opposite instantaneous pressure interacting with each other. In some of the examples of destructive interference, waveform shape changes, or wave amplitude decreases. In one case, in the fifth waveform down from the top, there is complete cancellation of the waves.

Another type of sound interference is *sound reverberation*. Sound reverberation is produced when sound waves reflect off of the walls of a room. Reverberated sound reaches the

 ClinicalConnection

In an audiology clinic, the problem of sound wave interactions is known as *standing wave interference*. Sounds from loudspeakers are sometimes used to test hearing while a patient is sitting in a sound-treated room. Interference problems can occur under such conditions if testing is performed with pure tone sounds. Pure tone sound reflecting off the sound booth wall may interact with pure tone sounds leaving the loudspeakers. Interference changes the intensity level of the sounds reaching the patient and affects the accuracy of hearing measurements. Audiologists use special tonal sounds that constantly fluctuate slightly in frequency when testing with loudspeakers in a sound-treated room. These special sounds, called *warble tones*, eliminate potential problems with standing wave interference.

FIGURE 2.15

Constructive interference (reinforcement) of waveforms (**A**) that increase in amplitude as they interact, and destructive interference (cancellation) of waveforms (**B**) that are cancelled out when their sum is zero. *Source:* Mullin, William J.; Gerace, William J.; Mestre, Jose P.; Velleman, Shelley L., *FUNDAMENTALS OF SOUND WITH APPLICATIONS TO SPEECH AND HEARING, 1st Ed.,* © (2003). Reprinted and Electronically reproduced by permission of Pearson Education, Inc., Upper Saddle River, New Jersey.

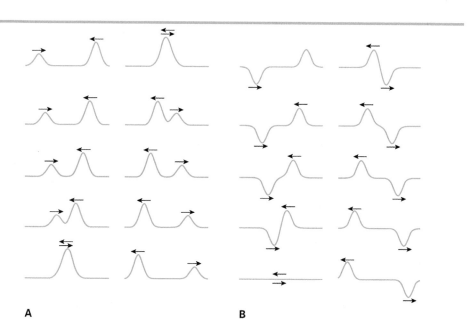

A   B

FIGURE 2.16

Examples of complex waveforms formed by adding together two sets of pure tones. One wave represents a pure tone of 200 Hz and the other is a pure tone of 400 Hz. Looking closely you'll see that the phase of the 400-Hz wave is different for each example. A difference in the phase of the wave changes the sum of the two waves. *Source:* Mullin, William J.; Gerace, William J.; Mestre, Jose P.; Velleman, Shelley L., *FUNDAMENTALS OF SOUND WITH APPLICATIONS TO SPEECH AND HEARING, 1st Ed.,* © (2003). Reprinted and Electronically reproduced by permission of Pearson Education, Inc., Upper Saddle River, New Jersey.

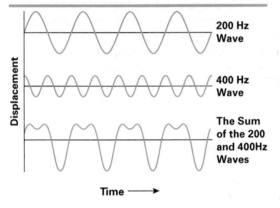

200 Hz Wave

400 Hz Wave

The Sum of the 200 and 400Hz Waves

Displacement

Time ⟶

listener's ears after a slight delay. Some of the sound travels directly from the source to the listener's ears, but other sounds first bounce off the walls of the room and are delayed slightly before they reach the listener's ears. Reverberation of sounds in a sound booth or in a school classroom interferes with a person's ability to perceive and understand speech.

Complex Sounds

We have already discussed in some detail the simplest of sounds . . . sinusoidal or pure tone sounds. Pure tone sounds are called *periodic* because the amplitude repetitively and predictably changes from positive to negative. Most sounds we encounter in the environment are not sinusoids and not periodic. Instead, most real world sounds are complex, consisting of many different frequencies. In the real-world acoustic environment there are infinite combinations of frequencies within complex sounds and also myriad combinations of frequency, phase, amplitudes, and temporal characteristics.

Figure 2.16 shows how complex sounds result from the combination of two or more waves with different frequencies, specifically, a complex waveform created by adding a 200-Hz and a 400-Hz wave. Complex waveforms are also formed from hundreds of waves at different frequencies. Complex sound, such as speech sounds or music, also consists of specific frequencies and specific temporal or timing characteristics.

Think for a moment about the many hundreds of different languages in the world or the untold thousands of songs written, sung, and played from ancient times to the present. Each is an example of an original and even unique sequence of complex sounds that can be used to convey meaning and emotion. The following review considers a variety of types of sound, with a focus on sounds that audiologists use in hearing assessment.

Properties of pure tone sounds and combinations of sinusoids are often displayed in figures that consist of two dimensions. You've already viewed figures showing the amplitude of sound plotted as a function of time. The graph is in the *time domain* when amplitudes of a sound or sounds are shown over a period of time. Most of the waveforms you've viewed in this chapter were plotted in the time domain.

Sound can also be shown in the frequency domain, with amplitude of sound plotted across a frequency range. The graph of the range of amplitudes at different frequencies is called a *spectral display*. Figure 2.17 shows examples of a spectral display in the frequency domain for a vowel speech sound. Spectral display with analysis of speech is a technique that speech pathologists sometimes use in the diagnosis of speech and voice disorders.

There is no simple way of showing simultaneously in a single two-dimensional graph or figure all of the properties of complex sounds, such as amplitude, frequency, phase, and temporal properties. Sometimes three properties of sound are displayed in a single three-dimensional figure. Speech sound is often graphed with time represented on the horizontal (X) axis, frequency on

 ClinicalConnection

Every day in the clinic audiologists analyze information in the time domain. In some hearing tests, a patient's response to sound is recorded over a period of time. Analysis of test results involves a calculation of how quickly the response occurred. Audiologists also measure the amplitude of sound over a specific time period in determining how much benefit a patient with a hearing loss will receive from a hearing aid, or some other assistive device for hearing. In contrast, speech pathologists analyze amplitude and other characteristics of more complex speech sounds at different frequencies.

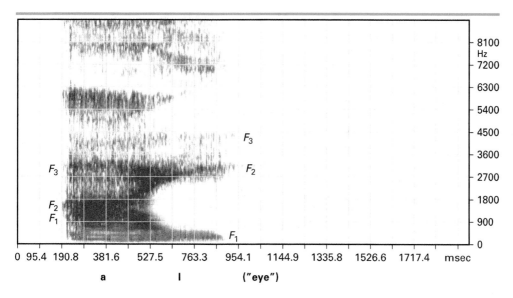

a   I   ("eye")

FIGURE 2.17

The frequency characteristics (spectrum) of an adult female voice saying the word "eye." The formant energy is indicated by the abbreviations F1, F2, and F3. *Source:* Mullin, William J.; Gerace, William J.; Mestre, Jose P.; Velleman, Shelley L., *FUNDAMENTALS OF SOUND WITH APPLICATIONS TO SPEECH AND HEARING, 1st Ed.,* © (2003). Reprinted and Electronically reproduced by permission of Pearson Education, Inc., Upper Saddle River, New Jersey.

the vertical (Y) axis, and the relative amplitude or intensity of the sounds represented by the shading of the print with darker shades representing more intense sound and lighter shades less intense sound. Speech sound amplitudes are sometimes depicted by differences in color.

Transient Sounds

Extremely brief sounds with durations of milliseconds or even a brief portion of just one millisecond are called transient sounds, or simply transients. The click sound is a common example of a transient. You were introduced to the click sound in our earlier discussion of the relation between sound duration and spectrum. The relation was illustrated in Figure 2.10. Other transient sounds lasting a handful of milliseconds include short segments of pure tone sounds called tone bursts, which often consist of less than 4 or 5 cycles of the sound.

 ClinicalConnection

Audiologists use transient sounds like clicks and short bursts of tones to measure auditory function with several clinical procedures. Some of the procedures are used to detect or to diagnosis hearing loss in newborn infants because very brief sounds often produce a clear response from the ear and hearing parts of the brain.

Noise

Noise is sometimes appropriately defined in a negative way as undesirable acoustical energy that disturbs or interrupts an activity or causes displeasure, discomfort, or even potential danger. There are many examples of undesirable acoustic noise in everyday life, from the sound of a motorcycle with straight exhaust pipes racing down a street very early in the morning to dogs barking late at night.

In reality, it's impossible to entirely escape background noise here on earth. Even the constant and inevitable movement of air molecules produces a small amount of noise throughout the audiometric frequency range of 250 to 8000 Hz. Brownian motion or movement was described earlier in the chapter. Hearing scientists in the 1930s calculated the spectral level of the energy produced by normal motion of air molecules (e.g., Sivian & White, 1933). At typical temperatures and atmospheric pressures, the level of background sound caused by Brownian movement at frequencies important for hearing is defined by the equation: Noise $= 10^{-16}$ Watts/cm^2. Fortunately for audiologists, this level of noise energy is very low on the hearing spectrum. It is inaudible and does not affect the accuracy of hearing measurements, even for persons with better-than-average hearing sensitivity.

Types of Noise in Hearing Testing. Noise is a valuable tool in clinical audiology and also in hearing research. Various types of noise are applied in hearing testing. Usually a specific type of noise is best suited to a specific test procedure. *White noise* is a good example. White noise is often called broadband noise. It consists of sound at about the same intensity level over a wide range of frequencies. The term *white noise* is derived from the meaning of the color white, which really consists of many colors.

Narrowband noise (NBN) is another type of noise used often in hearing testing. NBN includes frequencies within a more limited region, such as from 900 to 1100 Hz. *Speech spectrum noise* includes energy approximately within the frequency region that encompasses the energy found in speech. *Octave band noise* is noise that falls within a single octave range of frequencies, such as between 1000 and 2000 Hz or between 500 and 1000 Hz.

ClinicalConnection

Audiologists often use different sounds in hearing testing, in addition to pure tone sounds. Noise plays an important role in a number of hearing tests. In some hearing tests, noise is used to increase the accuracy of hearing testing with pure tone sounds. In certain specialized tests noise is combined with other sounds, like speech, to evaluate hearing in difficult listening conditions. You'll learn in later chapters about the many uses of noise in the assessment of hearing.

Speech

Speech is a highly complex sound. Speech sound consists of many different frequencies, intensity levels, and durations. Speech sounds are highly important for humans as they form the basis for oral communication. A full discussion of speech is far beyond the scope of this book. Indeed, many published studies and entire textbooks are devoted to a review of speech and speech perception (e.g., Pisoni & Remez, 2005; Raphael, Borden, & Harris, 2006). Each of the properties of sound that we've reviewed up to this point is essential for describing speech sounds. Here you'll be introduced to just a few concepts underlying speech sound that are important for audiologists and speech pathologists.

Fundamental Frequency. One important characteristic of human speech or voice is known as the *fundamental frequency* or F_0. The fundamental frequency of a voice is determined by the rate at which the vocal folds vibrate. For any given person, the fundamental voice frequency depends on a variety of factors, such as age, gender, and specifically the size of the vocal folds.

Some generalizations about the frequency of the human voice are important in understanding the impact of hearing loss on speech perception. For example, the fundamental voice frequency is typically lowest for males. The average male voice fundamental frequency is 125 Hz, with a range from 85 to 180 Hz. Fundamental frequency of voice is generally higher for females, falling within the region of 170 to 250 Hz. For young children, fundamental frequency is above 300 Hz.

ClinicalConnection

Speech pathologists evaluate how well children and adults produce speech and the impact of speech disorders on communication. Audiologists, on the other hand, often use speech signals like words and sentences to test hearing and to evaluate the impact of hearing loss on communication. An audiologist must have a good grasp of the properties of speech in order to determine how hearing loss affects communication. In later chapters, you'll learn about how speech is used in the hearing test process and about the effects of hearing loss on the ability to perceive speech.

Formants. In addition to fundamental frequency, the human voice contains multiple higher frequencies that are determined by the acoustic properties of the vocal tract from the throat to the mouth. Peaks of energy above the fundamental frequency in vowel sounds are called *formants*. Formants are regions of energy in speech that are related to resonance of the vocal tract.

The acoustic properties of speech are displayed visually in a *speech spectrogram* as shown earlier in Figure 2.17. A speech spectrogram is an image of the frequency information in speech plotted over a time period of one or two seconds. Changes in the size and shape of vocal tract during speech related to the lips, tongue, and teeth produce changes in speech sounds and variations in the speech spectrogram. For example, formant energy in the image is identified with darker regions that shift to higher or lower frequencies. The energy in speech extends up to frequencies of 4000 Hz and higher. As a general rule, vowels are dominated by lower-frequency energy whereas consonants consist of higher frequencies.

Music

Music is another form of complex sound that is used for communication. Each of the properties of sound already reviewed in the chapter is used in the description of music. The terminology used in audiology resembles to some extent the terminology used by musicians and scientists who conduct research on music and music perception. Music is described in terms of frequency and pitch, intensity and loudness, and temporal properties such as the duration and sequence of sounds. Often, however, the terminology of music differs from the terminology used in audiology, though many of the concepts are shared.

Persons with hearing impairment who have difficulties understanding speech also may express concerns about problems hearing music. Some knowledge of the musical scale is useful in evaluating and helping patients with hearing loss that express problems with music perception or reduced enjoyment of listening to music.

Figure 2.18 shows the frequencies associated with notes on a piano keyboard. The frequencies within the human range of hearing most important for perceiving and understanding speech within the range of 250 to 4000 Hz overlap with the frequencies on the piano keyboard.

 ClinicalConnection

It is important for audiologists and speech pathologists to have a general understanding of the properties of music, especially frequency characteristics. Auditory problems that disrupt speech perception and communication can also affect the ability to hear and enjoy music. Music is also used in therapy for some types of communication disorders. In later chapters you'll learn about how hearing is tested and about different patterns of hearing loss. Then you'll begin to appreciate the impact of hearing loss on listening to and enjoying music.

FIGURE 2.18   Piano keyboard relating musical notes to the frequencies in Hertz included in an audiogram.

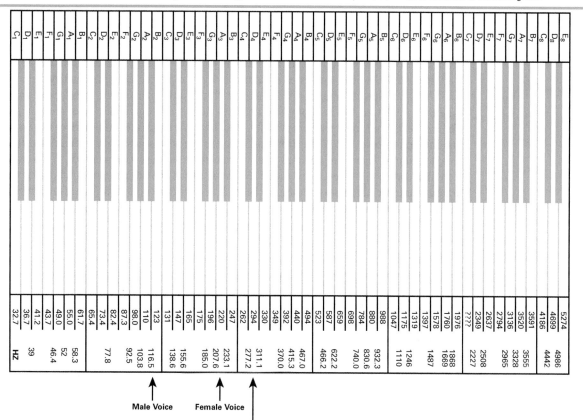

Environmental Sounds

It's almost impossible to avoid daily exposure to an incredibly wide variety of environmental sounds. As already noted, the term *noise* is usually used for environmental sounds that are irrelevant, do not convey meaning, and sometimes actually interfere with communication or quality of life. Sound levels of some typical sources were summarized earlier in Table 2.2. One of the most common causes of hearing loss results when a person is exposed to very high-intensity levels of sound. The sound may be noise or even high levels of music. In fact, hearing loss due to exposure to excessive levels of sound is a serious public health problem.

Many sources of sounds are sufficiently intense to damage hearing. There is a long list of potential damaging sounds associated with recreational activities, including riding noisy motorcycles, hunting, target shooting, attending concerts, and extended high-volume use of personal radios and MP3 players. Excessive sound exposure may also occur during work-related and vocational activities. Work activities include employment in a factory or a mine, driving heavy equipment or tractors, use of power tools, exposure to amplified music, and military service. Importantly, most sound-induced hearing loss is preventable. Audiologists and other professionals such as occupational health personnel are very interested in limiting and preventing permanent hearing loss caused by exposure to high-intensity levels of sound.

 ClinicalConnection

Hearing loss caused by exposure to high levels of sound is theoretically preventable. Audiologists play an important role in this effort. Later in the book, you'll learn about the damage that can occur to the ear with exposure to excessive sound and patterns of hearing loss that result from the damage. You'll also be introduced to hearing conservation strategies and devices that are used to minimize hearing deficits due to noise exposure.

PULLING IT ALL TOGETHER

You learned many new concepts and dozens of new terms in this chapter. We defined and discussed physical properties of sound and vibration, including frequency, intensity, and duration. Special attention was devoted to the unit of intensity, the decibel or dB. Then, we reviewed for each physical property the psychological attribute, such as pitch for frequency and loudness for intensity. You were introduced to sound level meters and the important topic of sound calibration. Diverse types of sounds were mentioned in the chapter, among them simple sinusoidal or pure tone sounds, various types of noise, and complex sounds like speech and music. Sound is one of the critical tools of the audiology trade. Therefore, an understanding of the information presented in this chapter forms the foundation for understanding audiology.

READINGS

Beyer, R. T. (1998). *Sounds of our times: Two hundred years of acoustics*. New York: Springer.

Durrant, J. D., & Feth, L. L. (2013). *Hearing sciences: A foundational approach*. Boston: Pearson.

Green, D. M. (1976). *An introduction to hearing*. Hillsdale, NJ: Erlbaum Associates.

Moore, B. (2003). *Introduction to the psychology of hearing*. San Diego: Academic Press.

Mullin, W. J., Gerace, W. J, Mestre, J. P., & Velleman, S. L. (2003). *Fundamentals of sound with applications to speech and hearing*. Boston: Allyn & Bacon.

Yost, W. A. (2007). *Fundamentals of hearing: An introduction* (5th ed). San Diego: Academic Press.

3 Anatomy and Physiology of the Auditory and Vestibular Systems

LEARNING OBJECTIVES

In this chapter, you will learn:

- New terminology for describing the anatomy of the auditory and vestibular systems
- Functions of the outer ear
- How sound energy is shaped by the outer ear and the middle ear before it reaches the inner ear
- Structures and processes within the inner ear that are important for converting mechanical energy from sound vibrations to electrical activity
- The role of the auditory nerve in coding the properties of sound and conveying electrical activity from the inner ear to the brain
- About auditory structures and regions in the brain that are specialized for hearing
- About the complexity of the central auditory nervous system and the role it plays in processing complex sound, like speech
- How the vestibular system helps us to maintain a stable position in space
- That peripheral vestibular structures detect different forms of movement
- About structures and regions in the brain that contribute to vestibular function and balance

CHAPTER FOCUS

A general and up-to-date understanding of the structure and function of the auditory system and the vestibular system is essential for the practice of audiology. Knowledge about the auditory and vestibular systems contributes in many ways to the identification, accurate diagnosis, and effective management of persons with hearing loss or vestibular disturbances. This chapter introduces terminology used to describe structures in the auditory and the vestibular systems from the *outer ear* to the highest levels of the brain. Critical concepts of functional anatomy involved in hearing are reviewed simply. We begin with structural features of the outer ear, *middle ear,* and *inner ear* that contribute to amplification of energy. The review also includes current auditory neuroscience explanations of how sound is represented and processed by the brain. Similarly, the *vestibular system* is reviewed, from structures in the ear to the *central nervous system* pathways. Throughout the chapter information about auditory and vestibular

KEY TERMS

Apex
Auricle
Brainstem
Central auditory nervous system (CANS)
Cerebral cortex
Cochlea
Concha
Cortilymph
Decussation
Efferent auditory system
Endolymph
Eustachian tube
External ear canal
Incus
Inner hair cells
Labyrinth
Malleus
Organ of Corti
Outer hair cells
Oval window
Perilymph
Peripheral auditory system
Pinna
Round window
Stapedius muscle
Stapes
Temporal bone
Temporal lobes
Thalamus
Traveling waves
Tympanic membrane
Vestibular system

CHAPTER FOCUS *Concluded*

system anatomy and physiology is related to clinical procedures employed by audiologists for hearing assessment and management of hearing loss.

Louis Henri Sullivan (1856–1924) famously noted that "form ever follows function." Structure always follows function within the amazingly complex auditory system. Anatomical structures found in each region of the auditory system are well designed to optimize hearing function. You'll be introduced in this chapter to many examples of this principle. Extensive processing of sound takes place in the ear and the auditory regions of the brain.

New terms in the chapter are listed alphabetically in the Glossary at the end of the book. The origins of many terms are also given in the Glossary, to help you understand and remember the meaning of the words.

General Anatomical Terms

The names of pathways and centers in the central nervous system include terms indicating the general location or orientation of the structures. At least ten general anatomical terms are used to describe the location of structures within the central auditory nervous system. Two different sets of terms describe the vertical anatomical dimension and the general location of structures that are relatively lower or higher within the central nervous system. The meaning of the terms *inferior* and *superior* requires no explanation. You can be certain that whenever the name of a structure includes the word *inferior* there is a similar structure just above it and vice versa. The terms *caudal* and *rostral* are also used to describe the general location of structures within the central nervous system. The term *caudal* refers to a direction toward the tail, whereas the meaning of term *rostral* is toward the head. For example, the spinal cord is caudal to the brain and the brain is located rostral to the spinal cord.

The terms *ventral* and *dorsal* are also used with the names of auditory structures. The word *ventral* refers to the front side of the brain, whereas *dorsal* means toward the backside of the central nervous system. Anatomic structures in the auditory system are also described with familiar terms like *anterior* and *posterior*. The final two anatomical terms that are used in naming auditory structures are *medial* and *lateral*. The word *medial* describes a location toward the middle or inside, whereas *lateral* means toward the side or outside. Each of these ten general anatomical terms permits more accurate description of the location of structures, or a portion of a structure, within the auditory system. We'll use and illustrate the terms throughout the chapter.

Peripheral Auditory System

The **peripheral auditory system** consists of the outer ear, the middle ear, the inner ear, and the auditory nerve that leads from the ear to the brainstem within the **central auditory nervous system (CANS)**. Figure 3.1 shows a simple diagram of the peripheral auditory system with each of the major structures identified.

Outer Ear
Auricle. The most obvious part of the auditory system is the outer ear. The technical term for the outer ear is **auricle**. Words with the root "auri-," for "ear," are derived from Latin. The C-shaped portion of the outer ear that projects outward is the **pinna**, another word derived from Latin, meaning "wing."

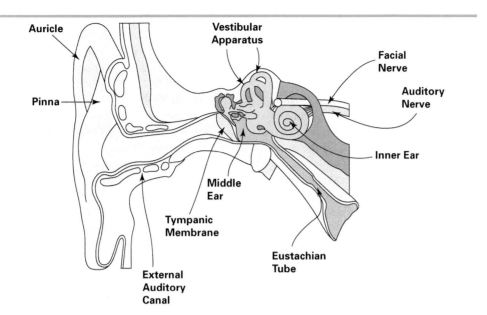

F I G U R E   3 . 1

The peripheral auditory system as seen from an anterior view.

Major components of the outer ear are identified in Figure 3.2. The photographs of the outer ear of a female adult (Figure 3.2A) and of a male infant (Figure 3.2B) illustrate the minor variations of normal auricular anatomy. Most variations in individual ear appearance have little or no impact on hearing function. Examples of variations include the appearance of the *triangular fossa,* the *scaphoid fossa,* the *anti-helix,* and the *intertragal notch or incisure.* Each of these structures is identified in Figure 3.2. Take a moment to casually inspect the outer ears of classmates, family members, or even strangers, and you'll also notice that outer ears vary considerably in appearance and size from one person to the next.

The main anatomic structures of the auricle are the *pinna,* the *helix,* the *lobe,* the *tragus,* and the *concha.* Each of these structures is also shown in Figure 3.2. In an adult ear, the distance from the top of the pinna to the lower end of the ear lobe is in the range of 6 to over 7 cm. The relatively flexible outer ear consists of *cartilage,* rather than bone, covered by skin. You've probably noticed that skull bones in a skeleton or a skull at Halloween lack outer ears.

F I G U R E   3 . 2   Photographs of the right outer ear of an adult female **(A)** and of a one-month-old male infant **(B),** showing major anatomical structures

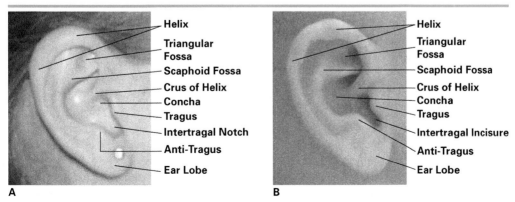

Function of the Auricle. Anatomy of the outer ear is easily visible to even a casual observer. The outer ear offers another clear example of form following function. Although differences among persons in the folds and crevices of the outer ear have no functional importance, the overall shape of the outer ear and its orientation on the head serves several purposes. The concave shape of the outer ear helps to collect and amplify sound and to funnel the sound into the external ear canal. The bowl-shaped **concha** increases sound levels by up to 10 to 15 dB in the frequency region of 4500 Hz. Orientation of a listener's outer ear toward the face contributes to better detection of a speaker's voice and speech. Sounds coming from behind must travel around the ear to be heard. So the outer ear enhances detection of sounds coming from the direction a listener is facing rather than irrelevant sounds behind the listener.

Localization is the process of determining where a sound is coming from. Many times each day we localize the source of sounds like a friend calling out to us, a bus coming down the road toward us, or an airplane flying overhead. We immediately turn our heads and eyes toward the general direction of the sound and then we more precisely determine the source of the sound. We are amazingly accurate in localizing sources of sounds. Of course, localization is an auditory process that has developed in most animal species over hundreds of thousands of years. Animals, including humans, would not survive in most environments without a highly refined ability to quickly and accurately localize sounds, especially sounds warning of danger.

External Ear Canal. The **external ear canal** is an S-shaped tube that carries sound from the auricle to the tympanic membrane. The external ear canal was shown in Figure 3.1. Walls of the lateral or outer two-thirds of the ear canal consist of cartilage, whereas walls of the medial or inner one-third of the external ear canal are formed of bone. On average, the length of the external ear canal in an adult is about 2.5 cm. Most external ear canals have a diameter of 0.5 to 0.75 cm. The canal makes a turn backward and then straightens out within the bony portion leading to the tympanic membrane. The curvy course of the external ear canal helps to protect the delicate tympanic membrane located at the medial end of the canal.

The volume of the adult external ear canal is about 1.0 cc (1.0 mL). The external ear canal is essentially a tube with effective acoustic characteristics. The acoustic characteristics vary somewhat among different persons, especially for adults versus children. The adult ear canal amplifies sound at a resonance frequency within the region of 2500 to 3000 Hz, depending on the diameter and length of the canal. The concept of resonance was reviewed in Chapter 2. Interestingly, this frequency region is very important in the perception of consonants in speech sounds. Resonance frequencies are considerably higher for the smaller ear canals of infants and young children.

Sebaceous and *ceruminous glands* lining the external ear canal secrete a substance called *cerumen,* commonly called earwax. Cerumen is a sticky, unpleasant-smelling (and -tasting!) substance that helps to protect the ear by catching debris before it reaches the delicate tympanic membrane. Cerumen also helps to minimize bacteria and fungus from infecting the ear canal. Too much cerumen can cause problems. Accumulation of cerumen in the external ear canal can block the miniature earphones sometimes inserted into the ear canal during hearing screening and assessment. Excessive cerumen may eventually block or occlude the opening of the external ear canal and interfere with sound from traveling from the outer ear to the middle ear. Blockage of the external ear canal with too much cerumen

ClinicalConnection

Audiologists are very familiar with anatomy of the external ear because the pinna and the ear canal are usually involved in hearing measurements or other clinical procedures. An audiologist examines the ear of almost every patient closely. Audiologists often place earphones over a patient's pinna or a soft tip into a patient's external ear canal during hearing testing. You'll learn about many hearing test procedures in Chapters 5 through 9.

ClinicalConnection

Removal of cerumen or earwax from the ear canal is within the scope of practice of audiologists. The American Academy of Audiology Scope of Practice includes the statement: "Audiologists conduct otoscopic examinations, clean ear canals and remove cerumen, take ear canal impressions, select, fit, evaluate, and dispense hearing aids and other amplification systems." (www.audiology.org)

produces hearing loss. Fortunately, the hearing loss is usually temporary and eliminated with removal of the cerumen.

Middle Ear

Borders of the Middle Ear. The middle ear consists of the tympanic membrane and a space behind it. The middle ear space is enclosed within the temporal bone, one of the strongest bones of the head. In adults the middle ear space has a volume of about 2 cc (cm^3). Figure 3.3 is a simple diagram that shows the borders of the middle ear space.

Laterally, the tympanic membrane separates the middle ear space from the external ear canal. In the other direction, the medial border of the middle ear space includes the *promontory,* the **round window**, and the **oval window**. These structures separate the middle ear from the inner ear. Lying on the surface of the promontory is the *tympanic nerve plexus,* a branch of the eleventh or spinal accessory cranial nerve.

Up above are two air-filled spaces called the *aditus ad antrum* and the *epitympanic recess* also known as the *attic.* The *hypotympanum* bone forms the inferior floor of the middle ear space.

The posterior region of the middle ear space consists of air cells within the mastoid region of the temporal bone and the *pyramidal eminence.* The pyramidal eminence is a hollow structure containing the **stapedius muscle**. Finally, the **Eustachian tube** is located toward the inferior and anterior border of the middle ear, as shown in Figure 3.3. The Eustachian tube connects the middle ear space to the back of the nose and mouth, a region called the nasopharynx. The Eustachian tube is named after a person. Table 3.1 includes a brief biographical sketch of some people whose names are attached to structures within the auditory system, including the namesake of the Eustachian tube.

The Eustachian tube is normally the single entrance to and exit from the middle ear space and the only route for outside air to ventilate the middle ear space. A mucous membrane lines the Eustachian tube. The membrane then continues with a different cellular composition into the middle ear space where it covers the walls of the mastoid bone. The bony portion of the Eustachian tube is closest to the middle ear. It accounts for about one-third of the overall length of the Eustachian tube, and it always stays open. In contrast, the remaining cartilaginous portion of the Eustachian tube near the mouth is normally closed. The Eustachian tube opens with contraction of several muscles.

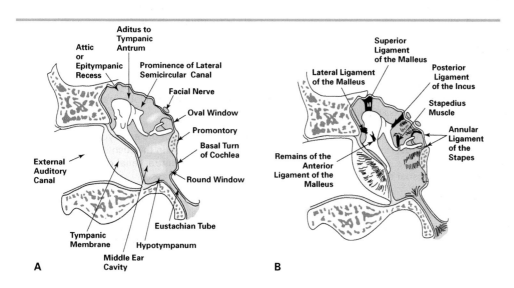

A   **B**

FIGURE 3.3

Schematic diagrams of the middle ear space on the right side of the head as viewed looking back from the face, showing the structures within and forming the borders of the middle ear space: borders of the middle ear space **(A)** and ligaments and muscles attached to the ossicular chain **(B)**. Adapted from *ZEMLIN, SPEECH and HEARING SCIENCE: ANATOMY and PHYSIOLOGY, 1st Ed.,* ©1968. Reprinted and Electronically reproduced by permission of Pearson Education, Inc., Upper Saddle River, New Jersey.

T A B L E   3 . 1   Brief biographies of a dozen persons who are honored by names of structures within the auditory system (arranged alphabetically).

Arthur Boettcher (1831–1889) was a German pathologist who identified cells in the cochlea located beneath Claudius cells. Boettcher cells are located only in the basal region of the cochlea. Resting on the basilar membrane, they definitely play a supporting role in cochlear structure. However, the cells also appear to have a functional role in regulating calcium activity and in the movement of ions.

Friedrich Matthias Claudius (1822–1869) was a German anatomist who described in 1856 what are now known as Claudius cells. Located above Boettcher cells and next to Hensen's cells, Claudius cells provide structural support in the organ of Corti. His name is also associated with Claudius fossa in the pelvic region.

Alfonso Giacomo Gaspare Corti (1822–1876) was an Italian anatomist who earned his medical degree and then conducted anatomical research in Vienna, Austria. His career began with investigations of the cardiovascular systems of reptiles. He later conducted research on cochlear anatomy in Germany and during a brief period at a laboratory in The Netherlands. Corti's descriptions of cochlear hair cells, the spiral ganglion, the tectorial membrane, and the stria vascularis within the inner ear resulted from careful study of at least 200 cochleas. His name is appropriately attached to the region of the cochlea where some of these structures are located ... the organ of Corti. Interestingly, Antonio Scarpa was a friend of Corti's father. Scarpa also has an auditory structure named after him as summarized later in this table.

Otto Friedrich Karl Deiters (1834–1863) was a German anatomist who devoted much of his career to microscopic research of the brain and spinal cord. Two structures in the auditory-vestibular system are named after him. Deiters' cells in the cochlea consist of tiny filaments and tubules that extend from the basilar membrane to the reticular formation. The cells provide support to the organ of Corti and perhaps contribute to ion regulation in the cochlea. Deiters has another structure named after him: The lateral vestibular nucleus is known as the nucleus of Deiters. Toward the end of his short life, Deiters provided a thorough description of nerve cells, including the axons and dendrites of nerve cells. Deiters died from typhoid fever when he was only 29 years old.

Bartolomeo Eustachi or Eustachius (1500, 1510, or 1513–1574) was an Italian anatomist during the Renaissance period. He was one of the earliest scientists to formally study human anatomy. The son of a physician, he spoke and read Italian, Greek, Hebrew, and Arabic languages. Eustachius was one of the first to make use of magnification in microscopic examination of human structures. Many of Eustachius' studies focused on the ear, including descriptions of the stapes, the stapedial muscle, the tensor tympani muscle, the cochlea, and the tube connecting the ear with the pharynx in the back of the mouth that bears his name. Interestingly, Eustachius prepared a classic textbook entitled *Anatomical Engravings* but did not publish it due to religious rules about human anatomy research and his concerns about excommunication from the Catholic Church. The book became very popular when it was published many years after Eustachius died.

Christian Andreas Victor Hensen (1835–1924) was a German zoologist and anatomist. Multiple structures in the auditory system bear the name Hensen. In the cochlea, Hensen's cells are tall supporting column-like cells arranged in several rows. Like Deiters' cells, Hensen's cells play a role in ion (calcium) regulation within the inner ear. Hensen's duct is a passageway from the saccule in the vestibular system to the cochlea duct in the inner ear. Hensen's stripe is a curvature in the gel substance on the surface of the tectorial membrane that plays a role in frequency disperision in the cochlea. Victor Hensen had diverse scientific interests. He received his doctorate for a study of epilepsy and urinary secretions. During his career, he was a strong proponent of marine biology and ecology. Among other accomplishments in biological oceanograpy, Hensen coined the term *plankton*.

Richard Ladislaus Heschl (1824–1881) was an Austrian anatomist. He published a textbook on pathological anatomy. In the book Heschl described the transverse temporal gyrus on the superior portion of the temporal lobe in the brain. The primary auditory cortex is known commonly as Heschl's gyrus.

Ernst Reissner (1824–1878) was a German anatomist. He conducted important early studies of the embryological development of the inner ear, mostly in birds. His name is honored by Reissner's membrane in the cochlea, separating the scala media from the scala vestibuli. He is also recognized by a long nerve fiber in the central canal of the spinal cord known as Reissner's fiber. Ernst Reissner's brilliant scientific career was cut short by illness.

Friedrich Christian Rosenthal (1780–1829) was a German physician and anatomist. His early research focused on olfaction (smell) but his anatomical studies also include the ear and the brain. Rosenthal described a narrow and spiral-shaped canal in the cochlea that encircles the modiolus. Afferent auditory fibers travel away from the cochlear within Rosenthal's canal. A vein in the brain is also named after him. Rosenthal died at an early age from tuberculosis.

Antonio Scarpa (1752–1832) was an Italian physician and anatomist. Midway through his career Scarpa conducted intensive studies on anatomy of the ear and particularly the nerves carrying information about hearing, vestibular stimulation, and smell. Scarpa's ganglion is a collection of cell bodies in the vestibular nerve that runs from the hair cells in the vestibular sensory organ to the brainstem. Remarkably, the head of Antonio Scarpa is preserved to this day in a museum in the University of Pavia in Italy.

Theodor Schwann (1810–1882) was a German physiologist. He is known for important contributions to cellular physiology of nerves and muscles and also the digestive system. Schwann cells, named after him, are specialized glial cells that encircle the axons of nerve fibers in the peripheral nervous system, including the auditory nerve. Reportedly, Schwann coined the term *metabolism*.

Franciscus Sylvius (1614–1672) was born in Germany but lived his life in The Netherlands. Although he began his career practicing medicine, Sylvius also studied and taught chemistry, physiology, and anatomy. His research on brain anatomy led to a detailed description of a deep fissure dividing the cerebrum into an upper and lower portion that later became known as the Sylvian fissure. Sylvius is also recognized as the person who invented an alcoholic drink called Holland or Dutch gin.

Tympanic Membrane. The **tympanic membrane** is the outermost structure of the middle ear system, separating the external ear canal from the middle ear space. Figure 3.4A shows the tympanic membrane as viewed from the ear canal with an otoscope or a microscope, and Figure 3.4B is a diagram of the tympanic membrane with major structures labeled. The normal tympanic membrane appears shiny and pearly in color. With illumination it typically reflects a *cone of light*. The normal tympanic membrane is only about 0.1 mm in thickness and weighs only 14 mg. The tympanic membrane consists of three different layers of tissue that contribute to integrity and strength. The outer epidermal layer of the tympanic membrane is distinguished from the other two layers because it renews itself, like skin on the body, with old cells migrating outward through the ear canal and new cells forming in their place.

The diameter of the tympanic membrane from one edge to the other is a little less than 1 cm, and the total area of the tympanic membrane ranges from 0.5 to 1 cm². The dimensions of the middle ear structures and other parts of the ear vary considerably depending on age and also gender. The outer rim of the tympanic membrane, where it connects with the bony wall of the external ear canal, is called the *annulus*. The tympanic membrane is not oriented vertically. Rather, the tympanic membrane angles in an inward direction from the top to the bottom. Also, the tympanic membrane is concave or slightly cone shaped and not flat. The center portion of the tympanic membrane extends further inward toward the middle ear than the annulus portion.

Regions on the tympanic membrane are usually defined by quadrants along the vertical axis from posterior to inferior and in the horizontal dimension from anterior to posterior. The four quadrants of the tympanic membrane are often used to describe the location of abnormalities. As seen in Figure 3.4A and B, the most flexible region of the tympanic membrane, called the *pars flaccid*, is near the edge in the anterior-superior quadrant. Another region of the tympanic membrane called the *pars tensa* is the largest and tightest portion and contributes mostly to hearing. The extent of vibration or displacement of the tympanic membrane is very small. Tympanic membrane movement is on the order of 5 to 7 *angstrom* or Å, even for moderate levels of sound intensity such as 70 to 75 dB SPL. One

 ClinicalConnection

The external ear canal is not straight. Even though the external ear canal is quite curvy, it is still possible for a rigid object to get around the bends to the tympanic membrane at the end. Unfortunately, from time to time audiologists encounter patients who have punctured their tympanic membrane by inserting an object into the ear canal like a cleaning stick or even a pen or pencil. The technical term for a hole in the tympanic membrane is a *perforation*. Perforations are discussed in Chapter 11. The old adage "never put anything into your ear canal smaller than your elbow" is good advice indeed.

FIGURE 3.4   Tympanic membrane as viewed from the external canal during otoscopic examination of the ear **(A)**, and a diagram of the tympanic membrane **(B)**. Labels identify major structures of the tympanic membrane that are visible from the external ear canal. Image **(A)** courtesy of Science Photo Library/Custom Medical Stock Photo.

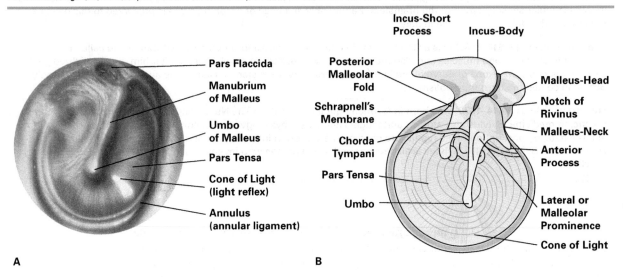

A   B

angstrom is equal to one ten-billionth (1/10,000,000,000) of a meter. Thus, vibrations of the tympanic membrane for a comfortable intensity level of sound are on the order of only about 0.0000005 millimeters!

FIGURE 3.5

Each of the three ossicles in the middle ear including the: **(A)** malleus, **(B)** incus, and **(C)** stapes. The stapes is the smallest bone in the body. It is slightly smaller than Franklin Delano Roosevelt's left ear as depicted on a US dime.

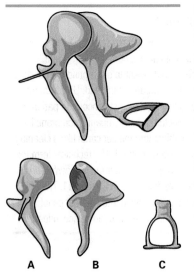

A   B   C

Ossicles. The ossicles are three tiny bones that form a chain connecting the tympanic membrane to the inner ear. The location of the ossicles in the middle ear was depicted earlier in Figures 3.1 and 3.3. Figure 3.5 shows each of the ossicles. The word *ossicle* ("little bone") is derived from Latin. Indeed, the ossicles are the smallest bones in the human body. The everyday words for the ossicles are hammer, anvil, and stirrup. We'll refer to them by the proper anatomical terms used by audiologists and other hearing healthcare professionals.

The first of the three ossicles is the **malleus** (Figure 3.5A). It is usually visible through the tympanic membrane, as illustrated earlier in Figure 3.4. The *manubrium* of the malleus rests against the inner portion of the tympanic membrane. The head of the malleus connects with the *short process* of the **incus**, the next ossicle (Figure 3.5B). The *lenticular process* of the incus is connected to the head of the **stapes**, the innermost stirrup-shaped ossicle. The stapes is the smallest bone in the body (Figure 3.5C). It consists of a neck and two arch-shaped structures, called the anterior crus and the posterior crus. The medial portion of the stapes is called the *stapes footplate*. The footplate is a flat structure that fits within the oval window. The ossicles are remarkably lightweight. The malleus and incus each weigh less than 35 mg, or 0.001234 oz. The stapes is the lightest bone in the body, weighing as little as 2 mg. The ossicles are often referred to collectively as the *ossicular chain* since they're connected one to another.

Middle Ear Muscles. Two very small muscles and several associated tendons are attached to the ossicles within the middle ear space. Several ligaments also support the ossicular chain. Figure 3.3B included one of the middle ear muscles and ligaments. Another middle ear muscle, the *tensor tympani muscle*, is connected to the malleus and is innervated by the fifth or trigeminal cranial nerve. Approximately 25 mm in length, the tensor tympani muscle contracts during self-generated sounds, like chewing. Contraction of the tensor tympani muscle reduces the interference of self-generated sounds with hearing of external sounds.

The stapedius muscle originates from a little projection on the medial wall of the middle ear space called the *pyramidal eminence.* As shown earlier in Figure 3.3, the stapedius muscle inserts into the neck of the stapes and is innervated by a branch of the seventh or facial cranial nerve. Approximately 6 mm in length, the stapedius muscle is the smallest skeletal muscle in the human body. The stapedius muscle stabilizes the stapes bone in quiet conditions (Hall, 2010; Mukerji, Windsor, & Lee, 2010).

Function of the Middle Ear. The middle ear system serves the important function of matching the low impedance of the air in the external ear canal to the high impedance of the fluid within the inner ear. This concept might be easier understood if you substitute the term *resistance* for impedance. That is, less energy is needed to move the air molecules in the external ear canal than the fluid within the inner ear. About 30 dB would be lost on the route from the external ear canal to the inner ear without a mechanism for transforming energy to overcome the resistance mismatch. The middle ear system, consisting of the tympanic membrane and the three ossicles working together, provides this increase in energy.

Three factors contribute to increased energy related to sound pressure as it passes from the ear canal through the middle ear to the inner ear. Figure 3.6 illustrates that the tympanic membrane is considerably larger in area than the stapes footplate. The ratio of the area difference is about 17 to 1. As a result, vibration of the tympanic membrane concentrates pressure where the footplate makes contact with the fluid of the inner ear. In considering the concentration of pressure from a larger to smaller area surface, it might be helpful to think of a hammer hitting a nail. Pressure exerted by the hammer on the nail head is increased markedly at the sharp tip of the nail.

Also, the ossicles connecting the tympanic membrane to the inner ear fluid function as a lever. The lever action of the malleus, incus, and stapes produces an increase of pressure by a factor of approximately 1.3. The actual lever factor varies for different sound frequencies. The tympanic membrane vibrates in a complex fashion for high frequency sounds. The response of the ossicles has a steadying effect, minimizing these highly variable movements of the tympanic membrane before they reach the inner ear.

Finally, the shape of the tympanic membrane contributes to an increase in the sound pressure reaching the inner ear. As noted already, the tympanic membrane is not flat but, rather, cone-shaped. Increased force upon movement of the malleus, due to the shape of the tympanic membrane, slightly enhances the impedance-matching property of the middle ear system. Overall, the middle ear system increases energy by about 26 to 30 dB. The transformer function of the middle ear system is essential for normal hearing. Patients with abnormal middle ear function inevitably have abnormal hearing test results.

 ClinicalConnection

The stapedius muscle is the smallest muscle in the body, but it plays a big role in a very popular auditory test procedure. The stapedius muscle contracts when a person hears sound exceeding about 80 dB HL. Contraction of the stapedius muscle to sound is part of a bodily reflex that occurs automatically, without conscious effort. This reflex is called the "acoustic reflex" because it is elicited with sound. Using devices found in most clinics, audiologists record the acoustic reflex of patients of all ages, including infants and young children. You'll learn more about the stapedius muscle and the acoustic reflex test in Chapter 8.

FIGURE 3.6

Concentration of sound pressure from the larger tympanic membrane to the small stapes footplate, and increased pressure produced by the lever action of the ossicular chain.

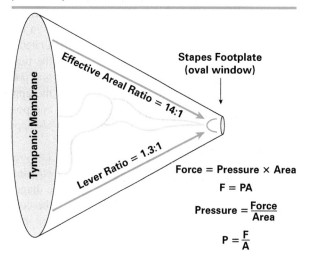

ClinicalConnection

Infections can be transmitted from the mouth along the membrane of the Eustachian tube into the middle ear space. Middle ear infection is very common in children. In fact, each year the costs associated with medical treatment of ear infections add up to billions of healthcare dollars. Ear infections can also cause hearing loss. You'll read in Chapter 8 about tests that measure how well the middle ear functions. Then, in Chapter 11 you'll learn about different types of ear infections and how they are treated medically and surgically.

Inner Ear

One of the most important processes in hearing occurs deep within the inner ear. The inner ear is surrounded by skull bones. Within the inner ear, mechanical activity related to sound vibrations is converted into electrical activity. The vibrations from sound waves were reviewed in Chapter 2. Energy from sound waves in the ear canal that is amplified by the middle ear is then transmitted as vibrations into the inner ear. The vibrations produce little waves in the fluids that fill the inner ear. The waves within these fluids in turn vibrate a very thin membrane within the inner ear. Vibrations travel along the membrane from the portion closest to the middle ear to the region furthest from the middle ear.

Thousands of tiny and delicate hair cells are activated as the membrane moves up and down rapidly in response to sound. The term *hair cell* is a little misleading because there are really no hairs in the inner ear. Each hair cell has many delicate hair-like *cilia* projecting upward. Each cilium consists of a thin strand of protein. You may be surprised to know that more than 100 cilia project from the top of each hair cell. High-pitch sounds activate hair cells in the *base* of the inner ear toward the stapes footplate. Lower-pitch sounds progressively activate hair cells toward the other end of the inner ear, called the **apex**. The normal human ear responds to frequencies over a remarkable range, from sounds with a frequency as low as 20 Hz to frequencies as high as 20,000 Hz.

The two general types of hair cells within the cochlea are called inner and outer hair cells. The terms refer to whether the hair cells are located in the inner or medial portion of the cochlea or in the outer or lateral portion of the cochlea. There are three to four times more outer hair cells than inner hair cells. **Inner hair cells** communicate with auditory nerve fibers. They release a chemical that produces a response in auditory nerve fibers when activated by vibrations. The electrical activity within auditory nerve fibers is transmitted quickly to the brain. **Outer hair cells** differ in many ways from inner hair cells. Importantly, outer hair cells change shape when activated. The movement produces energy in the inner ear that enhances hearing.

We will now review in a little more detail the inner ear and its essential role in hearing.

Temporal Bone. The inner ear is located within the temporal bone. Figure 3.7A shows the temporal bone in relation to three other bones of the skull. Specifically, the inner ear is within a triangular-shaped portion called the *petrous* portion of the temporal bone. This is also an appropriate term. It is derived from the word for "rock" or "stone." The temporal bone is one of the hardest bones in the body. The strength of the temporal bone helps to protect the inner ear from trauma-related damage. Figure 3.7B shows the closely connected segments of the **temporal bone** called the *squamous*, the *tympanic*, and the *mastoid bones*. The squamous portion of the temporal bone contributes to the upper border of the external ear canal. The floor and the anterior and posterior walls of the external ear canal consist of the concave or U-shaped tympanic bone.

  ClinicalConnection

Audiologists are very familiar with the mastoid portion of the temporal bone, which is located just behind the lower part of the pinna. The mastoid bone is a typical site for placement of a bone vibrator for hearing tests that involve the presentation of sounds to the ear through bone conduction. The bone conduction technique for hearing testing is described in Chapter 5.

Labyrinth. The proper anatomical term for the inner ear is the **cochlea**. The word is of Greek origin and means "snail." Figure 3.8 is a diagram showing one view of the cochlea. Even a quick glimpse at the cochlea in Figure 3.8 or earlier in Figure 3.1 confirms the reason for the origin of the word. The outer bony structure of the cochlea

FIGURE 3.7   The temporal bone viewed from the right side of the skull **(A)** and shown in relation to other major skull bones (frontal, parietal, and occipital bones). Portions of the temporal bone are shown in **(B)** including the mastoid and squamous segments.

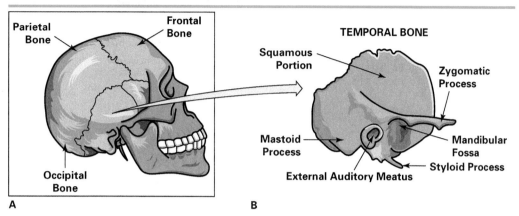

does look very much like a snail. It consists of two or three turns from the base or basal end, near the middle ear, to the apex or apical end.

Within the bony walls of the cochlea is a complex network of delicate membranes. The technical term for this portion of the inner ear is the membranous **labyrinth**. It is a Greek word that means "maze," or an intricate network of connecting passages. The middle ear connects with the inner ear where the stapes footplate fills the oval window. Behind the oval window is a space called the *vestibule*. You are probably familiar with the word *vestibule*. It is a space just inside the door of a building that leads to different hallways and rooms. The anatomical vestibule is a space that leads to the hearing part of the ear, the cochlea, and also to the vestibular part of the ear.

Cochlear Structure. The cochlea is tube-shaped and separated into three sections by thin membranes, as shown in Figure 3.8. From the beginning of the cochlea at the *base* to the *apex* at the other end, the tube curves several times around a structure called the *modiolus*. Two membranes separate the cochlea into three portions, or scala. The word *scala* is derived from the Latin for "ladder" or "staircase." A delicate partition called the *Reissner's membrane* separates the *scala vestibuli* from another wedge-shaped portion of the tube, named the *scala media*. The scala vestibuli is filled with a thick fluid called **perilymph**, whereas the scala media contains a different fluid called **endolymph**. The scala vestibuli continues from the oval window in the base of the cochlea to the apex or apical end of the cochlea, whereas the scala media begins at the round window in the base and extends to the apical end of the cochlea.

The scala media is appropriately named because it is located between the scala vestibuli and a third duct called the scala tympani. The scala media is sometimes referred to as the *cochlear duct*. The lower border of the scala media consists mostly of the basilar membrane, whereas the medial extreme is the *spiral limbus*. The thin and flexible basilar membrane is very important for hearing. Figure 3.8 shows how this complex structure separates the scala media from the scala tympani. The scala tympani is filled with perilymph, the same type of fluid that is within the scala vestibuli.

At the apical end of cochlea, far away from the base, is a small opening called the *helicotrema*. As shown also in Figure 3.8, the helicotrema forms a connection between the scala

FIGURE 3.8

Major structures within the cochlea or inner ear, including the three ducts (the scala vestibuli, scala media, and scala tympani), the organ of Corti, and membranes separating the different sections. Adapted from *ZEMLIN, SPEECH and HEARING SCIENCE: ANATOMY and PHYSIOLOGY, 1st Ed.,* ©1968 and *MUSIEK, FRANK E.; BARAN, JANE A., THE AUDITORY SYSTEM: ANATOMY, PHYSIOLOGY, AND CLINICAL CORRELATES, 1st Ed.,* © 2007. Reprinted and Electronically reproduced by permission of Pearson Education, Inc., Upper Saddle River, New Jersey.

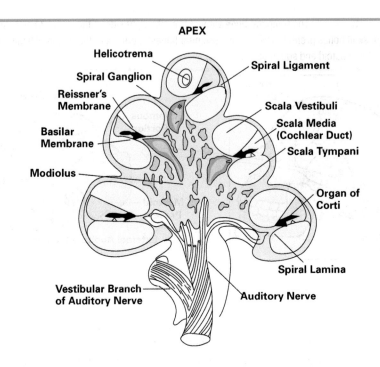

tympani and the scala vestibuli. In turn, the scala tympani duct is connected via the cochlear aqueduct with regions of the brain that contain the cerebrospinal fluid that surrounds the brain and spinal cord. Indeed, of the periplymph fluid within the ear has a composition similar to cerebrospinal fluid.

Form Follows Function. Now that you've been introduced to the general structure of the cochlea, we'll shift the emphasis to function and how the ear responds to sound. Figure 3.9 illustrates the functional anatomy of the cochlea. It's a more detailed view of a portion of the cochlea shown in Figure 3.8. The *stria vascularis* forms the lateral border of the scala media. It is a complex auditory structure that contributes importantly to cochlear function. As the term suggests, the stria vascularis receives a generous supply of blood. It also has a high rate of metabolism. The stria vascularis serves as a pump for transporting electrically charged ions like potassium (K+) ions into *endolymph,* the cochlear fluid within the scala media. By means of the ion pump mechanism, the stria vascularis plays a crucial role in producing energy used by other structures in the cochlea, particularly the outer hair cells. The stria vascularis contributes to generation of the *endocochlear potential.* The endocochlear potential is sometimes called the "cochlear battery." It is a sizable positive electrical charge within the scala media in comparison to the electrical state in other portions of the cochlea.

Mechanical properties of the basilar membrane change along the 25- to 35-mm length from its base to the apical end. Figure 3.10A shows the relative difference in width that's associated with a corresponding change in stiffness from the base to the apex of the cochlea. The basilar membrane is considerably narrower at the base than at the apical end. The base in humans is less than 0.15 mm in width, whereas at the apical end the width is 0.5 mm on the average.

Sound energy reaches the inner ear when the stapes footplate at the end of the ossicular chain moves in and out. Each movement of the stapes footplate produces vibration of the basilar membrane that travels away from the footplate. Motions of the basilar membrane in

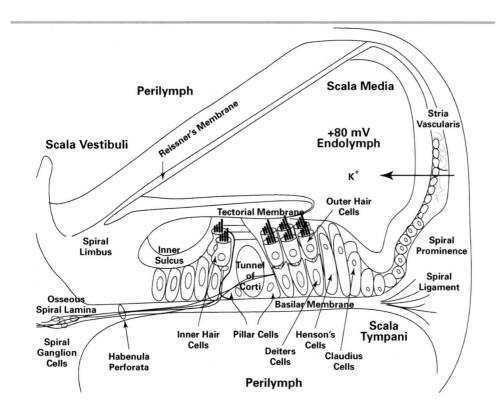

FIGURE 3.9

Cross-section of the cochlea, including the organ of Corti, other major cochlear structures, and the electrical potentials within the different ducts. The figure is an enlarged view of the cochlear ducts shown in Figure 3.8. Adapted from *MUSIEK, FRANK E.; BARAN, JANE A., THE AUDITORY SYSTEM: ANATOMY, PHYSIOLOGY, AND CLINICAL CORRELATES, 1st Ed.,* ©2007. Reprinted and Electronically reproduced by permission of Pearson Education, Inc., Upper Saddle River, New Jersey.

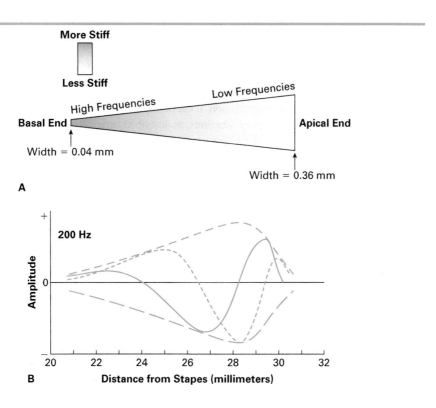

FIGURE 3.10

A diagram showing the inverse relation between width and stiffness of the basilar membrane from the base to the apex of the cochlea **(A)**. **(B)** is an illustration of a low frequency traveling wave along the basilar membrane moving from near the base toward the apex of the cochlea.

response to sound are referred to as **traveling waves**. Figure 3.10B shows the concept of a traveling wave on the basilar membrane. Traveling waves begin at the base of the cochlea and move toward the apex of the cochlea. Amplitude of the traveling wave varies as it moves along the basilar membrane. Importantly, amplitude or size of the traveling wave at different places along the basilar membrane depends on the frequency of the stimulus.

Mechanical properties of the basilar membrane contribute to the tonotopical organization of the cochlea. Tonotopical organization of the cochlea describes processing of sounds of different frequencies at different locations along the membrane (Hudspeth, 1989). Responsiveness to higher-frequency sounds occurs toward the relatively tight and stiff basal end of the basilar membrane. In contrast, lower frequencies are represented toward the apex where the basilar membrane is looser and less stiff.

Spectral or frequency analysis of sound is also dependent on other structures within the cochlea, which will be discussed next. Spectral analysis of sound by the inner ear is closely related to perception of pitch, as reviewed in Chapter 2. The difference in width and stiffness of the basilar membrane from the base to the apex is an excellent example of the previously cited principle that "form follows function."

ⓘ **Web**Watch

A massive collection of published scientific papers in the U.S. National Library of Medicine can be easily accessed at the website: www.nlm.nih.gov. A literature search on the topic of interest is an important part of scientific study. After you reach this website, select the PubMed/MEDLINE link. Next, enter key words that will direct the search. For example, if you're interested in reading more about inner ear function, you might enter the key words "inner ear" or "cochlea" plus "physiology." To narrow down the search to articles that review this topic, just add the key word "review." You can then review for each article a brief summary called an abstract.

Cochlear Fluids.   The entire cochlea is filled with fluid but the composition of the fluid differs among the three sections. This point was also illustrated in Figure 3.9. The fluid in the cochlea is not water but, rather, a more viscous substance. Perilymph within the scala vestibuli and scala tympani contains a high concentration of sodium (Na^+) ions and a low concentration of potassium (K^+) ions. Figure 3.9 included a summary of the chemical and electrical properties of the cochlear fluids. Perilymph is very similar in composition to the cerebrospinal fluid that surrounds the spinal cord and brain.

The scala media contains *endolymph* that shares features of fluids within most cells in the body. Produced by the stria vascularis, endolymph consists of a high concentration of potassium ions and a low concentration of sodium ions. Endolymph has a significant positive ion charge (+80 mV) in comparison to the essentially neutral ionic charge of the perilymph. The difference or gradient in ion composition and concentration of endolymph versus perilymph serves as an inner ear battery, supplying power for cochlear functions, as described earlier. The electrochemical potential difference in the cochlea is critical for powering the ongoing active processes within the cochlea.

Organ of Corti.   The **organ of Corti** is a complex of structures located on the basilar membrane of the cochlea. The organ of Corti plays a critical role in hearing. The rods or pillars of Corti form the main supporting framework for the organ of Corti and enclose the tunnel of Corti. The top of the organ of Corti, or its superior border, is the *tectorial membrane.* The tectorial membrane, shown in Figure 3.9, is a gelatinous complex extending laterally from the *limbus.* The limbus attaches to a thin shelf of bone called the *osseous spiral lamina* that projects from the modiolus. Within the organ of Corti is a third type of cochlear fluid called **cortilymph**.

In addition to the structures just mentioned, the organ of Corti contains a variety of different cell types that serve different functions, including support and structural strength. Some of the structures were depicted in Figure 3.9. Beginning at the lateral end of the basilar membrane toward the stria vascularis and moving medially toward the spiral

ClinicalConnection

Audiologists can record activity from the cochlea with clinical tests that can be performed even with infants, who cannot be tested any other way. In Chapters 8 and 9 you'll learn about these procedures and how they are used to diagnose and describe auditory problems in children and adults.

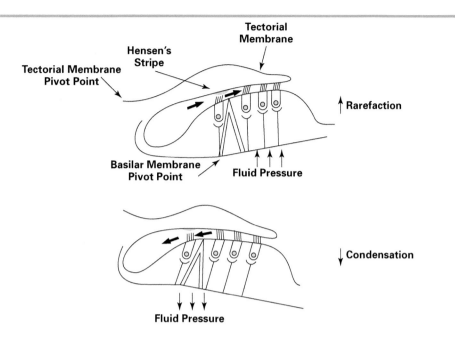

FIGURE 3.11

Upward and downward movement of the basilar membrane in response to rarefaction and condensation sound stimulation producing shearing and bending of the stereocilia of inner and outer hair cells. Adapted from *MUSIEK, FRANK E.; BARAN, JANE A., THE AUDITORY SYSTEM: ANATOMY, PHYSIOLOGY, AND CLINICAL CORRELATES, 1st Ed.,* ©2007. Reprinted and Electronically reproduced by permission of Pearson Education, Inc., Upper Saddle River, New Jersey.

lamina are *Claudius cells, Hensen's cells, and Deiter's cells,* . On the medial side of the organ of Corti are *inner sulcus cells.* You may wish to refer back to Table 3.1 for information on persons with names attached to selected inner ear structures, including Alphonso Corti and Drs. Claudius, Deiter, and Hensen. We'll now review the most important of the cochlear structures, the hair cells.

Inner versus Outer Hair Cells. As noted earlier, the term *hair cell* is used because many delicate cilia or strands resembling hairs project from the top of each cell. The term *stereocilia* is used to describe these structures because the cilia move together in a coordinated fashion when deflected by movement of the basilar membrane. Up to 150 stereocilia arranged in a V or a W pattern are found on the top or apex of each outer hair cell.

Unified movement of stereocilia is enhanced by tiny connections between the cilia strands called *tip-links.* Figure 3.11 shows the coordinated back and forth shearing of stereocilia on top of hair cells. Movement of stereocilia plays an important role in converting mechanical energy from sound vibrations into chemical and electrical energy within hair cells, which is essential for hearing.

There are about 3500 *inner hair cells* in the human cochlea. In contrast, there are approximately 12,000 *outer hair cells,* or roughly three times the number of inner hair cells. Figure 3.12 shows stereocilia for inner hair cells that are arranged in a single row on the medial side of the organ of Corti. Outer hair cells are arranged in either three or four rows on the lateral side of the organ of Corti. The figure shows photographs of the stereocilia of actual hair cells taken from above through a microscope.

Figure 3.13 illustrates some additional distinctions between inner versus outer hair. Inner hair cells are shaped like a goblet or flask with a nucleus toward the center of the cell. Mitochondria that are involved in metabolism are scattered throughout the cell. Outer hair cells in

FIGURE 3.12 Photomicrographs of one row of inner and three rows of outer hair cells in the cochlea, as viewed from above. Image courtesy of Steve Gschmeissner/Science Source/Photo Researchers, Inc.

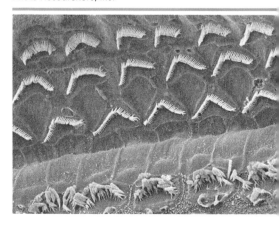

FIGURE 3.13 An example of an inner **(A)** and an outer hair **(B)** cell, illustrating some of the many structural differences. Adapted from *MUSIEK, FRANK E.; BARAN, JANE A., THE AUDITORY SYSTEM: ANATOMY, PHYSIOLOGY, AND CLINICAL CORRELATES, 1st Ed., ©2007.* Reprinted and Electronically reproduced by permission of Pearson Education, Inc., Upper Saddle River, New Jersey.

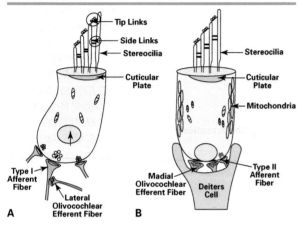

contrast have a cylinder or tube shape with a nucleus near the base and with mitochondria arranged along the walls. Each outer hair cell is extremely small, measuring only 5 μm wide and 20 μm long in the basal end of the cochlea and 50 μm long at the apex. To put the tiny size of the outer hair cells in perspective, 50 μm is only 0.001968 inch.

Another difference between inner and outer hair cells involves the relation of their stereocilia to the tectorial membrane. The tallest stereocilia on the top of outer hair cells are imbedded within the soft undersurface of the tectorial membrane. Stereocilia on the inner hair cells, in contrast, do not make contact with the tectorial membrane. Each of these structural differences between inner and outer hair cells is associated with equally clear distinctions in function. We'll now review the unique roles of outer and inner hair cells in hearing.

Hair Cell Regeneration. Most hearing loss is due to dysfunction of hair cells within the inner ear. Damage to hair cells caused by diseases or by exposure to very high intensity sounds is usually irreversible and results in permanent hearing loss. Hearing research involving chickens in the 1980s led to a remarkable discovery. Hair cells can regenerate (Cotanche, 1987; Ryals & Rubel, 1988). Chickens were exposed to high-intensity sound that severely damaged their hair cells. Before long new and normally functioning hair cells appeared and replaced the damaged ones.

As you can imagine, this discovery generated a great deal of excitement because it offered a potential approach for eliminating noise-induced hearing loss in millions of persons. Interest in hair cell regeneration is a specific example of the dramatic increase in stem cell research within the past few decades. A stem cell is a rather unique type of immature cell that can differentiate and develop into various specialized cells in the body, such as blood, nerve, or even hair cells.

Since the early research with birds, more recent studies carried out in mammals have led to the discovery of genes and mechanisms that play a role in hair cell development and regeneration (Brigande & Heller, 2009; Edge & Chen, 2008; Grove, 2010). Hair cell regeneration in humans may be possible with genetic manipulations and therapy in the future. Meanwhile, consistent use of proper hearing protection like earplugs and avoidance of exposure to high-intensity sound whenever possible is the best strategy for preventing permanent hearing loss due to noise exposure.

Outer Hair Cell Motility. Vibration of the basilar membrane produced by sound activates outer hair cells. Movement of the outer hair cells with basilar membrane vibration is enhanced because the tops of the tallest stereocilia on the cells are imbedded within the tectorial membrane. The tectorial membrane was illustrated earlier in Figures 3.9 and 3.11. Differences in movement of the basilar membrane below the outer hair cells and the tectorial membrane above the hair cells increase the bending motion of the stereocilia.

Outer hair cells are highly unusual because they are capable of changes in length and shape These changes are referred to as outer hair cell motility. Scientific understanding of hearing and of cochlear function changed dramatically in the 1980s with the discovery that outer hair cells change shape when the ear is stimulated with sound (e.g., Brownell et al., 1985). When activated, outer hair cells alternatively become longer and skinnier and then shorter and fatter. The rapid up-and-down movements of activated outer hair cells increase basilar membrane motion with sound stimulation. Even though outer hair cells are very small, simultaneous movement of many outer hair cells within a limited region in the normal cochlea generates a remarkable amount of energy. Outer hair cell motility adds to movement of the basilar membrane and contributes importantly to normal hearing.

Active Processes in the Cochlea: Solving the Case of the Missing Amplifier. For many years, researchers suspected a source of energy or an "amplifier" somewhere in the inner ear (Gold, 1948; Davis, 1983). Important clues in solving the case of the missing cochlear amplifier were reported in the scientific literature beginning in the late 1940s. First, experimental animal research on cochlear physiology suggested the presence of a "mechanical resonator" that contributed to active processing of sound rather than simple passive response to sound within the ear (Gold, 1948).

Later investigations in humans produced proof that stimulation of the ear with two closely spaced tones yielded the perception of other non-stimulus sounds (Hall, 1972; Zwicker & Harris, 1990). That is, a person listening to two simultaneous sounds with similar frequencies actually heard not only the two sounds but also one or more additional sounds. The additional sounds were referred to as "combination tones" or "distortion tones." The cochlea generated energy over and above the energy of the stimuli, or output of the cochlea exceeded input. Processing is linear when output is equivalent to input. A system producing output that exceeds input is described as nonlinear. Production of distortion or extra energy in the cochlea was a sure sign of active processing.

In the mid-1970s, David Kemp demonstrated in a very clever experiment that the human ear actually produces sounds (Kemp, 1978). The ear does not only convert sound into electrical energy. Stimulation of the ear with sound leads to new sources of energy that can be detected in the external ear canal. This dramatic discovery clearly supported the concept of active processes within the cochlea. The ear doesn't simply react passively to sound. Extensive studies over the years have confirmed many of the details underlying active processes and amplification of energy within the cochlea (e.g., Ashmore et al., 2010; Dallos, 2008).

Recent research on structure and function of the outer hair cells has revealed the presence of a specialized motor protein known as *prestin* (Ashmore, 2008; Ashmore et al., 2010; Zheng et al., 2000; Dallos, 2008). Rapid elongation and shortening of prestin molecules within the walls of outer hair cells is the mechanism underlying motility of the outer hair cells.

Inner versus Outer Hair Cell Differences in a Nutshell. You've just learned about the contributions of inner and outer hair cells to cochlear function and hearing. The rapid and coordinated up and down movement of outer hair cells adds energy to the movement of the basilar membrane in the very limited frequency region of the stimulus sound, but not in other frequency regions. The energy supplied by outer hair cell motility helps overcome the loss of energy that occurs as the basilar membrane moves within the thick cochlear fluids. Outer hair cell motility improves our hearing sensitivity by about 40 to 50 dB and contributes to our ability to precisely distinguish among specific frequencies (Ryan & Dallos, 1975). However, we cannot hear with outer hair cells alone. Inner hair function is essential for hearing. The additional energy in the cochlea associated with outer hair cell motility adds to vibration of the basilar membrane and increases activation of the inner hair cells.

 WebWatch

An Internet search with key phrases such as "outer hair cell motility" reveals websites containing video clips of cochlear functions including demonstrations of "dancing" outer hair cells. Also, a display of experimentally stimulated outer hair cell motility with a brief written explanation is available on the website for the House Ear Institute.

L E A D E R S   A N D   L U M I N A R I E S

Peter Dallos

Peter Dallos studied at the Technical University in Budapest, Hungary, and earned a bachelor's degree in electrical engineering from the Illinois Institute of Technology. He completed his master's degree and PhD in electrical (biomedical) engineering at Northwestern University. For almost fifty years, Dr. Dallos has explored the structure and function of the cochlea, with an emphasis on inner and outer hair cells in mammals. Along with colleagues in his laboratory at Northwestern, Dr. Dallos proposed and confirmed that outer hair cells function as amplifiers in the cochlea and contribute importantly to sensitivity of the ear to faint sounds and the ear's capacity to distinguish small frequency differences in sound. In 2000 Dr. Dallos and his research team discovered a special protein called prestin that powers the movement of outer hair cells. Using genetically engineered mice, they demonstrated that prestin-based amplification is essential for normal mammalian hearing. Throughout his illustrious career, Dr. Dallos has disseminated new research findings in scientific articles but also in readable review papers and remarkably understandable lectures to audiologists.

Dr. Dallos devoted most of his productive career to the study of why we have outer hair cells. A symposium was held at Northwestern University in 2010 to honor Dr. Dallos. A quote from an article about the symposium offers a glimpse at the impact that this hearing scientist has had on our understanding of how the ear works. In an interview Dr. Dallos explained: "Outer hair cells have clearly shown what makes the mammalian ear so wonderful. It turns out that they are local mechanical amplifiers. They feed mechanical energy back onto the vibrating substrate upon which they're located and boost its amplitude so that we hear better and hear more sharply."

You can read the entire interesting interview of Dr. Dallos at the Northwestern University website.

 ClinicalConnection

One common auditory test procedure measures indirectly how well the outer hair cells are functioning. It's called the otoacoustic emissions (OAE) test. If we break down the term *otoacoustic emissions*, the meaning will become clear. "Oto" means ear and "acoustic" means sound. So, *otoacoustic emissions* are sounds emitted from the ear. Measurement of otoacoustic emissions is a valuable clinical tool. OAEs are used for identification of hearing loss in newborn infants and along with other tests for precise diagnosis of hearing loss in patients of all ages. In Chapter 8 you'll learn more about the OAE procedure and its clinical applications.

This is a very simple description of a complicated process. Cochlear physiology is quite complex and the topic of intense ongoing research investigation (see Ashmore et al., 2010, for a review). Here's a very short version of the fascinating story of cochlear function: *We hear with our inner hair cells, but we hear much better because of our outer hair cells.*

Neural Innervation of the Cochlea. There are distinct differences in the way auditory nerve fibers innervate inner versus outer hair cells. Figure 3.13 showed some of these differences at the base of the hair cells. *Afferent* neural pathways in the auditory system carry information from the ear to the brain and in a rostral direction through the brain. Up to 95% of the afferent auditory nerve fibers leading from the ear to the brain communicate directly with inner hair cells. In contrast, relatively few afferent nerve fibers communicate with outer hair cells. Only about 5% of afferent auditory nerve fibers make some type of connection with outer hair cells.

In addition to ascending *af*ferent auditory pathways carrying information from the ear to the highest auditory regions in the brain, another system of pathways runs downward from the brain to the ear. The descending pathways form the **efferent auditory system**. The final portion of the efferent auditory system consists of nerve fibers originating in the lowest region of the brain that travel downward through the internal auditory canal to the cochlea.

There are two sets of efferent fibers. Fibers in one set originate in the *lateral superior olive nucleus* and then travel outward through the internal auditory canal to innervate the inner hair cells. A *nucleus* is a collection of nerve cell bodies in the central nervous system. The lateral efferent fibers don't make contact directly with the inner hair cells but, rather, with afferent nerve fibers leading away from the inner hair cells. The other set of efferent nerve fibers originates in the *medial superior olive nucleus* in the brainstem. The medial efferent fibers travel outward through the internal auditory canal to directly innervate the outer hair cells at their base.

How Hair Cells Communicate with Nerve Fibers. You just learned that inner and outer hair cells play very important roles in hearing. Hearing is also entirely dependent on transmission of electrical activity from the inner hair cells to auditory nerve fibers. Hair cells communicate with nerve fibers through a *synapse*. The word *synapse* is of Greek origin and means "point of contact." Figure 3.14 shows a diagram of a synapse permitting communication between an inner hair cell and an auditory nerve fiber.

Activation of inner hair cells, specifically movement of stereocilia at the top of the cells, results in the flow of potassium ions into stereocilia and produces an increase in calcium ions (Ca^{2+}) within the hair cells. The increased Ca^{2+} in turn triggers the release of an *amino acid* biochemical near the base of the cell (Oestreicher, Wolfgang, & Felix, 2002; Fuchs, Glowatzki, & Moser, 2003). The amino acid is called *glutamate*. It travels the short distance across the synaptic junction or cleft to post-synaptic receptors in a membrane at the end of the afferent auditory nerve fibers. Multiple afferent auditory fibers communicate via synapses with a single inner hair cell.

Figure 3.14 illustrates this process of synaptic transmission of information in the auditory system. The auditory nerve fibers are depolarized as glutamate reaches the post-synaptic membrane. Depolarization results in electrical potentials in the nerve fibers that convey information from the cochlea to the brainstem.

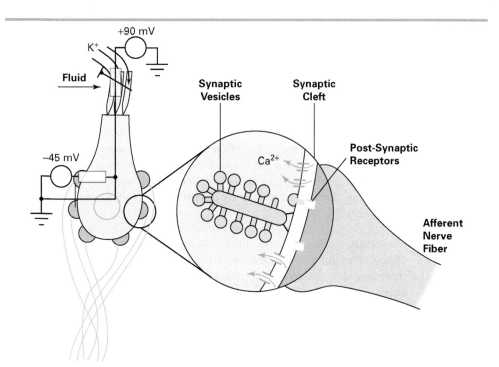

FIGURE 3.14

Diagram of a synapse between the inner hair cells and auditory nerve fibers.

F I G U R E   3 . 1 5

Structures within the internal auditory canal, including the auditory nerve, the facial nerve, two divisions of the vestibular nerve (superior and inferior), and the internal auditory (labyrinthine) artery.

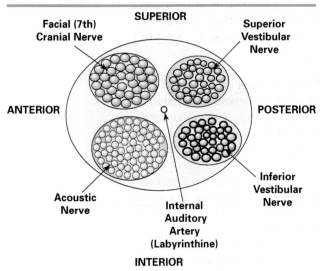

F I G U R E   3 . 1 6

The different courses of the type I (radial) fibers innervating the inner hair cells (IHC) and type II (longitudinal) fibers innervating the outer hair cells (OHC). Adapted from *MUSIEK, FRANK E.; BARAN, JANE A., THE AUDITORY SYSTEM: ANATOMY, PHYSIOLOGY, AND CLINICAL CORRELATES, 1st Ed., ©2007.* Reprinted and Electronically reproduced by permission of Pearson Education, Inc., Upper Saddle River, New Jersey.

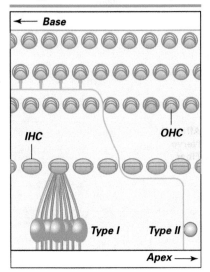

As noted earlier in our discussion of the differences between cochlear hair cells, the outer hair cells do not connect directly to the auditory nerve fibers that lead to the brain. Instead, direct neural connections with outer hair cells mostly involve efferent fibers from the brain that travel to the cochlea. A variety of neurotransmitters contribute to efferent auditory system function. One of the most common neurotransmitters in the efferent system called *acetylcholine*. Efferent neurotransmitters released by neurons near the bases of outer hair cells influence the function of outer hair cells, including the extent of their motility (Schwander, Kachar, & Muller, 2010).

Eighth Cranial Nerve

General Structure. The *eighth cranial nerve* transmits auditory and vestibular information from the ear to the brain. One of twelve cranial nerves, it is sometimes known as the auditory, acoustic, or *audiovestibular nerve*. We'll focus here on the auditory portion of the eighth cranial nerve. The auditory nerve in humans is approximately 25 mm in length and consists of over 30,000 individual nerve fibers. The auditory nerve is enclosed within a narrow passageway in the temporal bone called the *internal auditory canal (IAC)*. The adjective "internal" is an important part of the term, as it distinguishes this passageway from the external auditory canal (EAC) leading from the outer ear to the tympanic membrane.

Figure 3.15 is a very simple diagram showing how the auditory nerve shares limited space in the internal auditory canal with the facial nerve and the superior and inferior divisions of the vestibular nerve. The *facial* or *seventh cranial nerve* is important in controlling muscles of the face, including the concentrated collections of muscles around the mouth and the eyes. The two vestibular nerves are involved in maintaining balance and posture. We'll talk more about vestibular structures toward the end of the chapter.

Other structures important for auditory function are also enclosed within the internal auditory canal. The efferent auditory pathways already discussed extend downward within the internal auditory canal from the lower region of the brain to cochlear hair cells. And blood supply to the cochlea is carried through the internal auditory artery after it branches off larger blood vessels near the brain.

Structural Differences in Auditory Nerve Fibers. As already noted, almost all of the afferent auditory nerve fibers connect via a synapse with the inner hair cells. Indeed, ten to twenty afferent fibers make a synapse with a single inner hair cell. Auditory neurons are bipolar. That is, they consist of a cell body with two axons projecting from the cell body in opposite directions. The afferent neurons are called *type I cells* (Liberman, 1982). Figure 3.16 shows cell bodies of the type I neurons. The collection of auditory nerve cell bodies is called the *spiral ganglion*. The auditory nerve fibers pass from the inner hair cells through the dense bone that encloses the inner ear. The nerve fibers exit through small openings in the osseous spiral lamina called the *habenulae perforata*. The location of the habenulae perforata was shown earlier in Figure 3.9. The fibers then travel medially into the modiolus part of the ear through a passageway within the temporal bone named *Rosenthal's canal*.

Type I auditory nerve fibers innervate the inner hair cells. Type I auditory fibers are also called *radial fibers* because they extend in a radial fashion like bicycle spokes from the inner hair cells to the modiolus. Figure 3.16 illustrates the radial arrangement of the nerve fibers. Most type I auditory nerve fibers in older children and adults are surrounded with a specific form of *myelin* called *Schwann cells*. Myelin is a fatty covering or sheath around the nerve fibers. Myelin has two main functions. It protects the nerve fibers and also serves as insulation to increase their efficiency. Nerve fibers from the apical or low-frequency portion of the cochlea are located mostly within the central region of the auditory nerve. In contrast, nerve fibers arising from the basal high-frequency region of the cochlea are located more toward the outer portion of the auditory nerve.

Outer hair cells are innervated by *type II nerve fibers*. The type II nerve fibers are also known as *longitudinal fibers* because each fiber runs in a line parallel to the rows of outer hair cells before branching off to connect with multiple outer hair cells (Robertson, 1984). Figure 3.16 also shows the longitudinal arrangement of type II nerve fibers. In contrast to the type I fibers innervating the inner hair cells, the type II fibers reaching the outer hair cells generally have little or no myelin. Also, type II fibers mostly connect with the outermost of the three rows of outer hair cells in the basal region of the cochlea. The middle row and then the inner row of outer hair cells are innervated progressively more toward the apical end of the cochlea. The difference in the communication between cochlear hair cells and auditory nerve fibers is one of the numerous distinctions between inner and outer hair cells.

General Neural Function. Activity within auditory nerve fibers is important in coding or representing each of the properties of sound discussed in Chapter 2, including frequency, intensity, and temporal characteristics of sound (Meyer & Moser, 2010). Auditory nerve fibers have ongoing spontaneous activity even when an animal or human is in a quiet environment and there is no sound stimulus. The normal spontaneous nerve activity in auditory nerve fibers is known as the *resting potential* of the nerve.

Activation of inner hair cells results in a release of neurotransmitter into the synapse between the hair cells and auditory nerve fibers, as already noted. Stimulation of an auditory neuron via the neurotransmitter produces an abrupt increase in auditory fiber activity. The sudden increase in nerve activity is called *firing*. Nerve fiber firing appears as a sharp *spike* when plotted over a time period such as a second.

Spikes in auditory nerve activity are described in three ways: (1) the time interval, or latency, between the stimulus and the spike in activity, (2) the rate at which the auditory fibers fire, and (3) the probability of a spike occurring. Activity of many thousands of auditory nerve fibers after many stimulus presentations is sometimes displayed over a period of time like 1 second in graph called a *post-stimulus histogram*.

Coding of Frequency. *Frequency of sound* is coded by activation of a specific group of nerve fibers. You'll recall that as many as twenty nerve fibers make contact with a single inner hair cell. Remember also that the cochlea has tonotopic organization. If an inner hair cell is located in the basal region of the cochlea, then the nerve fibers from that particular inner hair cell are activated only by a high-frequency sound. In other words, that group of auditory nerve fibers is tuned to high-frequency sound stimulation. Each auditory nerve

ClinicalConnection

An understanding of the auditory system is necessary for interpretation of hearing test results and for accurate diagnosis of patients with hearing loss. Knowledge of auditory anatomy and physiology is particularly important for the diagnosis and management of patients with a relatively newly identified category of hearing impairment called *auditory neuropathy spectrum disorder (ANSD)*. You'll learn about the identification, diagnosis, and management of auditory neuropathy spectrum disorder in later chapters.

fiber has a *characteristic frequency (CF)* at which activation is greatest and the auditory nerve fiber is activated with the lowest sound intensity.

Tonotopic organization, or representation of different frequencies of sound by specific groups of neurons, is maintained throughout the auditory system from the cochlea to the highest auditory regions in the brain. A relatively low intensity sound activates a nerve fiber at its characteristic frequency, whereas much higher sound intensity levels are required to activate a nerve fiber for frequencies slightly higher or lower than its characteristic frequency. The responsiveness of auditory neurons to sounds at specific frequencies and not for sounds at other frequencies is called *frequency selectivity*.

Coding of Intensity. Intensity of sound is coded in at least three different ways in the auditory nerve. Intensity of sound is partly represented as the number of spikes per second for nerve fibers. As intensity of sound increases there is a corresponding increase in the average firing rate of spikes per second. For example, auditory nerve fiber activity may increase from a resting or spontaneous firing rate of 50 or 75 spikes per second to a rate of 300 spikes per second or even faster.

Firing rate of most auditory nerve fibers increases only over a range of about 20 to 50 dB of sound intensity. In other words, any single neuron is not capable of responding with a progressively higher firing rate to sound over a wide range of intensity levels, like 0 to 90 dB. Neurons in the auditory system usually respond over a specific limited range of intensity. Some neurons fire mostly for low intensity sounds, whereas other neurons are most responsive to mid- or high-level sound intensities. In combination, a collection of auditory neurons that includes those that are sensitive to different levels of sound effectively codes intensity over a wide range.

Intensity of sound is also related to the spread of excitation along the basilar membrane in the cochlea. To explain briefly, the intensity level of a sound determines the extent of activation along the basilar membrane. Higher-intensity sounds produce activation across a wider region of the cochlea. Consequently, at higher intensities more hair cells and more nerve fibers are activated.

In addition to these two intensity-coding mechanisms, activity of neurons also becomes more correlated or synchronized as stimulus intensity increases. The increase in probability that a spike will occur with increased stimulus intensity is sometimes described as *phase locking*. You were introduced to the concept of stimulus phase in Chapter 2. At higher-intensity levels there is higher correspondence between the phase of a stimulus and the phase of an auditory fiber response to the stimulus.

Coding of Timing Characteristics. Temporal characteristics of sound are faithfully represented by the activity of auditory neurons. Examples of temporal characteristics are duration of a sound and the time interval between two sounds. Specific neurons respond in different ways to temporal features of sound. For example, some neurons produce a spike in activity only at the onset of a sound. Then, soon after the sound begins the neural activity decreases to the baseline or resting level. Other neurons continue to keep firing for the duration of a stimulating sound before returning to their resting or spontaneous firing rate when the sound is no longer present. Another neuron type produces a spike in activity only at the end or offset of a sound. There are seven or eight different functional types of neurons in the auditory system based on their response patterns to sound. In addition to these different patterns of nerve response to temporal features of sound, timing properties of sound are coded when the discharge of auditory neurons is synchronized to the phase of the sound. In other words, the phase of the stimulus in part determines the phase or timing of the nerve fiber response.

Central Auditory Nervous System (CANS)

Ascending Auditory Pathways and Centers

General Layout. The end of the peripheral auditory system and the beginning of the central auditory nervous system is the point where auditory nerve fibers make connections with neurons in the *brainstem*. Figure 3.17 is a very simple diagram showing the location of major structures within the central auditory nervous system. The **brainstem** is the lowest portion of the brain located just above the spinal cord within the central nervous system. Auditory neurons form pathways of nerve fibers traveling from one region of the brain to the next. Neurons also are grouped together in brain centers called *nuclei*. Auditory pathways and centers are duplicated on both sides of the brain and communicate by means of bundles of nerve fibers that cross from one side of the brain to the other. The crossing fibers are called **decussations**.

There are a number of resources for readers interested in learning more about the central auditory nervous system and the processing of information by the brain. A recent textbook entitled *The Auditory System: Anatomy, Physiology, and Clinical Correlates* is a good starting point (Musiek & Baran, 2007).

Auditory nerve fibers enter the central nervous system in a region of the brainstem called the *pons*. Figure 3.17 shows the point of entry of eighth cranial nerve fibers into the brainstem. The word *pons* is derived from the Latin word for "bridge." The pons region of the brainstem is just above the *medulla* at the caudal portion of the brainstem. The medulla is in turn just above the spinal cord. The pons includes important auditory centers and pathways (Mukerji, Windsor, & Lee, 2010). Also within the brainstem are centers that control bodily functions essential for life, including breathing and heart activity.

The *cerebellum* is another important part of the brain found at the same level as the pons. In fact, the pons forms a bridge connecting the two sides of the cerebellum. The cerebellum plays an important role in balance and the coordination of movement. Continuing upward in the central nervous system we encounter another portion called the *midbrain,* which contains the largest collection of neurons within the brainstem.

The **thalamus** is found between the brainstem and the cerebral cortex. The thalamus is a major structure in the central nervous system, where information from the auditory, visual, and touch senses is coordinated. The *medial geniculate body* is a region of the thalamus specialized for processing auditory information. Several pathways lead from the thalamus to the **cerebral cortex**. The cerebral cortex is the most complex region of the brain and the highest level of the auditory system.

Concept of Complexity. Complexity in anatomy of the auditory system increases dramatically from the auditory nerve to the brainstem and to the cerebral cortex. Several rather general observations about anatomy highlight the complexity of the auditory system. One simple index of complexity is the *number of neurons*. There are about 90,000 neurons in the lowest regions of the auditory brainstem in comparison to the 30,000 fibers in the human auditory nerve. Proceeding upward, there almost 400,000 neurons in rostral regions of the auditory brainstem and over 10 million neurons in the auditory cortex.

Complexity is also reflected by the presence of *multiple types of neurons*. As already noted in the discussion of auditory nerve fibers, neurons within the auditory regions of the

FIGURE 3.17

Diagram of the central
auditory nervous
system pathways and
structures. Structures
and pathways are
described in the text.

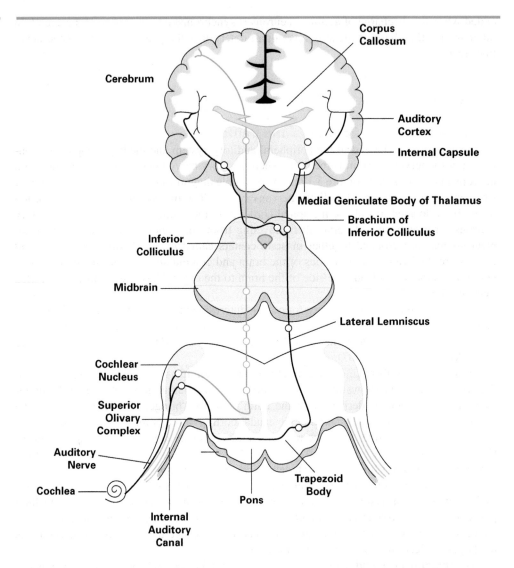

FIGURE 3.17

Diagram of the central auditory nervous system pathways and structures. Structures and pathways are described in the text.

brainstem can be differentiated based on their appearance and also how they respond when stimulated. The distinct structural and functional types of neuron play different roles in processing auditory information. Additional types of neurons are found in the different layers of the auditory cortex.

Tonotopic organization is also maintained throughout the auditory system from the cochlea and auditory nerve through the brainstem and to the highest regions in the auditory cortex. You already learned that tonotopic organization is the specialization of neurons in processing information for different stimulus frequencies.

Complexity is also reflected by the *multiple centers* or *nuclei* containing many neurons even within a rather limited region of the auditory system. Sometimes the collections of neurons consist of subdivisions. Examples include ventral and dorsal cochlear nuclei and posterior ventral cochlear nucleus. Another example is the inferior colliculus, which consists of a number of divisions and subdivisions, each containing thousands of specialized neurons.

Another indication of auditory system complexity is the *multiple crossings* or *decussations* of pathways from one side of the auditory system to the other. Figure 3.17 shows several examples of decussating fiber tracts connecting the two sides of the central auditory nervous system. Crossing fibers play an important role in quickly conveying large amounts of auditory information upward through the central nervous system. Decussating pathways within the auditory system also provide an alternative route for information when the usual pathways are not functioning normally or adequately. The *corpus callosum* is the most rostral and the largest decussating pathway. It permits communication between auditory regions in the left and right cerebral hemispheres.

Finally, complexity in the central auditory nervous system is reflected in the variety of *neurotransmitters*. As noted already, neurotransmitters are specialized brain chemicals permitting communication of information from neuron to neuron and from nucleus to nucleus. Neurotransmitters and their importance vary somewhat from one region of the central auditory nervous system to the next. The main neurotransmitters are categorized by their action in exciting or inhibiting neuron activity.

 ClinicalConnection

An appreciation of functional differences among neurons is useful for the interpretation of the findings of certain clinical auditory procedures. For example, some brain responses elicited by abrupt transient auditory stimulation arise from neurons that are activated only by the onset of the stimulus. Audiologists also apply knowledge of decussating pathways within the auditory system in analyzing the results of various hearing tests.

Auditory Brainstem

Auditory nerve fibers from the right ear and the left ear enter into the brainstem at the junction of the medulla and the pons on each side of the brainstem. This region is referred to as the *cerebellopontine angle (CPA)* since it is in a corner between the pons and the cerebellum.

Following activation of neurons in nuclei within the pons, some auditory pathways travel upward on the same side to higher centers whereas other pathways cross over from one side to the other before traveling to higher centers. In addition, there are crossing or decussating fibers that connect identical structures located on the right and left halves of the brainstem. Major and complex sets of crossing fibers are referred to as *commissures*. At every level of the brainstem and throughout the entire central auditory nervous system, different pathways lead from one structure to multiple other structures. In other words, auditory information can ascend through the central nervous system via many varied routes.

Cochlear Nucleus. Auditory nerve fibers make their initial synapse with neurons in the brainstem in a center called the *cochlear nucleus*. The cochlear nucleus in the brainstem is anterior to the cerebellum and cannot be visualized unless the cerebellum is moved out of the way. Communication from each inner ear to the cochlear nucleus is always along ipsilateral pathways. That is, auditory nerve fibers from the right ear lead directly to the right cochlear nucleus and those from the left ear lead to the left cochlear nucleus.

The cochlear nucleus on each side of the brainstem is subdivided into two regions, called the *ventral cochlear nucleus (VCN)* and the *dorsal cochlear nucleus (DCN)*. Some of the auditory nerve fibers

 ClinicalConnection

The cerebellopontine angle (CPA) is a site of a rare but very serious form of auditory abnormality. Tumors arising from the vestibular or auditory nerves may expand into the cerebellopontine angle. If undetected and undiagnosed, the expanding tumors often press upon the facial nerve and even against the brainstem. Growth of the tumor can lead to paralysis and other neurological abnormalities. Audiologists are ever alert for signs of auditory nerve tumors, particularly in patients with more pronounced auditory abnormalities on one side than the other.

leading from the ear terminate in the dorsal cochlear nucleus, while other fibers branch off to the ventral cochlear nucleus. The ventral cochlear nucleus is further divided into *posterior* and *anterior* portions, abbreviated *PVCN* and *AVCN*. Figure 3.17 shows the location of the cochlear nuclei. Neural connections within the cochlear nucleus allow for communication among the three subdivisions.

ClinicalConnection

Analysis and interpretation of test results for different clinical procedures in audiology requires an understanding of the anatomy of the brainstem. One common test procedure known as the acoustic stapedial reflex was mentioned earlier. Acoustic reflex pathways include multiple structures within the brainstem. The same statement is also true for an auditory brainstem response elicited by sound that is a valuable procedure for diagnosis of hearing loss in infants and young children. You'll learn about these and other test procedures in Chapters 8 and 9.

Large nerve fibers surrounded by myelin lead out of the cochlear nuclei. Myelinated nerves conduct impulses quickly from one center to another. Relatively few pathways lead from the cochlear nuclei to more rostral structures on the same side of the brainstem. There are three major neural pathways exiting the cochlear nuclei and carrying information from one side of the brainstem to more rostral auditory centers on the other side. The three pathways crossing from one side to the other in the brainstem are the *dorsal acoustic stria, ventral acoustic stria,* and *intermediate stria.* Portions of these pathways branch off to other important auditory brainstem nuclei like the *superior olivary complex.* Other nerve fibers form a major pathway called the *lateral lemniscus.* The lateral lemniscus carries information through the brainstem to the *inferior colliculus,* which is a major nucleus in the auditory system. Figure 3.17 illustrates the course of some of the crossing and ascending auditory pathways in the brainstem.

Superior Olivary Complex. The superior olivary complex (SOC) is located in the pons region of the brainstem. The structure is aptly named. Figure 3.17 shows the location of the superior olivary complex within the brainstem. The complex consists of groups of nuclei with the appearance of an olive when viewed from the surface of the brainstem. The superior olivary complex plays an important role in *localization* and *lateralization* of sound (Grothe, Pecka, & McAlpine, 2010). Localization is the ability to determine the source of sound in space, whereas lateralization is identifying whether sound is coming from the right or left side.

The superior olivary complex also plays a role in the fusion of two sounds heard separately in the right ear and the left ear into an image of one sound in the middle of the head. We've all had a sound fusion experience when using a headset or a set of earphones. The SOC is the first center in the auditory system that receives binaural input, from fibers entering the central nervous system from both ears. The ability to very precisely determine where a sound is coming from using binaural hearing helps us to perceive speech and other sounds in noisy listening environments.

Lateral Lemniscus. The *lateral lemniscus* is a large auditory fiber tract coursing upward through brainstem from more caudal centers like the cochlear nucleus and superior olivary complex to the inferior colliculus. Tonotopic organization of the cochlea is maintained within the lateral lemniscus and also throughout other auditory centers in the brainstem. All fibers within the lateral lemniscus terminate in the inferior colliculus.

Inferior Colliculus. The inferior colliculus is a major nucleus in the auditory system and the biggest structure within the auditory brainstem. Figure 3.17 identifies the location of the inferior colliculus on each side of the brainstem. The two large inferior colliculi are easily visible as bumps on the dorsal surface of the upper brainstem. Each inferior colliculus is not a single uniform structure. The inferior colliculus consists of three distinct sections, specifically a central nucleus, a dorsal cortex, and a lateral area. The *commissure of the inferior colliculus* connects the inferior colliculus on one side of the midbrain with the corresponding structure on the other side.

Tonotopic organization is quite distinct within the inferior colliculus. Ribbon-like regions known as *iso-frequency sheets* are dedicated to processing sound frequencies within specific ranges. Intensity coding is also maintained by changes in the firing rates of neurons in the inferior colliculus. The inferior colliculus plays an important role in the coordination of auditory information from both ears and in localizing the sources of sound in space. The inferior

L E A D E R S   A N D   L U M I N A R I E S

Frank Musiek

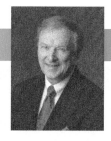

Frank E. Musiek earned his bachelors degree from Edinboro University in Pennsylvania, his master's degree from Kent State University, and his PhD from Case Western Reserve University. For many years, Dr. Musiek was Director of Audiology at Dartmouth-Hitchcock Medical Center and a professor in the Department of Otolaryngology and the Department of Neurology at Dartmouth Medical School. He is now Professor and Director of Auditory Research in the Department of Speech, Language and Hearing Sciences and in the Department of Surgery (Otolaryngology) in the School of Medicine at the University of Connecticut.

Dr. Musiek is the recipient of the James Jerger Career Award for Research in Audiology and the ASHA Honors for contributions in Audiology and Auditory Neuroscience. He has published over 150 articles in peer-reviewed journals and has edited or authored eight books. Many of these publications focus on the assessment central auditory disorders and underlying neurologic, neuroanatomic or neurophysiologic mechanisms for abnormal auditory function. He and colleague Marilyn Pinheiro developed some of the most widely used tests for central auditory assessment including the frequency patterns test, the duration patterns test, the dichotic digits test, and the Gaps in Noise (GIN) test. You will see a number of Dr. Musiek's books and published articles cited in the readings and the reference list for this book.

colliculus includes neurons specialized in detecting differences in the intensity, timing, and phase of sounds arriving from each ear.

Pathways from multiple auditory structures lower in the brainstem converge in the inferior colliculus. Auditory information passing upward from the inferior colliculus, however, travels along only two routes. One is a large ascending fiber tract called the brachium of the inferior colliculus. The word *brachium* is from the Latin word for "arm." The other route away from the inferior colliculus is the horizontal commissure that leads to the inferior colliculus on the other side of the brainstem.

Thalamus

The *brachium of the inferior colliculus* leads to the thalamus. Figure 3.17 illustrates the location of the thalamus within the central nervous system. The thalamus is located above the brainstem and below the auditory cortex. Pathways from the inferior colliculus specifically terminate in the medial geniculate body within the posterior portion of the thalamus plus several other thalamic nuclei. The medial geniculate body consists of ventral, medial, and dorsal sections.

At this juncture it is appropriate to comment on three types of pathways that carry auditory information from one center to the next in the brain. We'll focus the brief discussion on pathways leading to and from the thalamus. There are tonotopic pathways in each lateral lemniscus that contribute to clearly organized representation of frequencies within the medial geniculate body. These pathways are designed for fast and effective delivery of critical information. There is also a diffuse collection of pathways within the central portion of the brainstem. The diffuse pathways contain many neurons and synapses that result in relatively slow transmission of auditory information. Neurons and neuronal connections within the diffuse pathways

 ClinicalConnection

Recent research findings confirm that the ear and auditory regions in the brain play a role in the perception of bothersome *tinnitus*. Tinnitus is a ringing or buzzing sound that's heard even in a quiet setting. Perception of tinnitus can be very distressing for some people. In Chapter 15, you'll learn about how audiologists evaluate and treat persons with bothersome tinnitus.

probably undergo changes with auditory experience. Finally, there are polysensory pathways that convey visual, tactile, and auditory information. Indeed, the thalamus is an important center for coordinating and integrating these three distinctive types of information.

Auditory Cortex

The *auditory cortex* is within the *cerebrum* at the highest level of the central nervous system. It's often referred to as the cerebral cortex. The word *cortex* refers to the outer layer of any organ in the body. Here the term is used to describe a rather thin outer layer of tissue of less than 4.5 mm that covers the brain. The important auditory centers in the cerebrum are found in the **temporal lobes**. There is a temporal lobe on each side of the brain.

Information from the thalamus reaches the primary auditory cortex via several major *thalamocortical pathways.* The primary auditory pathway from the thalamus to the cerebral cortex is located within the posterior portion of the *internal capsule.* The internal capsule is a rather complex and prominent set of auditory and nonauditory pathways.

Figure 3.18 is a diagram of the cerebral cortex, showing the location of the temporal lobe on one side of the brain. A region known as the *primary auditory cortex* in the temporal lobe region of the cerebrum is essential for hearing. All information reaching the cerebrum from lower pathways and centers arrives first in the primary auditory cortex and specifically in a part of the temporal lobe referred to as *Heschl gyrus.* Heschl's gyrus sits on the superior surface of the temporal lobe cortex.

The *planum temporale* is immediately posterior to Heschl gyrus, on the horizontal surface of the temporal lobe in humans. The planum temporale portion of the temporal lobe plays an important role in hearing and also in language.

Another important auditory cortical region called the *insula* is located medially and deep within the *Sylvian fissure.* The Sylvian fissure is a deep groove separating the temporal lobe from the parietal

ClinicalConnection

You've already learned that the capacity for complex processing of auditory information increases in different regions from the ear to the brain due a variety of structural and functional features in the central auditory nervous system. Auditory processing is a hot topic in hearing science research and also in clinical hearing assessment. In later chapters, you'll read about clinical tests of auditory processing, causes of auditory processing disorders, and management of children and adults who are diagnosed with auditory processing disorders.

FIGURE 3.18

Lateral view of the cerebral cortex showing the temporal lobe, containing auditory centers and other lobes of the brain. Primary auditory cortex in the temporal lobe is known as Heschl gyrus.

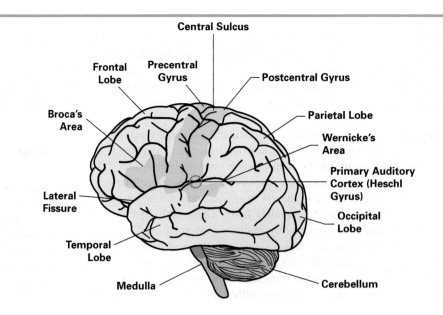

and frontal lobes on each side of the brain. Finally, Figure 3.18 also shows three other regions of the brain, including a frontal lobe, a parietal lobe, and the occipital lobe.

Additional Auditory Regions

If asked to describe the auditory system, most audiologists or speech pathologists would mention what we've reviewed up to this point. And, if asked also to sketch out the auditory system they would draw a diagram similar to the ones depicted earlier in Figures 3.17 and 3.18. Without question, the traditional auditory pathways are essential for hearing. However, two other major regions of the nervous system are also involved in a person's response to sound. In fact, sounds would be meaningless and uninteresting without the involvement of these two additional areas. And, importantly, sounds indicating danger would be ignored without activation of the additional auditory regions.

Limbic System. The *limbic system* is one of the additional regions of the nervous system that plays a role in hearing and our response to sounds. Functions served by the limbic system include emotion, long-term memory, and other aspects of behavior. One limbic system structure called the *amygdala* is important in a person's emotional response to sounds.

Some sounds like music or the voice of a friend generate positive "feel good" emotions. We like to listen to our favorite music because it gives us pleasure, making us feel happy and upbeat. An older favorite song may remind us of good times and events we experienced in years past. Other sounds, however, may produce negative emotions. Listening to a certain song or a person's voice may make us feel sad or lonely. Sound, especially voices and music, can trigger powerful emotions in people. The strong connection between the traditional auditory regions and the limbic system makes life interesting. In fact, it's hard to imagine life without the emotional richness derived from sound.

Autonomic Nervous System. The *autonomic nervous system* is another part of the brain that has strong connections with the auditory centers, including those in the limbic system. The highly complex autonomic nervous system controls vital bodily functions such as homeostasis. Homeostasis is maintenance of bodily stability, such as a steady body temperature of 98.6^{0}F (37^{0}C). The autonomic nervous system is activated when we hear potentially dangerous sounds.

Everyone at some time has heard a sound that signifies danger. Examples include the growl of a big dog as we walk along a dark street or a siren from a police car behind us as we drive too fast down the highway. Danger sounds activating the autonomic nervous system produce a "flight or fight" response. Adrenaline begins to flow and we quickly decide whether to confront the danger or try to escape. If your heart starts to beat very fast, if you begin to sweat and your legs feel rubbery when you hear a specific sound, you can be sure the autonomic nervous system is involved.

 ClinicalConnection

Brain imaging studies show that additional regions of the brain, including limbic structures and the autonomic nervous system, are usually involved in the negative reaction of some persons to the perception of *tinnitus*. Tinnitus is a phantom-type perception of sound that is not produced by an external sound. Post-traumatic stress disorder (PTSD) is also associated with activity within these regions of the brain.

Efferent Auditory System

You were introduced already to pathways descending from the brainstem to the inner and outer hair cells, comprising the efferent auditory system. In contrast to extensive research on afferent auditory pathways, much less is known about the efferent system (Berlin, 1999; Musiek, 1986; Musiek & Baran, 2007). The efferent system begins in the auditory cortex and includes pathways within each of the major auditory centers just described for the afferent auditory system.

Most investigation of the efferent auditory system has focused on the final pathways leading to the cochlea. The efferent fibers from the olivary complex in the brainstem that descend to the inner ear are known as the *olivocochlear bundle (OCB)*. One set of fibers called the *medial OCB* leads directly to the outer hair cells, whereas *lateral OCB* pathways have indirect connections with inner hair cells. The function of the efferent auditory system is poorly understood. However, the medial OCB is clearly involved in the inhibition or reduction of outer hair cell activity. Thus, the efferent auditory system plays a role in controlling function of the ascending afferent auditory system. Recent research evidence also suggests that the efferent auditory system may help to improve the detection, localization, and perception of speech in a setting of background noise (deBoer & Thornton, 2008; Andéol et al., 2011). Efferent auditory system function may also be related to auditory disorders like tinnitus in persons who have been exposed to excessive levels of noise (Attias, Bresloff, & Furman, 1996; Lalaki et al., 2011).

Vestibular and Balance Systems

The **vestibular system** contributes importantly to our ability to maintain a stable position in space. One of the most common examples is the ability to steadily stand upright on two feet. Coordination of vestibular system and visual system function is also necessary for us to maintain a stable view of the environment even when the head is moving constantly as we walk or run.

The auditory and vestibular systems both include sensory structures within the ear, including specialized hair cells. Auditory and vestibular neural pathways travel closely together within the internal auditory canal from the ear to the brain. And auditory and vestibular pathways and centers occupy nearby locations in the brainstem.

There are also several clear differences between the anatomy and physiology of the auditory system and the vestibular system. For example, vestibular system structures are mostly located in the brainstem, whereas important centers in the auditory system are located in the cerebral cortex, much higher in the central nervous system. Also, the vestibular system specializes in detection, coding, and processing of movement and not sound stimulation.

Disorders of the vestibular system result in what most people call dizziness, imbalance, lightheadedness, or vertigo. Among these disorders, *vertigo* is a main feature of a vestibular disorder. Vertigo is the sensation that the environment is spinning around a patient. Persistent or even occasional vertigo can seriously disrupt daily activities and quality of life. During a vertiginous episode a patient often must lie down and remain immobile until the spinning sensation diminishes. In some patients, a complete diagnostic medical assessment and balance evaluation reveals that the patient's dizziness, imbalance, or lightheadedness is not the symptom of a vestibular disorder but, rather, a nonvestibular illness such as a vascular or neurological abnormality.

 ClinicalConnection

You'll learn in Chapter 11 about diseases associated with vestibular abnormalities. And in Chapter 16 you'll discover that audiologists effectively treat a specific type of vestibular abnormality with relatively simple procedures performed in the clinic.

Audiologists must have a good working knowledge of the *vestibular system*. Assessment of the vestibular system and vestibular function is within the scope of practice of audiologists. Audiologists are trained to perform a variety of clinical procedures in the assessment of vestibular and balance function. In fact, some audiologists specialize entirely in vestibular assessment and the nonmedical management of persons with vestibular disorders. As noted in Chapter 1, graduate programs leading to the Doctor of Audiology degree now include one or more courses devoted to the vestibular system and management of vestibular disorders.

Peripheral Vestibular Apparatus

The vestibular system, like the auditory system, includes peripheral and central portions. Figure 3.19 shows that the *peripheral vestibular apparatus* is located in the temporal bone near the cochlea. The vestibular system consists of two specialized groups of structures for detecting different types of movement. The peripheral vestibular system also includes two vestibular nerves, mentioned earlier. The central nervous system portion of the vestibular system consists of nuclei in the brainstem and also pathways that lead from the nuclei to different muscle groups. Vestibular pathways from the brainstem connect with the tiny muscles controlling eye movements and larger muscles controlling the head, neck, torso, and arms and legs.

Receptor Organs. The locations of major structures in the peripheral vestibular system are shown in Figure 3.19. Two of the structures are the *saccule* and the *utricle*. Each structure detects movement in a straight line, or linear acceleration, and also the force of gravity. The saccule and utricle are referred to as *otolith organs* because they contain tiny rock-like crystals called *otoconia,* The saccule and utricle also each contain a special sense organ called the *macula*. There are two different types of hair cells in the vestibular system. *Type I* and *type II* cells are located within the macula. Forces of gravity and inertia bend the stereocilia on vestibular hair cells. Movement of the heavier otoconia that are located above the stereocilia increases displacement of the stereocilia on the hair cells and enhances vestibular function.

F ! G U R E 3 . 1 9 Diagram of the major vestibular structures and pathways. The insert shows the location of peripheral vestibular structures within the temporal lobe. Important vestibular structures in the enlarged view include the semicircular canals, the utricle, the saccule, and the two vestibular nerves.

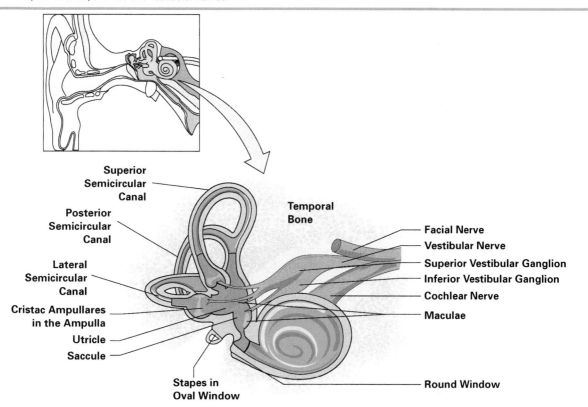

Figure 3.19 also shows the three *semicircular canals* within the vestibular apparatus. Each of the semicircular canals is oriented in a different position and at right angles to the others. One of the semicircular canals, aptly named the *lateral canal,* is in a horizontal plane. The *superior* and *posterior semicircular canals* are oriented in two different vertical planes. Angular or rotational movement of the head that is horizontal or vertical is detected by sense organs located at the base of the three semicircular canals. The wider portion of each semicircular canal is called the *ampulla.* A complex sense organ containing hair cells called the *crista* is located within the ampulla. Resting on top of the crista is the *cupula.* The cupula is a gelatinous structure that enhances movement of the hair cells in the crista with movement of the head.

Vestibular Nerves. A two-part vestibular nerve within the internal auditory canal runs from the vestibular apparatus on each side through the internal auditory canals to the brainstem. Figure 3.15 showed the *inferior vestibular nerve* and the *superior vestibular nerve.* There are about 18,000 vestibular nerve fibers with cell bodies located in a structure called *Scarpa's ganglion.*

The inferior division of the vestibular nerve originates at the macula of the saccule and the crista of the posterior semicircular canal. The superior division of the vestibular nerve innervates the macula of the utricle and the crista within the lateral and superior semicircular canals. Three different types of fibers in each of these nerves innervate the hair cells within the peripheral vestibular apparatus. In contrast to the auditory nerve, the vestibular nerves are distinguished by a very high rate of spontaneous activity. Movement producing a response from the vestibular sense organs typically produces increased rates of firing in the nerve fibers on one side of the head and decreased rates of firing in the nerve fibers on the opposite side.

Central Vestibular Nervous System

The central vestibular nervous system consists of a complex of nuclei in the brainstem and pathways leading to a variety of muscle groups. A vestibular complex on each side of the lower brainstem is composed of four sub-nuclei: the lateral vestibular nucleus, the medial vestibular nucleus, the superior vestibular nucleus, and the inferior vestibular nucleus.

Information from different structures within the peripheral vestibular apparatus, including each otolith organ and each semicircular canal, is conveyed to different regions of the vestibular nuclei in the brainstem. Many pathways lead away from the vestibular nuclei in the brainstem to a variety of destinations. Tracts from the vestibular nucleus on each side of the brainstem travel to the cerebellum, to visual and motor centers in the brainstem, to eye muscles, and to large muscles of the neck and trunk.

Vestibular-Oculomotor Reflex. An important set of pathways in the vestibular system contributes to the *vestibulo-oculomotor reflex* or *VOR.* The VOR is involved in the coordination of eye movements that compensate for the almost constant movement of the head during waking hours. Other long fiber tracts leave the vestibular nuclei in the brainstem, enter spinal cord, and then course downward to the muscles of the neck. Some of these long fiber tracks continue onward to the trunk and limbs. The long fiber tracts are important in the maintenance of balance.

The vestibular pathways and centers are mostly within the lower regions of the central nervous system, with few connections to the cerebral cortex. Nonetheless, vestibular function is quite complex and absolutely essential for our ability to move about and perform daily activities. Connections and coordination between the vestibular system and muscle groups allows us to maintain balance and equilibrium.

PULLING IT ALL TOGETHER

You now have a general understanding of the structure and function of the auditory system and the vestibular system. This information is directly applicable to diagnostic assessment of auditory and vestibular function, and the appropriate management of persons with auditory or vestibular disorders.

Our review began with an introduction to the structure of the outer ear and the middle ear, and their various contributions to auditory function. Then you learned about the complex anatomy of the cochlea, and the distinctly different roles that inner and outer hair cells play in hearing.

Our discussion followed the route taken by the auditory information we hear, from the auditory nerve to various pathways and centers in the central auditory nervous system. Three often-overlooked aspects of the auditory system, the efferent pathways, the limbic structures, and the autonomic nervous system, were recognized to have influence on hearing. Along the way, you were introduced to recent research developments that have considerably advanced our understanding of hearing and auditory processing.

Throughout the chapter you also learned about connections between auditory anatomy and the clinical procedures used by audiologists. Finally, we reviewed vestibular system anatomy and its importance in maintaining balance. Later, before learning in Chapter 11 about disorders affecting the outer, middle, and inner ear, and in Chapter 12 about dysfunction within the retrocochlear pathways and central auditory nervous system, you may wish to return to this chapter for a quick review.

READINGS

Ashmore, J., Avan, P., Brownell, W. E., Dallos, P., Dierkes, K., Fettiplace, R., Grosh, K., Hackney, C. M., Hudspeth, A. J., Jülicher, F., Lindner, B., Martin, P., Meaud, J., Petit, C., Sacchi, J. R., & Canlon, B. (2010). The remarkable cochlear amplifier. *Hearing Research, 266,* 1–17.

Berlin, C. I. (1999). *The efferent auditory system.* San Diego: Singular Publishing.

Brownell, W. E., & Oghalai, J. S. (2009). Cochlear biophysics. In J. B. Snow & P. A. Wackym (Eds.), *Ballenger's otorhinolaryngology—head and neck surgery* (17th ed., pp.101–106). Shelton, CT: B. C. Decker.

Clark, W. W., & Ohlemiller, K. K. (2008). *Anatomy and physiology of hearing for audiologists.* Clifton Park, NY: Thomson Delmar Learning.

Cristobal, R., Pepper, P., & Pereira, F. A. (2009). Hair cell regeneration. In J. B. Snow & P. A. Wackym (Eds.), *Ballenger's otorhinolaryngology—head and neck surgery* (17th ed., pp. 89–99). Shelton, CT: B. C. Decker.

Dhar, S., & Hall, J. W., III. (2011). *Otoacoustic emissions: Principles, procedures, and protocols.* San Diego: Plural Publishing.

Dallos, P., Pepper, A. N., & Fay, R. R. (Eds.). (1996). *The cochlea.* New York: Springer.

Lonsbury-Martin, G. K., & Hannley, M.T.G. (2009). Physiology of the auditory and vestibular systems. In J. B. Snow & P. A. Wackym (Eds.), *Ballenger's otorhinolaryngology and head and neck surgery* (17th ed., pp. 45–79). Shelton, CT: B. C. Decker.

Musiek, F. E., & Baran, J. A. (2007). *The auditory system: Anatomy, physiology, and clinical correlates.* Boston: Allyn & Bacon.

Schwander, M., Kachar, B., & Muller, U. (2010). Review Series: The cell biology of hearing. *Journal of Cell Biology, 190,* 9–20.

Yost, W. A. (2007). *Fundamentals of hearing: An introduction* (5th ed.). San Diego, CA: Academic Press.

4 Preparing for Hearing Assessment

LEARNING OBJECTIVES

In this chapter you will learn:

- About patient consent, confidentiality, and privacy
- What is meant by "professional liability"
- About medical errors in audiology and how they can be avoided
- What constitutes an "environment of care"
- About clinical etiquette—good clinical manners and habits
- The importance of a proper test environment for accurate hearing assessment
- What masking is and why it's important in hearing testing
- About equipment calibration in hearing testing, including why and how it is done
- How a patient is instructed for hearing assessment
- What is required of a patient who is undergoing hearing assessment
- Different ways a patient can respond to sounds in hearing testing
- About otoscopic ear inspection prior to auditory tests
- How earphones and bone vibrators are placed on a patient for hearing assessment

CHAPTER FOCUS

You might suspect that the delivery of hearing services begins when an audiologist first presents a stimulus sound to a patient and the patient responds. In fact, many important clinical activities take place before this.

In this chapter, you will learn about obtaining consent from patients undergoing hearing assessment and how patient confidentiality is protected. We will briefly review steps and policies that enhance patient safety and minimize the chance of errors in the diagnosis and management of auditory disorders. We will describe maintenance of an appropriate test environment. All of these factors create an "environment of care."

Preparing for hearing assessment also includes taking a thorough history from the patient (and sometimes family members), carefully inspecting the ear, escorting the patient to a test room, adequately instructing the patient for the upcoming tests, and finally properly placing the patient earphones that will be used for hearing testing. You'll be introduced to each of these clinical events.

We will follow the typical sequence of events that occurs after a patient arrives in an audiology clinic for a hearing assessment. In reading this chapter, you may have the sense that you are "shadowing" an audiologist who is preparing a patient for hearing assessment.

KEY TERMS

Ambient noise
Artificial ear
Artificial mastoid
Attenuate
Behavioral audiometry
Bone conduction
Bone vibrator
Calibration
Cerumen
Chief complaint (CC)
Conditioned play audiometry
Coupler
Cross hearing
Ear specific
Foreign objects
Gestation
Informed consent
Insert earphones
Listening check
Localization to sound
Masking
Otoscope and otoscopy
Patient history
Psychosocial
Supra-aural earphones
Transducers
Video otoscopy
Visual reinforcement

Patient Rights and Consent

Adults

In a single day, an audiologist in a busy clinic may conduct many test procedures on many patients. An audiologist knows from clinical experience that the procedures are simple for most adult patients to perform. Hearing test procedures pose little risk for pain and usually don't even produce mild discomfort.

Patients scheduled for a clinic visit with an audiologist are usually aware that they will be participating in hearing tests. However, a person who has never undergone hearing assessment may not appreciate what is involved in the testing. Sometime in the past, the patient may have undergone a painful invasive medical procedure. Without a clear and complete explanation of the testing process, the patient may be anxious or fearful. In greeting a new patient, therefore, an audiologist usually provides a simple explanation of the test process, to put the patient at ease as much as possible.

All patients have a right to know what procedures will be performed and what is expected of them during an assessment. Consent requirements vary from one institution to the next and from one state to another within the United States, as well as by procedure. Institutional policies and regulations usually require adult patients to give written *consent for treatment,* that is, the patient signs a form indicating agreement to the test procedures that will be administered to them. An *assumed consent,* rather than a formal written consent, may apply for certain common noninvasive procedures (such as a patient history). An **informed consent** form is a special type of consent document read and signed by patients who are serving as subjects in a research study. If the patient is incapable of understanding the nature of the assessment, including the procedures to be performed, a legally approved representative, such as a caregiver or guardian, signs the consent.

A patient about to undergo any procedure, like a hearing test, can rightfully expect that discomfort or pain will be minimized as much as possible. In hospital clinical facilities, an audiologist is now usually required to document in the clinical record the patient's pain status prior to administering any procedure.

Children

Parents or legal guardians must consent to hearing testing for younger individuals (in most states persons under the age of 18). Infants and young children, of course, are not able to understand even simple verbal explanations of hearing tests. Before a hearing test procedure is performed with a child, the parent or caregiver is given a verbal description of what will be done and also an opportunity to ask questions about the procedure. Many clinics give the parent or caregiver a simple yet complete written description of the procedures that are likely to be performed on the day of the clinic visit. Preschool and school-age children are less likely to be anxious about the testing if they can be told in advance what to expect in the audiology clinic.

On the day of the procedure, an experienced clinician often puts a child at ease with a pleasant, very simplified, and age-appropriate description of the upcoming test. For example, a 3-year-old may be told, "O.K., now we're going into this quiet room to play some listening games. You'll hear some very tiny little birdie sounds. Every time you hear a little sound, you need to put this block into the bucket. Let's give it a try. I think you're going to be very good at this game."

Professional Liability and Responsibilities

The Hippocratic Oath Adapted to Audiology

The Hippocratic Oath is a traditional promise given by healthcare providers to be ethical in their practice and dealings with patients. The Oath is named after Hippocrates, a Greek who lived in the 5th century BCE. The Oath first appeared many years after the death of

Hippocrates, so it was really written by someone else. Over the years, the Hippocratic Oath has been updated and revised to be more medically and politically correct.

Many themes of the Hippocratic Oath are highly relevant for audiologists, as well as physicians. For example, the Oath encourages healthcare professionals to share knowledge with those who follow them, such as less-experienced persons and students. According to the Hippocratic Oath, healthcare providers should use their knowledge and skills for the benefit of those who are not well while avoiding harm to the patient. The updated and modern version of the Oath also encourages healthcare professionals to treat patients with warmth, sympathy, and understanding, and to respect the privacy of patients. Healthcare problems should be prevented whenever possible, as prevention is preferable to a cure. Finally, healthcare professionals are encouraged to call on colleagues with more experience or skills for help as necessary.

 WebWatch

Hippocrates is sometimes referred to as the "father of medicine." With an Internet search you'll find many links devoted to information about the Hippocratic Oath, including some controversy about whether it's still relevant and adequate in the modern era of healthcare.

Preventing Medical Errors

Prevention of medical errors is a high priority in healthcare. The goal of preventing medical errors extends to all healthcare professions, including audiology. You have just learned that one of the principles underlying healthcare, as stated in the Hippocratic Oath, is to do no harm.

The phrase *medical errors* often brings to mind images of patients who receive the wrong drug or an overdose of the correct drug. Drug-related medical errors do account for a high proportion of adverse healthcare outcomes. In fact, one possible adverse medical outcome is hearing loss due to the administration of one or more drugs that are used in treating patients with serious illnesses, such as a severe infection or a brain tumor. Certain drugs can damage structures within the inner ear. Audiologists are sometimes asked to test patients who are at risk for drug-induced hearing loss.

Some medical error incidents occur in the operating room during surgical procedures. Audiologists may play a role in the prevention of surgically related medical errors. Consider, for example, the problems that could arise when an audiologist reverses the right and left ear when plotting the hearing test results for a patient who is a candidate for surgical management. Operating room personnel consulting the audiogram in the medical records immediately before ear surgery might prepare the wrong ear for the procedure.

Regular continuing education on the prevention of medical errors in audiology is required for renewal of professional licenses in some states and by some healthcare institutions. Prevention of medical errors is the most effective strategy for avoiding professional malpractice and minimizing professional liability. Professional liability dictates that healthcare professionals, including audiologists, by virtue of their advanced knowledge, training, and skill, have a responsibility to adhere to certain standards of conduct and protect patients from unreasonable risks and either intentional or unintentional injury.

Prevention of medical errors in audiology and speech pathology is best accomplished by maintaining proper professional credentials, consistently following various standards and guidelines for clinical services, communicating effectively with patients and their families, and maintaining very good written documentation.

Patient Privacy, Security, and Confidentiality

Patient privacy and security are top priorities in the modern healthcare system. Patient privacy includes the right to control personal information, the freedom from intrusion or observation, and the expectation that other persons will respect an individual patient's rights. Security, in the context of healthcare, involves the administrative, physical, and technical safeguards that limit and control access to patient related information and prevent either accidental or intentional disclosure of the information to unauthorized persons or entities.

Audiologists, physicians, and other healthcare professionals have an obligation to assure that *protected health information (PHI)* of patients remains strictly confidential. PHI includes information typically recorded in a medical or health history; physical examination and diagnostic test results; details about the patient's injury, illness, diagnosis, or surgery; and other displays of health findings, such as photographs, radiographs, and hearing test results.

Privacy rules also apply to any general information that could possibly reveal the identity of the patient, such as the patient's name, birth date, hospital or medical record number, social security number, telephone number, street mailing address, or email address. Health information should not go beyond a patient and her/his healthcare provider, unless the patient gives written consent for a release of information to other persons or parties or the information is required for treatment purposes.

WebWatch

You can read more about the Health Insurance Portability and Accountability Act (HIPAA) at the Internet link www.cms.gov. Audiologists and speech pathologists must be familiar with current HIPAA regulations. Regulations are revised and updated on a regular basis.

Federal and state laws pertaining to privacy and security of PHI were strengthened considerably between 2003 and 2005 with the widespread implementation of the *Health Insurance Portability and Accountability Act (HIPAA)*. HIPAA rules are designed to maintain patient privacy and security. Patient information in all formats must be kept confidential at all times. This includes verbal and oral communications, like discussing patient test results in person or over the telephone, and paper and electronic reports and records, including emails. Healthcare professionals can, with a patient's authorization, use PHI to provide appropriate care and treatment and for payment purposes. Healthcare professionals and all other persons who fail to maintain patient information confidentiality can face very serious penalties, among them civil or criminal sanctions such as substantial fines and prison time.

Penalties may be imposed whether the disclosure of PHI was incidental, accidental, or unintentional. An incidental disclosure of PHI might be when a passerby overhears an audiologist or speech pathologist talking with a patient about test results in a waiting room setting. An example of an accidental disclosure would be an email with test results that goes to the wrong person. Even an unintentional breach of confidentiality can happen surprisingly easily. For example, a healthcare provider leaves a vacant work area that contains unsecured PHI and an unauthorized person views the patient data. Most audiologists and speech pathologists are required by their employers to regularly review HIPAA rules and regulations and to complete training modules.

As you might expect, maintaining privacy and security of personal health information is important in any work setting, not just in hospital clinics. Audiologists, speech pathologists, and teachers who work in educational settings, from elementary schools to universities, must also adhere to institutional and federal rules and regulations regarding privacy and security of student personal information. The *Family Educational Rights and Privacy Act (FERPA)* was passed to ensure that student personal information is properly safeguarded and used only for legitimate purposes and only when necessary.

An audiology or speech pathology student or any other person who wishes to observe patient care for educational or training purposes must first comply with specific institutional requirements regarding patient privacy and security. Before being permitted into the patient care area of a health facility like a hospital or outpatient clinic, an observer must usually be sponsored by an employee of the institute, such as an audiologist. In most states, the patient care observer must be at least 18 years old. Depending on the specific policies of the institution, the observer may also be required to sign a confidentiality and security agreement, to complete a patient care observer health screening form, and/or participate in HIPAA training, including a brief post-test. Finally, each patient must consent to the observer's presence, with the patient's agreement documented in writing.

Patient Safety Is Priority #1

An audiologist's or a speech pathologist's primary professional responsibilities include diagnosis of speech, language, hearing, and related disorders; the implementation of appropriate intervention; and referral to other professionals when appropriate. The ultimate objective for audiologists and speech pathologists is improvement of a patient's communication and quality of life. As healthcare providers, however, audiologists and speech pathologists also have other very important professional duties and obligations.

Universal Precautions. Infection control and prevention are always foremost in a healthcare facility. Along with other healthcare providers, audiologists and speech pathologists receive inoculations for diseases that can be transmitted from one person to another, such as tuberculosis and hepatitis B. Direct patient contact is usually not permitted without documentation of the inoculations. In addition, educational modules must be periodically completed to assure basic knowledge of blood-borne pathogens, microorganisms that cause disease, and general components of infection prevention. Finally, audiologists and speech pathologists must closely comply with infection control policies and procedures.

Photographs in Figure 4.1 highlight some examples of universal precautions. As illustrated in Figure 4.1A and Figure 4.1B, hand washing between patient contacts, the availability of hand sanitizer throughout the facility, and the use of hospital-grade protective gloves are all fundamental forms of infection control. Current procedures for infection prevention in an audiology clinic include as shown in Figure 4.1C the use of disposable rather than reusable probe tips and insert earphones with disposable foam tips whenever possible for the different hearing tests.

Infection control includes disinfecting equipment and objects that come into contact with patients after each use, as shown in Figure 4.1D. Infection prevention policies and procedures are especially rigorous when caring for vulnerable patient populations, among them infants

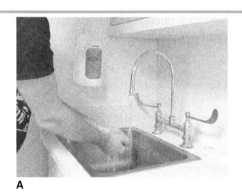
A

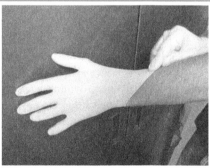
B

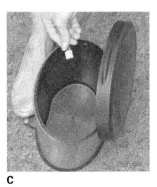
C

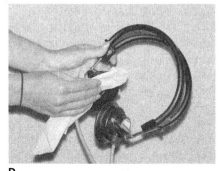
D

FIGURE 4.1

Examples of universal precautions, including hand washing before patient contact (**A**), the use of protective gloves (**B**), proper disposal of a foam tip used for hearing testing with insert earphones (**C**), and disinfecting a set of supra-aural earphones (**D**).

in an intensive care nursery and patients at risk for human immunodeficiency virus (HIV) and autoimmune diseases.

Patient safety efforts also include compliance with isolation policies to prevent the spread of infection. In a hospital setting, patients with certain infections are kept in isolation from healthcare staff and other patients. Isolation strategies include the use of protective clothing and gloves during any contact with the patient, and isolating the patient in a separate hospital room. Audiologists and speech pathologists working in a hospital setting also are also trained to deal with medical emergencies, including cardiopulmonary resuscitation (CPR).

Fall Prevention. *Fall prevention* is another important duty of modern-day healthcare providers, including audiologists. Healthcare costs associated with patients who fall are enormous, exceeding $2 billion annually in the United States alone. An estimated 11 million elderly persons fall each year, resulting in 2 to 3 million injuries, approximately 1 million hospitalizations, and 18,000 deaths annually. At least 70 percent of hospital patient accidents are due to falls.

Audiologists care for patients who are at high risk for falling, including the elderly and those with vestibular or other balance disturbances. Typical steps to reduce the likelihood of patient falls include regular education of clinic staff on fall prevention, questions for the patient about fall risk on the initial history form, written patient information about fall prevention, and adequate signage in the clinic, such as signs alerting patients to exercise special caution when stepping down as they exit a sound-treated room.

These general healthcare responsibilities, such as the protection of patient privacy, universal precautions for infections, prevention of patient falls, and basic knowledge of CPR techniques, are important for all audiologists and speech pathologists, but especially those working in medical settings such as multi-specialty clinics and hospitals.

Environment of Care. The phrase *environment of care* is often used in hospitals and other healthcare facilities. Physical and social factors affect the overall environment of care in any setting where healthcare is provided, including audiology and speech pathology facilities. In an audiology clinic, examples of physical factors in the environment of care include structural features, such as approved ramps to assure that patients safely enter a sound-treated room, proper containers for disposal of soiled supplies used in hearing testing, and hand sanitizer in each room where services are provided. Social factors include the education, training, and daily activities of persons providing healthcare services, including audiologists and speech pathologists. Research shows that the environment in which healthcare is provided can have a major impact on minimizing patient risk and improving patient safety and health outcome. Nationally recognized groups establish guidelines for environment of care that are followed by accredited healthcare organizations, such as hospitals.

Initial Patient Encounter

Importance of the First Impression

First impressions are often lasting impressions. This adage applies to the initial encounter with a patient scheduled for a hearing or speech-language assessment. Audiologists and speech pathologists strive to follow a humanistic approach in providing clinical services. Humanistic care is focused and centered on the patient and family, and not based primarily on the preconceptions and protocols of the healthcare provider. As DeBonis and Donohue (2004) note, humanistic care is provided in the context of a patient's "values, beliefs, history, needs, abilities, culture, and social network" (p. 5). Furthermore, a humanistic caregiver provides services with empathy and compassion, making every effort to understand the effect of the patient's hearing loss on **psychosocial** functioning and quality of life.

The term *psychosocial* describes a patient's conscious and unconscious psychological adjustment and adaptation to the social environment. (This is also referred to as mental health.) Healthcare in the past three to four decades has moved away from the traditional medical model focused on a physician and a patient to a bio-psychosocial approach that empowers the patient and family members, with the goal of improving health outcome and quality of life (Bandura, 1969; Branch et al., 2001; Engel, 1977). Common psychosocial responses to hearing loss and other communicative disorders include sadness, anxiety, frustration, irritability, a sense of loss, and depression. Later, in Chapter 14, you'll learn about the important role of audiologists and speech pathologists in counseling patients to effectively address the psychosocial consequences of hearing loss and other communication disorders.

Figure 4.2 shows major components and steps in the preparation for hearing assessment. In an outpatient setting, effective diagnostic hearing assessment of most patients really begins with a friendly greeting and a clear explanation of the purpose of the clinic visit. Whenever appropriate, the patient's family members are included in the initial encounter. Often it is not feasible to include family members at every step of the hearing assessment process. However, family members are typically summoned at the end of the hearing assessment for an explanation of test findings, counseling regarding the findings, and an explanation of recommendations for management.

Patient History

Before beginning the assessment process, an audiologist generally acquires and/or reviews the relevant **patient history**. In clinical settings, the phrase *patient history* is used to describe information about the patient's past and present health status, including complaints, symptoms, diagnosed diseases, family history of diseases and causes of death, medical test results, and previous medical treatments. The audiologist is most interested in discovering information about the patient's health status that is likely to influence which test procedures should be administered, how the testing will be conducted, and how the results will be interpreted. We'll focus here on the patient history of persons who might have hearing loss or a related disorder.

In some clinical settings, such as a busy medical clinic, a newborn intensive care unit, or a specialty floor in a hospital, the audiologist may have easy access to a detailed written summary of the patient's symptoms, past health problems, medical test results, and current medical status. The patient history has been obtained earlier by some other health professional, such as a physician, a physician's assistant, or a nurse. In such cases, the audiologist may simply verify the patient's **chief complaint (CC)**, that is, the main reason the patient presents for hearing testing. The brief discussion might take place in a private location such as a medical examination room or even in a sound-treated room immediately prior to hearing testing. Common examples of a chief complaint are hearing loss in one or both ears, ear pain, dizziness, or a bothersome ringing sound in the ears.

An audiologist might initially ask a simple question to elicit the chief complaint, such as: "What brought you to see us today?" By asking this open-ended question, the audiologist can often quickly and effectively discover why the patient is scheduled for the hearing assessment and what test strategy is most appropriate. The audiologist may then also ask a few very

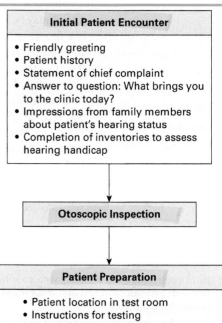

FIGURE 4.2

Sequence of events in the preparation for a hearing assessment beginning with the initial patient encounter and ending with patient instructions for testing and placement of earphones

Initial Patient Encounter

- Friendly greeting
- Patient history
- Statement of chief complaint
- Answer to question: What brings you to the clinic today?
- Impressions from family members about patient's hearing status
- Completion of inventories to assess hearing handicap

Otoscopic Inspection

Patient Preparation

- Patient location in test room
- Instructions for testing
- Placement of transducers
- Consideration of listener variables
- Determination of test strategy
- Selection of tests
- Troubleshooting as indicated

specific hearing-related questions. For example, "Do you think you hear better out of one ear or the other?" or "Have you noticed a change in your hearing recently?"

In an outpatient audiology clinic or a private practice office that is not associated with a medical facility, an audiologist often has full responsibility for acquiring all necessary information about the patient's health and hearing status. Before coming to the clinic, the patient may complete a detailed multipage history form that was mailed by clinic clerical staff. Or, the patient may be asked to complete the history forms upon arrival at the clinic.

In either case, before beginning the hearing assessment, an audiologist typically takes a few moments to review the responses on the form and to question the patient in more detail about certain responses. Case history or patient history forms may be brief, but they may also be quite lengthy. In clinics that offer services to special patient populations, the history form may include a number of questions focusing in considerable detail on the particular disorder of interest. Examples of special populations would be patients with profound hearing loss or deafness, a balance disorder, or very bothersome ringing noises in their ears.

Some of the questions commonly asked by an audiologist in a patient history are summarized in Table 4.1. While taking a patient history, experienced audiologists can quickly

TABLE 4.1   Questions often included on a history form for a patient visiting an audiology clinic.

Questions for Older Children and Adults

- What brought you here today?
- Have you noticed any difficulty with your hearing? Can you describe the problem for me? When do you think the problem with your hearing first began? Did your difficulty with hearing come on gradually, or was there a sudden onset of the problem?
- Is your hearing problem in both of your ears or just one ear?
- Do you have more difficulty hearing women's, men's, or children's voices? Do you have more difficulty in hearing people speak when there is background noise (like a restaurant, driving in a car, or at a party)? Do you frequently have to ask people to repeat what they said?
- Have you ever worn a hearing aid?
- Is there a family history of hearing loss? Has anyone in your family had a hearing loss from birth in one or both ears? Do or did your parents have a hearing loss in later years?
- Have you ever had ear infections, even as a child? Did a doctor ever treat you for the ear infections? Have you ever had ventilation tubes placed in your eardrums, or any other ear surgery?
- Have you experienced any pain in your ears or any type of discharge from your ears?
- Do you have ringing or other sounds in your ears?
- Do you experience dizziness, imbalance, or the sensation of spinning?
- Have you been exposed to loud noise in recreational activities (such as shooting, hunting, or listening to personal audio players), at work, or in military service?

Additional common questions for children (directed to the parents or caregivers)

- Are there any concerns about speech and language development? Has the child ever been evaluated by a speech-language pathologist?
- Does the child recognize and respond to familiar sounds?
- Has the child ever had any illnesses? Ever been hospitalized? Ever had a head injury?
- Was the child in an intensive care nursery after birth?
- Was the child's hearing screened in the hospital after they were born? Do you know the results of the screening?
- Has the child had previous hearing screening or a hearing assessment?
- How is the child doing in school (for older children)?

and efficiently (1) determine why the patient is scheduled for a hearing or balance assessment, (2) identify test procedures most likely to yield diagnostic information about hearing or balance function, and (3) develop an efficient strategy for completing the hearing assessment. Even though a history may begin with rather general questions, such as those in Table 4.1, the actual history-taking process varies from patient to patient, depending on the patient's initial responses to questions and the audiologist's interpretation of responses.

Physical Examination of the Ear

An audiologist almost always inspects the pinna and external ear canal before performing any test procedure. Otoscopic inspection is one of the main components in the flowchart shown in Figure 4.2. Ear inspection includes close observation of the pinna and the region around the ear to detect any evidence of abnormality.

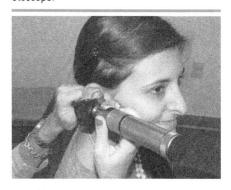

FIGURE 4.3

An audiologist inspecting an ear with an otoscope.

Otoscopy. Visual inspection of the ear canal is usually made with an **otoscope** (Figure 4.3), which is a handheld device equipped with a bright light that illuminates the ear canal and tympanic membrane. The meaning of the word *otoscope* is "instrument to examine the ear." The term *otoscopy* is used for careful visual inspection of the pinna and ear canal with an otoscope. A *speculum,* a funnel-shaped piece, is attached to the otoscope before it is inserted into the ear canal. Since the speculum makes direct contact with the skin of the external ear canal, it must either be properly disinfected before and after use or disposed of after single use with a patient.

Although the otoscope is adequate for visual inspection of the ear, a number of manufacturers now offer special equipment for **video otoscopy**. During video otoscopy, images viewed through an otoscope-type earpiece are displayed on a computer monitor. The larger image improves visualization of the external ear canal and tympanic membrane. Also, the image can be stored and/or printed for documentation of the findings and later analysis. With video-otoscopy technology, patients may view images of their own ears.

 ClinicalConnection

Audiologists sometimes observe abnormalities during visual inspection of the ear. A wide variety of diseases and pathologies may affect the ear. In Chapter 11, you'll learn about many diseases and pathologies that involve the external ear, the middle ear, and the inner ear.

Common Abnormalities. During the ear inspection, an audiologist looks for and makes note of **foreign objects**, debris, and **cerumen** within the ear canal. *Cerumen* is the technical term for earwax. The phrase *foreign objects* refers to anything seen in the ear canal that is not either part of the body or produced by the body. Otoscopic inspection, particularly in children, may reveal a variety of unexpected objects, including pebbles, small parts of toys, bits of food, pieces of cotton swabs, and even insects. Otoscopy also provides clues about the possibility of ear canal collapse and may reveal evidence of external or middle ear pathology.

In some cases, the patient history or results of hearing testing suggest the possibility of a perforation. *Perforation* is the technical term for a hole in the tympanic membrane. Causes for perforations include trauma and prolonged ear infections. Otoscopic inspection of a patient with a history of ear infections might also show a ventilation tube in the tympanic membrane. A *ventilation tube,* sometimes simply called a "tube," is a tiny cylinder inserted into the tympanic membrane by an ear specialist to improve hearing and prevent infection. When inspecting the tympanic membrane, the audiologist documents the presence and location of the ventilation tube or perforation.

 ClinicalConnection

In Chapter 11, you'll learn more about perforations, what causes them, and how they are treated medically. In Chapter 11, you'll also view photographs of tympanic membranes with perforations and with ventilation tubes.

ClinicalConnection

Collapsing ear canals should be suspected in any patient who shows a high-frequency hearing loss that appears to be due to a problem in the outer ear or middle ear. Suspicion of collapsing ear canals is highest in elderly patients. The possibility of collapsing ear canals is eliminated with the regular use of insert earphones with soft foam plug-type cushions placed into the external canals rather than rigid headset-type earphones that put pressure on the external ear. Techniques for hearing assessment with pure tone sounds and for detection of collapsing ear canals are reviewed in the next chapter, which is about pure tone audiometry.

Collapsing Ear Canals. Collapsing ear canals can interfere with presentation of sounds during hearing tests and can lead to an erroneous finding of hearing loss. The relatively soft cartilaginous portion of an external ear canal sometimes collapses under the pressure of conventional earphones that fit over the external ears. The likelihood of ear canal collapse is increased in certain patient populations, such as infants and elderly adults. Fortunately, patients at risk for collapsing ear canals are usually identified during visual inspection of the ear. The audiologist can then take steps to prevent ear canal collapse during hearing test procedures.

The audiologist notes findings observed during visual inspection of the ear and later records them in the formal written report of the hearing assessment. For example, the results section of an audiology report often begins with a sentence such as: "Otoscopy revealed clear ear canals and intact tympanic membranes bilaterally." If abnormalities are discovered during otoscopy, the patient is invariably referred to a physician for medical examination and possible treatment.

Hearing Test Environment

Noise Requirements for Hearing Testing

Accurate measurement of hearing requires a sufficiently quiet test setting. Background sound during audiometric testing is referred to as **ambient noise**. There are internationally recognized standards for maximum acceptable levels of ambient noise in rooms used for hearing assessment. For example, in the United States, audiometric sound-treated booths, rooms, or suites are designed to be in compliance with standards such as those of the American National Standards Institute (ANSI, 1999).

LEADERS AND LUMINARIES

Roger A. Ruth (1950–2009)

Roger Ruth earned his Bachelors, Masters, and PhD degrees in audiology from The Ohio State University. Roger Ruth's first and only position was in the Department of Otolaryngology at the University of Virginia. For over thirty years until his untimely death, Dr. Ruth taught multiple generations of Doctor of Audiology and PhD students in the classroom, clinic, and research laboratory. He was also a popular speaker at professional conferences, seminars, and workshops in the United States and around the world.

Much of Dr. Ruth's illustrious career was devoted to practical instruction in hearing testing. As the director of a busy audiology clinic in a major medical 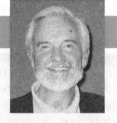 center, he was also responsible for assuring that patient services were of the highest quality. In the 1980s, Dr. Ruth was among the first audiologists to introduce and personally provide then-new audiology services such as newborn hearing screening, intra-operative monitoring, rehabilitation of cochlear implant patients, and the assessment and management of persons with bothersome tinnitus or hyperacusis (Holmes, Kileny, & Hall, 2011). In 2008, Dr. Ruth received the Distinguished Achievement Award from the American Academy of Audiology in recognition of his many contributions to our profession.

Acceptable noise levels vary, depending on whether the ears are covered or uncovered. Ears are covered when hearing testing is conducted with earphones. Ears are uncovered when sounds are delivered with a loudspeaker in the test booth. All devices that deliver sound during hearing testing are called **transducers**. The term *transducer* refers to the conversion of electrical signals to sound by the earphone or some other device. Figure 4.4 shows examples of four major types of transducers, including an insert earphone, a conventional earphone, a bone vibrator, and a loudspeaker.

With **insert earphones** (Figure 4.4A), the stimulus is delivered into the ear canal by means of a soft compressible foam plug inserted well within the external ear canal. **Supra-aural earphones** are another common type of transducer used in hearing testing, as shown in Figure 4.4B. The earphone itself fits within a soft rubber donut-shaped cushion. As the term suggests, a supra-aural earphone rests on the pinna of the ear. Stimulus sounds can also be delivered to the inner ear by vibrating the bones in the skull using a bone vibrator or oscillator (Figure 4.4C). Finally, sounds are sometimes delivered to a patient with loudspeakers that are located a few feet away from the ears, as depicted in Figure 4.4D.

In a sound-treated room, both types of earphones reduce the amount of ambient noise that reaches the inner ear. Properly fitted insert earphones are most effective in reducing or attenuating the background noise that reaches the inner ear. In audiology, the term **attenuate** is commonly used instead of the word *reduce*, and the phrase *attenuation of sound* describes a reduction of sound. Values in Table 4.2 provide clear evidence of greater attenuation of ambient sound with insert earphones than with supra-aural earphones. There is no attenuation of ambient sound when stimulation is presented via loudspeakers, with the ears uncovered.

FIGURE 4.4

Major types of transducers used in hearing testing, including insert earphones with soft tips that fit within the external ear canal **(A)**, supra-aural earphones that fit over the ears **(B)**, a bone vibrator that rests on the skull **(C)**, and a loudspeaker **(D)**.

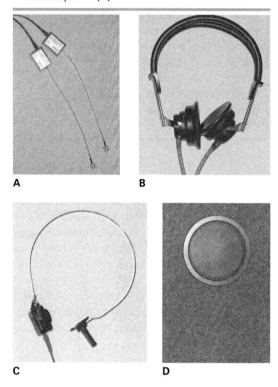

A   B

C   D

TABLE 4.2
Acceptable ambient noise levels for hearing testing (ANSI, 1999).

Frequency in Hz (Octave Band)	Transducer*		
	Insert Earphone	**Supra-Aural Earphone**	**Sound Field/Bone Vibrator (Ears Uncovered)**
125	59.0	35.0	29.0
250	53.0	25.0	21.0
500	50.0	21.0	16.0
1000	47.0	26.0	13.0
2000	49.0	34.0	14.0
4000	50.0	37.0	11.0
8000	56.0	37.0	14.0

* Over the frequency range of 125 to 8000 Hz. Noise in dB SPL (re: 20 µPa) are rounded to the nearest 0.5 dB

Acceptable noise levels in the test room also depend on the frequencies of sound used to assess hearing. Table 4.2 shows acceptable sound levels at various audiometric test frequencies for two different earphones and for uncovered ears. Inspecting the table, you'll see that the maximum permissible level of background noise for a 500-Hz frequency band is 50 dB SPL with insert earphones, but only 21 dB SPL for supra-aural earphones. Maximum permissible noise levels are even lower, 16 dB SPL, with no earphones. The condition with no earphones applies when hearing is tested with loudspeakers.

Even the highest level of acceptable noise for sound-treated rooms is considerably less than noise levels encountered in everyday settings. For example, background noise in a typical office is, on the average, about 50 dB SPL. And noise produced by various sources in a relatively quiet car is usually in the range of 60 to 75 dB SPL, depending on road conditions, speed, whether the windows are open or closed, and other factors.

🎧 **Clinical**Connection

A sufficiently quiet test environment, meeting accepted standards, is especially crucial for accurate assessment of persons with relatively good hearing abilities who can detect soft sounds. A modest level of ambient noise is less likely to affect the accuracy of findings for hearing testing conducted with stimulus sounds at high intensity levels.

Sound-Treated Rooms

Hearing testing is usually conducted in a quiet room specially designed for the purpose. Hearing test rooms are sometimes inappropriately referred to as "sound-proof" booths or chambers. The term *soundproof* is not accurate since outside sound is only reduced in the rooms, not entirely eliminated. *Sound-treated* is a better way of describing hearing test rooms. Sound-treated rooms range in size from small enclosures for single persons, about the size of a phone booth, to large rooms that accommodate multiple people, chairs, and audiology test equipment.

Figure 4.5 shows a typical sound-treated room used for hearing testing. The patient is inside the sound-treated room during hearing testing, whereas the tester who operates an audiometer is located outside of the test room. Referring to Figure 4.5, the tester would be located on the opposite side of the window in the wall of the sound-treated room.

An *audiometer* is a piece of equipment designed specifically for hearing assessment. With this equipment, an audiologist can select certain types of sounds, like tones, noise, or words, and can present the sounds to the patient at precise intensity levels. In the next chapter you'll learn more about the features and operation of an audiometer.

Sound-treated rooms for audiology clinics are available for purchase from several manufacturers. Prefabricated panels are shipped from the manufacturer to the clinical setting and then assembled in the audiology clinic by a crew of workers with special skills for the job. The panels, once assembled, form the floors, ceilings, walls, and doors of the room. As seen in Figure 4.5, sound-treated rooms typically include one panel consisting of receptacles and conduits so that wires from the audiometer can reach the transducers (earphones, bone vibrators, and speakers) inside the test room. Wires from a microphone and from a patient response button in the sound room run through the same panel back to the audiometer. A sound-treated room almost always includes a sound-attenuating window so the tester and patient can maintain visual contact.

The audiologist, audiometer, and other test equipment are often enclosed within an adjoining quiet but non-sound-treated room. The room outside the sound-treated chamber

FIGURE 4.5

A sound-treated room in an audiology clinic, used for hearing testing. The photograph was taken from the door that leads into the sound-treated room. The door is always closed for hearing testing.

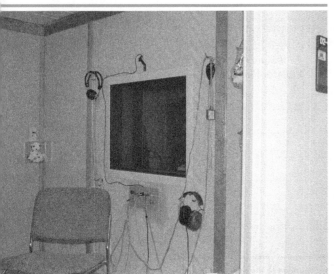

sometimes serves as an additional test setting or even office space for the audiologist. Or, two sound-treated rooms can be connected to form a sound room suite, with one room for the audiologist and the other serving as the test room for the patient.

When sound-treated rooms are installed in an existing space and not within a recessed area in the floor of the building, there is inevitably an 8" to 10" step up into the enclosure. Sound-treated rooms with a step require a ramp meeting certain specifications so that patients who are not ambulatory and who cannot negotiate the step can be wheeled into the test environment. For audiology clinics in a hospital setting where there are non-ambulatory patients, sound-treated rooms can be installed with oversized sound room doors and adequate space for maneuvering wheelchairs or gurneys.

Equipment Calibration

Calibration Equipment and Standards

The accuracy of hearing test results depends on precise **calibration** of equipment, including the audiometer and the transducers. *Calibration* is verification that the equipment is performing properly and that the stimuli produced by the audiometer and the sound levels produced by the transducers are accurate. In the United States, regulations require calibration of audiometers and transducers with special equipment at certain time intervals. Occupational Safety and Health Administration (OSHA) regulations state that: "Audiometer calibration shall be checked acoustically, at least annually, according to the procedures described in this appendix. The equipment necessary to perform these measurements is a sound level meter, octave-band filter set, and a National Bureau of Standards 9A coupler. In making these measurements, the accuracy of the calibrating equipment shall be sufficient to determine that the audiometer is within the tolerances permitted by American Standard Specification for Audiometers, S3.6-1969."

WebWatch

Dozens of standards pertaining to hearing and hearing testing are available on the website for the American National Standards Institute.

Records of equipment calibration are maintained on file in the clinic. The calibration includes verification of the accuracy of the frequency of different pure tones and the intensity level of each of the types of sound used in hearing testing, including pure tones, noise, and speech signals. Calibration is also performed for each of the transducers connected to the audiometer, including earphones, bone vibrators, and speakers. Equipment is calibrated according to well-accepted standards for audiometers and other test devices used in audiology.

In the United States, the American National Standards Institute (ANSI, 2010) defines standards for output levels in dB SPL that correspond to audiometric zero, or 0 dB HL, for each test signal. *Audiometric zero is defined as the median hearing level for a large number of normal-hearing persons.* Hearing test equipment, such as an audiometer, is calibrated with a sound-level meter using a physical reference for decibels (dB) sound pressure level (SPL) even though hearing testing is conducted using the dB HL unit of intensity. Units for describing the intensity of sounds, like SPL, and sound-level meters were reviewed in Chapter 2.

The Calibration Process

Regular calibration of audiometers according to ANSI standards is conducted with a sound-level meter connected to the earphone or bone vibrator with a device called a **coupler**. You were introduced to sound-level meters in Chapter 2. Figure 4.6 shows a sound-level meter in a laboratory coupled (connected) to a supra-aural earphone, an insert earphone, and a bone vibrator. The sound level meter is to the left and identified with an arrow. An acoustic coupler for an earphone is sometimes referred to as an **artificial ear**, whereas a coupler used with a bone vibrator is called an **artificial mastoid**. In Figure 4.6, the artificial ear coupler is connected to a supra-aural earphone just to the right side of the sound level meter whereas the

FIGURE 4.6

A sound-level meter coupled to supra-aural earphones that are connected to a diagnostic audiometer (not shown in the figure). A coupler just to the right of the sound level meter is connected to a supra-aural earphone. Further to the right a bone vibrator is coupled to an "artificial mastoid" device.

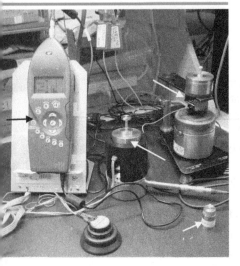

artificial mastoid and bone vibrator is further to the right in the figure. Each of the couplers is also identified with an arrow.

As you would expect, design and construction of couplers used in equipment calibration also comply with standards. Supra-aural earphones are coupled to a sound-level meter with a precisely defined coupler that encloses a cavity of 6 cm³, in accordance with ANSI standards. Standardized 6-cm³ couplers include the *NBA-9A coupler*, used in the United States, and the IEC 60318-3 coupler, used in Europe and elsewhere. During the calibration process, an earphone is pressed down onto the coupler with a specified amount of weight. This process is also shown in Figure 4.6. A pressure of 500 grams is used for coupling an earphone to the microphone of the sound level meter because it's comparable to the pressure of earphones against an ear during hearing testing. Insert earphones are calibrated using a 2-cm³ coupler, specifically an *HA-2 coupler*, which is also used for measuring the output of hearing aids.

If the output level in dB SPL for any of the combinations of transducers and types of sound does not equal the expected value, then a certified technician calibrates the audiometer. In calibration, the output level of sound is adjusted internally in the audiometer so that it corresponds with the standard for each type of sound and each transducer.

Biological Calibration

Problems with the output of an audiometer or with a defective transducer may develop any time and unexpectedly. Regularly scheduled physical calibration of hearing test equipment with a sound-level meter is typically performed only three or four times each year. Between formal scheduled calibration sessions, the output of audiometers should be monitored on a daily basis with a **listening check**. The listening check is also referred to as *biological or psychoacoustic calibration*. The listening check is performed with a person who is known to have normal hearing. Because the person serving as the listener has very good and stable hearing, audiologists sometimes informally refer to their ears as "golden ears." Usually this listener is an audiologist, a Doctor of Audiology student, or a clinic support staff member.

If careful listening checks are not conducted for each audiometer and transducer each workday, there is a possibility of inaccurate audiometric findings for patients seen in the clinic. The clinical consequences of inaccurate test findings are very serious, including misdiagnosis and mismanagement of auditory dysfunction. Failure to maintain properly calibrated equipment might also result in liability issues and legal consequences.

The daily listening checks are really a simple verification that the equipment is operating as intended, not an actual calibration. If any change in biological threshold measurements is detected from one day to another, and verified after appropriate troubleshooting to rule out simple technical problems, a formal physical calibration is scheduled as soon as possible. Examples of technical problems that might affect proper equipment function include a damaged earphone or bone vibrator, a break in an earphone cable, or an earphone that is not completely plugged into the panel in the sound room.

Importance of Calibration

Results of hearing assessment contribute importantly to the medical, educational, and audiological management of patients, as well as treatment outcome. Accuracy of hearing test findings is essential. Regularly scheduled physical calibration of audiology equipment, along with daily biological calibration, provides reasonable assurance that test results meet a consistent criterion for accuracy.

Imagine for a moment that one person makes a coast-to-coast trip across the United States, stopping along the way for hearing testing at ten randomly selected audiology clinics.

A comparison of hearing test results obtained at each of the ten different audiology clinics should reveal no clinically important differences even though the testing was carried out in different clinics, in different cities, with different equipment, and by different audiologists. Cross-country hearing test results should be consistent because equipment in each of the clinics is regularly calibrated using the same standards and because the audiologist in each of the different clinics follows the same methods for hearing testing. You'll learn in the next chapter about methods used for determining how well a patient can hear pure tone sounds.

Patient Responsibilities and Requirements in Hearing Testing

Behavioral Hearing Testing Is Subjective

Traditional hearing assessment is described as **behavioral audiometry**. This term is used because the person being tested responds to sound with some type of behavior that can be observed by the tester. Examples of behavioral responses include a head turn toward a loudspeaker producing a sound, pressing a button when a tone is heard, pointing to a picture representing a word that is heard, or repeating a word that is heard during testing.

Behavioral audiometry techniques are sometimes categorized as *subjective* measures. That is, the response is dependent on the perception and experiences of the particular person being tested. Also, the tester's detection of the patient's response is dependent on perception and experience. In most cases, particularly with cooperative adult patients and older children, hearing can be accurately tested using behavioral techniques. However, there is always a possibility that unexpected variables and factors will influence the test process and invalidate the results. For example, the patient's behavioral response to a sound may suggest a hearing problem when hearing is really normal. Or, the patient's behavioral response to sound may lead to an overestimation of actual hearing loss. In some cases, a tester may interpret certain behavior, like head turning in a child, as a response to sound when in fact the behavior is random and unrelated to the stimulus sound.

 ClinicalConnection

Objective hearing test procedures are available to most audiologists for accurate auditory assessment. Objective tests do not depend on a behavioral response from the patient. With objective hearing assessment, measurements are made directly from the ear or the brain, often while the patient is sleeping. You'll learn about common objective auditory tests in Chapters 8 and 9.

Factors Influencing Behavioral Test Results

General Listener Variables. A variety of patient factors can influence the assessment of hearing using behavioral techniques. Patient factors (listener variables) affecting behavioral hearing assessment are summarized in Table 4.3. Some of the factors—for example, the patient's chronological age—are quite easy to document, and the effect of this factor on hearing testing is relatively well defined. However, even the effect of age on hearing performance is not always simple or straightforward.

Other factors listed in Table 4.3 are not easy to measure or describe. The influence of factors such as motivation or attention may vary considerably among patients or even in one patient during the course of hearing testing. To a large extent, an audiologist's clinical skill and expertise in hearing assessment is reflected by the ability to recognize which factors are likely to influence a specific patient's response to sound. The audiologist then uses test techniques and strategies most appropriate for the patient. The overall goal is to obtain valid measures of hearing performance. Of course, an audiologist's knowledge and skill grow with acquired clinical experience and ongoing continuing education.

Adults. For many types of hearing tests, the patient's task is to listen closely for sounds, including very faint ones, and to respond with some kind of motor activity whenever they hear a sound. Typical responses given by adult patients during hearing testing include pressing a response

TABLE 4.3

Listener variables affecting behavioral hearing assessment in children and adults.

Patient age

- Chronological age
- Developmental age

Maturation

Motor development

Cognitive factors

- Attention
- Processing speed
- Memory
- Cognitive level

Motivation

Emotional state

State of arousal

- Alert
- Sleepy or lethargic
- Asleep

Speech and Language

- Articulation skills
- Language level
- Native language

button or raising a finger, hand, or arm. Any adult who is undergoing a hearing test must (1) understand the task and what response is expected, (2) remember the task until testing is completed, (3) attend to and listen carefully for the sounds throughout testing, (4) be motivated to cooperate and do his or her best for the duration of testing, and (5) produce the requested response to sound.

An audiologist is responsible for instructing the patient adequately on the test process and for verifying that the patient understands the instructions. The level of difficulty of the instructions and the way instructions are given must be modified for certain patients. Information gleaned from the case history and from initial observations of and interactions with the patient will guide an experienced audiologist in selecting the most effective approach for instructing an adult patient. The audiologist must sometimes substantially modify the instructions and the test approach for the patient to assure that the result will be a valid and accurate measure of hearing.

Consider for a moment two separate patients on the clinic schedule one morning. The same primary care physician has referred both patients to the clinic because they are having difficulty understanding conversational speech, especially in noisy settings. One patient is a 35-year-old male, married, with two children, who works at a local post office. He has driven to the clinic by himself and correctly completes the history form and other necessary paperwork when he arrives at the reception area. His history includes years of exposure at work and during recreational activities to high-intensity noise. When greeted by the audiologist in the waiting room and during the walk back to the test area, the patient engages in an appropriate and friendly conversation with the audiologist, clearly stating his hearing concerns and his hope that something can be done to help him.

Now, let's consider another patient, also a 35-year-old male. A volunteer from a local rehabilitation facility transports the patient to the audiology clinic in a wheelchair. With some help from the patient and notes from the rehab facility, the volunteer completes the history form and other necessary clinic documents. According to the clinic history, the patient first demonstrated communication problems following a severe head injury suffered in a motor vehicle accident. History indicates that the patient is right-handed. Upon reaching the patient in the waiting room, the audiologist notices that the patient awkwardly extends his left hand and is unable to clearly express a greeting. As you suspect, the entire testing process is likely to be quite different for these two patients even though the outcome—the hearing test results—might be the same.

Adults undergo hearing testing for various reasons. And among adult patients there are considerable differences in intelligence, educational level, processing speed, stamina, energy, and general motivation and enthusiasm related to the test process. Nonetheless, with proper instruction, occasional verbal reinforcement, and reinstruction as needed, valid pure tone hearing test results are obtained rather quickly for the vast majority of adult patients.

Children. There is a saying in pediatric medicine that children are not just little adults. The auditory system and the child's capacity to respond to sounds are immature at birth and throughout childhood. The age of a child has a well-appreciated influence on the performance of behavioral hearing tests. The child's ability to respond to sounds is constantly changing as he or she develops physically and mentally.

In clinical hearing assessment, not only is a child's behavioral response dependent on maturation of the auditory system, it is also affected by cognitive function and motor function. Cognitive factors in hearing testing include memory, attention, and the time required to process sounds, and motor function affects the child's ability to respond to sound with some kind of physical movement. In understanding the influence of maturation on hearing performance, the important concept is not a child's chronological age but, rather, developmental age. A child's level of physical, neurological, and auditory system maturation may not be consistent with expectations based on chronological age. A child who is 5 years old with developmental delay, for example, may function more like a child who is only 3 years old.

The audiologist must always take developmental age and ability into account in pediatric hearing assessment. The child's developmental status will influence which strategy is used for estimating hearing thresholds, test instructions, whether one or two persons are needed to test the child, and the analysis and interpretation of test results. Indeed, based on a child's developmental status, an audiologist may begin the assessment process with objective test procedures rather than with behavioral audiometry.

Preparing the Patient for Testing

Introducing the Patient to the Test Room

Let's assume the audiologist we're shadowing has completed a patient history and otoscopy. Following the history and visual inspection of the ear, the patient is escorted to a clinic room where hearing test procedures are performed. The initial portion of the hearing assessment may or may not take place in a sound-treated room. Certain tests, particularly objective tests, are usually carried out in a quiet but non-sound-treated room, with equipment and chairs for the tester, patient, and one or two others.

For most hearing test procedures, the patient is escorted to a sound-treated room and asked to sit in a comfortable and stable chair. Entry into most sound-treated rooms requires a step up. The audiologist must point this out and remain close to the patient to assure his or her safety. If the patient ambulates with a walker or is confined to a wheelchair or gurney, the audiologist may need to place a portable ramp in front of the door. Tall patients may need to be cautioned to avoid hitting their head as they enter the room.

A potential deviation in the usual routine for positioning a patient in the sound-treated room should be noted at this juncture. Occasionally, audiologists encounter patients who become anxious about being placed in a relatively small room, particularly a sound-treated room with thick walls and tightly fitting doors. Upon entering the room, patients might even acknowledge that they have claustrophobia, a fear of being confined in a small space. Most patients will assent to remaining in the sound-treated room for a brief test once they are assured that the audiologist will be nearby, on the other side of the sound booth window, and that communication is possible anytime during the test session. Anxious patients are always comforted when they realize that the door is easily opened and they can exit the sound-treated room on their own. If a patient continues to express concern about being enclosed in the sound-treated room, the problem is often resolved by allowing a family member, or someone else, to remain in the room during the testing.

Once the audiologist and patient are inside the sound-treated room, it's important for the audiologist to direct the patient to the test chair, since there may be other chairs in the sound-treated room for family members, or for audiologists assisting in the hearing test. Family members accompanying a patient to the audiology appointment often ask to remain in the sound-treated room during the testing. For adult and older pediatric patients, it's generally advisable for family members to sit outside of the sound-treated room, possibly in a designated waiting area, until the testing is complete. The sounds produced by family members, such as talking or coughing, or the ringing of cell phones, may interfere with the accuracy of the test results. Also, the patient may be distracted by the presence of another person or persons in the room. For young children, and sometimes elderly patients, a family member should be allowed to remain in the sound-treated room with the patient. The family member is given a brief explanation about the importance of being as quiet as possible during the testing.

Location of Patient in the Sound Room

Older Children and Adults. For adult patients, and children of school age and older, the patient chair is usually located near the window of the sound booth, with the audiologist located on the other side of the window. Figure 4.7 shows an adult patient ready for hearing testing in a sound-treated room with insert earphones (Figure 4.7A) and with supra-aural earphones (Figure 4.7B). The window between the test room and the control room is on the patient's left side. The patient is not directly facing the window, where the audiologist will be located in front of the audiometer. Instead, the patient is facing slightly away from the window. In this position, the audiologist has a clear view of the patient's face, but the patient cannot directly observe the audiologist. In this position, the patient will be less likely to be distracted by the audiologist's activities, such as operation of the audiometer or recording of test results. Also, the patient will be less likely to detect unintentional cues given when the audiologist presents signals.

Infants and Young Children. Young children often need to sit in a caregiver's lap during pure tone audiometry. In addition, young children do not always comply with wearing earphones. In such cases, the child is seated in a location a specific distance from the loudspeakers that are used to present sounds. There are nearby toys for **visual reinforcement**. *Visual reinforcement* is a technique used to reward a child's participation in hearing testing. An interesting mechanical toy near the loudspeaker is activated whenever the child hears a sound and turns toward the loudspeaker.

Figure 4.8 shows a child sitting in a sound-treated room, with loudspeakers and visual reinforcement toys in the background. An "X" on the floor or the ceiling of the sound-treated room often marks the proper location for the child. It's important to maintain the proper distance between the loudspeakers and the patient to assure accurate calibration of intensity levels. The child is generally positioned facing straight ahead with an ear toward each of two speakers, as depicted in Figure 4.8. In such a position, the child is most likely to turn the head or move the eyes away from the midline and toward the loudspeaker source of the sound.

Audiologist-Patient Communication. During behavioral hearing test procedures, an audiologist often communicates with the patient, and the patient with the audiologist. The audiologist needs to give the patient instructions for test procedures and to answer patient questions that arise during the testing. It is impractical for an audiologist to enter the sound-treated room whenever communication with the patient is necessary. Communication with the patient is accomplished easily with a *talkback system*.

FIGURE 4.7   An adult patient sitting in a sound-treated room, ready for hearing testing with insert earphones **(A)**, and with supra-aural earphones **(B)**.

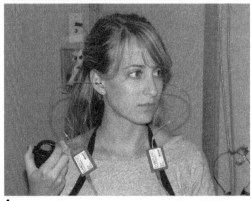
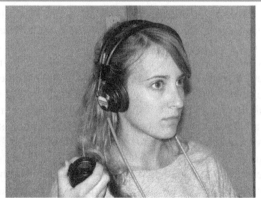

A   **B**

In the sound-treated room, the patient is positioned near a talkback microphone that is mounted on the wall and connected to a special speaker in the audiometer. Sometimes, the audiologist affixes a talkback microphone on the patient with either a lanyard placed around the neck or with a clip that can be attached to the patient's clothing. The audiologist can then hear anything the patient says during testing. The audiologist also has a microphone that enables quick and easy communication with the patient. The output of that microphone is easily adjusted so that the loudness of the audiologist's voice can be raised and lowered, depending on the patient's hearing status.

Patient Instructions

Older Children and Adults. There is no standardized script for reciting instructions for hearing testing, even with adult patients. Although the exact words and the length of instructions differ from one audiologist to the next, and for each audiologist depending on the patient, the message almost always includes the following points and types of statements:

- The patient should listen carefully for certain types of sounds, such as tones or words.
- Some of the sounds will be easy to hear, whereas others will be very faint.
- The patient is told to "press the button" or "raise your hand" when "you hear a tone," or "repeat each of the words," even if are very faint and hard to hear.
- The patient should "release the button" or "put your hand down" when the sound goes away.
- The patient is advised, "Don't pay attention to any rushing water sound you may hear during the testing. Just listen for the tones or the words."
- Often, the audiologist will also assure the patient: "There's a microphone here in the room, so I can hear you if you have any questions or concerns."
- Finally . . . "Do you have any questions before we get started?"

With certain patients, the audiologist may include a few additional statements, like: "Be sure to respond even when you barely hear the sounds. It's O.K. to press the button even if you're not sure you heard the sound." After hearing simple instructions one time, the majority of patients quickly understand what is required of them and hearing testing proceeds smoothly. However, preschool and schoolage children, elderly adults, and persons with cognitive impairments often require reinstruction and even periodic reminders about their role in the test process.

Infants and Young Children. When testing an infant or young child, the audiologist gives instructions to the parent or caregiver rather than the patient. The test process should be explained in simple and clear terms to the caregiver or parent. The audiologist especially needs to verify that the parent or caregiver understands his or her role in the test process and what is expected of him or her. Parents and caregivers may be nervous or anxious about the test process and the outcome, particularly if they suspect that the child might have a hearing loss.

A parent or caregiver naturally wants the child to perform well during hearing testing. If sounds are presented to the child through loudspeakers, a normal-hearing parent or caregiver sometimes intentionally or unintentionally encourages the child to respond to the sound or to

FIGURE 4.8

A child seated in a high-chair within a sound-treated booth during hearing testing. Loudspeakers and visual reinforcement toys are visible behind the patient. A toy is on the highchair tray in front of the patient.

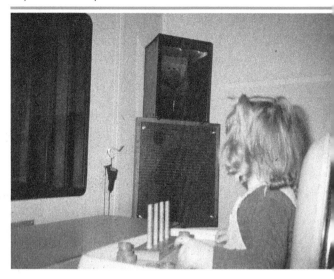

 WebWatch

You'll find many videos on YouTube showing young children undergoing hearing testing using the visual reinforcement technique.

listen more carefully. The audiologist usually explains to the parent or caregiver the importance of obtaining accurate test findings, pointing out that sometimes they will hear sounds that the child does not hear. The audiologist may also urge the parent or caregiver to refrain from giving any indication to the child when a sound is presented.

The Art of Earphone Placement

Placement of earphones (or a bone vibrator, addressed below) on the patient is the final step before testing begins, and obviously a very important one. Audiologists usually delay earphone placement until the after the patient is given instructions about the test procedure. Patients have difficulty hearing with earphones on their ears or insert earphones in place. Even normal-hearing patients may struggle to understand test instructions under these circumstances.

Red Is Right. It is essential to place the right earphone on the right ear and the left earphone on the left ear. Right earphones versus left earphones are distinguished by red versus blue markings on the outside of each earphone, and often there are color markings on the cord for each earphone. Although the technique seems simple enough, inadvertent reversal in earphone placement occasionally occurs in clinical hearing testing. Unrecognized placement of the right earphone on the left ear, or vice versa, leads to misrepresentation of hearing test results for the two ears. If not detected, the error may contribute to misdiagnosis and mismanagement of the patient. A tester placing earphones while facing a patient must be mindful that the right earphone will be held in the left hand and vice versa.

Supra-Aural Earphones. As noted already, the term *supra-aural earphone* refers to an earphone that fits over the ears with a soft round cushion resting on the pinna of each ear. Supra-aural earphones are placed on the patient's ears by grasping the cushion and earphone assembly firmly with each hand, expanding the headband slightly, and sliding the headband over the patient's head until the earphones are directly over the ears. This technique is shown in Figure 4.9A. Care is taken to ensure that the diaphragm of each earphone, that is, the opening in the earphone cushion, is aligned with the opening of the external ear canal. Also, the patient's hair is pushed back so the earphone cushion fits directly over the pinna. As the headband is gently allowed to return to its neutral position, the earphones are held in place with the pressure of cushions against the ears. The headband can then be adjusted up or down until it is resting on the patient's head.

Before placing supra-aural earphones over the ears, the audiologist sometimes must ask the patient to remove jewelry, clothing, or headgear that might interfere with an accurate fit. This step in earphone placement should be modified as necessary to accommodate religious or cultural conventions regarding clothing covering the head, and even the ears. Occasionally, when a patient readjusts the earphones before testing, the audiologist will need to again verify their placement.

Insert Earphones. A different technique is required for placement of insert earphones. As shown in Figure 4.9B, an insert earphone consists of a cable leading to a small transducer box where electrical signals are converted to sound. Sound then travels down a tube and through a foam tip that is inserted within the external ear canal. Each of the small transducers must be located on the correct side. The earphone for the right ear has red coding, and the left earphone is marked with blue. Insert earphone boxes are usually held in place with either a clip to the patient's clothing or a Velcro strap around the patient's neck. Clean unused foam tips are inserted onto the acoustic tubes connected to the transducer box, as shown in Figure 4.9B and earlier in Figure 4.4A. The tubes are 280 mm in length. Yellow foam tips with a 13-mm diameter are appropriate for most adult ears, whereas beige-colored 10-mm tips fit patients with smaller ears, including some females and most children. As noted already, otoscopy always precedes insert earphone placement to verify that the external ear canals are clear of debris and excessive cerumen.

The foam tips of insert earphones are rolled firmly between the thumb and index finger for a few seconds until compressed. Then, each compressed foam tip is immediately inserted into

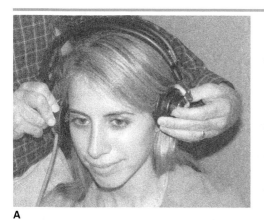
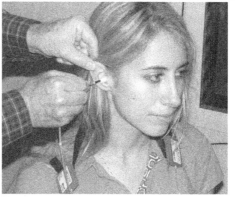

A   B

FIGURE 4.9

Placement of two types of earphones on a patient for hearing testing, including supra-aural earphones **(A)** and insert earphones **(B)**.

the appropriate ear canal. Audiologists sometimes gently pull the pinna upward and backward to straighten the external ear canal in order to more deeply insert the foam tip. This technique is illustrated in Figure 4.9B. For young children, the external ear canal is straightened by gently pulling the earlobe back and out.

For insert earphones, two additional steps are important when testing is complete. First, the insert foam tips must be gently withdrawn from the ear canal and carefully removed from the acoustic tubing so that the tiny plastic adaptor or "nipple" remains in the tubing. Without the adapter, it's impossible to connect the insert foam tips to the acoustic tubing. Finally, as already shown in Figure 4.1C, it's important to properly dispose of used insert foam tips so they are not inadvertently used on another patient.

Double-Checking Earphone Placement. Immediately after earphones are placed on the patient, it's important to verify that they are in place and on the correct ears. Most audiology students, and sometimes even experienced audiologists, occasionally forget to place earphones on the patient. Perhaps thinking ahead to the next steps in the test process or being distracted in some way, the audiologist upon finishing instructions to the patient immediately leaves the test booth, closes the test booth door(s), and settles down in front of the audiometer at the sound booth window. It is good clinical practice to gaze briefly through the sound booth window and closely inspect the patient to be sure that the earphones are on the patient and that each earphone is on the correct ear.

Bone Vibrator Placement

Supra-aural earphones or insert earphones are almost always used in hearing testing. Sound from these earphones travels through the air in the ear canal to the tympanic membrane. Then, vibrations of the tympanic membrane are conveyed through the middle ear system to the inner ear where hair cells are activated. The term **air conduction** is used to describe hearing tests conducted with earphones since the ear is stimulated by sound waves traveling through the air.

Hearing can be tested also with bone-conducted sounds. You'll recall from our review of anatomy in Chapter 3 that the inner ear is located within the temporal bone in the skull. Vibrations transmitted through the temporal bone generate movement of fluids within the inner ear and activate outer and inner hair cells. **Bone conduction** hearing testing is important in the diagnostic assessment of hearing disorders. Three different mechanisms for bone conduction hearing are further explained in the next chapter. Here we'll focus only on the placement of the **bone vibrator** used in bone conduction hearing testing.

Figure 4.10A shows a typical bone vibrator placed on the mastoid portion of the temporal bone. The headband is opened slightly and then gently brought into place over the top of the head. Releasing tension on the headband, an audiologist positions the bone vibrator on the mastoid process located just behind and toward the lower portion of the pinna.

As shown in Figure 4.10B, a bone vibrator can also be located on the forehead during hearing testing. The audiologist is responsible for placing the bone vibrator, not the patient. If the bone vibrator or headband moves out of place, the audiologist must reposition it. Care is taken to assure that no hair interferes with contact between the bone vibrator and skin. The side of the bone vibrator that makes contact with the head is often concave. The entire surface of the bone vibrator rests against the gently curving shape of the mastoid process.

The bone vibrator headband expands to accommodate variations in average-sized heads. However, the metal headband is typically too big for the small heads of young children and sometimes too small for adult patients with large heads. In such cases, the audiologist must take special steps to ensure adequate and consistent bone vibrator contact with the skull.

At this juncture it is appropriate to comment again on maximum permissible ambient sound levels for bone conduction hearing testing. Bone conduction hearing assessment is almost always conducted with the test ear uncovered. Looking again at Figure 4.10, you'll notice that there is no earphone on the ear that is being stimulated via bone conduction. As confirmed by values in Table 4.2, maximum permissible ambient noise levels in a sound-treated room are considerably lower when hearing is tested using a bone vibrator than when testing with either supra-aural earphones or insert earphones.

Patient Response Mode

Adults. As described above, an adult patient produces an overt behavioral response to sounds such as pure tones or words. The patient is instructed to respond in one of three ways: (1) pressing a response button at the onset of the stimulus and releasing the button when the stimulus is turned off; (2) raising a finger, hand, or arm for the duration of the sound heard; or (3) making a vocal response, such as saying "yes," when a sound is heard. Each of the three response modes has advantages and disadvantages.

A button-pressing response is unequivocal in that there is either a response or no response. The patient presses the button when the stimulus is heard and then immediately releases the button. If the stimulus is a pulsing tone (a rather brief continuous tone), the patient presses the button only one time as the tone is first heard. When a patient presses the button after hearing a pure tone signal, the audiologist can visually detect the response by viewing a light or visual display on the audiometer. Also, using the microphone located in the test room and the audiometer talkback system, an audiologist can typically hear a clicking sound each time the patient presses the response button.

Monitoring a patient's response through visual or auditory indicators on the audiometer offers two related advantages. Because the audiologist doesn't need to watch the patient to detect a response, there's little likelihood that the patient will detect any visual clue that a

FIGURE 4.10

Two different placements of a bone vibrator on a patient for bone conduction hearing testing, including on the mastoid portion of the temporal bone **(A)** and on the forehead **(B)**. The test ear is not covered during bone conduction testing.

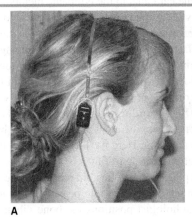
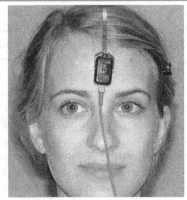

A   B

signal has been presented. Also, rather than watching the patient during the test procedure, the audiologist can focus on the audiometer controls and on recording test results.

The button-pressing response does lead to a problem with certain patients, particularly patients who have difficulty understanding and carrying out the task and persons with deficits in attention. Patients who experience difficulty with the task are typically young children or persons of any age who have reduced cognitive function. These patients sometimes press the button but then do not release it when the stimulus is turned off. Some patients do not consistently press the button when they hear the stimulus sound. In such cases, the audiologist must repeatedly remind the patient of the task required.

Raising a finger, hand, or arm in response to sound was often relied upon in the past and is still sometimes used in hearing testing with older children and adults. This rather simple response mode has several readily apparent advantages. Raising a finger, hand, or arm is "low tech" and doesn't require a button or a response indicator on the audiometer. The relatively greater activity required to raise a hand, in comparison to pressing a small button, sometimes helps to keep the patient engaged in the task of listening carefully for faint sounds.

However, there are also drawbacks to this conventional response mode. The audiologist must look closely at the patient to detect the response. The audiologist may inadvertently cue the patient that a signal was presented by momentarily turning attention from the patient to the audiometer or by looking at the response form used to record test results. Also, when a patient becomes fatigued during testing or is unsure about the presence of a sound, the hand-raising response may be slower and less obvious. A very small movement may contribute to doubt about whether the patient heard the signal. Uncertainty about whether the patient responded is a good example of the limitation of any subjective hearing test procedure. (On the other hand, the change in speed and distance of a finger, hand, or arm as it is raised may provide some additional qualitative information. For example, a brisk response suggests that the patient clearly heard the sound.)

Children. In contrast to the rather limited number of response modes just reviewed for adult patients, pediatric hearing assessment utilizes many types of responses. To a large extent, a child's behavioral response to sound depends on developmental age. As you would expect, infants and young children cannot be instructed to respond in a specific way.

Within the first six months after full-term birth, an infant's response to sound consists of mostly eye opening or eye blinking. (*Full-term birth* follows the typical forty weeks of *gestation.*) An infant who is sleeping during hearing testing may awaken when a sound is presented. The response to sound of a newborn infant depends not only on whether he or she is awake or asleep, it also may vary depending on depth of sleep. Hearing assessment of newborn infants using behavioral techniques is challenging in part because infants spend much of their time sleeping. Also, young infants do not respond to faint levels of sound. Rather, responses are only observed at moderate levels of sounds, about the intensity level of conversational speech.

With maturation of the auditory system and neurological and physical maturation, a child's response to sound also matures and becomes more purposeful. Infants begin to respond to sound by turning their head from side to side toward the source of the sound. Children between about 7 months and 2 years of age yield a more precise head turn response for softer sounds, including sounds that originate above and below the head. The term for an eye opening or head turning response is **localization to sound**.

As shown earlier in Figure 4.8, a child typically sits in a caregiver's lap or perhaps in a highchair in a position midway between two sound speakers. An effort is made to keep the child facing forward until a sound is presented through one of the speakers. Upon hearing a sound from one of the speakers, the child automatically turns toward the location of the sound. An audiologist repeatedly presents sounds at gradually lower intensity levels, closely watching the child's response at each level.

Before too long, most children become disinterested in the sounds from the speakers. To maintain the child's interest long enough to permit an assessment of hearing threshold, often for several different types of sounds, presentation of the sound is paired with a visual activity that appeals to a young child. For example, when the child turns to one of the speakers as the sound is presented, the child sees a toy animal, like the one in Figure 4.8, doing something funny. The technical term for this pediatric testing technique is *visual reinforcement audiometry*.

With maturation a child can participate in a technique called **conditioned play audiometry**. The process of reinforcing response behavior is described as *conditioning,* a term borrowed from psychology. Sounds are presented to the child through speakers, earphones, or a bone vibrator. The child is taught to respond to hearing the sound by performing some simple play task, such as dropping an object into a bucket or putting a peg into a pegboard. Teaching the task involves repeatedly demonstrating to the child how to respond to the sound, and then immediately reinforcing the child's behavior with praise. As children reach 4 to 5 years of age, they can often be tested with slight variations of the techniques and procedures used with adults.

An Introduction to Masking

Hearing testing is based on the premise that the patient's response is due to sound stimulation of the test ear. For example, if sound is presented to the patient's right ear, an audiologist presumes that the patient's response to the sound is due to activation of the right ear. Under certain test conditions, however, there's a possibility or even a probability that sound presented to the test ear actually activates the other ear, the non-test ear. We'll take a moment now to briefly discuss **masking**. *Masking* involves presentation of sound to the non-test ear, that is, the ear opposite the test ear. The goal of masking is to assure that the patient's response is due to sound stimulation of the test ear (Sanders & Hall, 1999).

We reviewed different types of noise sounds in Chapter 2. The type of noise used in masking depends on the stimulus that is being used during a hearing test procedure. If a tone stimulus is presented to a patient, the masking sound is usually a narrow band of noise centered on the frequency of the tone. In contrast, if hearing is being tested with speech signals, like words, then the masking sound will be noise that includes all of the frequencies found in speech. Masking is necessary in any hearing test procedure where there is a chance of **cross hearing**, that is, a possibility that the stimulus sound might cross over from the test ear to the non-test ear.

Why Is Masking Needed? It's very important with any hearing test procedure to verify that responses are **ear specific**. That is, responses attributed to the right ear should only reflect auditory function of the right ear and responses attributed to the left ear only function of the left ear. Accurate diagnosis of hearing loss and appropriate management of patients with hearing loss is based on the assumption that the test results are ear specific. An audiologist must be confident that the responses the patient is producing are due to stimulation only of the ear that is being tested.

The ability to efficiently and effectively perform masking during hearing testing is one of the most important skills in clinical audiology. You'll learn more about masking techniques and challenges in Chapter 7.

Good Clinical Etiquette

We'll conclude the chapter with a few comments about what might be called "clinical etiquette," that is, good clinical manners and habits. You learned in this chapter about the importance of a positive, professional, and safe environment for delivery of hearing health care services. Good clinical manners and habits contribute importantly to the ongoing maintenance of an environment of care and to an appropriate environment for hearing services. For example, a good clinical habit is to regularly tidy up all spaces used for patient care. Documents with patient health information should be kept out of sight and used supplies should be properly disposed of. Good clinical manners also include consistently positive interactions with patients and their families, as well as clinic professional and support staff.

Clinical etiquette includes good habits in the direct provision of services, such as hearing testing. Just three of many examples include (1) taking the time to write a patient's name and the test date on clinic forms before the test process begins to prevent later confusion about patient identify, (2) returning equipment controls and switches to their original settings after completion of a hearing test to minimize errors in the next hearing test, and (3) taking a moment to untangle wires and cords connected to earphones, bone vibrators, and patient response buttons in a sound-treated room. Development and consistent practice of good clinical habits will result in fewer mistakes in hearing testing, more efficient use of test time, and, perhaps most importantly, improved quality of care to patients.

PULLING IT ALL TOGETHER

Were you surprised by anything you read in this chapter? Perhaps you were unaware of the many professional responsibilities that audiologists and speech pathologists have, in addition to assessing and managing children and adults with communicative disorders. Audiologists and speech pathologists are responsible for the general safety and wellbeing of their patients. Or maybe you didn't realize that modern-day patients seeking healthcare services have very important and legally protected rights to privacy and security.

You learned in this chapter how audiologists establish a positive and professional working relationship with patients and their family members.

You now have an appreciation for diverse aspects of the environment for provision of audiology services, from the general importance of an "environment of care" to very specific noise requirements for sound-treated rooms used for hearing testing. You also learned about different types of devices that are essential for hearing testing, along with how they are calibrated. You were introduced to the different ways patients can respond to sounds, to various factors that can influence patient responses, and to the important technique of masking.

Finally, you now have a better understanding of the value of patient-related activities that occur before hearing testing formally begins, such as review of the patient history, visual inspection of the ear, effective instruction about hearing testing, and the proper placement of earphones and bone vibrators.

READINGS

DeBonis, D. A., & Donohue, C. L. (2004). *Survey of audiology: Fundamentals for audiologists and health professionals.* Boston: Allyn & Bacon.

Hall, J. W. III, & Mueller, H. G. III. (1997). *Audiologists' desk reference, Volume I. Diagnostic audiology principles, practices and procedures.* San Diego: Singular.

Mueller, H.G. III, & Hall, J. W. III. (1998). *Audiologists' desk reference, Volume II. Audiologic management, rehabilitation and terminology.* San Diego: Singular.

5 Pure Tone Audiometry

LEARNING OBJECTIVES

In this chapter you will learn:

- What an audiometer is and the features of an audiometer
- About earphones and other transducers used in hearing testing
- About techniques used to measure pure tone hearing thresholds
- How we hear by bone conduction stimulation
- How pure tone hearing thresholds are used to describe hearing loss
- What the pure tone average is, and how it's calculated
- About the audiogram, a graph of pure tone hearing test results
- How pure tone hearing test results are plotted on an audiogram
- The ways an audiogram provides information about the degree, configuration, and type of hearing loss

KEY TERMS

Air-bone gap (ABG)
Ascending technique
Audiometer
Audiometric zero
Automated audiometry
Audiometric frequencies
Bone-air gap
Bone vibrator
Configuration of hearing loss
Degree of hearing loss
Descending-ascending method
Distortional bone conduction
Ear-specific
Flat (hearing loss configuration)
Inertial bone conduction
Insert earphones
Osseotympanic bone conduction
Preferred method
Pure tone audiometry
Pure tone average (PTA)
Rising (hearing loss configuration)
Sloping (hearing loss configuration)
Sound field
Sound-field testing
Supra-aural earphones
Talk Back
Test-retest reliability
Transducer
Vibrotactile response
Warble tones

CHAPTER FOCUS

Most of us have experienced a simple hearing test. We were asked to sit quietly and to listen carefully for very faint beeping sounds. Then, a nurse or some other health professional gently placed earphones over our ears, adjusted them carefully, and the testing began. The phrase *pure tone audiometry* is used to refer to hearing tests that involve tones of different frequencies presented with earphones and sometimes with a bone vibrator. In this introduction to pure tone audiometry, you will first learn about the audiometer, an instrument specially designed for hearing assessment. The pure tone hearing test process is explained next, with a step-by-step discussion of techniques for air conduction and bone conduction testing.

Later in the chapter, you'll be introduced to the audiogram. The *audiogram* is a graph for plotting the results of air and bone conduction hearing testing. You'll learn about the symbols used for the right and the left ear and for air conduction and bone conduction testing. By the end of the chapter, you'll be able to plot an audiogram using the correct symbols. You'll also begin to develop the ability to analyze audiograms and to recognize some common audiogram patterns.

What Is Pure Tone Audiometry?

Pure tone audiometry is the measurement of hearing thresholds for pure tone sounds. A hearing threshold is the softest sound that a person can hear. Measurement of pure tone thresholds is one of the oldest forms of hearing testing, dating back to early in the twentieth century, before audiology was a profession. Hearing thresholds for pure tone signals, and other types of sounds, are measured with an *audiometer*. The **audiometer** is an electronic device, now sometimes computer based, that allows the operator to choose a specific type of sound and then to present the sound to the patient at a specific intensity level. Audiologists rely on audiometers to test hearing. They are a "tool of the trade" in audiology.

Use of an audiometer involves three general steps. First, the audiologist decides how the sounds will be delivered to the patient. The usual options for presenting sounds to the patient are earphones, a bone vibrator, or a loudspeaker. Second, the audiologist selects a particular sound, such as a pure tone, speech signals like words or sentences, or some type of noise. In this chapter we'll focus on hearing testing with pure tone sounds. Finally, an audiologist uses an audiometer to present sounds to the patient at specific intensity levels.

The results of pure tone audiometry help to define a person's hearing abilities for sounds in the frequency region that is important for understanding speech. The results of pure tone hearing testing contribute importantly to the diagnosis of hearing impairment and to decisions regarding patient management.

Test Equipment

Audiometers

Audiometers have changed remarkably during the past seventy to eighty years as a result of advances in electronics technology. The changing appearance of audiometers is readily appreciated in Figure 5.1. The audiometers represent technology from years before audiology was a profession to modern times. A glimpse inside the audiometers depicted in Figure 5.1 would reveal even more substantial advances in technology. Audiometers in the early years of audiology were almost always encased in wood and, like radios of the same era, were powered by vacuum tube technology.

The Western Electric audiometer shown in Figure 5.1A is actually enclosed in what looks like a suitcase. Examine the photograph closely and you'll see an earphone in the top portion, a turntable and stylus that are used to present recorded numbers and words, and even a handle on the front of the case to crank the machinery that powers the turntable.

The vintage Maico audiometer and Grason Stadler Incorporated (GSI) audiometers shown in Figure 5.1B and Figure 5.1C are good examples of audiometers available in the early years of audiology. Each of them is powered by large vacuum tubes. The device in the lower portion is a GSI Békésy E800 audiometer, which played an important role in diagnostic testing. The upper portion of Figure 5.1C shows a GSI 162 audiometer sitting on top of the E800 device. The GSI 162 was used for a variety of hearing tests in early years of the profession of audiology.

In time, with the advent of electronic circuits, audiometers became smaller and lighter but more powerful. The audiometer shown in Figure 5.1D is an audiometer representing the latest generation of technology for hearing testing.

Technological advances have resulted in increased flexibility and features. Modern computer-based audiometers use a wide array of acoustic signals, from pure tones to synthetically produced speech signals. An acoustic signal is a specified type of sound used in hearing testing. Audiometers also vary considerably in complexity. Audiometers range from relatively

FIGURE 5.1   Audiometers over the years, including a Western Electric 4-A audiometer, first introduced in the 1920s (**A**), a Maico audiometer from the 1940s (**B**), a Grason Stadler Békésy E-800 audiometer (below), and 162 audiometer (top) from the 1950s (**C**), and a modern-day GSI AudioStar diagnostic audiometer (**D**). Courtesy of Grason Stadler Inc.

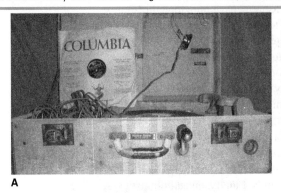

A

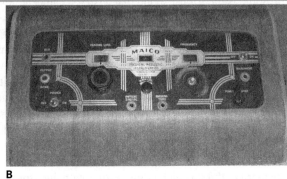

B

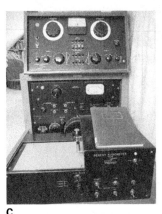

C

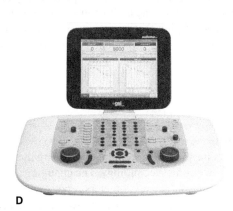

D

FIGURE 5.2   Small, lightweight, and easily portable audiometers are available with the capacity to perform a wide range of diagnostic procedures in different settings (**A**). Computer-based audiometers (**B**) offer many features for efficient and comprehensive hearing testing. Courtesy of Maico Diagnostics and GN Otometrics.

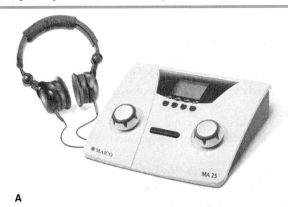

A

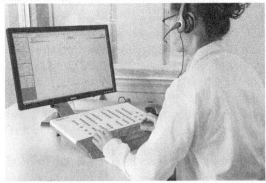

B

small, simple, and portable devices designed for simple hearing screening to larger more sophisticated audiometers that can be used to perform a variety of test procedures in the diagnosis of hearing loss.

The distinction in features between small simple hearing screening devices and larger diagnostic audiometers is becoming less obvious. Figure 5.2A shows an example of a relatively small, lightweight, and portable audiometer. This type of portable audiometer offers the option for conducting pure tone audiometry and other important hearing test procedures in settings far removed from a clinic. Finally, Figure 5.2B shows an example of recent audiometers that utilize computer platforms with an almost unlimited capacity for generating a wide variety of acoustic signals. Computer-based audiometers are also ideal for storage, formatting, printing, and transmission of audiometric data.

Features of an Audiometer. Despite advances in audiometer technology over the years, a handful of general features have remained essentially unchanged. The diagram in Figure 5.3 shows the features common to most audiometers. Each feature is indicated in the text with italic font. Although the layout and design of control panels vary among audiometer brands and models, the overall appearance and buttons, knobs, dials, and pads shown in Figure 5.3 are representative of many clinical audiometers. You will probably find it helpful to refer back to this figure from time to time during the following description of the audiometer.

The *power on/off* switch for the audiometer, and most other clinical devices, is usually not located among other controls on the front panel shown in the figure. Rather, the power switch is often found in a location that is not easily accessed, such as the side or the back of the device. The hard-to-get-to location for the on/off switch minimizes the likelihood that the audiometer will be inadvertently turned off during use.

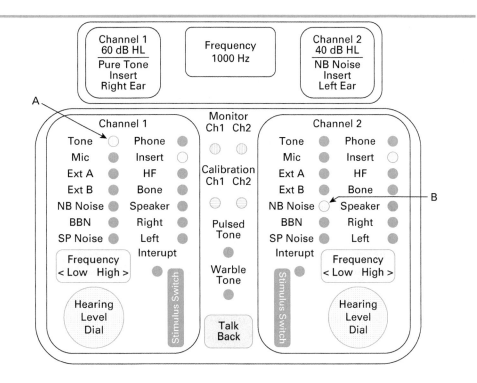

FIGURE 5.3

Features common to most audiometers. The diagram represents the control panel of a typical clinical audiometer. Each of the controls is described in the text.

As you will readily notice, the control panel of the audiometer illustrated in Figure 5.3 contains an array of buttons, knobs, dials, and keys for selecting and presenting different types of sounds to the patient. During pure tone audiometry, a tester will consistently use a handful of these controls, whereas some of the other controls may be used only rarely, if at all.

We'll now review briefly the features and functions of the most commonly used controls on an audiometer. You may be a little bewildered by the layout of the control panel and by many new terms used in describing the audiometer. We've all experienced similar confusion when first encountering new technology, such as the latest model car, a complicated remote control for an entertainment center, or even a smart phone. Reading about the operation of a new machine like an audiometer is a good starting point. However, operation of the machine will really begin to make sense only when you have used it a few times. Skill in operating any new device increases with practice. Before long you will probably have some first-hand experience with an audiometer, practicing by yourself and with classmates or friends. You might find it helpful to refer to these pages during your the first encounter with an audiometer.

Like many diagnostic audiometers, the device illustrated in Figure 5.3 has two channels, labeled *Channel 1* and *Channel 2*. With two channels, it is possible to send two sounds independently and simultaneously to two earphones, or even to one earphone and one ear. You'll notice that there are duplicate sets of most knobs and buttons, a set on each side of the control panel. Let's begin our review with the section of the panel labeled *Channel 1,* containing fifteen round buttons, two different rectangular-shaped pads, and a big dial.

The operator of an audiometer can select the type of sound that is presented to the patient using buttons labeled *Tone, Mic, Ext A, Ext B, NB Noise, BBN, or SP Noise.* A pure tone signal is selected with the *Tone* button, identified by A in Figure 5.3. We will talk about the other types of signals shortly. For pure tone signals, frequency is selected with the rectangular pad below labeled *Frequency.* Notice at the top of the control panel diagram that the frequency in this example is 1000 Hz. The tester may select from a set of frequencies ranging from a frequency as low as 125 Hz up to 8000 Hz and even higher frequencies. Test frequency is increased or decreased by pressing the high or low part of the frequency control. When frequency is changed from 1000 Hz in our example, the new frequency is displayed in the same place on the audiometer.

The tester controls the intensity level of a pure tone or any other sound by turning the *Hearing Level* dial located toward the bottom of the figure. By convention, turning the dial to the right increases the intensity of the sound and turning the dial to the left decreases the sound intensity. By manipulating the hearing level knob or key, the tester can precisely control the intensity of signals in decibels (dB). As you learned in Chapter 2, the decibel scale utilized in clinical hearing assessment is dB HL (dB hearing level), with 0 dB as the reference value for normal hearing. That is, the average threshold for people with normal hearing is 0 dB HL. Intensity of a signal can be increased or decreased from low levels to high levels. With most audiometers, intensity can be manipulated in increments of 1, 2, or 5 dB and over a range of intensity from less than 0 dB HL up to levels of 110 dB HL or higher.

In pure tone hearing assessment of a patient, the tester changes the intensity level of each pure tone many times. Each time the stimulus intensity level is increased or decreased, the signal is presented to the patient by turning it on for a second or two and then turning it off again. The tester manually presents pure tone signals to the patient by pressing on the stimulus pad, indicated in the diagram as the vertical rectangle labeled *Stimulus Switch.* The control for switching the signal on and off is typically used together with the hearing level dial. The two controls are usually located near each other on any audiometer. The three controls—the frequency pad, the intensity dial, and the stimulus switch—are all in the lower portion of the panel for each channel. Each of the control knobs is manipulated almost constantly during pure tone hearing testing.

Speech sounds can be presented via the tester's voice or via recorded speech materials. You'll learn more about speech audiometry in the next chapter. By pressing the *Mic* button located just below the *Tone* button in Figure 5.3, the tester activates a microphone in order to speak to the patient and to present a speech signal, such as a one- or two-syllable word. The *Mic* button is also used to talk with the patient anytime during the assessment. The tester selects the *Ext A* or *Ext B* option to present speech materials from an external source, such as a tape recorder, a CD player, or even an iPod. On some audiometers, these knobs are identified as *Tape A* or *Tape B,* since a tape recorder used to be the most common external device connected to an audiometer. Techniques for hearing testing with speech signals are reviewed in the next chapter. At that time we'll return to the diagram of an audiometer.

Just below the *Ext A and Ext B* buttons are additional controls that allow an audiologist to choose among several types of noise, such as narrowband noise *(NB noise or NBN),* broadband noise *(BBN),* or speech noise *(SP Noise).* Noise controls are identified by B in Figure 5.3. During pure tone audiometry or any other test procedure, noise is sometimes presented to a specified ear. One type of noise is called *masking noise,* which prevents the patient from hearing the test signal in the nontest ear. You were introduced to the concept of masking in the previous chapter and you'll learn about masking noises and masking techniques in Chapter 7.

Now, let's move from the types of sounds or signals that are available on an audiometer to a review of the destination of the signals, that is, where they'll be sent by the audiologist. You'll probably need to refer back to Figure 5.3 from time to time as we discuss each control. For Channel 1, the controls for transducers are located to the right side of the buttons we have just reviewed for type of signal. Remember, in audiology a transducer is a device for converting an electrical signal to a sound. If supra-aural earphones are employed in presenting sound, the tester selects *Phone,* whereas *Insert* is chosen if the patient is fitted with insert earphones. Some audiometers also include the possibility of using special earphones that are designed especially for delivering very high frequency *(HF)* pure tone signals, for frequencies between 8000 Hz and 20,000 Hz. Other transducers that can be selected from the control panel include a bone vibrator *(Bone)* or a loudspeaker *(Speaker).*

Finally, with a two-channel audiometer each sound type can be routed to the transducer for the right side or to that for the left side. You will notice that the panel for each channel in the Figure 5.3 diagram includes buttons labeled *Right* and *Left.* For pure tone audiometry with earphones, one earphone is designated for the right ear and one for the left ear. As you learned in the previous chapter, the right earphone is color coded red, whereas the left earphone is blue. On some audiometers, all of the controls related to the right and left ears are also indicated with red or blue.

Audiologists sometimes evaluate hearing using bone conduction stimulation. The tester first places a bone vibrator on the patient in the sound-treated room. You learned in Chapter 4 about two different placements for the bone vibrator. The locations were shown in Figure 4.10A and B. An audiologist selects the *Bone* (the bone vibrator) control on the audiometer panel once the bone vibrator is in place on the patient. Important points about pure tone audiometry for bone-conducted signals are reviewed in another section later in this chapter. Sounds may also be presented to the patient via one or more loudspeakers located in the sound test room, without using either earphones or a bone vibrator.

The audiometer includes a few other knobs and buttons that play an important role in pure tone audiometry, in addition to controls for the type of sounds, for the destination of sounds, and for the frequency and intensity of sounds. In the center and toward the top of the diagram in Figure 5.3, you'll see for each channel a knob labeled *Monitor.* Throughout the hearing assessment, the tester must be able to monitor, or listen to, sounds presented to the patient. The tester controls the intensity of the monitored signals with these two knobs. The audiometer also typically includes a knob for controlling the intensity level of sounds detected by a microphone located in the test room. The tester is most interested in hearing the patient's voice. Just below the monitor knobs are others labeled *Calibration*. The precise intensity level of sounds from an external source, such as a CD player or an iPod, must be adjusted manually before they are presented to the patient.

Four other controls on the diagram of the audiometer have not yet been mentioned. The *Pulsed Tone* button in the lower center portion of the diagram is sometimes used with certain patients. Pure tone signals are easier to detect by some patients when they are presented in a pulsing fashion, that is, on and off repeatedly several times per second, rather than as a single presentation lasting one to two seconds.

 ClinicalConnection

Pulsed pure tones rather than continuous tones are typically used in testing patients with bothersome tinnitus. Patients with tinnitus hear "phantom" sounds like ringing, buzzing, or cricket-like sounds, especially in quiet settings like a sound-treated room. During hearing testing, a pulsing tone increases a tinnitus patient's awareness of the signal and distinguishes it from the often-continuous tinnitus sound. Also, to provide more precise information in the evaluation of persons with tinnitus, 1- or 2-dB-intensity increments are sometimes used, rather than the typical 5-dB increments.

The next button, labeled *Warble Tone*, modifies the pure tone signal so that its frequency varies slightly and rapidly. The use of **warble tones** minimizes the likelihood of sound interference problems and inaccuracies in hearing assessment when pure tones are presented to the patient via loudspeakers in a sound-treated room. You learned about interference in sound propagation in Chapter 2, including reinforcement of sound or constructive interference and cancellation of sound, also called destructive inference. The two concepts were illustrated in Figure 2.15. Acoustic interference between the stimulus and possible reflections of the stimulus is likely to affect the intensity level of the stimulus sound and the accuracy of test results.

Looking closely at the diagram in Figure 5.3, you'll find a button labeled *Interrupt* located just to the top and side of the stimulus switch control, below the *SP Noise* label. The *Interrupt* button is used to control whether a stimulus is consistently on or consistently off during testing. For example, when an audiologist communicates with a patient via microphone (*Mic*), the *Interrupt* button is toggled to keep the microphone on until it's no longer needed. On the other hand, during hearing threshold testing the *Interrupt* button is typically in the off position so that only the pure tone stimulus is presented when the audiologist presses the *Stimulus Switch* control.

Finally, you will note a control located at the bottom center of the audiometer diagram labeled **Talk Back**. From time to time during a hearing assessment, the tester will need to speak briefly with the patient, for example, to encourage the patient or to explain a particular test procedure. The *Talk Back* button permits quick and convenient communication between the tester and the patient. It eliminates the need for an audiologist to use the microphone button or to repeatedly enter the sound-treated room to talk face-to-face with the patient.

When an audiologist operates an audiometer, some information about the test settings is displayed on the control panel. In the audiometer diagram in Figure 5.3, the main controls selected for each channel are shown at the top of the panel. As you can see, the audiometer is set up for pure tone audiometry (*Pure Tone*). The display confirms that whenever the stimulus switch is activated, a 1000-Hz pure tone frequency is presented through Channel 1 at an intensity level of 60 dB HL with an insert earphone to the right ear. At the same time, a narrow band (NB) of noise centered around 1000 Hz at an intensity level of 40 dB HL is being presented via an insert earphone to the left ear.

The latest generation of audiometers that are based on a computer platform permit storage and direct access to files containing speech signals, in addition to the features just reviewed. There are also computer-based audiometers designed to carry out automated hearing testing. Once the earphones are placed on the patient, the automated device goes through the steps involved in pure tone audiometry without the need for manual control by a human operator. You'll learn more about automated devices later in this chapter.

Earphones

You were introduced to earphones and bone vibrators in Chapter 4. We'll now review these important devices in more detail. An earphone is a **transducer**, a term for an electronic device that changes a signal from one form to another. Two examples of transducers utilized everyday in audiology are earphones that convert an electrical signal to a sound and microphones that convert sound into an electrical signal. The three types of transducers used routinely for pure tone audiometry include (1) *supra-aural earphones* that fit over the pinna; (2) *insert earphones* that consist of a small transducer box, a flexible acoustic tube, and a soft tip that fits within the ear canal; and (3) a *bone vibrator* located on the skull either behind the ear or on the forehead. Loudspeakers are also used in hearing testing, but rarely with pure tone sounds. The four types of transducers were shown earlier in Figure 4.4 (Chapter 4).

Supra-Aural Earphones. For many years, **supra-aural earphones** were the conventional transducer option in pure tone audiometry. Unfortunately, adequate infection control is difficult with conventional supra-aural earphones, which fit within a soft rubber cushion. The rubber cushions on supra-aural earphones making contact with skin on the pinna are reused after each patient. Effectively disinfecting the supra-aural cushions after use is not feasible. Disposable and acoustically transparent covers for supra-aural earphone cushions that do not interfere with sound transmission are the next best for minimizing the possibility of infection.

Insert Earphones. Although supra-aural earphones are still widely used in hearing testing, **insert earphones** offer distinct advantages in certain patient populations. Table 5.1 summarizes the advantages of properly fit insert earphones. The last advantage in the list warrants special mention. Disposal of the part of the insert earphone that makes contact with the patient's ear is important for effective infection control. This important step in aural hygiene was illustrated earlier in Figure 4.1C.

Despite the compelling advantages of insert earphones, there are some drawbacks for their universal application in clinical audiology. Insert earphones cannot be used to test patients with certain abnormalities of the pinna or external ear canal. The use of insert earphones with disposable ear tips also modestly increases the cost associated with hearing testing. Finally, unexpected pure tone hearing test findings are occasionally encountered when using insert earphones with select patients.

Whenever the results of pure tone hearing testing are inconsistent with expectations or with findings on other tests, it is advisable to repeat the measurements with a different type of earphone. To close our discussion about earphones, it is important to keep in mind that transducers used for hearing tests must meet formal well-defined standards for performance

---

- Attenuation of background ambient sound that might interfere with the assessment of hearing thresholds
- Increased comfort during extended test sessions
- Greater inter-aural attenuation, that is, diminished likelihood that the stimulus sound will cross over from the test ear to the non-test ear
- Reduced possibility of problems with collapsing external ear canals, especially in infants and elderly patients
- More consistently precise placement than supra-aural earphones
- Improved aural hygiene, i.e., better infection control. The small tip that makes contact with the walls of the external ear canal is discarded after it is used with a single patient.

TABLE 5.1
Advantages of properly fit insert earphones in hearing testing of children and adults.

and must be periodically calibrated. You'll recall learning about standards and the calibration process in the previous chapter.

Bone Vibrators

Like earphones, bone vibrators are a very important type of transducer in clinical audiology. A **bone vibrator** is a small boxlike device consisting of electronic circuitry encased in plastic. A bone vibrator was shown in the previous chapter (Figure 4.4C). The portion of the bone vibrator that is placed against the skull may be round or rectangular in shape. The part that contacts the skull may have a concave surface or a flat surface. Bone vibrators must meet certain design standards and must be properly calibrated.

Loudspeakers

In most audiology clinics, sound-treated rooms are equipped with loudspeakers that are also controlled by the audiometer. Each type of sound used to evaluate hearing, including tones, speech, and noise, can also be presented to the patient via one or more loudspeakers. There are clinical indications and advantages associated with the use of loudspeakers rather than earphones.

Loudspeakers in Hearing Testing. With adults, loudspeakers are typically used to assess hearing performance of patients who use hearing aids or other devices. Loudspeakers are also often the transducer of choice for hearing testing of infants and young children who do not tolerate wearing earphones or a bone vibrator. Infants and even some older children may not allow proper placement of a set of earphones over the ears or placement of insert cushions into the ear canal. If a child or any other patient does not tolerate earphones, or if problems with earphone acceptance are anticipated, hearing assessment is carried out by presenting sounds in the sound-treated booth or room through one or more loudspeakers.

The distance between a patient and a loudspeaker is important. The distance affects the intensity level of the stimulus reaching the patient and also proper calibration of the stimulus. The space enclosed within the sound-treated room is referred to as a **sound field**. Hearing assessment with loudspeakers is called **sound-field testing**. Sound-field testing can be conducted with warble tones, narrow bands of noise, or some type of speech signal.

Drawbacks of Loudspeakers. The main disadvantage of hearing assessment with loudspeakers instead of earphones is the lack of **ear-specific** information. In other words, sound presented with a loudspeaker will reach both ears, even if the speaker is located on one side of the patient. With sound-field testing, it is not possible to determine whether a response to a sound reflects the hearing status of one better-hearing ear, of both ears, or of one ear for some sounds and the other ear for other sounds. Sound-field test outcome in children is usually interpreted while taking into account findings from other tests that provide information for each ear separately, that is, ear-specific findings.

Automated Audiometers

In the typical clinical setting, hearing testing is performed manually by a trained tester, usually an audiologist. The tester controls the audiometer, presents the pure tone signals to the patient, analyzes the patient's responses, and makes ongoing decisions about the test strategy. However, automated hearing testing offers advantages in certain settings and with certain patient populations.

Some degree of automation in hearing testing is not new. Békésy audiometry was one of the earliest techniques for hearing testing. You've already read the name von Békésy several times in the book. In Chapter 1, you learned about Georg von Békésy and his contribution to research on how the ear functions. Figure 5.1C depicted a vintage audiometer named after von Békésy. The Békésy audiometer automatically changed the test frequency while the patient controlled the stimulus intensity level by pressing or releasing a button. Békésy audiometry was not fully automated. The audiologist was responsible for determining the test ear, and also for analysis of test results.

Automated Audiometer Features. Research since the 1970s has led to fully automated devices for hearing screening of newborn infants with various test techniques. The term *microprocessor audiometer* is sometimes used to describe a device that is connected to or incorporated within a computer with special software for hearing testing. More recently, sophisticated computer-based automated systems were introduced for measurement of air and bone conduction hearing thresholds, for hearing screening or assessment with certain objective test procedures, and even for the measurement of speech perception in many different languages.

Figure 5.4A shows a modern system for automated hearing threshold assessment permitting air and bone conduction testing without a sound-treated room. With this particular device, ambient noise in the ear canal during testing is effectively attenuated with a combination of insert earphones enclosed within sound-attenuating earmuffs. Figure 5.4B shows this earphone arrangement. Testing is automatically stopped temporarily whenever ambient noise levels exceed a specified criterion.

Applications. Automated hearing test equipment is widely used for hearing testing in the military and in industry. **Automated audiometry** offers the only feasible testing option in an industrial setting where large numbers of persons at risk for noise-induced hearing loss are required to undergo hearing screening or assessment on a regular basis, perhaps annually. A high proportion of the workers undergoing testing will have reasonably good hearing and will cooperate in the test process. Only a relatively small number of the workers will have an unusual pattern of hearing loss or ear disease that will complicate the test process. Anytime the volume of persons needing to be tested is high and the likelihood of hearing loss is low, automated technology and techniques are probably more efficient and cost effective than conventional manual audiometry.

For a variety of reasons, the use and acceptance of automation in routine hearing assessment are rapidly increasing. Automated devices permit efficient, cost-effective, and consistently high-quality hearing test services for populations not served by audiologists and other properly trained

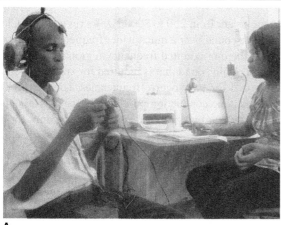

A

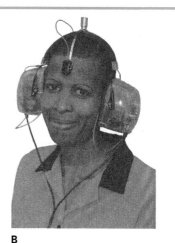

B

FIGURE 5.4

An automated KuduWave audiometer system for hearing threshold assessment with air conduction and bone conduction sounds (**A**) with a special headset that features with insert earphones within sound attenuating enclosures and a bone vibrator (**B**). Courtesy of GeoAxon.

personnel. The automated audiometers use artificial intelligence and sophisticated algorithms that consistently control the test process for most types and degrees of hearing loss, while minimizing mistakes associated with operator error. Automated technology offers a practical means of expanding hearing services globally and increasing accessibility of hearing assessment in underserved populations (Maclennan, Swanepoel, & Hall, 2013; Swanepoel et al., 2010).

Limitations of Automated Audiometry. It is important to point out here that automated clinical devices are designed for use with persons who can comply with and cooperate during the test process, such as older children and adults. Automated hearing testing is not appropriate for difficult-to-test patients, such as infants, young children, or persons with cognitive deficits. Automation in testing cannot take the place of an experienced clinician who skillfully incorporates information from a case history, clinical observation, and other test findings to reach an accurate diagnosis of auditory dysfunction and develop an effective management strategy.

Principles of Pure Tone Audiometry

Definition of Hearing Threshold

Hearing threshold levels are defined as the faintest intensity levels in dB that generate a response from the patient approximately 50 percent of the time. That is, for a given pure tone frequency, the patient usually detects the presence of the sound for higher-intensity levels than the threshold level and rarely detects the sound for lower-intensity levels. The increment or "step size" for clinical hearing threshold estimation is 5 dB. Smaller intensity increments are sometimes used in auditory research.

Audiometric Zero

The average person in a large normal-hearing population has hearing threshold levels of 0 dB HL, sometimes called **audiometric zero**. The standard deviation for hearing threshold levels is 5 dB (Studebaker, 1967) for testing using 5-dB-intensity increments. For any given test ear and pure tone frequency, about two-thirds of the normal-hearing population will have hearing threshold levels of either -5 dB, 0 dB, or 5 dB. From a statistical perspective, almost all normal-hearing people (more than 99 percent) have hearing thresholds of 15 dB or better. How is the concept of normal variability applied in clinical hearing testing? A patient with a hearing threshold of greater than 15 dB has hearing sensitivity that is outside of the normal region. Auditory dysfunction should be suspected.

Test Frequencies

The conventional **audiometric frequencies** are from 250 to 8000 Hz. As reviewed in Chapter 3, a young normal-hearing ear can perceive sound over a much wider frequency range, from a low of 20 Hz up to 20,000 Hz. However, the more limited frequency region for clinical hearing assessment encompasses all of the energy in sound that is required for speech perception. Hearing thresholds are also often measured for inter-octave frequencies, such as 3000 and 6000 Hz. In certain test situations, such as bone conduction pure tone hearing assessment or hearing testing of young children, pure tone hearing thresholds are measured only for a frequency range of 500 Hz to 2000 or 4000 Hz.

Preferred Method for Pure Tone Threshold Measurement

The goal of standardized methods for pure tone audiometry is to maximize consistency of results across testers and clinical facilities. Methods currently used for finding pure tone hearing thresholds are quite similar to those initially described and recommended over seventy years ago (Bunch, 1943; Hughson & Westlake, 1944) and later further defined by formal studies (Carhart & Jerger, 1959). In 1959, two of the important figures in the early years of audiology, Raymond Carhart and James Jerger, published rather detailed recommendations for performing pure tone audiometry. You may recall from the historical overview of audiology in Chapter 1 that Raymond Carhart was instrumental in the development of audiology as a formal profession. He is sometimes referred to as the "Father of Audiology." James Jerger, one of Carhart's early students, went on to make important contributions to diagnostic audiology.

The Carhart and Jerger article entitled "Preferred Method for Clinical Determination of Pure-Tone Thresholds" (Carhart & Jerger, 1959) has largely guided clinical measurement of hearing thresholds for the past fifty years. In this classic paper, Carhart and Jerger summarize and reinforce the main features of the **preferred method,** or what is sometime called the Hughson-Westlake method, including (1) determining hearing thresholds with ascending series of tones, progressing from lower- to higher-intensity levels; (2) separating successive stimuli lasting a second or two by periods of silence; and (3) stopping each ascending sequence of sounds when the patient responds. The authors also provide data confirming that with a 5-dB step or increment, rather than smaller intensity increments like 1 or 2 dB, there is really no difference in the hearing thresholds obtained with ascending and descending techniques.

Guidelines for Pure Tone Hearing Threshold Measurement

The Carhart and Jerger "Preferred Method for Clinical Determination of Pure-Tone Thresholds" is a systematic clinical method for determining hearing threshold levels. With minor variations, the preferred method is still used today for pure tone audiometry. A comprehensive and more recent source of practical information on the topic is *Guidelines for Manual Pure-Tone Threshold Audiometry* developed by the American Speech Language and Hearing Association (ASHA, 2005). These guidelines provide useful information on pure tone audiometric testing with air and bone conduction signals in cooperative patients and also information about multiple related topics, including audiometer equipment and calibration, the test environment, infection control, ear examination, and record keeping.

Published standards for pure tone audiometry are also available from the American National Standards Institute in a document entitled *Methods for Pure Tone Threshold Audiometry* (S3.21-2004). In a clinical setting, it is not always possible to follow exactly all components of the guidelines or to apply the same techniques with every patient. Deviation from the recommended approach is sometimes necessary in the clinical setting with certain patients, such as young or difficult-to-test children and persons with developmental or neurological problems.

Guidelines for pure tone audiometry differ from one country to the next. There are also international differences in standards for calibration and performance of equipment, the test environment, the graphs and symbols used to plot hearing test findings, and even the definitions of the degree of hearing loss.

Techniques for Pure Tone Hearing Threshold Measurement

We reviewed in the previous chapter four important steps that usually precede pure tone audiometry: (1) taking a patient history, (2) visually inspecting the ears, (3) properly positioning the patient in the sound-treated room, and (4) instructing the patient about the test process and what is expected of him or her. You may wish to review information in Chapter 4 on preparation of the patient (pages 92 through 108) before reading further.

Two accepted techniques for estimating a person's hearing for pure tone signals differ based on whether the test tones are initially increased in intensity or initially decreased in intensity. The starting intensity level really distinguishes the two techniques. The **ascending**

technique relies on ascending rather than descending intensity levels, beginning at an intensity level that is so low that the tone is probably inaudible. For example, if normal hearing sensitivity is expected for a patient, the starting intensity level with the ascending technique may be as low as −10 dB HL. If the patient fails to respond, intensity level is increased by 5 dB and the tone is presented again.

Perhaps the most common strategy for measurement of pure tone hearing thresholds involves a combination of descending and ascending changes in the intensity level of stimulus sounds. With the **descending-ascending method** the starting level is well above the patient's expected threshold. Then the test tone is decreased. We'll now review this approach for pure tone hearing threshold testing in a step-by-step fashion. Keep in mind that the actual steps and the order of steps may vary somewhat among different audiologists and from one patient to the next.

Air Conduction Thresholds First. We'll assume in the following discussion of pure tone hearing threshold measurement that sounds are presented first via air conduction. You learned in the previous chapter that earphones of some type are almost always used in hearing testing. Sound from the earphones travels through the air in the ear canal to the tympanic membrane. Vibrations of the tympanic membrane are conveyed through the middle ear to the inner ear, where outer and inner hair cells are activated. Hearing testing with earphones, therefore, involves the entire auditory system from the external ear to the inner ear. Since the ear is stimulated by sound waves traveling through the air, the term *air conduction* is used to describing hearing tests performed with earphones.

Which ear should be tested first via air conduction? If the patient indicates a difference in hearing between ears, the better-hearing ear is usually tested first. Before hearing testing begins, an audiologist often asks the patient a question like: "Do you notice any difference in hearing between the right and left ears?" Then hearing testing begins with the better-hearing ear. As you would expect, it is not feasible to ask infants or young children about how they hear in each ear. Sometimes, however, the better-hearing ear is clearly identified before pure tone audiometry begins, based on information in the patient history or the results of other auditory test procedures.

Air conduction pure tone hearing testing typically begins with a test frequency of 1000 Hz. Application of the descending-ascending technique for a person who probably has reasonably good hearing sensitivity is illustrated in Figure 5.5.

You'll notice in the left portion of the graph that a 1000-Hz tone is first presented at an intensity level within a typically comfortable intensity range of 30 to 40 dB HL. The patient responds to the tone, so the intensity level is decreased by 10 dB and presented again. The patient responds at the lower level, so the intensity level is decreased another 10 dB step and presented again.

This process is continued until the patient no longer responds to the tone. In our example, the patient didn't respond to the tone at 0 dB HL. Then the intensity level is increased by 5 dB. The tone intensity is alternately increased in 5 dB increments and decreased in 10 dB increments until hearing threshold is found.

Threshold is defined as the lowest intensity level in dB at which the patient responds for at least one-half of ascending tone presentations. Criterion for hearing threshold is sometimes defined as the intensity level that results in two responses out of three stimulus presentations. In our example, hearing threshold for the 1000-Hz tone is 5 dB HL. The patient consistently hears tones for higher-intensity levels but never hears tones for a lower-intensity level. When a hearing threshold is established in the range of 0 to 10 dB HL for the first test frequency of 1000 Hz, the starting intensity level for remaining frequencies is often lower to save time, as shown in the right portion of Figure 5.5.

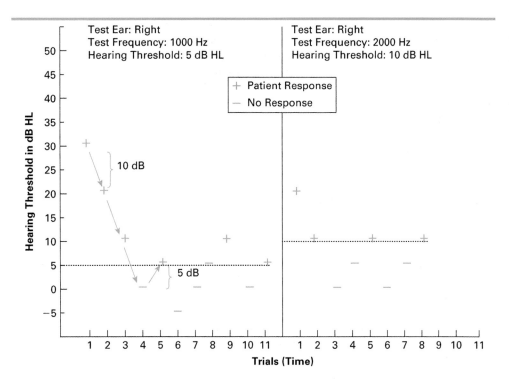

FIGURE 5.5

The descending-ascending technique used in measurement of pure tone hearing thresholds.

If the patient doesn't respond at a starting point of 30 dB HL, then the tone is presented at an intensity level 20 dB higher. If there is still no response at the higher level, stimulus intensity is again increased 20 dB, and the tone is presented to the patient. The 20-dB ascending process is continued until the patient responds or until the maximum intensity level for the equipment is reached. A higher-intensity level is then used for subsequent audiometric test frequencies, with the assumption that the patient has a hearing loss at other frequencies.

After hearing threshold is established for the 1000-Hz tone, thresholds are measured for other test frequencies as indicated in Figure 5.5. Sometimes the hearing threshold will be rechecked at the 1000-Hz threshold after measurements are complete for other frequencies. Then the same process is repeated for the other ear.

Variations in Techniques. The process of finding pure tone thresholds, as just reviewed, is straightforward. In most cases, threshold measurement is successfully completed without difficulty. Occasionally, however, the process must be modified to ensure that accurate results are obtained in a timely fashion.

Some common alterations in the usual test procedure include the use of (1) pulsed tones rather than continuous tones of 1 to 2 seconds for persons with tinnitus, to enhance the detection of the stimulus, (2) insert earphones rather than supra-aural earphones to prevent ear canal collapse in infants or elderly adults, (3) an ascending technique for presenting signals (beginning at a low-intensity level, so the sound cannot be heard) rather than the combination descending-ascending technique, for persons who are suspected of demonstrating a false or exaggerated hearing loss, and (4) a low-frequency start, such as 250 Hz rather than 1000 Hz, for persons with very severe hearing loss for high-frequency sounds.

Hearing Threshold Measurement in Young Children. As noted earlier, the term *hearing threshold* refers to the softest sound a person can hear. Modification of the procedures just described is often necessary to effectively assess hearing thresholds in certain patient populations. With younger children, a second tester may remain in the sound booth to work directly with the child to ensure that the test process is successful. An audiologist or an assistant may serve as the second tester.

Also, loudspeakers are often used to deliver the signals to a young child who simply won't wear earphones. In pediatric hearing assessment, the signals are often different, with narrow bands of noise or warbled tones used instead of pure tones. Rarely is it possible to determine hearing thresholds in young children across the frequency range of 250 to 8000 Hz. Rather, the goal is to estimate hearing thresholds with tones or bands of noise within the frequency region most important for hearing speech, that is, between 500 and 4000 Hz.

Test-Retest Reliability

Some variability in hearing threshold testing is unavoidable, even when a very specific testing technique is performed carefully and consistently. Variability in hearing testing can be described with measurement of test-retest reliability. **Test-retest reliability** is determined by the change in hearing thresholds obtained with repeated measurements for the same patient under identical test conditions. Identical test conditions include the same test environment, the same test ear, and the same test, such as measurement of air hearing thresholds. Typical test-retest reliability is within ±5 dB. In other words, if pure tone audiometry is repeated two or more times for a patient, hearing thresholds at any given pure tone signal are expected to vary or differ by only ±5 dB.

As an example, let's assume that a patient yields a hearing threshold of 20 dB HL for a pure tone signal of 1000 Hz in the right ear. If hearing threshold measurement is repeated, either immediately, later that day, or even days, weeks, or months later, we would anticipate that the patient's subsequent hearing threshold levels at 1000 Hz for the right ear would most likely again be 20 dB HL. However, the patient's right ear hearing threshold might be 15 dB HL or 25 dB HL, even though hearing is unchanged. What is the clinical implication of the concept of test-retest reliability? If hearing thresholds do not differ by more than ±5 dB from one test to the next, we assume that there has been no change in hearing sensitivity.

Bone Conduction Pure Tone Audiometry

Everyday listening in the world almost always begins with sound entering the external ear canal. You learned about ear anatomy in Chapter 3. Briefly, sound reaching the tympanic membrane produces vibrations that are transmitted through the ossicles in the middle ear space to the inner ear. When the vibrations reach the base of the inner ear, they produce tiny waves in the thick inner ear fluid that produce an up-and-down movement of the thin basilar membrane in the cochlea. The vertical basilar membrane movement and the horizontal movement of cochlear fluid activate the outer and inner hair cells on the basilar membrane. The end result of these various actions is increased activity in auditory nerve fibers and then in auditory regions of the brain.

The inner ear is also activated more directly by vibration of the bones surrounding it. The membranous labyrinth consists of fluids, membranes, hair cells, and other structures within the cochlea. A part of the temporal bone called the bony labyrinth encloses the membranous labyrinth. During bone conduction hearing testing, a bone vibrator placed on the temporal bone produces vibrations at specific frequencies and intensity levels. The earlier discussion of bone vibrators and brief summary of bone conduction hearing will now be augmented with a review the anatomical pathways that play a role in stimulation of the ear via bone conduction. Then, we'll go over bone conduction techniques audiologists employ in hearing testing.

Anatomy of Bone Conduction Hearing

You'll recall from Chapter 3 that the skull or cranium consists of a small number of major bones. Some of the bones are unpaired, that is, there is one bone extending from one side of the head to the other. Two of the major unpaired bones are the frontal bone, located at the front of the head, and the occipital bone in the back of the head. Two major paired bones are the parietal bones that form the upper sides of the head and the temporal bones that form the lower sides of the head. The inner ear is enclosed within the temporal bone.

The mastoid bone is the portion of the temporal bone that's important in bone conduction audiometry. As illustrated in Figure 3.7 (Chapter 3), the mastoid bone is located behind the pinna and projects downward as the mastoid process. For older children and adults, the four major cranial bones vibrate almost as a single unit. Vibrations beginning on any part of the skull travel from bone to bone and quickly reach the temporal bone and the inner ear on each side of the head. In fact, even stimulation causing vibration of bony structures connected indirectly to the skull will generate a bone conduction response.

You can do a simple experiment to demonstrate the phenomenon of indirect bone conduction hearing. All you need is a tuning fork or a bone vibrator. First, clean and thoroughly disinfect the tuning fork or bone vibrator. Then activate either device and place it on your front teeth. You may be quite impressed with the quality and intensity of the sound you hear.

Here's another interesting and clinically practical fact about conduction of vibrations through the skull. In young infants, under the age of about 6 months, the four major skull bones are not yet fused together. Vibrations cannot cross effectively from one part of the skull to another because the connections or sutures among the bones are still forming. Bone conduction stimulation presented anywhere on an infant's temporal bone on one side of the head only activates the ear on that side. Sound cannot be transmitted via the skull to the other ear because the infant temporal bone is not yet firmly connected to surrounding bones.

How We Hear by Bone Conduction

In bone conduction audiometry, an electronic device generates precise vibrations in the skull. The bone vibrator is designed specifically for the purpose of hearing testing. Energy from the bone vibrator reaches and stimulates the inner ear in three ways, with three distinct mechanisms (Tonndorf, 1964).

Distortional Bone Conduction. Vibration of the temporal bone surrounding the membranous inner ear directly transmits energy to the fluids within the inner ear. Direct activation of the cochlear hair cells by temporal bone vibration is referred to as **distortional bone conduction**. This is illustrated in Figure 5.6. The vibration or distortion of the walls of the bony labyrinth creates little waves within the fluid of the inner ear. The energy from the vibration in turn produces movement of the basilar membrane and activation of the outer and inner hair cells on the basilar membrane.

Inertial Bone Conduction. The second mechanism for bone conduction hearing involves the connection between the middle ear and the inner ear. This mechanism for cochlear activation via vibration is called **inertial bone conduction**. It is also shown in Figure 5.6. The stapes bone is the innermost of the three ossicles linking the tympanic membrane with the cochlea. The oval base of the stapes bone (the stapes footplate) fits within an opening in the bony wall of the cochlea called the *oval window*.

When vibrations of the skull and the temporal bone reach the bony walls of the cochlea surrounding the oval window, the movement is not transmitted to the stapes footplate. As a result of inertia, the stapes footplate movement lags behind the vibration of the bony walls of the cochlea. In effect, the stapes footplate moves inward and outward relative to the cochlear

FIGURE 5.6

Mechanisms of bone
conduction hearing,
including a distortional
bone conduction (**A**),
inertial bone conduction
(**B**), and osseotympanic
bone conduction (**C**).

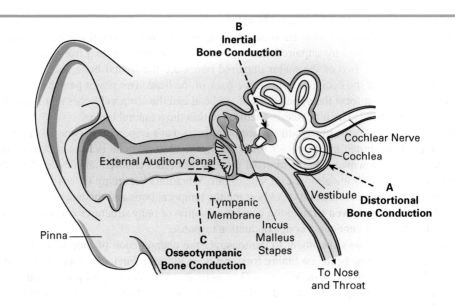

walls and fluids. Energy produced by the relative difference between movement of the stapes and movement of the bony walls of the cochlea is transmitted through the cochlear fluids to the basilar membrane, causing activation of the outer and inner hair cells.

Osseotympanic Bone Conduction. The third mechanism for bone conduction hearing involves the bony wall of the external ear canal and the tympanic membrane. It is called **osseotympanic bone conduction**. The medial or deepest portion of the external ear canal wall consists of bone, whereas the lateral portion of the ear canal is lined with cartilage. As depicted in Figure 5.6, vibration of the bony wall of the inner ear canal produces sound waves in the ear canal. If the ear canal is open, and not occluded by an earphone, some of the sound waves escape out of the ear canal. The remaining energy, however, travels further into the ear canal, vibrating the tympanic membrane. The vibrations are transmitted through the ossicular chain to the inner ear much as they are with air conduction hearing.

Technique for Bone Conduction Hearing Threshold Measurement

Mastoid Bone Vibrator Placement. As already noted, the cochlea can be stimulated with vibrations originating anywhere on the skull. However, clinical measurement of bone conduction responses is conducted with the bone vibrator located on either the mastoid process of the temporal bone or on the forehead.

For routine bone conduction pure tone hearing threshold measurements, audiologists tend to rely on mastoid placement of the bone vibrator rather than forehead placement. The primary advantage cited for mastoid placement is an enhancement in effective stimulus intensity level. Even a 5- to 10-dB increased in maximum intensity level for mastoid versus forehead placement contributes more accurate determination of bone conduction hearing thresholds in certain patients.

A bone vibrator is usually coupled to the mastoid bone with a flexible metal headband. This arrangement was described in Chapter 4 and shown in Figure 4.10A. The bone vibrator is a rectangular plastic box that encases electronics designed to produce vibration. It is held in place on the mastoid process with tension from the springy metal headband and a swivel mechanism that allows the bone vibrator to adjust to the shape of the skull. The conventional metal band is too large for infants and young children with smaller heads. Alternative methods like Velcro straps are often used to keep the bone vibrator in place in such cases.

Forehead Bone Vibrator Placement. For forehead placement, the bone vibrator can be coupled to the skull with a metal band (shown in Figure 4.10B) or with an adjustable headband. An adjustable headband usually consists of either leather or soft plastic, and sometimes a metal receptor in the front, where the vibrator is attached. The size of the headband can be adjusted so that it closely matches the circumference of various head sizes by means of Velcro.

The bone vibrator is placed at the midline of the forehead an inch or two above eyebrow level, with hair pushed aside. Hair between a bone vibrator and the skin may affect the intensity level of bone conduction stimulation and compromise the accuracy of hearing thresholds. Cochlear activation produced by vibration originating at the forehead is dominated by a combination of distortional and inertial bone conduction, but not osseotympanic bone conduction.

Placement of the bone oscillator on either the mastoid or forehead is acceptable clinical practice. The major advantage of forehead placement is less variability from test to test. Accuracy in measurement of bone conduction thresholds is enhanced if variability is lower. This advantage is probably related to greater consistency in the pressure exerted by the bone vibrator on the skull. The traditional reason cited for mastoid placement in clinical hearing assessment is a greater maximum-intensity level than that for forehead location. However, modern audiometers and bone vibrators often produce adequate intensity levels with forehead placement bone conduction testing.

Which Ear Is Tested First?

There are no firm criteria or consistent protocols for determining which ear to test first in bone conduction audiometry. When a patient has an air conduction hearing loss in one ear and hearing thresholds are within normal limits for the other ear, bone conduction testing is generally performed first for the ear with hearing loss. In fact, if hearing thresholds are entirely normal for one ear, bone conduction may only contribute useful information for the abnormal ear. However, findings from other test procedures also influence the decision about which ear is tested first with bone conduction.

L E A D E R S   A N D   L U M I N A R I E S

Jerry Northern

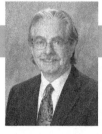

The following is a brief summary of Dr. Northern's professional background in his own words: "A lifetime as an audiologist, working with hearing-impaired children and adults, was the perfect career for me. I had an undergraduate major in experimental psychology. My deaf grandparents raised me from the age of two. Looking back over my forty-five years of working in this profession, I can't imagine any other working environment that would have provided me with such a wonderfully wide variety of opportunities and experiences. There is great self-satisfaction in providing hearing services that impact the lives of patients and their families. My audiology career has been both fun and exciting. It has included extensive teaching and clinical activities, military audiology, medical-legal work, scientific research, writing articles and books, consulting with manufacturers, and being actively involved with leadership responsibilities in our professional organizations."

You can learn more about the many accomplishments of Dr. Northern and his important contributions to audiology at the Colorado Hearing Foundation website.

Bone Conduction Hearing Testing Step-by-Step. The process for measuring hearing thresholds with bone conduction stimulation in many ways is similar to that for air conduction pure tone audiometry (Carhart, 1950; Hood, 1960). Therefore, the steps reviewed for air conduction also apply to bone conduction pure tone hearing testing. Bone conduction hearing threshold levels are recorded for intensity levels that yield a response from the patient approximately 50 percent of the time. Thresholds are measured with 5-dB-intensity increments.

The range of test frequencies is more limited for bone conduction stimulation than for air conduction hearing testing. Bone conduction hearing thresholds are regularly measured for frequencies of 500, 1000, 2000, and 4000 Hz, but never for higher frequencies and not always for lower frequencies. Assessment of bone conduction thresholds for a 250-Hz pure tone is feasible, but test results may be influenced by ambient noise in the test setting. For persons with reasonably good hearing sensitivity, and with the test ear uncovered, ambient noise can interfere with detection of low-frequency bone conduction pure tone signals.

As with air conduction pure tone audiometry, bone conduction testing begins with a test frequency of 1000 Hz and then proceeds upward to the highest test frequency of 4000 Hz. Thresholds are measured last for the lower frequency or frequencies. With certain patients, hearing thresholds are also measured via bone conduction for a test frequency of 3000 Hz.

There is one very distinct difference between bone conduction and air conduction pure tone measurements. High-intensity low-frequency bone conduction stimulation may produce a **vibrotactile response**, rather than an auditory response (Nober, 1970). This statement requires some explanation. For low-frequency pure tone stimulation of 250 and 500 Hz, the highest intensity level that can be produced by a bone vibrator is approximately 50 to 60 dB HL. At this intensity level for bone conduction sound, a patient may respond to a tactile sensation and not an auditory sensation. In other words, the patient feels a vibration rather than hearing a sound. The patient usually announces spontaneously or upon questioning by the tester that he or she felt a vibration rather than hearing a sound. In such cases, a vibrotactile response is noted on the audiogram.

Introduction to the Audiogram

"One picture is worth more than a thousand words."   (CHINESE PROVERB)

What Is an Audiogram?

An audiogram is a graphic summary of the results of hearing testing. An example is shown in Figure 5.7. The audiogram is a graph showing hearing thresholds in dB HL on the vertical Y-axis, plotted as a function of pure tone signals at different frequencies in Hz, shown on the horizontal X-axis. The intensity level corresponding to hearing threshold is usually shown in 5-dB increments, beginning at −10 dB in the topmost part of the graph and continuing down to approximately 110 or 120 HL. Soft sounds on the audiogram are represented near the top edge of the graph and loud sounds are represented near the bottom (Jerger, 2013).

Audiometric frequencies are pure tones spaced an octave apart. An octave is an interval between two different frequencies in which one frequency is either twice or one-half the other. So, for example, a frequency of 2000 Hz or a frequency of 500 Hz is an octave interval from 1000 Hz. Test frequencies usually extend from a lower limit of 125 or 250 Hz up to a high-frequency limit of 8000 Hz. Testing at two inter-octave test frequencies of 3000 and 6000 Hz is also recommended in pure tone hearing testing, as already noted.

Variations in audiogram format are not uncommon. In most formats test frequency in Hz is shown on the horizontal axis and intensity in dB hearing level is shown on the Y-axis. Some audiogram formats place the frequency labels at the bottom of the graph rather than the top, and the intensity labels are to the right of the graph instead of the left. Also, the hearing level

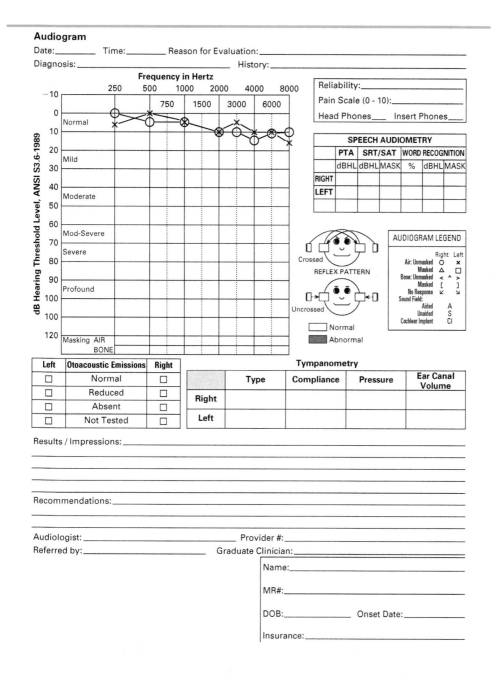

FIGURE 5.7

An audiogram format showing hearing thresholds in dB HL on the vertical (Y) axis plotted as a function of pure tone signals at different frequencies in Hz shown on the horizontal (X) axis. Hearing thresholds for the right ear (O) and left ear (X) are plotted at audiometric frequencies on the same graph. The audiogram form also includes a key to symbols as well as space to record demographic, health, and other information.

scale on the audiogram in some figures extends from −10 dB to 130 dB. The upper limit for intensity on other audiograms is 110 dB.

Audiogram Formats

There are two main options for representing the results of pure tone hearing testing. One is the audiogram. The audiogram typically includes hearing thresholds for the right and the left ear on air conduction stimulation, and often on bone conduction stimulation. Hearing test results can also be reported in a numerical format. Both the graphic and the numerical formats have a high degree of consistency within one test facility. Although formal standards for audiogram format do not exist, similarity in the way hearing thresholds are plotted facilitates accurate analysis and interpretation of test results nationally and internationally.

Any form for displaying hearing test findings includes important demographic information, such as the patient's name, date of birth, gender, and often a clinic identification or medical record number. An audiogram or numerical table with hearing test results almost always contains other general information like the date of testing and the audiologist's name and license number. In most hospital settings, all clinic forms used to report patient findings are reviewed and approved by a special hospital committee to ensure consistency and compliance with regulations established by the hospital and national healthcare organization accreditation groups.

Traditional Audiogram. Let's return to the traditional audiogram format displayed in Figure 5.7. The exact layout and organization of the audiogram form and the data found in specific sections of the audiogram vary from one clinical facility to the next. However, the information included on this audiogram example is typical of current trends and reflects requirements for reporting the results of hearing testing and related patient information in a healthcare setting.

In a traditional audiogram format, pure tone hearing thresholds for both ears are plotted on a single graph always with intensity in dB HL on the vertical axis and frequency in Hz on the horizontal axis (ASHA, 1990). Symbols are used to plot hearing threshold levels. Pure tone thresholds with air conduction signals are often indicated with a circle ("O") for the right ear and an "X" for the left ear. At least eight different symbols are sometimes required to distinguish on a single graph the results for the right and the left ears in four test conditions involving either no masking of the non-test ear or masking of the non-test ear. These are (1) air conduction with no masking, (2) air conduction with masking, (3) bone conduction without masking, and (4) bone conduction with masking.

Additional symbols are also occasionally needed to specify certain test conditions. For example, symbols are required to indicate forehead versus mastoid placement of the bone vibrator. In addition, a symbol is needed to indicate that the patient did not respond to the sounds even at stimulus intensity limits for the equipment.

Somewhere on the audiogram each of the symbols is described in a *key to symbols* or *audiogram legend*. The audiogram legend is located toward the center right side of the audiogram form in Figure 5.7. Each of the symbols used on a traditional audiogram, including those for the right and left ears and for the unmasked and masked test conditions, is described briefly in Table 5.2. If you have not yet seen an audiogram form, you'll need to take a few minutes to become familiar with the symbols used for each ear under each test condition.

On the audiogram form shown in Figure 5.7, patient demographic information, including name, medical record (MR) number, and date of birth, is entered in the lower right hand corner of the sheet. Demographic information may be located on the top of the form on other audiogram formats. Other information may be required by some healthcare facilities, such as the date of onset of the hearing problem or reference to the health insurance carrier. In the example of the audiogram shown in Figure 5.7, additional features are sometimes found to the left of the demographic information, including the logo for the healthcare facility, documentation of formal approval of the form, and a bar code for tracking the patient information electronically.

Just above the patient demographic and healthcare facility information is a line for the name of the audiologist who performed the procedure. There is usually also a space for the audiologist's signature and sometimes a license or provider number, if required by a hospital or some other entity. Nearby on most audiogram forms is a line for the name of the person who referred the patient to the audiologist. Typical referral sources are physicians, other audiologists, or speech pathologists.

TABLE 5.2   Conventional audiogram symbols used to designate hearing thresholds with air- and bone conduction stimulation in different test ears and under conditions with no masking of the non-test ear versus masking of the non-test ear. With the conventional audiogram, test results for the right and left ear are plotted on the same graph. Therefore, a different symbol is required for each test condition to differentiate findings for the right versus left ear. Most audiogram forms include a key or summary of symbols to facilitate analysis of test findings, often using the abbreviation AC for air conduction and BC for bone conduction.

Symbol	Test Ear	Mode Stimulus	Masking Presentation
○	Right ear	Air conduction	No masking of non-test ear
×	Left ear	Air conduction	No masking of non-test ear
Δ	Right ear	Air conduction	Masking of the non-test ear
□	Left ear	Air conduction	Masking of the non-test ear
<	Right mastoid	Bone conduction	No masking of the non-test ear
>	Left mastoid	Bone conduction	No masking of the non-test ear
⊏	Right mastoid	Bone conduction	Masking of the non-test ear
⊏	Left mastoid	Bone conduction	Masking of the non-test ear
⌐	Forehead	Bone conduction	Masking of the left ear (Right)
Γ	Forehead	Bone conduction	Masking of the right ear (Left)
∨	Forehead	Bone conduction	No masking (Unmasked) (Either ear)
S	Sound field	Air conduction	No masking (Either ear) (No hearing aid)
●	Sound field	Air conduction	No masking (Either ear) (Hearing aid)
↘	No response symbol attached to any of the above symbols as appropriate		

General information about the assessment is entered in spaces located at the top of the audiogram form shown in Figure 5.7. General information includes test date and time, a brief patient history, the reason for the evaluation, and the patient's diagnosis. This information may be located in various places on the audiogram form. Information on the general health status of the patient, currently required by the Joint Commission (formerly known as the Joint Commission on Accreditation of Healthcare Organizations, or JCAHO) is included in the upper right portion of the Figure 5.7 audiogram. There are questions in this section regarding patient identification, pain, and fall risk, as well as patient acknowledgment of receipt of basic information about the procedure.

Separate Ear Audiogram. When the separate ear audiogram was first introduced in 1976, colored pencils or pens were invariably used to plot by hand color-coded hearing threshold levels, using red for the right ear and blue for the left ear (Jerger, 1976). The consistent use of distinct colors for the right and left ears contributed importantly to quick and accurate audiogram interpretation. There was less value in color-coding audiograms with increasing use of copy machines that rendered all documents black and white.

A different audiogram version displays the results for the right ear and the left ear on two separate graphs. Some separate ear audiogram forms simply plot the symbols from the traditional audiogram on the graphs for the right ear and the left ear. Circles are used for the right ear and "X" symbols for the left ear. This approach produces a cleaner display of test findings, as the number of potential symbols on each graph is one-half the number that occurs when results for both ears are plotted on a single graph. As many as four different symbols for air and bone conduction thresholds and for the right and left ears are sometimes clustered on one hearing level for one test frequency with the traditional audiogram format.

Most separate ear audiogram formats use a combination of traditional and newer symbols plotted on the separate graphs for each ear. Figure 5.8 shows an example of an audiogram for with a single set of symbols for both ears. For our discussion, we'll focus only on the top set

FIGURE 5.8

Hearing thresholds for the right and left ear plotted at audiometric frequencies on a separate-ear audiogram with one graph for the right ear and one for the left ear. The audiogram form also includes a key to symbols as well as space to record demographic, health, and other information. Hearing thresholds plotted for the right and left ear are the same values as those shown in Figures 5.7 and 5.9.

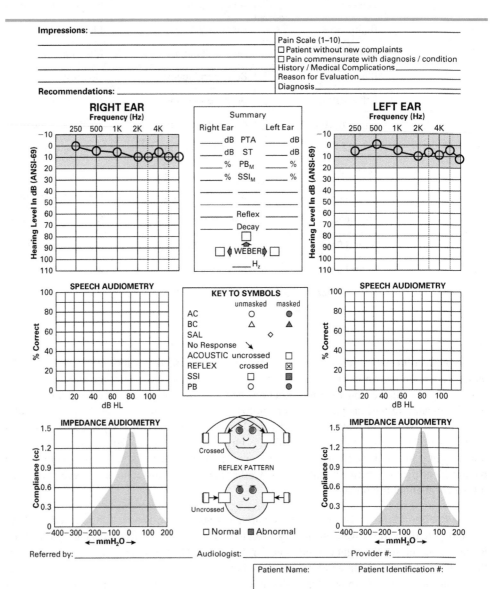

of graphs on the form, where the hearing thresholds for air and bone conduction stimulation are plotted. The key to symbols is located in the center of the form. Thresholds obtained without masking of the non-test ear are always represented by open symbols (e.g., ○) and thresholds obtained with masking of the non-test ear are represented by filled symbols (e.g., ●).

Simplicity is the major practical advantage of the separate ear audiogram. Since the same set of symbols is used to plot results for each ear on a separate ear audiogram, the number of different symbols required is one-half the number for the traditional audiogram. Ease and speed in audiogram interpretation by non-audiologist healthcare professionals who are less familiar with hearing testing are enhanced by the simpler symbol system. Persons who may not be familiar with audiograms include primary care physicians, patients, and parents of patients.

The separate ear audiogram form shown in Figure 5.8 also includes space for symbols describing test findings other than air and bone conduction hearing thresholds. We'll return to those parts of the audiogram form when we review speech audiometry in Chapter 6, masking and audiogram interpretation in Chapter 7, and some special objective auditory tests in Chapter 8. The summary box located between the right and left ear audiogram graphs includes a line for the pure tone average or PTA (discussed in detail below), as well as other test findings.

Numerical Tabular Format. In some settings, such as audiology clinics in Veterans Administration Medical Centers, results of hearing testing are often displayed as numbers in a tabular audiogram format. As illustrated in Figure 5.9, the tabular format includes sections for the right ear and left ears. Columns in the table are available for each pure tone frequency from 250 up to 8000 Hz. Hearing threshold values are represented by numbers rather than symbols, as on an audiogram. There are rows in the table for the numerical values obtained for pure tone hearing thresholds as measured by air conduction and bone conduction stimulation. Rows may also be designated for the intensity levels of masking noise presented during the measurement of pure tone thresholds. In addition, findings for other hearing test procedures are usually included in the table.

Current Audiogram Requirements. Audiology clinics located in hospitals and certain other healthcare facilities in many states in the United States must adhere to requirements established for voluntary accreditation by the Joint Commission. Healthcare facilities in the United States, such as hospitals, are motivated to maintain accreditation by the Joint Commission to ensure quality healthcare, and because accreditation is linked to licensure and to reimbursement for clinical services set by the Centers for Medicare and Medicaid (CMS).

Audiologists employed in medical and healthcare settings are expected to be familiar with, and comply with, Joint Commission regulations. Among the requirements is documentation of certain information on the audiogram or in the formal report of findings. The required information includes confirmation of patient identity and documentation of the patient's pain and risk of falls. Other general information may also be required on the audiogram form, such as the patient's history, diagnosis, reason for evaluation, and the date of onset of the auditory or vestibular problem.

Pure Tone Average (PTA)

An audiogram reveals details of hearing loss across a wide range of frequencies. Accurate analysis and interpretation of hearing test findings requires a frequency-by-frequency inspection of thresholds

ClinicalConnection

Audiologists working in a hospital setting are aware of the Joint Commission. The mission of the Joint Commission is "to continuously improve health care for the public, in collaboration with other stakeholders, by evaluating health care organizations and inspiring them to excel in providing safe and effective care of the highest quality and value." Joint Commission guidelines influence a variety of important clinical policies including the professional responsibilities reviewed in Chapter 4.

FIGURE 5.9

Tabular format used for reporting the results of hearing testing with air and bone-conduction hearing testing in Veterans Administration Medical Center audiology clinics. The numbers on the form represent the same hearing thresholds shown in Figure 5.7.

VA Department of Veterans Affairs   **AUDIOLOGICAL EVALUATION**

REASON FOR REFERRAL   REFERRAL SOURCE

AIR CONDUCTION

EXAMINER INITIALS	RIGHT									EXAMINER INITIALS	LEFT								
	250	500	1000	1500	2000	3000	4000	6000	8000		250	500	1000	1500	2000	3000	4000	6000	8000
	O	5	5		10	10	15	10	10		5	O	5		10	5	10	10	15
MASKING LEVEL										MASKING LEVEL									

RIGHT PURE TONE AVERAGE			TRANSDUCER TYPE		LEFT PURE TONE AVERAGE		
2 FA	3 FA	4 FA	☐ EARPHONE ☐ INSERT		2 FA	3 FA	4 FA

BONE CONDUCTION

EXAMINER INITIALS	RIGHT							EXAMINER INITIALS	LEFT						
	250	500	1000	1500	2000	3000	4000		250	500	1000	1500	2000	3000	4000
MASKING LEVEL								MASKING LEVEL							

ACOUSTIC IMMITTANCE

	RIGHT							LEFT					
PROBE (RIGHT)	PEAK PRESSURE daPa	V_ea	PEAK STATIC IMMITTANCE 226 Hz / 678 Hz		TYMPANOGRAM TYPE		PROBE (LEFT)	PEAK PRESSURE daPa	V_ea	PEAK STATIC IMMITTANCE 226 Hz / 678 Hz		TYMPANOGRAM TYPE

STIMULUS (LEFT)	CONTRALATERAL AR THRESHOLDS					REFLEX DECAY		STIMULUS (RIGHT)	CONTRALATERAL AR THRESHOLDS					REFLEX DECAY	
	500	1000	2000	4000	BBN	500	1000		500	1000	2000	4000	BBN	500	1000

STIMULUS (RIGHT)	IPSILATERAL AR THRESHOLDS					HALF-LIFE		STIMULUS (LEFT)	IPSILATERAL AR THRESHOLDS					HALF-LIFE	
	500	1000	2000	4000	BBN	500	1000		500	1000	2000	4000	BBN	500	1000

OTHER TESTS (RIGHT)	WEBER	PT STENGER	RINNE	OTHER:	OTHER TESTS (LEFT)	WEBER	PT STENGER	RINNE	OTHER:

SPEECH AUDIOMETRY

	RIGHT SRT		RIGHT SPEECH RECOGNITION								LEFT SRT		LEFT SPEECH RECOGNITION						
	1	2	1	2	3	4	5	6	PBMAX		1	2	1	2	3	4	5	6	PBMAX
LEVEL										LEVEL									
LIST										LIST									
MASKING LEVEL										MASKING LEVEL									

INTER-TEST CONSISTENCY (RIGHT) ☐ GOOD ☐ POOR ☐ FAIR   INTER-TEST CONSISTENCY (LEFT) ☐ GOOD ☐ POOR ☐ FAIR

MATERIAL ☐ MARYLAND CNC ☐ CIDW-22 ☐ NU-6 ☐ OTHER, SPECIFY: PRESENTATION ☐ RECORDED ☐ MLV

COMMENTS

LAST NAME - FIRST NAME - MIDDLE INITIAL	AGE	CLAIM NO.	SOCIAL SECURITY NO.
NAME OF EXAMINING STATION OR CLINIC	SIGNATURE OF EXAMINING AUDIOLOGIST		DATE OF EXAM

VA Form oct 2004 **10-2364**

for air and bone conduction. In describing and reporting hearing loss for a patient, however, it is helpful to be able to summarize concisely the degree of hearing loss. Simple descriptions of hearing loss are useful in describing the results of hearing assessment to patients, to parents of pediatric patients, to physicians, and to other audiologists.

Imagine, for example, two audiologists reviewing the findings for a patient during a telephone conversation. It would be very cumbersome and possibly confusing for one audiologist to report to the other hearing thresholds for four to six individual test frequencies for each ear. The **pure tone average**, abbreviated **PTA**, is a single dB value for summarizing the overall degree of hearing loss. Although the PTA provides a handy glimpse of a patient's hearing status, it is not a substitute for the audiogram or more detailed verbal descriptions of hearing loss.

Traditional PTA. The traditional PTA is based on hearing thresholds for three frequencies: 500, 1000, and 2000 Hz. The PTA is calculated by adding the hearing threshold levels obtained at each of the frequencies and then dividing by three. For example, if hearing thresholds are 0 dB at 500 Hz, 10 dB at 1000 Hz, and 15 dB at 2000 Hz, the sum of the hearing thresholds is 25 dB. The PTA is calculated as 25/3 or 8.3 dB, and rounded off to 8 dB.

The PTA is a useful way to quantify with a single number hearing sensitivity in a frequency region that is important for hearing and perceiving speech information. The audiogram usually includes a box for noting the PTA. Closely examine Figures 5.7, 5.8, and 5.9 and you'll see a space on each graph in for recording the PTA. Audiologists often refer to the PTA when reporting the results of hearing testing. Since the PTA reflects hearing sensitivity for some of the frequencies that are important for detecting speech sounds, comparison of the PTA with the hearing threshold levels for speech sounds provides additional clinical information. The relation between the PTA and speech threshold and its clinical value is discussed further in the next chapter.

Fletcher Two-Frequency Pure Tone Average. When hearing thresholds are the same or at least similar for two frequencies, but considerably different (>20 dB) for the third frequency, a simple average of the hearing thresholds for all three frequencies may produce a value that does not accurately reflect hearing in the speech frequency region. A pure tone average calculated with only the two better hearing thresholds is referred to as a two-frequency or "Fletcher" pure tone average (Fletcher, 1950). It is named after Harvey Fletcher, a brilliant and highly productive researcher who made many important contributions to hearing science and to the development of audiology. You may recall that Harvey Fletcher was featured in Leaders & Luminaries in Chapter 2.

Degree of Hearing Loss

Categories of Hearing Loss. **Degree of hearing loss** is often categorized based on hearing threshold levels at different test frequencies. The degree of hearing loss is usually described with adjectives such as mild, moderate, severe, or profound. Figure 5.10 shows general categories of degree of hearing loss displayed on an audiogram form (Clark, 1981).

Determining the degree of hearing loss and its likely impact on communication is one of the important objectives of pure tone audiometry. Categorizing the degree of hearing loss facilitates this process. For adult patients, hearing sensitivity is considered normal if thresholds are better than 20 dB HL across the audiometric frequencies of 250 to 8000 Hz. A slight decrease in hearing sensitivity between 0 and 20 dB HL has no impact on communication for patients with fully developed speech and language abilities.

In contrast, for young children even a mild hearing deficit of 15 to 25 dB may interfere with speech and language acquisition, with school performance, and with communication. Any degree of hearing loss in a child may have consequences and may require some type of management. As a rule, greater degrees of hearing loss have a more significant impact on communication. The need for intervention with hearing aids or another management approach increases directly with the degree of hearing loss.

The pure tone average is often used for describing the amount of hearing loss at any given test frequency, using the terms defined graphically in Figure 5.10. So, in the earlier scenario involving two audiologists discussing a patient, the results of the hearing assessment could be quickly summarized with a description of the degree of hearing loss based on the PTA. For example, one audiologist might report: "Based on the PTA, the patient has a moderate hearing loss in the right ear and a severe hearing loss in the left ear." The other audiologist would immediately understand that hearing is substantially decreased in both ears but more so in the left ear. Recall that the PTA summarizes thresholds in the frequency region important for hearing speech. Thus, the concise description of the PTA in each ear in our example confirms

FIGURE 5.10

Criteria for hearing
thresholds within
normal limits and for
different categories of
hearing loss from mild
to profound.

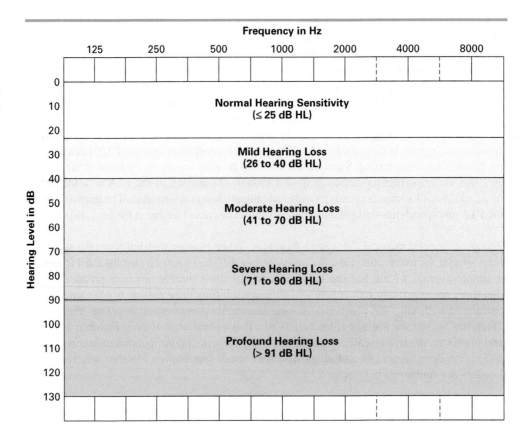

that the patient's hearing loss interferes with communication and may require hearing aids or
another intervention.

Limitations of Hearing Loss Categories. There are no universally accepted guidelines
for the categories used in describing degree of hearing loss. Not all audiologists use the exact
criteria given for each category of hearing loss in Figure 5.10. And, non-audiologists such as
patients, parents of patients, and physicians may not be familiar with terms used to describe
the degree of hearing loss.

There is another limitation to reliance on categories of hearing loss to describe test results.
The simple categories of degree of hearing loss may result in serious underestimation of
the impact of hearing loss in children. The terms *slight, mild,* and *minimal* suggest to non-
audiologists that a hearing loss is of little consequence. That is, the terms imply that the hearing loss is insignificant and not likely to affect communication or the acquisition of speech
and language in infants and young children. However, extensive long-term research clearly
shows that for young children any degree of hearing loss greater than 15 dB may interfere
with speech and language acquisition, with communication, and with academic performance
(e.g., Delage & Tuller, 2007; Yoshinago et al., 1998).

Why Is Hearing Loss Described in dB and Not Percentage?

Patients often ask about the percentage of their hearing loss. Also, physicians sometimes
describe the extent of hearing loss in terms of percentage rather than in decibels or with the
adjectives used by audiologists, such as mild, moderate, or severe. For example, a patient

might say: "I was told that I have a 20 percent hearing loss in my right ear and a 25 percent hearing loss in my left ear." Or, a physician might tell a patient: "Mr. Jones, you have a 60 percent hearing loss."

Limitations of Percentage versus dB. There are two major problems with quantifying the degree or extent of a hearing loss as a percentage. First of all, most patients and some physicians incorrectly equate the extent of hearing loss in dB directly with percentage. A 60 dB hearing loss in the higher-frequency region is described as a 60% hearing loss. As you'll recall from Chapter 2, the decibel is a logarithmic quantity, not a linear quantity like percentage. There is really no direct correspondence between a hearing impairment described in dB and that described as a percentage. Comparing hearing loss in percentage with hearing loss in decibels is inaccurate and misleading. To use a common phrase, it's like comparing apples and oranges.

A second and serious problem involves the approach typically used to calculate the percentage of hearing impairment. Hearing impairment can be precisely defined in percentage using longstanding methods defined by well-respected organizations, such as the American Medical Association (AMA, 2008). Quantification of the percent of hearing impairment is important for determining the amount of financial compensation for persons with hearing loss that can be attributed to noise exposure in work settings or military service. Percentage of hearing impairment is calculated with a formula based on the average hearing threshold levels for 500, 1000, 2000, and 3000 Hz. It's important to test a patient's hearing threshold for a 3000-Hz test frequency plus the other three test frequencies for calculation of the percentage of hearing impairment.

Types of Hearing Loss

What Is an Air-bone Gap? You learned in Chapter 4 that earphones and bone vibrators are calibrated periodically to assure accuracy in the intensity levels produced during hearing testing. At a given intensity level, the output for earphones should be equivalent to the output for a bone vibrator. For example, an intensity level of 10 dB HL with earphones is equal to an intensity level of 10 dB HL with a bone vibrator. Thus, a person with entirely normal hearing sensitivity is expected to yield very similar air and bone conduction hearing thresholds at each test frequency. In fact, any person with normal middle ear function is expected to have very similar hearing thresholds as measured by either air conduction or bone conduction stimulation. Approximately the same amount of energy reaches the person's inner ear whether sound is presented via air conduction or bone conduction.

An **air-bone gap** that is clinically important is defined as a difference of more than 10 dB between air and bone conduction pure tone thresholds (Studebaker, 1967). In other words, no air-bone gap is present if air and bone conduction hearing thresholds are the same or if they differ by no more than 10 dB. The absence of an air-bone gap is consistent with relatively normal middle ear function, whereas the finding of an air-bone gap suggests the likelihood of middle ear dysfunction. Let's take this reasoning one step further. If there is a hearing loss with air conduction testing and with bone conduction, and there is no air-bone gap, then the hearing loss is due to inner ear dysfunction. Again, the absence of an air-bone gap implies that the middle ear system is functioning normally.

 WebWatch

You can read more about air conduction and bone conduction hearing, and the air-bone gap, on websites such as AuDStudent. The website includes figures that help explain important concepts and also questions to assess your understanding of the concepts.

The Air-bone Gap and Types of Hearing Loss. The concept of air-bone gap is best understood when air conduction and bone conduction pure tone hearing thresholds are viewed on an audiogram. In the following discussion about the air-bone gap and types of hearing loss,

FIGURE 5.11

Audiogram with results of pure tone hearing testing for the right ear showing normal hearing sensitivity. Air-conduction thresholds for the right ear are plotted with an O. Bone conduction thresholds for the right and left ear are plotted with a < or > symbol as indicated in the legend to the right of the graph. There is no difference in hearing thresholds for air conduction versus bone conduction stimulation.

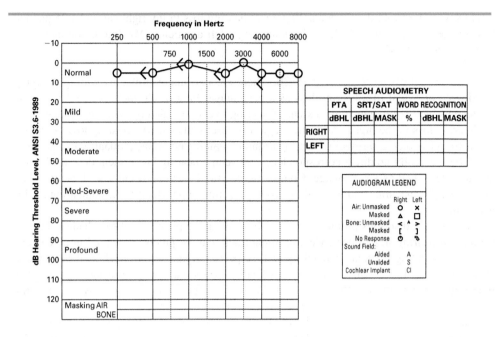

let's assume that test results always reflect a response of the test ear. In other words, we'll make the assumption that the right ear was tested when the earphone or the bone vibrator was placed on the right side and, conversely, the left ear was tested when the earphone or the bone vibrator was placed on the left side. These assumptions are not always valid in hearing testing of patients with hearing loss. You'll learn in Chapter 7 about masking techniques and their importance in obtaining results for air conduction and bone conduction testing that can be attributed to the test ears, without involvement of the other non-test ear.

You've already seen that most audiogram forms include a simple key to symbols. For audiograms with results for both ears on one graph, right ear results are identified with a circle (O) and left ear results are identified with an X. The caret symbols used for bone conduction hearing thresholds open to the right side (<) for the right ear and to the left side (>) for the left ear.

Figure 5.11 shows an audiogram for the right ear with equivalent hearing thresholds for air and bone conduction. There is no air-bone gap. The audiogram shown in Figure 5.11 indicates normal hearing sensitivity for air and bone conduction testing.

The audiogram in Figure 5.12 also reveals equivalent hearing thresholds for air and bone conduction and no air-bone gap. However, hearing thresholds are outside of the normal region, confirming a hearing loss. Since hearing threshold levels are abnormal and there is no air-bone gap, we presume that hearing loss in this audiogram is mostly likely due to inner ear dysfunction. The absence of an air-bone gap rules out abnormal middle ear functioning.

Hearing loss due to inner ear dysfunction is described as a sensori-neural hearing loss. The term combines the words *sensory* and *neural*. In fact, sensory etiologies for hearing loss due to inner ear dysfunction are far more common than neural etiologies involving the auditory nerve. However, the term *sensorineural hearing loss* is typically used to describe a hearing loss with no air-bone gap. With the information from pure tone hearing testing alone it is not possible to determine

ClinicalConnection

With a test battery that combines multiple different hearing tests and pure tone audiometry, it is usually possible to confidently differentiate inner ear or cochlear hearing loss from neural hearing loss. This topic is covered in Chapter 10, in a discussion of the diagnosis of auditory and vestibular disorders. Causes for cochlear and for neural hearing loss are reviewed in Chapter 11.

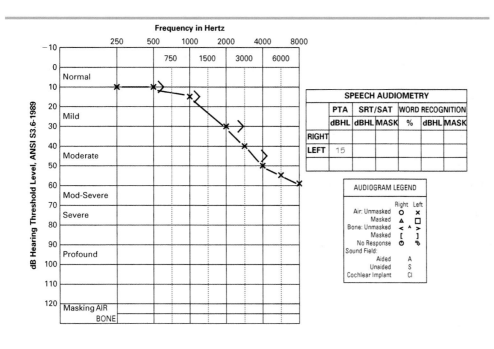

FIGURE 5.12

Audiogram with results of pure tone hearing testing of the left ear showing a high frequency hearing loss. There is no difference between air conduction and bone conduction pure tone hearing thresholds, that is, no air-bone gap, The findings are consistent with a sensorineural hearing loss.

whether hearing loss is due to inner ear dysfunction or to auditory nerve dysfunction. The term *retrocochlear auditory dysfunction* is sometimes used for neural abnormalities because the auditory abnormality is found beyond the inner ear, or cochlea.

Figure 5.13 shows an audiogram with a large air-bone gap. The term *conductive hearing loss* is used to describe a hearing loss for air conduction testing and normal-hearing thresholds for bone conduction producing an air-bone gap of more than 10 dB. You can clearly see a hearing loss by air conduction, yet bone conduction hearing thresholds are normal.

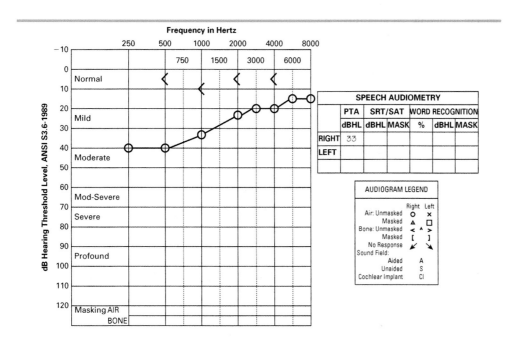

FIGURE 5.13

Audiogram with results of pure tone hearing testing of the right ear showing a conductive hearing loss. There is an air-bone gap between the thresholds for air conduction versus bone conduction stimulation. The size of the air-bone gap ranges from 35 dB in the lower frequency region to less than 20 dB for a test frequency of 4000 Hz.

We will take a moment here to review the explanation for the relationship between air-bone gap and conductive hearing loss. A blockage in the external ear canal or abnormal middle ear function interferes with the conduction of energy from earphones to the inner ear via the air conduction route. Energy from sound stimuli presented by air conduction must be transmitted through the external ear canal and the middle ear to activate the inner ear. In contrast, most of the energy produced by the bone vibrator activates the inner ear directly. Transmission of energy to the inner ear is not affected by a blockage in the external ear canal or by abnormal middle ear function. As a result, better hearing thresholds for bone conduction than for air conduction with an air-bone gap are characteristic findings for middle ear dysfunction and also for blockage of the external ear canal. Conductive hearing loss due to abnormal middle ear function is not uncommon, particularly in young children with ear infections.

It is important to point out that an air-bone gap is possible even though air conduction hearing thresholds are within normal limits. This combination of findings is sometimes encountered in children with air conduction thresholds of 10 or 15 dB HL and bone conduction thresholds that are better than 0 dB HL. Indeed, a patient with normal hearing sensitivity as defined by air conduction hearing levels of 15 dB and bone conduction thresholds of −10 dB would have a rather substantial 25-dB air-bone gap.

Bone conduction hearing testing is advisable in children even though hearing thresholds are generally within normal limits. The decision to perform bone conduction hearing testing in children is determined in part by a patient history of middle ear disorder and also by other test findings suggesting the possibility of middle ear abnormality.

Is it possible for a patient to have a hearing loss due to a combination of conductive hearing loss and sensorineural hearing loss? The answer to this question is a definite *yes*. The combination of the two forms of hearing loss is called a *mixed hearing loss*. Figure 5.14 shows an audiogram reflecting a mixed hearing loss. Test results are plotted on a separate-ear audiogram so the same symbols are used for the right and the left ears.

A mixed hearing loss is defined by abnormal hearing for bone conduction and a greater loss by air conduction, with an air-bone gap of more than 10 dB. In other words, an air-bone gap indicating a conductive hearing loss component is added to a sensorineural hearing loss. The conductive component in a mixed hearing loss may be due to blockage of the external ear canal or to middle ear abnormality.

Returning to Figure 5.14 you'll see that there is a clear discrepancy in the hearing thresholds for air and bone conduction stimulation. The size of the air-bone gap ranges from 35 dB in the lower-frequency region to 20 dB for higher test frequencies above 1000 Hz. However, even if the air-bone gap disappeared, a sensory hearing loss would remain.

FIGURE 5.14

An audiogram plotted on a separate-ear form showing a mixed hearing loss in both ears. Air conduction thresholds for each ear are plotted with an O whereas bone conduction hearing thresholds are indicated with a triangle symbol. Hearing thresholds are outside of the normal region for air conduction and for bone conduction stimulation. However, there is a greater hearing loss for air conduction stimulation. A clear air-bone gap is present for each ear at all test frequencies.

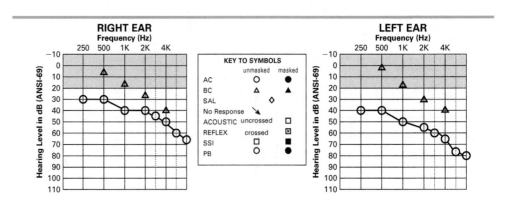

A mixed hearing loss may result from the combination of one cause for an outer or middle ear abnormality with a different cause for inner ear abnormality. A variety of diseases and pathologies can combine to produce mixed hearing loss. One explanation for a mixed hearing loss occasionally seen in clinical practice involves older patients. An older patient with long-standing sensorineural hearing loss due to the aging process may also have excessive cerumen (earwax) that blocks the external ear canal. The combination of these two unrelated forms of auditory dysfunction is a mixed hearing loss. The audiogram in Figure 5.14 is a good illustration of this explanation for mixed hearing loss.

The audiogram in Figure 5.15 depicts a severe sensorineural hearing loss. There is no clear or consistent air-bone gap. Air conduction and bone conduction thresholds differ by no more than 10 dB for the lower three test frequencies (250, 500, and 1000 Hz). Due to the severity of the hearing loss, bone conduction hearing thresholds at the highest test frequencies were measured at the intensity level limits of the bone vibrator. You'll note a little downward-pointing arrow indicating that the patient's hearing threshold exceeds the stimulus intensity level plotted on the audiogram.

The patient confirmed that he did not hear bone conduction pure tones that were presented at test frequencies of 1000 Hz and above. When the tester queried the patient about the bone conduction responses for the two lower test frequencies of 250 and 500 Hz, the patient acknowledged feeling a sensation of vibration rather than actually hearing the sounds. The letter "V" on the audiogram indicates a vibrotactile response at pure tone frequencies of 250 and 500 Hz.

Test-Retest Variability. One of the features common to both air and bone conduction audiometry is the certainty of test-retest variability. Given the precise calibration of stimulus intensity levels for earphones and bone oscillators, it is reasonable to expect absolutely no difference between air and bone conduction thresholds, and no air-bone gap. In clinical measurements, however, differences between air and bone conduction hearing thresholds in persons with normal middle ear function are commonplace, due to the inevitable test-retest variability

FIGURE 5.15

Audiogram showing a severe hearing loss for the left ear. Air-conduction thresholds for the left ear are plotted with an X. Bone conduction thresholds are plotted with a > symbol. The downward arrows indicate that the patient did not response to bone conduction stimulation. Hearing thresholds are abnormal for air conduction and for bone conduction hearing thresholds. The patient reported a vibro-tactile response for pure tone bone conduction stimulation at 250 and 500 Hz as indicated the "V" symbol. That is, the patient felt a vibration rather than hearing a sound at an intensity level of 60 to 70 dB HL.

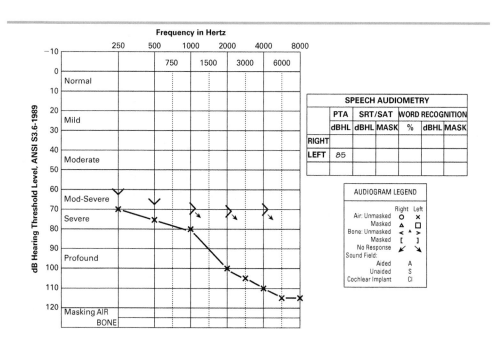

ClinicalConnection

An air-bone gap is not the only hearing test finding associated with middle ear dysfunction. Other hearing tests are typically performed to confirm or rule out the presence of middle ear dysfunction. Other behavioral tests will be discussed next in this chapter and the next chapter. Then, in Chapter 8, you'll learn about some objective auditory tests that are very useful in assessing middle ear function and detecting middle ear abnormalities.

of the measurements (Studebaker, 1967). Hearing thresholds will vary from one test to the next, or even with two separate measures of hearing sensitivity at the same frequency in the same test ear during the same test session. In other words, the hearing threshold for the second test may be better or worse than the hearing threshold for the initial test.

How much variation can be expected between air and bone conduction hearing thresholds? Variability of either air or bone conduction thresholds will often produce an apparent air-bone gap of 5 to 10 dB. Indeed, in citing the findings of a classic study done more than forty years earlier (Studebaker, 1967), Margolis (2010) commented, "Studebaker correctly warned that air-bone gaps of 10, 15 and 20 dB should be expected for a significant proportion of threshold measurements, and these should not be over-interpreted as evidence of middle ear dysfunction" (Margolis, 2010).

Is a Bone-Air Gap Possible?   The inherent variability in both air and bone conduction measurements predicts the likelihood of a **bone-air gap** in some patients (Barry, 1994; Margolis, 2010; Margolis & Saly, 2008). The term, a reversal of the phrase air-bone gap, is used when hearing thresholds are poorer for bone conduction than for air conduction stimulation. From an anatomical perspective, poorer hearing for bone versus air conduction is impossible. Assuming normal middle ear function, hearing should never be worse for bone conduction than for air conduction. However, given the normal variability in hearing threshold measurement with air and bone conduction stimulation we can expect to encounter some patients with hearing thresholds that are worse for bone conduction than for air conduction. Technical factors also may contribute to bone-air gaps, including problems with the placement or calibration of the bone vibrator.

Audiogram Analysis

Degree of Hearing Loss

When analyzing patient audiograms, audiologists can usually very quickly distinguish different patterns that describe various degrees, configurations, and types of hearing loss. You were introduced to the term *degree of hearing loss* earlier in the chapter during the brief review of the audiogram format and the pure tone average (PTA). As noted then, the degree or amount of hearing loss is often categorized and described with adjectives such as mild, moderate, severe, or profound. Categories of degree of hearing loss were shown earlier in Figure 5.10.

Combinations of the terms are sometimes used to describe hearing loss that falls between categories or hearing loss that falls into different categories for different test frequencies. Audiograms showing such patterns are often described with terms like *mild-to-moderate* or *moderately severe hearing loss*. Nonetheless, determining the degree of hearing loss and its likely impact on communication is one of the important objectives of performing pure tone audiometry.

Configuration of Hearing Loss

Degree of hearing loss often varies across a range of test frequencies from 250 Hz to 8000 Hz. The term **configuration of hearing loss** is typically used to describe how hearing thresholds change as a function of the test frequency. Six commonly encountered configurations of hearing loss are illustrated in Figure 5.16.

Three common hearing loss configurations shown in the top portion of Figure 5.16 are described with the terms *flat, rising*, and *sloping*. With a **flat** hearing loss configuration, hearing thresholds are similar for most test frequencies. The difference in hearing thresholds between any of the test frequencies does not exceed 10 to 15 dB.

Another basic audiogram pattern is called a **rising** configuration. It features poorer hearing thresholds for lower frequencies and better hearing at higher frequencies. Audiograms with a rising pattern are recorded most often in patients with conductive hearing loss.

The **sloping** audiogram configuration shown on the top right of Figure 5.16 is commonly encountered in hearing testing. Hearing thresholds are relatively better at lower frequencies and progressively decrease at higher frequencies. A sloping configuration is associated with some of the most common causes for sensorineural hearing loss, such as hearing loss associated with the aging process.

A variation of the sloping configuration is the *precipitous sloping* hearing loss, as depicted on the bottom left of Figure 5.16. Hearing thresholds are reasonably good for lower test frequencies. Then, hearing thresholds decrease very sharply as test frequency increases, often changing by more than 20 dB per octave.

The *notching* configuration shown next in Figure 5.16 is another variation of a sloping hearing loss. Hearing thresholds are relatively good for lower test frequencies. Thresholds then slope downward, usually reaching maximum hearing loss at one or more test frequencies within the region of 3000 to 6000 Hz. In distinct contrast to the typical sloping hearing configuration, however, hearing threshold levels improve for the highest test frequencies with a notching pattern. A 4000-Hz notching hearing loss configuration is quite common clinically, and associated with a history of exposure to excessive levels of noise.

The final configuration shown in Figure 5.16 is known as a *corner audiogram*. Hearing thresholds are recorded only for a few of the lowest test frequencies and only at very high-intensity levels. For higher-test frequencies, there is no response to pure tone stimulation even at the intensity output limits of an audiometer. The corner audiogram always reflects a profound hearing loss that has a major impact on communication.

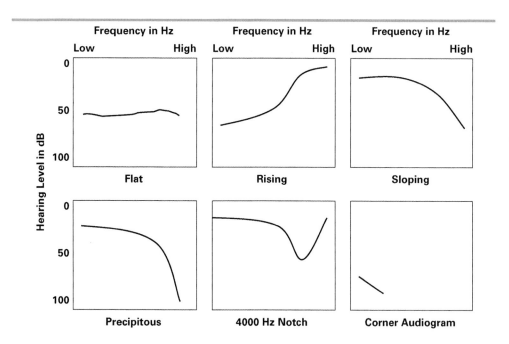

FIGURE 5.16

Six configurations of hearing loss commonly encountered in clinical hearing assessment. *Configuration* is the term used to describe the degree of hearing loss as a function of test frequency. Each configuration is described in the text.

PULLING IT ALL TOGETHER

At the beginning of the chapter you learned about the features of an audiometer, one of the most important pieces of equipment in an audiology clinic. The audiometer allows an audiologist to present different types of sounds to a patient at carefully controlled intensity levels. We reviewed the types of transducers used to present sounds to patients, including supra-aural earphones, insert earphones, bone vibrators, and loudspeakers. You also read about automated audiometers and their role in hearing testing.

Next, we reviewed important pure tone audiometry concepts, including hearing thresholds, audiometric zero, and accepted methods for estimating hearing threshold levels. You now understand how we hear via air conduction and bone conduction and how the information from air conduction and bone conduction pure tone audiometry contributes to the description of hearing loss.

In the second half of the chapter you were introduced to different formats for audiograms, graphs for plotting the results of pure tone hearing testing. You learned about the symbols used to plot hearing thresholds for air and bone conduction for the right and left ears. And, you recognize that in addition to hearing threshold values other important information is included on an audiogram form. The audiogram review led to a discussion of the pure tone average, categories for degree of hearing impairment, and why hearing loss is described in decibels rather than percentage.

Finally, you learned how analysis of an audiogram permits description of the degree and configuration of hearing loss. Importantly, you now can recognize audiogram patterns for normal hearing and three major types of hearing loss—conductive, sensorineural, and mixed hearing loss.

READINGS

American Speech-Language-Hearing Association. (2005). *Guidelines for manual pure-tone threshold audiometry*. [Guidelines]. Available from www.asha.org/policy

Valente, M. (2009). *Pure tone audiometry and masking*. San Diego: Plural Publishing.

6 Speech Audiometry

CHAPTER FOCUS

For most people, the ability to hear and understand speech is vital for communication. All day long, from the time we wake up in the morning until we go to sleep at night, our sense of hearing allows us to detect, perceive, and understand what others are saying. We may hear people speaking on the radio, on television, or via a cell phone. During much of the day we're use our hearing in face-to-face conversations with people. We rely on our ability to quickly and confidently recognize and understand speech at home, at work, in the classroom, and in social settings like at a restaurant, a sports event, or a party. Sometimes in our communication the demands on hearing are rather simple, like when we're carrying on a conversation in a quiet setting with one person who is nearby. Other times, in a noisy environment such as a crowded classroom or a busy restaurant, we may strain to understand what people are saying. Listening can be challenging and stressful under adverse conditions, even for people with entirely normal hearing.

Speech audiometry is the process used to evaluate a patient's ability to detect and recognize speech. It is a necessary part of comprehensive hearing assessment. In response to the question "What brings you to our clinic today?" almost all patients with hearing loss complain that they are having problems hearing speech. A common statement from someone seeking help from an audiologist is: "I can hear people talking, but I can't understand what they are saying."

CHAPTER FOCUS   *Concluded*

You were introduced to the audiometer in Chapter 5 in a discussion about pure tone audiometry. In this chapter, you'll discover that the same diagnostic audiometer is also used to evaluate the patient's ability to hear words and other speech materials. You'll learn in this chapter how audiologists present specially selected words to a patient at specific intensity levels, and you'll discover the different ways a patient may respond to the words. We will talk about techniques and strategies for conducting simple speech audiometry with children and adults. You'll be introduced to three commonly applied hearing tests that involve speech: the speech detection threshold test, the speech recognition threshold test, and the word recognition test. Then you will read about various factors that influence patient performance on these tests.

Building on the knowledge you acquired in the previous chapter, you'll learn about the relation between test findings for pure tone audiometry versus speech audiometry. The information in this chapter is central to clinical audiology. An audiologist has not truly evaluated a patient's hearing unless the assessment includes speech audiometry. Here you'll find out how that's done.

Overview of Speech Audiometry

Various stimuli used in speech audiometry are referred to as **speech materials**. The term *speech materials* refers to different kinds of speech, including consonant-vowel (CV) syllables like "da," single-syllable (monosyllabic) words such as "jar," and two-syllable words like "baseball." Materials used in speech audiometry also consist of more complex units of speech, such as sentences. Often, two or more different speech materials are used during hearing testing of a single patient.

Speech audiometry often begins with an audiologist asking the patient to repeat two-syllable words as the intensity level of the words is systematically decreased. The test yields a threshold that is reported in dB hearing level, like 5 dB HL. Then, later in the test session the patient may be asked to repeat single-syllable words or to point to pictures representing the words that are presented at a fixed intensity level, usually a comfortable listening level. The goal in this hearing test is to measure speech perception or, more accurately, how well the patient recognizes words. Results of a word recognition test are reported as percent correct value, such as 80 percent or 92 percent.

Speech audiometry also includes the assessment of more complex auditory processes. For example, an audiologist may present two different types of speech materials to the patient simultaneously or even two different speech materials to the same ear of the patient at the same time. A patient may be asked to repeat recorded single syllable words presented to one ear while also hearing a recording of many people talking at once in same ear.

Pure tone audiometry and other tests are certainly important in evaluating hearing sensitivity and other aspects of hearing. Speech audiometry, however, plays a special and essential role in hearing assessment. Most patients with hearing loss readily describe the difficulty they have with speech perception. An older married woman might give examples of how her husband doesn't seem to understand what she's saying, adding: "He only hears what he wants to hear." Grandparents relate the ongoing struggles they experience when listening to their grandchildren speak. A military veteran with a hearing loss may relate daily problems communicating with coworkers and supervisors in a noisy workplace while expressing concern about losing his job.

Speech audiometry allows the audiologist to validate these patient complaints, and to document the impact of a patient's hearing loss on communication. The results of speech audiometry contribute importantly to decisions about the need for further diagnostic hearing testing. Speech audiology findings also are very useful in determining which management strategies are most likely to be successful and for developing a management plan for the patient.

Test Equipment

Diagnostic Audiometer

In the previous chapter about pure tone audiometry, you were introduced to the general features of a typical diagnostic audiometer. Here we'll discuss how the same audiometer can be used to perform speech audiometry tests. Most audiometers like the one illustrated in Figure 6.1 have two *channels*. A channel on an audiometer allows an audiologist to select a signal like a pure tone or speech, to change the intensity level of the signal, and to direct the signal to either or both ears of a patient with earphones, a bone vibrator, or a loudspeaker. Each channel is almost like a separate audiometer.

With a two-channel audiometer, it is possible to independently select, control, and deliver to the patient at the same time two different types of signals. For example, words can be presented to the right ear with channel 1 while some type of noise is simultaneously presented to the left ear through channel 2. Or, different words can be presented at the same time to the right ear via channel 1 and to the left ear via channel 2. Only one channel on an audiometer is needed for relatively simple hearing tests. An audiometer with two independent channels is required for more sophisticated hearing testing, including administration of some speech audiometry procedures.

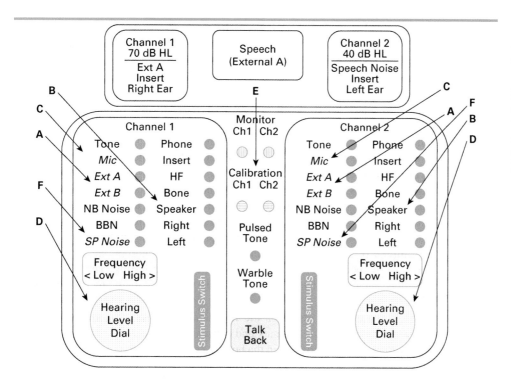

FIGURE 6.1

Schematic diagram of an audiometer highlighting controls used most often in performing speech audiometry. The controls identified with letters (**A, B, C, D, E, F**) are described in the text.

You'll notice in Figure 6.1 two duplicated collections of knobs and buttons, a set on each side of the control panel. The audiometer consists of a separate set of buttons for each channel. Now we'll focus on those controls and features of the audiometer that are used in performing various speech audiometry procedures. Let's begin with the sections of the panel labeled "Channel 1" and "Channel 2" that contain the same fourteen round buttons, two different rectangular shaped pads, and the large hearing level dial.

External and Internal Sources of Speech Signals.   First, locate the buttons identified with an "A" in Figure 6.1. An audiologist can select with the controls labeled *"Ext A"* or *"Ext B"* the *source* of sound that will be presented to the patient. *Ext* is an abbreviation for external, meaning the source of the signal is a device outside of the audiometer. The most common external source is a CD player, another audio player, or a computer tablet. Some older audiometers also have *Tape* controls, in addition to other buttons for external devices. For many years, tape recorders were the external device used most often for speech audiometry.

Modern computer-based audiometers generally have the capability for internal digital storage of unlimited types and quantities of speech audiometry test materials, such as words and sentences. Features of newer computer-based audiometers were discussed in Chapter 5. An example was shown in Figure 5.2B. Specific test materials are quickly and easily selected with a pull-down menu on the computer monitor. A computer-based audiometer also offers the option of customizing for each patient the presentation speed of the speech signals. In other words, the time interval between each word can be shortened for alert patients who respond quickly and then lengthened for other patients, like the elderly, who need a little more time to give a verbal response.

Prerecorded speech materials are recommended regardless of the audiometer used for speech audiometry. Various speech materials recorded in professional sound studios and validated in formal studies are available to audiologists. You'll learn more about the many benefits of recorded speech testing materials later in this chapter.

Speech Presentation via Microphone.   One control used at times during speech audiometry is the *Mic* button, shown as "C" in Figure 6.1. Mic is a common abbreviation for microphone. The microphone is usually part of a lightweight headset worn by an audiologist during the test session. By selecting the *Mic* button, an audiologist activates a microphone for presentation of a speech signal, like words, at a specific intensity level. With the microphone of the audiometer, the audiologist's voice is directed via earphones to one ear or both ears of the patient, or via loudspeakers into the sound-treated room.

An audiometer microphone can be used to communicate with the patient, to provide instructions for tests, or to actually present words during tests. The audiologist selects the desired voice intensity level in dB HL using the *Hearing Level Dial,* shown as "D" in the lower right and left corners of Figure 6.1. Audiologists can verify or monitor voice level by looking at a display, either a needle or digital meter, on the audiometer.

Recorded materials offer a number of advantages in speech audiometry, as you will soon learn. However, a microphone is sometimes an appropriate option for presenting speech signals to young children or elderly adult patients. When using a microphone, an audiologist can change the pace of speech presentation or even quickly stop testing. The *Mic* presentation mode also allows an audiologist to immediately talk with the patient any time during the assessment.

This is an appropriate point to mention the *Talk Back* option on an audiometer. A *Talk Back* feature on the audiometer offers a quick and convenient option for communicating with a patient. The *Talk Back* control is located in the bottom central portion of Figure 6.1. Pressing down on the *Talk Back* button activates the microphone so an audiologist can communicate with the patient for brief periods. For example, the *Talk Back* feature is used to alert a patient that testing is about to begin or that testing has concluded for one ear and is about to resume with the other ear. The *Talk Back* feature doesn't permit precise control of the intensity level of the audiologist's voice and is not used for formal testing with speech. The *Talk Back* system includes a microphone in the sound-treated room, so an audiologist can hear the patient speak at any time.

Control of Speech Intensity. Knobs for controlling the intensity level of speech materials are identified as "E," near the center of Figure 6.1. The knobs in the center of the figure labeled *Calibration* are used to make small adjustments in the intensity of the speech signals during the calibration process, to assure accuracy of the speech signal intensity presented to the patient. Similar-appearing knobs found just above, labeled *Monitor Ch 1* and *Ch 2,* control the intensity of the speech materials for each channel (*Ch*) that is monitored or listened to by the tester.

The intensity level of the speech signal is controlled by turning the *Hearing Level Dial* (attenuator control) located toward the bottom of Figure 6.1 and labeled "D." As usual, turning the dial to the right increases the intensity of the sound and turning the dial to the left decreases the intensity. By manipulating the hearing level knob or key, an audiologist can precisely control intensity of the speech signals presented to the patient. The decibel scale utilized in clinical hearing assessment with speech signals is dB HL, as it is in pure tone audiometry, with 0 dB as the reference for normal hearing. Intensity level can be increased or decreased in 5-dB or smaller steps, from low levels of less than 0 dB HL to levels up to 110 dB HL or higher.

Control of Speech Output. The destination of the signals is selected by buttons located to the right side of the controls for the type and source of speech signals, displayed as "B" in Figure 6.1. An audiologist can send speech signals to all of the usual transducers that you've already learned about, including insert earphones, supra-aural earphones, loudspeakers, or even a bone vibrator. The same output knobs are used for both pure tone and speech audiometry. If supra-aural earphones are employed in speech audiometry, the audiologist selects *Phone,* whereas *Insert* is chosen to present speech with insert earphones. Other transducers that can be selected from the control panel include a bone vibrator (*Bone*) or a loudspeaker in the sound-treated test room (*Speaker*).

To reiterate, with a two-channel audiometer various types of sounds can be routed to the earphone for the right or the left ear, a *monaural* listening condition, or to both ears at the same time for a *binaural* listening condition. Speech sounds may also be presented to a patient via one or more loudspeakers located in the sound-treated test room. Speech audiometry with loudspeakers, rather than earphones, is often performed with very young children and with patients who are wearing hearing aids or other electronic hearing devices.

Masking Noise. As with pure tone audiometry, masking noise may be needed during speech audiometry testing to keep the non-test ear from contributing to the patient's response. The masking sound called speech noise (*Sp Noise*) is selected with buttons toward each side in Figure 6.1. These controls are identified as "F." Speech noise includes energy within a frequency range that is typical of most speech signals. Masking in pure tone and speech audiometry is reviewed in the next chapter.

Devices for Presenting Recorded Speech Materials

Devices used for recorded speech materials in audiology have changed considerably over the years. Most of the devices employed in hearing testing for well over sixty years until quite recently are probably unfamiliar to most of the readers of this book. Former devices for recorded speech materials included turntables used to spin vinyl records, reel-to-reel tape recorders, and cassette tape recorders.

Speech materials in audiology clinics today are invariably stored in digital format, either on CDs or on relatively small external devices, such as iPods, MP3 players, and other personal digital players. The external device is connected to the audiometer with a typical audio cable. As noted already, on modern computer-based audiometers speech materials can be accessed quickly in digital format, without reliance on an external device.

Sources of Recorded Speech Materials

There is no single source or vendor for recorded speech materials. Several small companies sell recordings of selected tests developed by various researchers during the past fifty years. A number of speech audiometry tests on CDs can be acquired from an audiology service that is part of the Veterans Administration system. Given the widespread practice of downloading information, such as music, from the Internet, audiologists might also soon have ready access to online files of speech audiometry recordings. Meanwhile, an Internet search will reveal vendors who supply tests used in speech audiometry.

Test Environment

Sound Requirements

You learned in Chapter 4 that a quiet test environment is desirable for any type of hearing testing. Ambient background sound may interfere with accurate measurement of hearing thresholds when stimulus sounds are presented at faint intensity levels. Pure tone hearing testing is almost always adversely affected by ambient noise. In contrast, the influence of ambient background noise on speech audiometry varies, depending on what test is performed.

Threshold Measures. Speech audiometry procedures that measure the detection or the threshold of speech are often conducted at faint intensity levels, particularly for patients who have normal hearing sensitivity. Let's assume that a patient has an audiogram with hearing threshold levels in the range of 5 to 10 dB HL. You'll recall from reading Chapter 5 that the region of normal hearing sensitivity for adults is defined by thresholds of 20 dB HL or better, whereas for children normal hearing sensitivity is defined by thresholds of 15 dB or better. Speech thresholds are usually found at intensity levels close to the patient's pure tone hearing thresholds.

If testing were conducted in a typical sound environment and not in a sound-treated room, excessive ambient noise could interfere with the normal-hearing patient's ability to detect or recognize words presented at low intensity levels. The patient's difficulty hearing faint sounds in background noise would probably lead to invalid test results. A patient's speech threshold might be recorded at 15 or 20 dB HL due to interference from background noise, whereas better thresholds would have been obtained in an adequately quiet test setting.

Supra-Threshold Measures. Some speech audiometry procedures are performed at **supra-threshold** intensity levels. That is, words or sentences are presented at intensity levels considerably higher than the patient's hearing thresholds. For persons with normal or near-normal hearing sensitivity, a modest amount of ambient noise may not affect the outcome of supra-threshold tests. Ambient noise consists mostly of sound in the low-frequency region. Ambient noise interferes more with the ability to hear low-frequency speech than higher-frequency speech sounds. A person with normal hearing sensitivity can often use high-frequency hearing when responding to the words.

Earphones versus Loudspeakers. You may recall from our discussion of the test environment for pure tone audiometry in Chapter 4 that acceptable noise levels, the maximum levels of noise permitted during hearing testing, vary depending on the type of earphone used in testing. The level of ambient background noise reaching the inner ear is reduced considerably with properly fitted insert earphones when compared to supra-aural earphones that fit over the ear. Acceptable noise levels in the test setting are even lower for loudspeakers because there is nothing over the patient's ears to block ambient sound from reaching the inner ear.

The quiet test environment provided by a sound-treated room is always recommended for speech audiometry, but a quiet test setting is particularly important for measurement of the detection and threshold levels for speech and when the speech is presented via loudspeakers.

Control Room. A discussion of the sound environment for speech audiometry should also include mention of the room where the audiologist is located during testing. The term *control room* is typically used to describe the room adjacent to the sound-treated test booth where the audiologist and audiometer are located. Background sound in the control room has no impact on measurement of pure tones. The pure tone stimuli are generated by the audiometer and delivered directly to the patient in the sound-treated room, often with insert earphones that further attenuate ambient noise in the environment. There really is not a way for the pure tone stimuli to be affected by ambient sound within the control room. Similarly, noise in the control room is not a factor in the test process when recorded speech materials from an external device are delivered through an audiometer and then earphones or a loudspeaker to the patient.

In contrast, noise levels in the control room can have a very serious negative impact on testing when an audiologist presents speech to the patient via a microphone. Background sound, including unwanted noise produced by equipment or someone in the control room, is detected with the same microphone used to present speech materials. A patient will hear this background noise along with the speech stimuli.

Patient Responsibilities and Responses

We will now focus on patient responsibilities and responses during hearing assessment with speech materials. Since the patient's role in speech audiometry often differs considerably for adults and children, each patient population will be discussed separately

Adults

The responsibilities and responses are similar whether the adult patient is undergoing speech audiometry or pure tone hearing testing. For both types of testing, patients must listen closely for sounds, including very faint ones, and they must respond with some kind of motor activity whenever they hear a sound. Any adult who is undergoing a test of hearing thresholds must (1) understand the task and what is expected of him or her, (2) remember the task until testing is completed, (3) attend to and listen carefully for the sounds throughout the testing, (4) be motivated to cooperate and do his or her best for the duration of the testing, and (5) produce the requested response to sound. In both pure tone and speech audiometry, an adult patient may also need to ignore or not be distracted by non-test sounds, including noise presented to the non-test ear. The listener variables affecting a patient's performance during behavioral hearing testing in general that were summarized in Table 4.3 in Chapter 4 apply as well to speech audiometry.

In some ways the types of responses required of a patient during speech audiometry are distinctly different than responses required for pure tone audiometry. The patient undergoing pure tone audiometry usually responds to tonal sounds by either pushing a button or raising a hand. In contrast, the most common response mode during clinical speech audiometry is verbal, that is, the patient vocally repeats the speech test item, such as a word or a sentence. A verbal response is considerably more complex than pressing a button or raising a hand. It is also more challenging for the audiologist to judge whether the patient's verbal response is correct or incorrect. Other response modes during adult speech audiometry include identification of a word or sentence by pointing to a picture and, less often, writing down the test item.

As in any behavioral hearing testing, an audiologist must instruct the patient adequately on the test process before conducting speech audiometry. It is also important to confirm that the patient understands the instructions. In addition, before speech audiometry begins, the audiologist needs to informally assess the patient's speech quality and ability. The audiologist's accuracy in scoring the patient's spoken responses depends in part on how distinctly and clearly the patient produces the responses.

In most cases, speech audiometry proceeds quickly. Test items are presented every few seconds as the patient promptly produces a clear vocal response that is easily scored by the audiologist as correct or incorrect. The speed and accuracy of conventional speech audiometry using a verbal response mode can immediately diminish, however, with patients who have speech or language impairment. Examples of adult patients with speech and/or language impairment include those with serious cognitive deficits, patients who have suffered a stroke or traumatic brain injury (TBI), and patients with a disease or disorder affecting the vocal tract. Whenever the clarity of an adult patient's verbal response is poor, an audiologist must implement an alternative testing technique using a nonverbal response mode, such as a written or picture-pointing response.

Children

As you would expect, techniques and strategies used during speech audiometry with children are very much dependent on the patient's age, especially developmental age. A child's age is a performance factor during speech audiometry just as it is with pure tone hearing testing. An audiologist must always consider developmental age and ability during pediatric hearing assessment with speech audiometry. A child's ability to respond to speech changes with development and maturation of the nervous system. The child's language status, especially vocabulary level, is a particularly critical factor in the accuracy of test results, since words or sentences are used in speech audiometry.

Challenges associated with speech audiometry in children have long been recognized (e.g., Jerger, 1984; Lawson & Peterson, 2011). Audiologists can select from a variety of test procedures designed specifically for assessing speech thresholds and speech recognition in young children, including tests incorporating words that are within the vocabulary of preschool and young school-age children. The impact of immature speech production and articulation on the accuracy of speech audiometry in young children is also well appreciated. The typical solution is to rely on a picture identification response mode. In other words, the child points to a picture representing the test word when it is presented.

Speech Threshold Measures

Detection or Awareness of Speech

One of the simplest speech audiometry measures is the **speech detection threshold (SDT)**, also referred to as **speech awareness threshold (SAT)**. The recommended term is *speech detection threshold,* or *SDT* (ASHA, 1988). SDT is the lowest intensity level in dB HL at which a person is aware of or can detect the presence of a speech signal. Measurement of the SDT does not require the patient to repeat or understand speech. Only awareness is needed for a correct response.

With older children or adults, the SDT is often measured using words that are also incorporated in other speech tests, such as common two-syllable words like *toothbrush* or *baseball*. The patient is instructed to respond whenever he or she hears something by pressing the response button for the audiometer, or by saying "yes." The patient is reminded that he or she does not need to attempt to repeat the word.

When the SDT is measured in infants and young children, an audiologist typically does not use formal speech audiometry test materials and certainly cannot require a button or verbal response from the patient. Instead, an audiologist observes the child's head turning or localization response to the presentation of simple and often nonsense forms of speech that attract the child's attention. For example, using the microphone on the audiometer the audiologist may verbalize in an expressive voice: "Buh-buh-buh," "UH-oh," "Look here!" or "Look here [child's name]!"

Relation to Audiogram. For children and adults, the intensity level at which speech is detected generally agrees with the lowest pure tone hearing threshold in the test ear within the frequency region from 250 to 4000 Hz. In other words, the SDT is closest to the best threshold on an audiogram. And, the SDT can be up to 10 dB better than the speech recognition threshold in the same person (Chaiklin, 1959).

You might reasonably ask, "What is the value of the SDT if it only reflects hearing sensitivity for a very limited frequency region and it doesn't agree with speech recognition threshold?" and "Doesn't the SDT seriously misrepresent hearing thresholds at other frequencies?" These are good questions. Indeed, information from the SDT is limited. The SDT is typically measured only in patients who for a variety of reasons cannot produce valid responses in other speech audiometry tests. Whenever clinically feasible, speech recognition measurement is conducted, with the patient repeating words rather than simply responding to the presence of speech.

Clinical Value. In some patient populations, such as infants, persons with reduced cognitive functioning, and persons with profound hearing loss, only SDT measurement may be possible. Other speech audiometry procedures may not be feasible for auditory or nonauditory reasons. At the least, the SDT provides information on the minimum intensity level the patient requires for detection of speech. If, for example, an SDT of 50 dB HL is recorded in the sound field using loudspeakers rather than earphones, we can safely assume that the patient has at least a moderate hearing loss in the better-hearing ear.

Even though the SDT provides no information on how well a person perceives or understands speech, the relatively limited information gleaned from SDT measurement may be just what is needed to prompt further diagnostic hearing assessment. In our example, hearing loss of 50 dB or greater would interfere with communication and would interfere with speech and language acquisition in a young child. Additional diagnostic hearing assessment would be clinically indicated to define hearing threshold levels at different test frequencies for each ear. Information obtained from the diagnostic testing in turn usually leads to decisions about appropriate management, such as amplification of sound with hearing aids.

Threshold for Speech

Speech recognition threshold measurement is a common procedure in clinical audiology. Threshold for speech recognition is defined simply as the faintest or lowest intensity level in dB HL at which a person can correctly recognize or identify about 50% of words that are presented (ASHA, 1988). Recognition or identification of speech, such as specific words, is a more complex response than simple speech detection or awareness.

Different Terms for Threshold for Speech. Since the 1940s, various terms have been used to describe threshold for speech recognition. Also, different test materials have been introduced and sometimes debated. **Spondee words** are a common form of speech material used for measuring the threshold for speech recognition. Examples of spondee words are shown in Table 6.1. The term *spondee* refers to a meter in poetry consisting of two long or stressed syllables. Spondee words consist of two syllables that are presented to the patient with equal stress on each syllable.

Spondee words used in clinical measurement of the threshold of speech were first developed and used in clinical procedures during and immediately following World War II. Early research on spondee word materials was conducted by some of the pioneers in audiology, including Ira Hirsh, who conducted research in the famous Psycho-Acoustic Laboratory (PAL) at Harvard University (Formby & Musiek, 2011). Over thirty years ago, the term **spondee threshold (ST)** was recommended (ASHA, 1979) to describe measurement of the threshold of speech. The more general term *speech threshold* (also abbreviated ST) is preferable to spondee threshold as it is not limited just to spondee words.

Two other terms for describing measurement of the threshold for speech recognition are **speech reception threshold** and **speech recognition threshold**, both abbreviated as **SRT**. The term *speech reception* threshold has been criticized as too vague. That is, speech reception does not distinguish between speech detection, speech recognition, and speech discrimination.

The term *speech discrimination* has yet another meaning. In a discrimination task, the subject or patient must judge similarities or differences between two or more stimuli. A speech discrimination test assesses the patient's ability to distinguish between two or more words that usually sound very similar.

The term *speech recognition threshold (SRT)* is currently preferred for the measure of threshold of speech. We will use this phrase, abbreviated SRT, in the following discussion. Actually, Harvey Fletcher first used the phrase "speech recognition" more than eighty years ago. You may recall that Fletcher was featured in Leaders & Luminaries in Chapter 2.

TABLE 6.1
A sample of spondee words used for measurement of speech thresholds.

Word	Normal Threshold (dB SPL)
hot dog	15.2
whitewash	16.4
iceberg	16.5
airplane	17.1
hothouse	17.2
inkwell	18.5
birthday	18.8
woodwork	19.2
toothbrush	19.7
daybreak	20.3
farewell	20.3
sunset	21.3
greyhound	21.6

Measurement of Speech Recognition Threshold. In clinical audiology, SRT is typically measured with spondee words, although any type of speech can be used. Over the years, more than a dozen various techniques were reported for measurement of the SRT (Lawson & Peterson, 2011). A generally accepted method (ASHA, 1988) is described here.

Before SRT measurement is formally started, patients are instructed to repeat each word, even if the words are very faint, and to guess at words if necessary. Then, the patient may be given an opportunity to become familiar with the words to be used in SRT measurement by listening to them at a comfortable intensity level. We'll soon discuss further the influence of familiarization on SRT measurement outcome.

SRT testing generally begins at a comfortable intensity level. If normal hearing is suspected, the spondee words are initially presented at an intensity level of about 30 to 40 dB HL. An intensity of 30 to 40 dB HL is a comfortable listening level for most normal hearers, not too soft and not too loud. With young children an SRT is often determined first to provide some estimate of hearing sensitivity before pure tone hearing testing is attempted.

Steps in SRT measurement are similar to those used in pure tone audiometry. If the patient correctly repeats one or two spondee words at the initial comfortable level, the intensity level is decreased by 10 dB and one or two words are again presented. Intensity level is decreased in 10-dB steps with two words presented at each step until the patient no longer repeats two words correctly. Then, intensity level is increased 5 dB and spondee word recognition again assessed.

The SRT is defined as the intensity level at which the patient correctly repeats between 50 and 70 percent of the spondee words. As shown in Table 6.1, the actual threshold for spondee words in normal hearers varies among the different word items. In a group of normal hearers, the speech thresholds range from as low as 15.2 dB for the words *hot dog* to 21.6 dB for the word *greyhound,* a difference between items of more than 6 dB. A difference in thresholds among words, that is, lack of homogeneity, is a well-recognized finding (Curry & Cox, 1966).

Relation Between SDT and SRT. What is the relation between speech detection threshold (SDT) and the speech recognition threshold (SRT)? The answer to this question would be helpful in interpreting SDT findings in young children for whom SRT measurement is not feasible. The SDT is typically measured at intensity levels from 6 to 10 dB lower or better than the intensity levels for SRT, even when the same words are used for each measure (Chaiklin, 1959).

Several explanations have been offered for the difference between SDT and SRT (Wilson & Margolis, 1983). More energy is apparently needed to provide enough information for recognizing a specific word among a group of other words, with less energy required to simply detect the presence of a word. Also, within any single word the intensity level of different sounds may vary substantially. For example, a vowel sound may be 25 dB more intense than the energy associated with a consonant (Fletcher & Steinberg, 1929).

In addition, detection of a word requires only audibility of the vowel sound, whereas correct recognition of the word verified by repetition depends on adequate information for audibility plus recognition of both the consonant and vowel sounds. Again, the amount of energy associated with different vowels and consonants varies from one spondee word to the next. So, test words are not identical or homogeneous. Finally, physical characteristics, including the acoustic properties, are not exactly the same for the words.

Familiarization. Before beginning actual measurement of the SRT, some audiologists first present all of the words at a comfortable intensity level to assure that they are familiar to the patient. Although the familiarization process requires an extra minute or two, it is often included in clinical SRT measurement. Familiarization generally increases test-retest reliability and enhances the correlation between threshold of speech and the pure tone average. Interestingly, research shows that the effect or benefit of familiarization varies considerably among spondee words. It is possible to construct a list of words that yield an SRT unaffected by the familiarization process.

Findings of a study in 1975 of familiarization in SRT measurement are worth noting. Hearing test data were collected from forty-eight adult patients undergoing an an ear, nose, and throat examination. Pure tone hearing threshold levels were no greater than 30 dB HL in the speech frequency region of 250 to 4000 Hz, and none of the patients had ear disease. The study resulted in two clinically relevant points about familiarization in the measurement of SRT.

For some words, familiarization doesn't have any effect on the SRT (a 0-dB change). In addition, for some rather common spondee words, such as *baseball*, *armchair*, and *airplane*, the average improvement in SRT is minimal, less than 3 dB. Yet the threshold for some spondee words, such as *drawbridge*, *inkwell*, and even the common word *cowboy,* is improved by 11 dB or more when the subject is first introduced to or familiarized with the words. Put another way, first familiarizing the patient with these words will result in better thresholds, whereas elevated and inaccurate measures of threshold will occur if the familiarization process is not followed.

Based on the results of this study, it is possible to select words for measurement of SRT that are associated with little or no familiarization effect. By using only these words in SRT measurement, an audiologist can eliminate the familiarization process, thereby saving valuable test time.

Factors Influencing SRT. Familiarization is just one factor contributing to variability in measurement of SRT. Spondee words differ from each other in many ways. They are not homogeneous. The different effect of familiarization for various spondee words is an example of the heterogeneity of spondee words. Several other factors contribute to differences in thresholds among spondee words for persons with entirely normal hearing.

Differences in word thresholds for a single normal hearer are partly due to variations in the total amount of energy and other physical characteristics of the words. How the words are presented to the patient may also affect the measured SRT. SRT performance is enhanced when the interval between words is constant. The fixed interval, sometimes called the listening interval, alerts the patient to when another word will be presented.

Additional factors that influence the speech threshold variability include physical characteristics of the speech, such as the total amount of energy in each word. Soon you'll learn about another clinically relevant factor, the presentation mode. Whether the words are spoken by the tester using a microphone or presented from a research-based recording has an important influence on SRT.

Relation of SRT to Pure Tone Thresholds. You learned about the relation between the pure tone average (PTA) and the threshold for speech in Chapter 5. To review briefly, the conventional PTA is the average of hearing threshold levels for three frequencies: 500, 1000, and 2000 Hz. Calculation is as follows: PTA = (hearing thresholds for 500 Hz + 1000 Hz + 2000 Hz)/3. For example, if hearing thresholds were 10 dB for a 500-Hz tone, 20 dB for a 1000-Hz tone and 40 dB for a 2000-Hz tone, then the PTA would be: (10 + 20 + 40)/3, or 70/3, or 23.3 dB HL, rounded off to 23 dB HL.

The PTA provides a handy way to quantify hearing sensitivity for a central portion of the **speech frequency region**. However, it is very important to keep in mind that hearing for frequencies below 500 Hz and especially for higher test frequencies like 3000 or 4000 Hz is also essential for accurately perceiving speech in quiet and in noisy listening settings. In other words, neither the PTA nor the SRT reflect all of the frequencies required for optimal speech perception and speech understanding.

Research on the prediction of speech recognition thresholds from pure tone thresholds dates back to the 1940s, when audiology was just beginning as a profession (Carhart, 1946; Fletcher, 1950).Raymond Carhart was among the first to recommend the use of the three-frequency PTA for predicting the threshold of recognition for spondee words and other speech materials (Carhart, 1946).

The PTA predicts the SRT within about ±6 dB. For example, we would expect a SRT test outcome of no less than 10 dB and no more than 20 dB for a patient with a PTA of 15 dB. For a variety of reasons, substantial discrepancies between the PTA and SRT are sometimes found in certain auditory disorders (Wilson & Margolis, 1983). For patients with very poor speech recognition abilities, the SRT may be lower or worse than the PTA. This discrepancy can be explained by the fundamental difference in the auditory task for the two measures.

Also, pure tone hearing testing is a detection task requiring the patient to detect the presence of a very simple stimulus. As the term implies, speech <u>recognition</u> threshold requires the patient to recognize the speech signal, like a specific spondee word. The patient's accurate recognition of the word is typically confirmed by assessing the patient's ability to accurately repeat the word or to point to a picture that represents the word. Speech recognition performance may be markedly decreased in persons with neural auditory dysfunction, involving the eighth cranial (audiovestibular) nerve or the central auditory nervous system, even though hearing sensitivity for pure tones is normal.

Is the SRT Ever Better than the PTA? Lower or better thresholds for speech recognition testing than for pure tone testing are sometimes encountered clinically. In fact, better thresholds for speech than for pure tones is one of the characteristic findings for patients with *false* or *exaggerated hearing loss*. You'll learn more about this interesting clinical condition in Chapter 15.

Possible explanations for the difference in thresholds between speech and pure tone thresholds that need to be explored include technical problems, like improperly placed earphones and patient-related factors, such as with patient understanding of the task required for the test. At the least, a large discrepancy between thresholds for speech and pure tone signals should be critically examined, perhaps with an objective hearing test that does not rely on a behavioral response from the patient.

Picture-pointing SRT Testing. For older children and adults, SRT is typically measured by having the patient repeat the words as they are presented at gradually lower intensity levels. With younger children, however, more effective SRT measurement often involves a picture-pointing task rather than a verbal response.

With the nonverbal response mode, an audiologist instructs the child to point to a picture of the word that the child hears. An audiologist, an assistant, or perhaps the child's caregiver holds in front of the child a laminated sheet of paper containing four to six pictures representing different spondee words to be used during SRT measurement. Often the pictures or photographs are quite colorful and appealing to young children. The sheet in Figure 6.2 shows pictures or photographs of two-syllable spondee words that are in the vocabulary of a young child, for example, *toothbrush, airplane, cowboy,* and so forth.

FIGURE 6.2

Pictures of spondee words used for the measurement of speech recognition threshold using a picture-pointing task. The child points to the picture of the word that he or she hears, such as *ice cream, cowboy, toothbrush,* or *popcorn.*

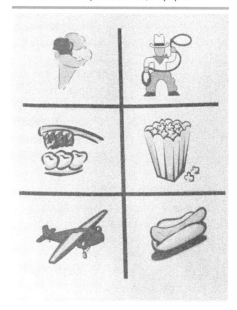

Before measurement of speech threshold begins, an audiologist remains in the sound room with the child for a few minutes to verify that the child is familiar with the words and the pictures, understands the task, and is capable of performing the task. An audiologist may say the words at a comfortable high-intensity level while encouraging the child to point to the picture of the word he or she hears, verbally reinforcing this behavior. An example of verbal reinforcement is, "That's right, Jason, you point to the picture of the word you hear, even if it's very soft. Good job!"

Body Part Identification SRT Testing. Another nonverbal response option is sometimes helpful in SRT testing of young children. When pictures representing children's spondee words are not available, or a child for any reason cannot or will not perform the picture-pointing task during the practice session, speech reception threshold can be estimated by simply asking the child to point to selected body parts. Pointing to body parts is a simple yet effective SRT test strategy. Let's review a typical scenario for the body parts response mode.

A young child sits on a caregiver's lap in a designated location within the sound-treated room. An audiologist sits at the audiometer in an adjacent control room speaking into a microphone while viewing the child through a window. Beginning at an intensity on the hearing level dial that is probably easily heard by the child, the audiologist says to the child "point to your MOUTH ... show me your MOUTH" (Note: The audiologist's emphasis in pronouncing the words is shown by the capital letters). The audiologist gives the child plenty of verbal reinforcement for a correct response, such as "Good job!," That's right!," "Good girl!" Once the child gives a response, the audiologist decreases the intensity level and says the name of another body part, such as "Point to your NOSE . . . show me your NOSE . . . Yes, that is your NOSE!" The process continues with words presented at different intensity levels until the child's SRT is defined for each ear with earphones or for the better-hearing ear with a loudspeaker.

Most older children and adults readily participate in a test requiring repetition of the test words. Young children, however, may not be similarly engaged in a task involving simple repetition of spondee words. The active participation required of the child in picture-pointing and body part identification tasks helps to maintain a young patient's interest and often permits adequate measurement of threshold for speech.

SRT Measurement by Bone Conduction. Although not routinely done during hearing assessment, it is possible to measure the SRT with the words presented by bone conduction rather than with the conventional air conduction technique via an earphone or loudspeaker. The bone vibrator is placed on the mastoid bone or the forehead, as it would be for pure tone testing. Spondee words are then presented through a bone vibrator to the patient with the intensity level systematically decreased until speech threshold is determined. Either live voice or recorded test materials may be used.

SRT measurement by bone conduction is sometimes helpful with young children. Due to their developmental age, young children may be unable to participate in the test process for the length of time required to obtain both air and bone conduction hearing thresholds for a number of pure tone frequencies. Bone conduction SRT measurement with words can be completed rather quickly while providing a reasonable estimate of hearing within the speech frequency region.

Since bone conduction stimulation may reach each inner ear, it may not be possible to determine which ear is contributing to the patient's response. The words presented via bone conduction might be reaching the right ear, the left ear, or both ears, regardless of where the

 ClinicalConnection

You'll learn in Chapters 8 through 10 about objective tests of auditory function and how behavioral and objective test procedures are combined into a test battery for accurate diagnosis of hearing loss and auditory processing in the central nervous system.

bone vibrator is located. Young children often don't comply with the placement of earphones, so it is not always possible to measure SRT with appropriate masking noise in the non-test ear in order to verify that the response is arising from the test ear.

Live Voice versus Recorded Techniques

We've not yet discussed exactly how speech is presented to patients during SRT measurement. There are two general approaches for delivery of speech signals to the patient when performing a speech audiometry procedure including SRT.

Monitored Live Voice. One presentation mode is referred to as the **monitored live voice (MLV)** technique. An audiologist speaks into a microphone that is connected to the audiometer. The phrase *monitored live voice* requires a brief explanation. We all appreciate the difference between a live music performance and a music recording. The same concept applies to monitored live voice versus recorded speech audiometry. MLV means that the tester is speaking directly to the patient, not using a recording of speech. During the test, the audiologist closely monitors voice level in dB with a meter on the audiometer.

With the MLV technique, an audiologist has complete control over the rate at which words are presented to the patient and the speed with which the test is performed. If the patient is slow to respond, words can be presented at a slower rate, with more time between any two words. In contrast, the words can be presented rapidly if the patient responds quickly to each one. Flexibility in managing the time interval between words is an advantage when performing speech audiometry in young children and also sometimes with elderly adults.

Despite the appeal of flexibility in presenting words, routine use of the MLV technique is not recommended in speech audiometry (ASHA, 1988). Reliance on the MLV technique increases variability in the intensity level of the test words and contributes to unpredictable inconsistencies in the patient's responses (Hall & Mueller, 1997; Kruel et al., 1968).

Some factors potentially influencing the consistency and accuracy of speech audiometry findings with the monitored live voice method are summarized in Table 6.2. In combination, the factors increase variability and reduce reliability of speech threshold measurement. The information in Table 6.2 explains why monitored live voice is generally not recommended in clinical measurement of speech threshold or for other speech audiometry procedures.

Recorded Speech. The other option for performing speech audiometry is to rely on *recorded speech* materials. Recordings used in speech audiometry are professionally made in commercial sound studios. The recordings consist of carefully selected words clearly spoken by a person without any distinct dialect. With recorded speech materials the tester can be confident of consistency each time they are used. In other words, there will be no difference in the acoustical features of the words from one test to the next for a patient, from one patient to the next in the clinic, or even from one clinic to other facilities that use the same recordings.

- Findings obtained with different talkers are not necessarily equivalent.
- Findings for the same talker at different test sessions may not be equivalent.
- Acoustic characteristics of the speech signal are highly variable from one speaker to the next. Speaker differences include pitch, articulation, rate of speech, and dialect.
- The difficulty of the words depends to some extent on who is talking.
- With an open microphone, background noise reaches the patient when examiner is not seated in a sound-treated room, or when examiner shares a control room with other persons.

TABLE 6.2
Factors potentially influencing the consistency and accuracy of speech audiometry findings with the monitored live voice method for speech audiometry.

In the early years of audiology, recorded speech materials were available on vinyl records that spun around on turntables mounted on or located near the audiometer. In the 1960s and 1970s, the record players gave way to tape recorders of various sizes and shapes and then, within the past ten years, to CD players. Now, some audiologists and audiology students connect the latest generation of digital audio devices to audiometers for presentation of speech materials developed and initially recorded over fifty years ago!

Until recently when performing speech audiometry with recorded materials there was an unavoidable trade-off between the advantage of consistency and the disadvantage of an inflexible and somewhat time-consuming presentation mode. When recorded speech materials are delivered to the patient, test time is typically prolonged by a fixed-time interval of two or three seconds between each item, such as each word. Let's say the time interval between words is three seconds. If a list of twenty-five words is presented to each ear, for a total of fifty words, then the sum of all the time intervals would amount to 150 seconds, or two-and-a-half minutes of test time.

Speech Audiometry with Computer-Based Audiometers. The introduction of computer-based audiometers within the past few years offers a solution to the problem of the fixed speed with which recorded words are presented to the patient. High-quality recorded speech materials, used for many years in clinical audiology, can be readily accessed from the computer. The rate of presentation for the items can be easily controlled and varied by an audiologist using several techniques. The words can be presented to any given patient at a consistent rate, or the rate can be adjusted as necessary for any patient. For example, the presentation rate can be slowed down to an interval of four or five seconds between words or sped up to one or two seconds between words, depending on how slowly or how quickly a patient responds.

Alternatively, with a computer-based audiometer patients can press a button to activate the presentation of each new word as soon as they have responded to the previous word and are ready for another one. Additionally, an audiologist can use the computer-based audiometer to keep a tally of correct and incorrect patient responses. Computer-based audiometer technology really offers the best of both worlds. That is, the new technology permits the speed and flexibility of the MLV method in speech audiometry, but the standardization and consistency of recorded test materials. Word presentation and test speed can be customized for each patient to optimize test efficiency without compromising consistency or accuracy.

Verification of Intensity Level. Verification of intensity level is an important step that must be taken before beginning speech threshold measurement. As you may recall from reading Chapter 5, an audiometer includes a display or meter that is used for fine-tuning intensity level. Intensity level is usually adjusted over a range of 10 to 15 dB with a knob and a VU (volume unit) meter located on the face of the audiometer. VU meters in older audiometers consisted of a needle and a meter, typically ranging from ⊠10 to +5 dB. Modern audiometers sometimes feature a VU meter with a digital display rather than a needle. When the VU meter indicates 0, the intensity level reaching the patient is accurately described with the intensity knob on the audiometer.

When speech signals are presented with a microphone using the MLV approach rather than with a recording, an audiologist must take care to constantly monitor vocal intensity level. Intensity of the tester's voice must be maintained as close as possible to "0 dB" on the VU meter. If an audiologist's voice is too soft and the VU meter registers below 0 dB, then the intensity level of the speech signals actually delivered to the patient will be below the intended level. For example, if an audiologist's voice is at –5 dB on the VU meter and the intended intensity level in speech threshold measurement is 60 dB, the actual intensity level of the words presented to the patient is 55 dB.

You can readily appreciate how the accuracy of intensity level on the VU meter directly affects the accuracy of speech threshold measurement. When the MLV approach is relied upon in conducting speech threshold measurement, tester experience, skill, and attention to the VU meter are factors affecting the accuracy of test results.

Verification of intensity for recorded speech materials is more straightforward and simple. Prior to actual presentation of recorded speech materials, an audiologist calibrates the recording using the VU meter on the audiometer. The recording itself begins with a calibration tone or "cal tone" of 1000 Hz. The duration of the calibration tone is usually a minute or more, giving the audiologist time to make fine adjustments in the intensity level until the VU meter registers "0 dB." Once calibration is completed, the intensity level for all of the speech materials on the recording corresponds to the intensity level presented to the patient.

Clearly, the major advantage of reliance on recorded speech materials in clinical audiology is consistency in test results. In theory, a patient tested with specific recorded speech materials presented after calibration via an audiometer should yield the same speech audiometer findings from one test session to another in a clinic or even from one clinic to another anywhere in the country.

Loudness Levels

Up to this point in the chapter, we've discussed the use of speech signals in measurement of hearing thresholds. Pure tone hearing threshold measurement was covered in the previous chapter. Audiologists also make supra-threshold hearing measurements at intensity levels considerably greater that those required for detection of sound. The term *supra-threshold measurement* is probably self-explanatory. It refers to assessment of auditory function at intensity levels well above hearing threshold. Much hearing testing done by audiologists is carried out not at a patient's threshold for the sound, but instead at higher intensity levels. Supra-threshold testing is conducted with pure tones and with speech signals.

Most Comfortable Level. One supra-threshold measure is the **most comfortable level** or **MCL**. As the term implies, MCL is the intensity level that a person perceives as comfortable to listen to: not too soft and not too loud. The MCL can be measured for pure tone signals (Kamm, Dirks, & Mickey, 1978) and for speech signals, like words or ongoing everyday speech (Cox et al., 1997).

First, an audiologist explains to the patient that the MCL is the range of loudness level that seems comfortable for everyday listening. Loudness levels are often measured while the patient holds a chart like the one shown in Table 6.3. Sample instructions are also indicated on the chart (Cox et al., 1997). Patients can indicate verbally when pure tones or words are heard at a comfortable level or they can point to each loudness level on the chart as an audiologist gradually increases the intensity of the pure tones or words.

Pure tones and speech signals can be easily heard at the MCL, and they are not uncomfortably loud. For example, a patient listening to a radio or television would probably want loudness of speech and music at MCL. Measurement of the MCL begins 5 to 10 dB above a patient's hearing threshold for pure tones, already available from his or her audiogram. Intensity of the pure tone or speech signal is gradually but progressively increased in 5-dB steps until the patient reports that it is at a comfortable level. Intensity level of the tone or speech is then decreased quickly.

Testing then continues with the presentation of a sound at progressively higher intensity levels until, once again, the patient reports that the sound is at a comfortable level. An average MCL is estimated from the comfortable intensity values as measured with a small sample of ascending and descending measurements. Most normal-hearing persons will report MCLs for pure tones or speech that are 40 to 50 dB HL higher than audiogram thresholds.

TABLE 6.3
A chart for estimating
most comfortable level
(MCL) and loudness
discomfort level (LDL).

Cox Contour Test Loudness Chart

7. Uncomfortably loud

6. Loud, But Okay

5. Comfortable, But Slightly Loud

4. Comfortable

3. Comfortable, But Slightly Soft

2. Soft

1. Very Soft

Instructions: The purpose of this test is for you to judge the loudness of different sounds. You will hear sounds that increase and decrease in volume. You must make a judgment about how loud the sounds are. Pretend you are listening to the radio at that volume. How loud would it be? After each sound, tell me which of these categories best describes the loudness. Keep in mind that an uncomfortably loud sound is louder than you would ever choose on your radio, no matter what mood you are in.

Source: Cox, R. M., Alexander, C. C., & Gray, G. A. (1997). The contour test of loudness perception. *Ear and Hearing, 18,* 388–400.

Loudness Discomfort Level. The **loudness discomfort level (LDL)** defines the intensity level at which sound becomes uncomfortable or causes discomfort. Other terms are also sometimes used to describe either the intensity level where sounds become uncomfortable or the upper limit for comfortable sounds. The terms include *uncomfortable level* (abbreviated as *UL* or *UCL*), *threshold of discomfort (TD), upper level of comfortable listening (ULCL), upper limit of comfort (ULC),* and *highest comfort level (HCL).* Here, we'll simply use the phrase *loudness discomfort level,* or *LDL.*

The intensity levels required for measurement of the LDL are considerably higher than those used for estimating the MCL. Precisely worded instructions are very important in measuring LDLs. Different instructions are likely to yield differences in measured loudness levels (Mueller & Hall, 1998). As with measurement of the MCL, pure tones or some type of speech signal are first presented at intensities above the patient's hearing threshold levels and then the intensity level is gradually increased. Measurement of the LDL can begin at the upper limit of the range of comfortable intensity levels if MCLs are already available for the patient,. The patient holds the same chart shown already in Table 6.3. The instructions in Table 6.3 are use for measurement of LDLs as well as MCLs.

 ClinicalConnection

Information on MCLs and LDLs plays an important role in fitting hearing aids to persons with hearing loss. Measurement of LDLs is also useful in the diagnosis and management of persons with intolerance to loud sounds, a problem known as hyperacusis.

Word Recognition Performance

Measurement of word recognition ability is a traditional hearing assessment procedure. The phrases *word recognition* and *speech discrimination* may not be clear to some readers. The meaning of the phrases will probably make sense following an explanation of the test process.

The phrase **word recognition** is used rather than *word understanding* because the patient can repeat the words without understanding or comprehending their meaning. The phrase **speech discrimination** (or the shortened "speech discrim") is sometimes used when referring to word recognition, especially by physicians. However, speech discrimination is not an accurate description of the patient's task. We reviewed the distinction between discrimination

NU6 (Northwestern University Auditory Test #6) Word List	
Ten Most Difficult Words	**Fifteen Remaining Words**
knock	fat
kite	yes
take	fall
keen	which
puff	sell
hash	king
tip	lot
pool	raid
burn	vine
sub	jail
	reach
	rag
	home
	goose
	love

TABLE 6.4
An example of a word list for efficient assessment of word recognition performance in which the words are arranged in order of difficulty with the 10 most difficult words listed first.

and a recognition task a little earlier in this chapter. With a discrimination test, the subject listens to and compares two or more sounds. Words in a speech discrimination task might be the same or they might differ slightly in some way. With word recognition testing, a patient simply repeats each word that is heard, or the patient points to a picture representing the word.

We will first go through typical steps in the word recognition process for a patient who is an older child or an adult. An audiologist presents single-syllable words one at a time, usually through earphones. Table 6.4 shows a sample of typical single-syllable words used to test word recognition. During word presentation, there is a long enough interval between successive words for the patient to respond by repeating the word before the next one is presented. An audiologist knows which words the patient is hearing and closely compares the words presented with the words repeated by the patient. If an audiologist concludes that the presented and the repeated words are the same, the response is scored as correct. Differences between the original and repeated words are scored as errors. An error occurs, for example, when the test word is *kite* but the patient responds with the word *bite*.

Development of Speech Recognition Materials

As noted already, the clinical importance of evaluating a person's ability to hear speech was recognized even before audiology became a profession (Fletcher & Steinberg, 1929). Early systematic investigation of the use of speech recognition materials for hearing assessment dates back to a period in the late 1940s and early 1950s. During that era, immediately

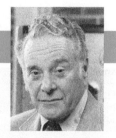

Ira Hirsh (1922–2010)

Ira Hirsh earned his BA degree in 1942 from the New York State College for Teachers (Albany). Upon graduation he accepted a scholarship to the Northwestern University School of Speech. Here, Raymond Carhart motivated him to move away from his initial pursuit of a broadcasting and drama career toward speech and hearing studies (Green & Watson, 1992). Hirsh completed his master's degree in 1944 and then served for two years as an instructor in the U.S. Air Force Communication Officers School. One of his supervisors and mentors was S. Richard Silverman, another well-known scientist and coauthor of a popular audiology textbook.

After World War II Hirsh was offered a position in the Psycho-Acoustic Laboratory (PAL) at Harvard University, where the famous psychoacoustics researcher S. S. Stevens was his mentor. Hirsh went on to earn a PhD in experimental psychology at Harvard. It was during this period, between 1948 and 1951, that he was involved in the development of early speech audiometry test materials and published his classic textbook, entitled *The Measurement of Hearing*. Ira Hirsh, the "Father of Speech Audiometry," spent most of his remarkably productive career at the Central Institute for the Deaf (CID) at Washington University in St. Louis, Missouri, working with other well-known hearing scientists, including Hallowell Davis (Formby & Musiek, 2011).

following World War II, a remarkable collection of hearing scientists at a then-prestigious facility called the Psycho-Acoustic Laboratory at Harvard University conducted a series of classic studies (Davis, 1948; Egan, 1948; Hirsh et al., 1952; Hudgins et al., 1947).

Development and investigation of word recognition materials continued through the 1960s at several other university laboratories (Boothroyd, 1968; Tillman, Carhart, & Wilber, 1963). Each group of investigators carefully selected hundreds of monosyllabic words and arranged them into lists, with each list usually containing fifty words. The researchers verified that a person's performance score, the percentage of words correctly repeated, was equivalent or very similar on each of the word lists. That is, the word lists were equally difficult. During the process of test development, words not in common usage and not familiar to most persons were eliminated from the lists.

There was also an attempt in the development of materials for word recognition to compile word lists composed of speech sounds or phonemes occurring with about the same frequency as they occurred in everyday conversation. That is, the frequency of occurrence of phonemes within a list of fifty words, and in the beginning, middle, and end of the single-syllable words, corresponded to the frequency of occurrence of the phonemes in conversational speech. This strategy in test development produced word lists that were *phonetically* or **phonemically balanced**, and the test materials were described as **PB word lists**.

Variables in Word Recognition Performance

A number of factors influence the outcome of word recognition testing. It is important for an audiologist to have some understanding of these factors and how they affect test results.

Live Voice versus Recorded Presentation. We've already reviewed in this chapter the advantages of recorded test materials in measurement of SRT, but the recommendation for avoiding the MLV presentation approach bears repeating in this discussion of word recognition testing. When the MLV technique is employed, especially with multiple speakers, variability in the presentation of words is always higher and reliability of the test results less than it would be if the same words were presented from recordings. Some variability in the words is associated with the speaking style and dialects of different speakers. However, even when a single experienced audiologist says the same word more than one time there are differences in the acoustic characteristics of the word, including variations in intensity and frequency.

Another variable affecting word recognition scores is the level of difficulty of each specific test. Over the years, as already noted, several research laboratories have independently developed separate word recognition tests. Research confirms that a single person with hearing loss will yield different word recognition scores on different recorded tests of word recognition. Some word recognition tests are more challenging than others for persons with hearing loss.

Carrier Phrase. Sometimes a short phrase called a **carrier phrase** precedes each word. A carrier phrase in a word recognition test usually consists of three words that come before the presentation of each word. The carrier phrase alerts the patient that the target word will soon be presented. The same carrier phrase is used for all of the words on the word lists of a specific recording. The carrier phrase preceding the test word is often: "Say the word _____" or "You will say _____," where the blank is the word the patient is expected to repeat. An audiologist conducting word recognition with a microphone using the live-voice technique controls the intensity level of the spoken test word by first monitoring the level of the preceding carrier phrase.

Although the use of a carrier phrase is a common procedure in word recognition assessment, the strategy does not necessarily improve test scores (Martin, Hawkins, & Bailey, 1962). Occasionally patients with hearing loss repeatedly recite an incorrect carrier phrase throughout the clinical assessment of word recognition. For example, in response to the carrier phrase "Say the word *tip*" or "Say the word *burn*" the patient might consistently say, "Saving birds *tip*" or "Saving birds *burn*." In such cases, the carrier phrase would appear to confuse the patient and may also diminish word recognition.

Nonmeaningful versus Meaningful Test Items. Materials for speech audiometry include nonmeaningful and meaningful test items. Nonsense syllables are a typical form of nonmeaningful test material. Nonsensence syllables generally consist of a consonant-plus-vowel (CV) combination, such as "fa," "ga," "zha," or a vowel-consonant (VC) combination like "uth," "ip," "ang."

In a clinical setting, word recognition is almost always evaluated with real words that have meaning for the patient. The rationale for using familiar words in the vocabulary of the patient is to minimize the effect of language factors on test results. The clinical goal is to assess the patient's word recognition abilities, not the extent of the patient's vocabulary or familiarity with the English language. As you already know, items for assessment of word recognition performance are invariably single-syllable words, in contrast to the two-syllable spondee words regularly used for measurement of SRT. Examples of single-syllable words used in assessing word recognition were shown earlier in Table 6.4.

It seems logical to describe how well a patient hears everyday speech if the goal of testing is to estimate communication-related hearing loss. You would think that recognition of real and meaningful words would provide a more accurate representation of the patient's ability to understand conversational speech. There is, in fact, little evidence in support of this assumption. Indeed, nonsense words might actually offer some clinical advantages over meaningful words.

Careful analysis of errors in a list of nonsense syllables consisting of a single consonant and a single vowel helps to identify patterns in the types of sound recognition errors a patient tends to make. Correct identification of nonsense syllables depends on correct recognition of consonant sounds. Nonsense syllable tests generallly have greater sensitivity to the effects of hearing loss on speech sound perception. Finally, reliance on CV or VC syllables eliminates concern about the influence of word familiarity or memory on test performance. Nevertheless, word recognition tests consisting of meaningful single-syllable words rather than CV syllables are used most often by audiologists and have enjoyed clinical popularity for over fifty years.

Number of Words in a List. The accuracy of word recognition testing is determined to a large extent by how many items are included in a word list. Put another way, word recognition scores are more variable for shorter word lists and more consistent for longer word lists (Dubno et al., 1995; Thornton & Raffin, 1978).

This concept can be easily demonstrated with a little experiment.

Let's say you first measure a patient's word recognition for the right ear by presenting a 100-word list at an intensity level of 60 dB HL. Suppose the patient's score is 90 percent. He missed ten of the words. Then, using a different 100-word list, but still at an intensity level of 60 dB HL, you again assess the patient's word recognition performance for the right ear. According to research findings (Dubno et al., 1995; Thornton & Raffin, 1978), we would expect the patient's score on the second test to be somewhere between 81 and 96 percent, a range of 16 percent.

Use of a 100-word list for each ear and maybe more than one list requires considerable test time. In a clinical setting, test time is often limited. It is reasonable, therefore, to ask: "Would variability in word recognition scores be affected with shorter word lists?" Let's assume that you evaluate word recognition for the right ear of the same patient, also at an intensity level of 60 dB HL, but you decide to use a list of twenty-five words instead of a 100-word list. Let's also assume that the patient had a score of 92 percent on the test. The patient incorrectly repeated two words. Now, you assess the patient's word recognition a second time using another twenty-five-word list.

According to research data, the patient's probable score would be somewhere between 72 to 100 percent or within a range of 29 percent. In other words, from a statistical viewpoint the patient's score would be the same whether he correctly repeated all twenty-five words, or he missed seven words. In our example, variability in word recognition scores was considerably larger for the shorter twenty-five-word list than for the 100-word list.

Variability in word recognition scores is clearly minimized with a 100-word list. Nonetheless, due to limited clinical test time for completion of comprehensive hearing assessment of each patient, most audiologists rely on twenty-five-word lists. Even with the shorter word lists, considerable clinical test time is required to assess word recognition performance for each ear, sometimes at more than one intensity level.

As noted already, recently introduced computer-based audiometer technology permits patient control of the presentation rate for words. Automated devices may also include features like voice recognition for computer scoring of word recognition performance. Technological advances may help to reduce the amount of time audiologists devote to assessment of word recognition.

Intensity Level. One of the major factors in word recognition performance is the intensity level of speech materials. The intensity level must exceed a patient's SRT. A patient will only respond to speech that is audible, that is, speech that is heard. The intensity level at which speech is just barely detected is greater for a patient with a hearing loss than for a normal hearer. The relationship between the intensity level of words and how well a patient performs on a word recognition test is often plotted on a graph called a **performance intensity function**, shortened to **PI function**.

Figure 6.3 shows a **PI-PB function**. This is a graph of performance on phonemically balanced (PB) word lists presented at different intensity levels. Speech intensity level in dB HL is indicated on the horizontal (X) axis, and the score in percent correct for word recognition is indicated on the vertical (Y) axis.

Figure 6.3 shows that scores in percent correct are lowest when speech is presented at a very soft level, close to a person's hearing threshold. For most normal-hearing persons, performance improves rapidly as the speech intensity level is increased up to a level of 30 to 50 dB above hearing threshold. The maximum or best score for word recognition scores is often found within an intensity region that the patient considers comfortable, or at a slightly higher intensity level. The abbreviation **PBmax** refers to the maximum performance score on a list of PB words.

In clinical hearing measurement, word recognition is sometimes measured for each ear with a single word list presented at a single comfortable intensity level. The motivation for this approach is to minimize test time. However, it is often necessary to assess word recognition at more than one intensity level to find the maximum score. Research confirms that the maximum score in word recognition testing is not always recorded when word lists are presented at a single intensity level, even at a comfortable loudness level for a normal-hearing person (Dubno et al., 1995; Guthrie & Mackersie, 2009; Ullrich & Grimm, 1976).

What intensity level should be used for word recognition testing? There is no short answer to this rather simple question. As just discussed, a typical goal in word recognition testing is to find the patient's best performance or maximum percent correct score. Yet it is not possible to predict which intensity level will produce the best performance on a word recognition task. In some cases, a word recognition score of 100 percent will be recorded quickly at the initial presentation level, such as an intensity level that is 30 to 40 dB above the patient's SRT.

The maximum word recognition score may also be found when words are presented at the patient's most comfortable level (MCL). However, the patient's MCL must first be determined by presenting words at different intensity levels, while at the same time asking the

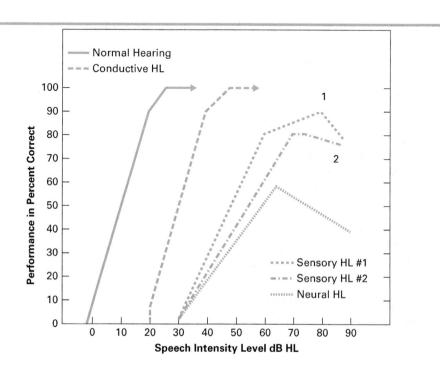

FIGURE 6.3

Performance intensity (PI) functions for single syllable ("phonetically balanced" or PB) words. Performance is reported in percent correct scores (Y-axis), whereas intensity is shown in dB HL (X-axis). Patterns of PI functions are shown for a normal hearer and patients with different types of hearing loss.

patient to judge the loudness level. For most patients, optimal word recognition scores are found at an intensity level higher than the MCL. Reliance on a single or fixed intensity level does not always result in a measure of optimal performance for word recognition, particularly for patients with sensory hearing loss. It is worthwhile to emphasize that a patient's maximum performance for each ear can only be verified by completing word recognition testing at two or more intensity levels.

PI-PB Functions in Hearing Loss. Examples of PI-PB function were shown in Figure 6.3 for normal hearers and also for patients with conductive hearing loss, cochlear hearing loss, and neural hearing loss. The term *sensory hearing loss* is appropriate for a patient with cochlear auditory dysfunction, whereas *retrocochlear* is often used to describe neural hearing loss. The PI function is shifted to the right for patients with conductive hearing loss because a greater intensity level is required for the patient to first detect the speech signal.

Figure 6.3 also shows an example of word recognition performance typical of a patient with conductive hearing loss. Word recognition scores begin to increase at an intensity level of about 20 dB HL, suggesting that the patient has a mild degree of hearing loss. Word recognition scores are typically quite good once the intensity level is high enough to overcome the degree of conductive hearing loss and the words reach the patient's normal inner ear at a comfortable level.

Variability in the intensity level producing maximum performance (PBmax) is greater for persons with a hearing loss than for normal hearers. In other words, it's harder to predict in advance what intensity level will produce the maximum percent correct score for word recognition. This point was illustrated in Figure 6.3 by PI functions for two subjects with typical sensory hearing loss. For sensory hearing loss #1, the maximum score is recorded for an intensity level of 80 dB HL. The maximum score for the PI function of sensory hearing loss #2, in contrast, occurs at an intensity level of 70 dB HL.

Now we'll consider the PI-PB function in Figure 6.3 labeled *neural hearing loss*. The results are for a hypothetical patient with confirmed tumor affecting the auditory portion of the eighth cranial nerve. We can assume that the degree of the patient's hearing loss is similar to that of the two patients with sensory hearing loss (#1 and #2) because the PI-PB function for all three patients begins at 30 dB. Two features of the PI-PB function are distinctly different for the patient with neural hearing loss from the two patients with the sensory pattern.

First, even though hearing sensitivity may be equivalent for the three patients, the maximum score for the patient with neural hearing loss is less than 60%, compared to 80 percent or higher for the patients with sensory hearing loss. The maximum score for the PB word recognition test, the PBmax, is evident by inspecting the highest point on the PI function for each patient.

Second, word recognition scores for the patient with neural hearing loss reach a maximum percent correct at a speech intensity level of about 65 dB HL, and then the scores decrease to almost 30 percent at the highest presentation intensity level of 90 dB HL. As seen in Figure 6.3, the normal-hearing PI-PB function in word recognition scores steadily increases as intensity level is increased until performance stabilizes at 100 percent. A paradoxical decrease or *rollover* in word recognition scores as intensity level increases is one of the characteristic signs of neural auditory dysfunction (Jerger & Hayes, 1977; Jerger & Jerger, 1971).

The abbreviation **PBmin** is used to describe the poorest or minimum word recognition score at the highest intensity level, at the end of rollover. Rollover can be specified and quantified by calculating the difference between PBmax and PBmin (Jerger & Jerger, 1971). There

 ClinicalConnection

Diagnostic tests and patterns of test findings that are valuable in distinguishing among types of hearing loss, including differentiation between cochlear and auditory nerve disorders, are discussed further in Chapters 8 through 10. You'll learn more in Chapters 11 and 12 about various diseases and disorders affecting the auditory system.

is even a simple equation for the calculation, the **rollover index**, that takes into account the amount of rollover relative to the maximum PB score: Rollover index = (PBmax − PBmin)/ PB max).

Configuration of Hearing Loss. Some variability in word recognition performance for persons with hearing loss is explained by the configuration, or shape, of the hearing loss. You will recall from our discussion of pure tone hearing testing in Chapter 5 that *configuration* is the term used for describing how hearing loss changes across a frequency region. Patients with a flat configuration have about the same amount of hearing loss across the range of test frequencies, whereas patients with other audiogram configurations have relatively greater hearing loss for lower or higher test frequencies or even notches or dips in hearing thresholds in certain frequency regions.

The **audiogram of speech sounds** illustrated in Figure 6.4 is one way to graphically display the distribution of speech sound energy across the range of audiometric test frequencies. You can see that a total of thirteen speech sounds have energy at frequencies slightly below 500 Hz and energy for another four speech sounds is found in a frequency region near 500 Hz. Also, the frequency region from 1000 to 2000 Hz is important for identification of a number of consonant sounds, such as *ch, sh, p,* and *k,* and hearing for even higher frequencies of 2000 to 4000 Hz contributes to correct identification of the consonant sounds *f, s,* and *th*. The communicative implications of hearing loss can usually be appreciated when a patient's pure tone hearing thresholds are plotted on a copy of the audiogram of speech sounds. Thus, the graph is useful when explaining the impact of hearing loss on communication to patients, parents of patients, and even physicians.

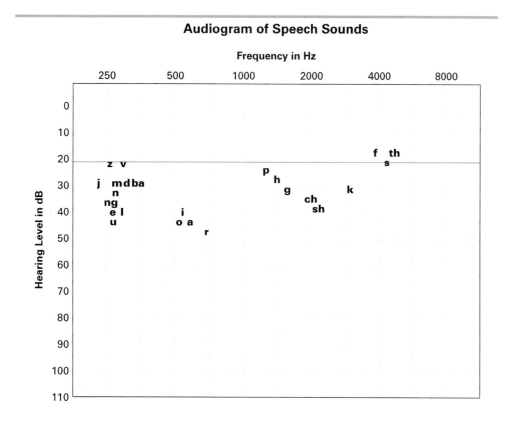

Audiogram of Speech Sounds

FIGURE 6.4

Audiogram of speech sounds showing the distribution of speech sound energy across the range of audiometric frequencies.

Appreciation of the importance of hearing sensitivity across the range of 500 to 4000 Hz on the correct identification of single-syllable speech sounds dates back to the 1940s (Carhart, 1946). Correct identification of speech sounds is particularly dependent on hearing in the region of 1900 to 2000 Hz (French & Steinberg, 1947). Word recognition scores are generally poorer as hearing thresholds begin to decrease in the high-frequency region of patients with a sloping hearing loss. The slope of the hearing loss, the overall degree of hearing loss, and intensity level of speech all interact in influencing word recognition test scores. Of course, factors other than the degree and slope of the hearing loss also contribute importantly to differences in word recognition. It is not surprising that word recognition scores vary widely in patients with hearing loss.

Speech Recognition and Pure Tone Hearing: The Count-the-Dots Method

The ability to detect speech or audibility of speech sounds is directly related to pure tone thresholds. A person with entirely normal hearing sensitivity as defined by pure tone hearing thresholds of 0 dB HL will detect without any difficulty even the faintest speech sounds. In contrast, speech at a typical *conversational level* is inaudible for someone with a severe hearing loss, who has pure tone hearing thresholds exceeding 60 dB HL. A person talking at a conversational level, not talking too softly but also not shouting, produces speech at an intensity level ranging from 20 dB up to about 50 dB HL. As you've already learned, recognizing and understanding speech is more difficult than simply detecting of speech sounds. However, if sound is not audible, there is no chance for adequate speech recognition and understanding.

Information in speech that contributes most importantly to its detection and perception is in a frequency range from 300 Hz up to about 4000 Hz. Recall from Chapter 2 that speech contains some energy above and below these frequency limits. For example, the fundamental frequency of male speakers is generally within the range of 85 to 180 Hz, whereas the fundamental frequency for a female voice is higher, usually between 170 and 250 Hz. Spectral information above 8000 Hz contributes to perception of high-frequency consonant sounds, and frequencies lower than 300 Hz also contribute to the quality of speech. However, the range of 300 to 4000 Hz contains the frequency information most important for detecting and perceiving speech. This point was evident from audiogram of speech sounds (Figure 6.4).

The Articulation Index. The impact of a hearing loss on speech detection is roughly estimated by taking into account this general information and by viewing an audiogram showing hearing threshold levels at different frequencies. The term **articulation index** is used to describe the percentage of speech that is audible. The articulation index ranges from 1.0 to 0. An articulation index of 1.0 indicates that 100 percent of speech is audible, whereas at 0 speech is not audible.

For over ninety years, hearing researchers have described variations on methods for determining the articulation index and the effect of hearing loss on the audibility of speech (Fletcher, 1921; French & Steinberg, 1947; Kryter, 1962; Mueller & Killion, 1992). In simpler forms of the articulation index, the spectrum of speech is represented on an audiogram form by a collection of 100 symbols. Gus Mueller and Mead Killion, two names well known in audiology, first reported the simple "count-the-dots" audiogram (Mueller & Killion, 1992).

Count-the-Dots Audiogram. Figure 6.5 depicts the latest version of the count-the-dots audiogram (Killion & Mueller, 2010). The figure shows dots at the various frequencies important in detecting speech, including inter-octave frequencies of 3000 and 6000 Hz. The numbers of dots on the audiogram indicate the relative importance of different frequency bands.

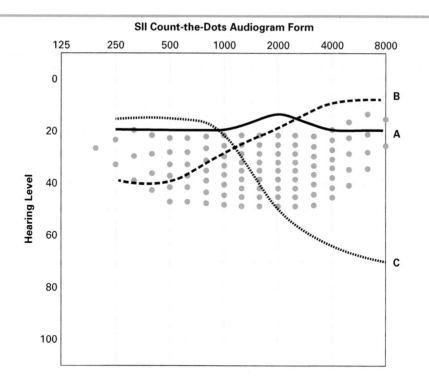

SII Count-the-Dots Audiogram Form

FIGURE 6.5

A "count-the-dots" audiogram form. Audibility of speech is illustrated for three patients each with a different audiogram pattern including: Hearing thresholds generally within normal limits **(A)**, a low-frequency hearing loss **(B)**, and a high-frequency hearing loss **(C)**. Courtesy of Mead Killion and H. Gustav Mueller.

Greater concentrations of dots reflect frequency regions more important for speech audibility, whereas fewer dots reflect less importance for speech audibility.

Calculation of the audibility of speech or the articulation index for persons with hearing loss is rather easily performed using the count-the-dots method. We assume that a person can always hear speech for dots at intensity levels greater than hearing threshold levels and, conversely, that speech information represented by dots at lower intensity levels is inaudible. With the count-the-dots method, the only mathematical skill required to calculate a patient's articulation index is the ability to count to 100. Remember, speech information is inaudible at fainter intensity levels that do not reach the patient's hearing threshold level.

The solid line labeled "A" in Figure 6.5 represents an audiogram for a listener with hearing sensitivity essentially within normal limits, with no pure tone hearing thresholds exceeding 20 dB HL. The dark horizontal line represents the listener's pure tone hearing thresholds. Hearing sensitivity would be entirely normal if thresholds were at 0 dB HL for all of the audiometric frequencies. Hearing threshold levels for audiogram "A" in Figure 6.5 are poorer than 0 dB HL, yet the intensity level of speech exceeds the patient's hearing thresholds for almost all of the different frequencies.

Three dots above 4000 Hz are at intensity levels less than hearing thresholds represented with line A in Figure 6.5, even though the patient's hearing sensitivity is within normal limits. This finding suggests that some high-frequency speech information is not audible to the patient. The articulation index for this hypothetical patient is 0.97. An adult listener with this audiogram would probably experience little or no difficulty with speech perception in quiet listening settings.

The dashed line labeled "B" in Figure 6.5 depicts a low-frequency hearing loss. By counting the dots reflecting speech that remains audible, we can calculate an articulation index of 0.80. Put another way, twenty dots are at intensity levels lower than the patient's hearing thresholds. The articulation index indicatest that speech information is fairly audible despite the hearing loss. Looking closely at the count-the-dots graph, you will see that there are fewer dots in the low-frequency region than in the high-frequency region. The higher concentration of dots in the high-frequency region reflects the relatively greater amount of speech information with the frequency region of 1000 to 4000 Hz. The patient's hearing loss is quite mild within that frequency region.

The high-frequency hearing loss indicated by the dotted line labeled "C" in Figure 6.5 exerts a rather substantial impact on articulation index and speech audibility. The articulation index for this audiogram is only 0.45. The articulation index is low even though hearing sensitivity is normal for test frequencies up to 1000 Hz. High-frequency hearing loss limits audibility of speech sounds in the important frequency region of 1000 to 4000 Hz.

According to Mueller and Killion (Killion & Mueller, 2010; Mueller & Killion, 1992), the articulation index calculated with the count-the-dots method helps to predict the difficulty a patient will have in perceiving conversational speech at a typical intensity level. The method is also useful in estimating a patient's possible benefit from the use of a hearing aid. It is important to remember, however, that the audibility score is a measure of how much speech a patient hears and not the percentage of speech the patient can understand.

Response Factors in Word Recognition

Method of Response. During clinical measurement of word recognition, a patient almost always responds verbally by repeating each word back to an audiologist. You can probably anticipate some limitations to this common clinical practice. An audiologist judges whether the patient responded correctly by comparing the word repeated to the word presented. Research confirms a 20% range of variability in word recognition scores, even when normal-hearing persons are judging patient responses on word recognition testing (Lawson & Peterson, 2011; Olsen & Matkin, 1979). Audiologists have a tendency to accept as correct responses that are really incorrect.

A variety of factors play a role in the accuracy with which an audiologist determines whether a patient's response is correct or incorrect. One factor is the quality of the audiometer system used to monitor the patient's speech. Audiometer variables include the microphone in the sound booth, the speaker system used by the audiologist, and background noise in the control room where the audiologist is located. An audiologist's hearing and auditory processing abilities are major factors affecting scoring on word recognition tests, particularly for audiologists who themselves have hearing impairment. For all of these reasons, a picture-identification or pointing task is an attractive alternative to a word repetition method of response. We will discuss this test format next.

Open- versus Closed-Set Response. The terms *open-set response* and *closed-set response* are often used in describing word recognition test materials. In an **open-set response test**, patients have no advance notice about which word they are about to hear (Olsen & Matkin, 1979; Wilson & Strouse, 1999). The test items can be any words in their vocabulary. As already noted, single-syllable word lists used for evaluation of word recognition include a relatively large number of different words, and there is no familiarization process before word recognition testing begins.

With a **closed-set response test**, in contrast, the patient responds to a test word within a limited collection of possible words. Since the 1960s, various closed-set tests with monosyllabic words have been described in publications (Kruel et al., 1968; Pederson & Studebaker, 1972; Schultz & Schubert, 1969). Some of these closed-set response tests utilize a multiple-choice format and/or a rhyming task, but none are routinely applied today in clinical hearing assessment.

Picture-identification closed-set response tests, on the other hand, are a common alternative to word recognition procedures requiring repetition of test items (Elliott & Katz, 1980;

Ross & Lerman, 1970). A drawing or photograph represents the test item on a picture-identification test. Figure 6.6 shows examples of response plates from a picture-identification procedure called the Northwestern University Children's Perception of Speech (NU CHIPS) test.

The drawing or photograph is on a laminated sheet of paper that also includes pictures of three to five other items. The patient identifies or recognizes the test item within the collection of pictures. Picture-identification word recognition tests are used most often for hearing assessment of young children, as we will discuss soon.

Errors in Word Recognition. Patients undergoing word recognition assessment will inevitably make errors, especially patients with hearing loss. A word recognition error occurs when the word repeated by the patient differs from the word presented. Interestingly, errors made by a person with a hearing loss on a word list are usually not consistent from one test to the next, even if the same word lists are used on each occasion. There are, however, some general patterns or trends in the types of incorrect responses made by patients (Olsen & Matkin, 1979).

Errors occur much more often for consonant sounds than for vowel sounds. In most cases, a patient substitutes an incorrect consonant for the correct consonant. For example, a patient may say the word *knot* for the test word *knock*. Final consonants in a word are frequently omitted from a response. A patient may say the word *you* for the test word *youth*. As you might expect, patients with greater hearing loss errors produce more errors in word recognition testing. The relation between errors in word recognition and hearing loss is strongest when hearing loss involves high frequencies. As you'll recall from our earlier discussion of the audiogram of familiar sounds and the count-the-dots audiogram, hearing for high-frequency sounds is most important for correct recognition of consonant speech sounds.

Efficiency in Word Recognition Measurement. We've already reviewed techniques for assessing word recognition and factors that do or do not influence test results. You've probably noted opportunities for enhancing the efficiency of the test process, ways to reduce test time without diminishing the quality of test results. Strategies for optimizing testing efficiency are particularly important given the ever-increasing demands on audiologists in clinical settings to provide diagnostic services for more patients, in less time, with diminishing reimbursement for services. Several simple techniques or strategies may help to minimize test time for some patients without sacrificing accuracy or losing clinically valuable information.

- Utilize twenty-five-word lists arranged in order of difficulty from most difficult to easiest, with the ten most difficult words first. As shown in Table 6.4, research has led to the construction of word lists with the words arranged in descending order of difficulty (Hurley & Sells, 2003). Word recognition testing is stopped if the patient gives a correct response for the first ten words and the score is 100 percent. The likelihood of any subsequent errors on easier words is very low.

- Perform word recognition testing with instrumentation that permits adjustment of the time interval between words or presentation rate, and/or that allows the patient to control the rate at which they listen to the words. You can readily appreciate how this simple technique will save test time. An audiologist who conducts word recognition testing on an alert patient

FIGURE 6.6

Example of a response plate from a clinically popular picture identification test called the Northwestern University Children's Perception of Speech (NU CHIPS) test. Courtesy of William Carver, PhD. Auditec of St. Louis.

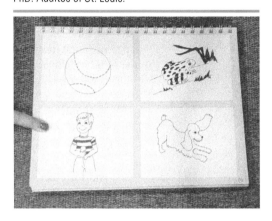

with a time interval of two seconds between words instead of the customary four-second interval will complete the testing in one-half the time without sacrificing test quality.

Word Recognition Testing in Young Children

Test Development. Test materials for assessment of word recognition performance in older children and adults are not appropriate for use with young children. The word recognition materials that we have reviewed so far were developed for use with school-age children or older persons. The lists consist of words that are not in the vocabulary of younger children. An apparent deficit in word recognition may be due to language factors rather than word recognition if the vocabulary level of a test is inappropriate for the child's age.

This point was well appreciated in the 1940s when initial word recognition materials were developed. Researchers at that time created lists of fifty words chosen especially for use with children. Words in each list were drawn from a pool of over 400 monosyllabic words, and all of the words were in the vocabulary of young children. These pediatric speech materials came to be known as *phonetically balanced kindergarten word lists,* or simply *PBK lists.* They are useful for word recognition assessment of children who have a developmental age of 4 to 5 years, and for older children. If there is no concern about developmental delay or cognitive deficit, then a child's chronological age is equivalent to the child's developmental age.

Word recognition assessment is more challenging to perform with children. Younger children respond more readily to an active and interesting visual task such as pointing to pictures rather than simply repeating words. Before testing begins, the pictures are reviewed with the child to verify that each can be accurately identified.

ⓘ WebWatch

You'll find videos of children undergoing speech audiometry testing on YouTube and other Internet sites.

Current Pediatric Word Recognition Tests. One of the earliest pediatric tests utilizing a picture-pointing task, rather than word repetition, is the Word Intelligibility by Picture Identification (WIPI). The WIPI was first reported in 1970 by two audiologists (Ross & Lerman, 1970), then at the University of Connecticut. A picture or photograph represents each of the monosyllabic words in the WIPI test. Six pictures are arranged on a laminated sheet. There are a total of twenty-five sheets, each with different pictures. The WIPI is another example of a closed-set or *closed-response* word test. Each word the child hears and responds to is among the limited set of six words represented by the pictures.

The Northwestern University Children's Perception of Speech (NU-CHIPS) is also a popular pediatric picture-pointing word recognition test (Elliott & Katz, 1980). You viewed the NU-CHIPS test earlier in Figure 6.6. There are a total of fifty different single syllable words with four words shown on each sheet. The NU-CHIPS test can be used for word recognition assessment of children who are 2.5 years old and older.

Another test for speech audiometry in young children is called the Pediatric Speech Intelligibility (PSI) test. Susan Jerger developed the PSI test when she was affiliated with the audiology department at Baylor College of Medicine in the early 1980s. The test differs in several important ways from other pediatric tests.

First, it includes both monosyllabic words and sentence test items. The words are nouns represented as colorful pictures. The child is instructed to "Show me _____," with the word inserted in the blank space. An example of the instruction for a word item is: "Show me *bear*." The sentences describe a simple action, with an instruction to the child such as "Show me *The bear brushing his teeth*." Second, the words and the sentences can be presented to the child in a quiet setting or when the child is also hearing speech in the background. The speech in the background is called a "competing message." Unlike other pediatric speech audiometry procedures, the PSI takes into account the child's receptive language abilities.

LEADERS AND LUMINARIES

Susan W. Jerger

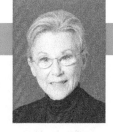

Susan Jerger earned a bachelor's degree in speech and hearing sciences from the University of Houston. She received a master's degree in speech and hearing sciences from Purdue University and a PhD in audiology and bioacoustics from Baylor College of Medicine. Dr. Jerger is Ashbel Smith Professor and Director of the Honors Program, School of Behavioral and Brain Sciences, University of Texas, Dallas. Her research studies lexical development in children with hearing loss. With colleagues, she developed the pediatric speech intelligibility test, the first audiovisual multi-modal picture word task, and the first children's versions of a cross-modal picture word task and an auditory Stroop task. Results with these innovative tasks provided new insights into how differences in auditory experiences affect the development of the phonological/semantic processes supporting speech perception. Her current research is defining a new auditory illusion, called the visual speech restoration effect, in which people report hearing missing auditory speech sounds when they are presented audiovisually. Dr. Jerger's research, supported by the NIH from 1989 to 2014, is helping us understand the large variability in speech perception characterizing children with the same degree of hearing loss.

Word Recognition in Background Noise

Throughout this chapter, we've reviewed speech audiometry procedures that involve the presentation of test items, usually words, in a quiet setting, without any background sound. When word recognition is assessed in quiet, the listening conditions are optimal. The patient is seated in a sound-treated room and words are presented with as little background noise as possible. In routine hearing assessment, the SRT and word recognition performance are almost always measured in a quiet condition. Many patients have no difficulty hearing and understanding people speaking in quiet settings. On the contrary, patients commonly report difficulty understanding speech in noisy settings, such as when they are dining in a busy restaurant or riding in a car on the freeway.

Over the years, a number of tests were developed in an attempt to evaluate word recognition performance in noisy listening conditions. The relation between the intensity level of the words and the intensity level of the background sound is described as the **signal-to-noise ratio**, or **SNR**. The noise might be rather simple, such as broadband noise or speech-spectrum noise that includes mostly frequencies found in speech. With some **speech-in-noise tests**, SNR is varied, to make the test easier with a larger SNR or more difficult with a smaller SNR.

However, in everyday listening situations patients don't usually encounter simple noises when trying to understand what someone is saying. To better estimate communication ability in real-world conditions, background noise in some tests is a recording of actual environmental noise from, for example, a restaurant or a cafeteria. In these test conditions, many people are talking in the background but it is not possible to follow any of the conversations. The noise is sometimes referred to as cafeteria noise or **multi-talker babble**.

Another type of background noise consists of a small group of speakers. With some effort, a normal-hearing listener can understand what each speaker is saying. The latter type of noise often produces what is called the **cocktail party effect**. Word recognition is more difficult and requires more effort due to the cocktail party effect, and word recognition performance deteriorates.

There are clinically compelling reasons to regularly evaluate word recognition performance in background noise, particularly when scores on tests of word recognition in quiet do not reveal a deficit. Information gained from the additional time required for assessment of speech perception in noise is often very useful in determining the most effective management strategy and whether additional diagnostic testing is needed.

Assessment of speech perception in noise and with meaningful competing speech signals also plays a critical role in the documentation of central auditory nervous system disorders. To a large extent, we hear more with our brain than our ears. Using a variety of speech audiometry tests that tap into hearing and listening abilities more effectively than simple tests of word recognition in quiet, audiologists can evaluate auditory function at the highest levels of the central nervous system.

Audiologists are increasingly supplementing simple word recognition testing with the assessment of speech perception in noise. Assessment of speech perception in noise is particularly useful for persons who experience considerable difficulty with day-to-day communication, including some persons with normal-hearing thresholds or hearing-impaired persons who already use hearing aids. Examples of such patient populations include school-age children who are experiencing listening difficulties in the noisy classroom setting and also adults with traumatic brain injuries who are unable to communicate effectively in the workplace.

 ClinicalConnection

Diagnostic speech audiometry procedures, in addition to word recognition tests, play an important role in assessment of central auditory nervous system function in certain patient populations. You'll learn about a variety of diagnostic speech tests in Chapter 9 and about disorders affecting the central auditory system in Chapter 12.

PULLING IT ALL TOGETHER

Measurement of a patient's ability to hear speech is a very important part of comprehensive hearing assessment. Using a diagnostic audiometer, an audiologist can measure speech detection threshold, speech recognition threshold, and word recognition performance. Speech audiometry is conducted with lists of two-syllable or monosyllabic words developed specifically for use in clinical hearing testing.

Whenever feasible, word recognition performance is assessed with recorded test materials rather than presentation of words via a microphone using the monitored live voice technique. Word recognition testing must often be conducted at different intensity levels to determine a patient's optimal, or maximum, score. In patients who cannot provide a clear verbal response, like very young children, speech recognition thresholds and word recognition performance are measured using a picture identification response mode.

In addition to providing information on how well a patient hears speech, word recognition testing can also help to distinguish type of hearing loss, including the difference between sensory hearing loss due to cochlear auditory dysfunction and that due to neural auditory dysfunction. With some patients, assessment of hearing for speech must go beyond measurement of speech threshold and word recognition performance. Diagnosis of auditory dysfunction with more sophisticated speech audiometry tests is reviewed in Chapter 9.

READINGS

Konkle, D. F., & Rintelmann, W. F. (1983). *Principles of speech audiometry*. Baltimore: University Park Press.

Lawson, G. D., & Peterson, M. E. (2011). *Speech audiometry*. San Diego: Plural Publishing.

Mueller, H. G. III, & Hall, J. W. III. (1998). *Audiologists' desk reference. Volume II: Audiologic management, rehabilitation, and terminology*. San Diego: Singular Publishing Group.

Wilson, R. H., & Strouse, A. L. (1999). Auditory measures with speech skills. In F. E. Musiek & W. F. Rintelmann (Eds.), *Contemporary perspectives in hearing assessment* (pp. 21–66). Boston: Allyn & Bacon.

7 Masking and Audiogram Interpretation

LEARNING OBJECTIVES

In reading this chapter you will learn:

- What masking is and why it is important in clinical audiology
- When masking is needed
- Principles important in the understanding of masking
- The meaning of *interaural attenuation, crosshearing, central masking, over-masking, occlusion effect,* and *masking dilemma*
- How masking is applied in air-conduction testing with pure tones
- How masking is applied in bone-conduction testing with pure tones
- About the use of masking in speech audiometry, including differences between masking for measurement of speech reception threshold and for word recognition
- How to perform the Weber test and the Bing test
- How to plot pure tone audiometry test results on an audiogram when masking is used
- More about analysis of audiograms showing air- and bone-conduction test results

KEY TERMS

Bing test
Central masking
Critical band
Cross hearing
Cross masking
Effective masking
Initial masking
Interaural attenuation (IA)
Masking dilemma
Maximum masking
Minimum masking
Occlusion effect
Over-masking
Sensorineural acuity level (SAL) technique
Speech noise
Transcranial hearing
Transcranial transmission loss
Under-masking
Weber test

CHAPTER FOCUS

The focus of this chapter is masking. One of the most important objectives in clinical audiology is to be certain that hearing test results are specific to the ear being tested. Confident analysis of an audiogram is based on the assumption that test results are "ear-specific." In other words, we assume that air-conduction and bone-conduction test results obtained with the earphone or bone vibrator on the right side accurately reflect hearing in the right ear, and vice versa. Effective masking of the nontest ear with an appropriate type and level of noise is often necessary in order to verify that air- and bone-conduction test results are ear specific.

Time-tested rules and principles guide audiologists as they apply masking in clinical hearing tests. The rules are based on extensive research findings and cumulative published clinical experiences. In this chapter, you'll be introduced to the rules of masking and to key principles underlying masking. You'll learn what masking is, why it's needed, and when it's needed. You'll also read about concepts like interaural attenuation for earphones, minimum and maximum masking, under- and over-masking, the role of the occlusion effect in masking decisions, and what is meant by the curious phrase "masking dilemma."

Our discussion about masking concludes with an explanation of clinical techniques that audiologists use to properly mask the nontest ear during

CHAPTER FOCUS *Concluded*

pure tone audiometry and during speech audiometry. In the final portion of the chapter your new knowledge about masking will be reinforced with a review of audiograms for two cases representing different types and patterns of test findings. The discussion of each case begins with a summary of the test findings. The case discussions conclude with comments about a possible cause for the hearing loss and appropriate options for managing the patient.

Overview of Masking

"If you can't explain it simply, then you don't understand it well enough."   ALBERT EINSTEIN

In Chapter 2 you learned about different forms of noise that can be used as masking sounds. Then in Chapter 4 you were introduced to the concept of masking and why it is needed in clinical audiology. It makes sense to learn about the concepts of and techniques for pure tone hearing testing and speech audiometry before trying to understand masking. You read all about hearing testing in the previous two chapters. The information in this chapter builds on the foundation of knowledge you acquired in the chapters on pure tone audiometry and speech audiometry. We will now discuss masking rules, concepts, and techniques.

Masking is a very important element of hearing testing. To appreciate the overall goal of masking and its importance in clinical audiology, it might be useful to first consider a basic element of vision testing. Everyone has at one time or another undergone a simple vision test. A nurse in school or a vision professional like an optometrist instructs you to identify selected block letters that are displayed in rows on a chart some distance in front of you. The size of the letters decreases from the top row to the bottom. During the test process you are asked to cover your left eye so vision for only the right eye can be tested, and then the sequence is reversed. Isolating one eye and then the other is an essential feature of a complete vision test.

Masking in hearing testing serves the same purpose as covering an eye in vision testing. The goal of masking in clinical audiology is to isolate the test ear and to eliminate any contribution of the nontest ear to the hearing test results. You'll soon appreciate that masking in audiology is more challenging that simply covering an eye in vision testing. A variety of factors contribute to increased difficulty associated with masking. However, you'll begin to understand masking and how it's applied with patients after reading about the concepts underlying masking and masking techniques used in clinical audiology.

What Is Masking?

The dictionary definition of the word *mask* includes, "To make indistinct or blurred to the senses" and "To cover in order to conceal or protect." Briefly, masking is the presentation of sound to the nontest ear that prevents the patient from hearing the test sound in that ear. The goal in masking is to ensure that the nontest ear is not contributing to the patient's response.

Why Is Masking Needed?

Accurate assessment of hearing depends on verifying that test results only reflect stimulation of the test ear, the ear that is being tested. When testing the right ear, an audiologist must be confident that the patient's response is due to activation of the right ear and not the left ear. Likewise hearing testing of the left ear should produce responses from the patient that are due only to activation of the left ear. Ear-specific test findings are always very important for pure tone audiometry with air-conduction and also for bone conduction hearing testing. In fact, correct analysis and meaningful interpretation of hearing test results is entirely dependent on an accurate description of the hearing status for each ear. Important decisions about management of patients with hearing loss are also made with test information that is specific to each ear. A number of serious mistakes in the interpretation of test results may occur without the proper use of masking. For example, a patient who appears to have a moderate hearing loss in one ear may in fact have no hearing at all in that ear. And, a patient with a sensorineural hearing loss due to inner ear damage may incorrectly appear to have a conductive hearing loss. Errors in hearing testing resulting from inadequate masking of the non-test ear can lead to inappropriate treatment for hearing loss or no treatment for patient's who really need it.

When Is Masking Needed?

Masking is necessary in any hearing test procedure if there is a chance that the stimulus might cross over from the test ear to the nontest ear. The term **cross hearing** is often used to describe detection of a stimulus sound in the nontest ear. The concept of interaural attenuation is key to determining the likelihood of cross hearing. *Interaural attenuation* is the phrase used to describe reduction of sound as it crosses the head from one ear to the other.

The amount of interaural attenuation varies depending on what type of earphone is used in hearing testing and also the use of earphones versus bone vibrators. We'll soon review interaural attenuation in a little more detail. Here we will stress the point that masking is needed whenever a hearing response from the nontest ear is suspected, or even possible.

Historical Perspective

Publications describing research about masking in pure tone hearing testing date back to the 1920s and 1930s (Fletcher & Munson, 1937; Wegel & Lane, 1924). However, the most intensive masking research was done in the 1950s and 1960s (Chaiklin, 1967; Coles & Priede, 1970; Denes & Naunton, 1952; Dirks & Malmquist, 1964; Egan & Hake, 1950; Hawkins & Stevens, 1950; Hirsh & Bowman,1953; Hood, 1960; Jerger & Tillman, 1960; Jerger, Tillman & Peterson, 1960; Liden, Nilsson & Anderson, 1959; Martin, 1966; Studebaker, 1962, 1967). Authors of the impressive number of publications on the topic of masking during that era include many well-known hearing researchers in the United States, the United Kingdom, and Scandinavian countries.

Audiology was emerging as a new profession during the two decades of intensive masking research. Also, manufacturers began to market clinical audiometers that included options for presenting masking noise during air- and bone conduction hearing testing. Figure 5.1 in the chapter on pure tone audiometry (Chapter 5) showed a few of these early audiometers. Information generated in the many early research investigations largely led to the rules of masking and masking techniques that are still used in clinical audiology today.

Challenges in Masking

In 1971 Ira Ventry, Joseph Chaiklin, and Richard Dixon edited a book of carefully selected readings that included seven previously published papers on masking. In an introduction, the authors concisely summed up the rationale for masking:

> The need for masking in clinical audiometry is based on two facts: (1) an intense stimulus delivered to an earphone placed over one ear may cross to the opposite ear via bone conduction, via air conduction, or via both routes; and (2) bone-conducted signals tend to stimulate both cochleas simultaneously and nearly equally, even at low-intensity levels. These two circumstances sometimes make it difficult to know which ear is actually being stimulated. A common approach to resolving this problem is to reduce or eliminate the participation of the ear not under test by using a masking noise to elevate its threshold. (Ventry, Chaiklin, & Dixon, 1971, p. 297)

The authors then went on to emphasize the challenges associated with masking, noting:

Clinical masking is one of the most complex audiometric procedures to understand and to execute. It is complex because it involves so many variables that operate simultaneously, some of them under very tenuous control. Masker spectrum, minimum masking levels, interaural attenuation, central masking, and occlusion effects are only some of the variables that must be considered. (Ventry, Chaiklin, & Dixon, 1971, p. 297)

Mastering Masking

You may be a little confused after reading about masking or talking about masking with graduate students in audiology who are struggling to grasp masking concepts and clinical skills. Mastering masking does require study, thought, and hands-on practice with other students and with devices that simulate clinical masking situations. Confident, consistent, and correct application of masking comes about only with clinical experience that involves testing many patients with different types and degrees of hearing loss.

Don't be discouraged. You'll discover in this chapter that masking becomes much more manageable with an understanding of a handful of closely related concepts along with the factors mentioned by Ventry, Chaiklin, and Dixon. Concerns about masking are also greatly reduced when insert earphones are routinely used in air conduction pure tone testing and for masking during bone conduction hearing testing. Insert earphones weren't yet invented when early researchers opined on the complexity of masking decisions.

Furthermore, masking is unnecessary with air-conduction and sometimes even with bone-conduction testing for some patients undergoing hearing assessment in an audiology clinic. Finally, worries about whether to mask or not to mask are essentially eliminated when you follow the adage: "When in doubt, mask." Put another way, when you're testing a patient and questions arise about how to verify ear-specific air- and bone-conduction thresholds, "don't ask . . . just mask!"

General Rules of Masking

Masking in clinical audiology follows certain rules. The rules are simply stated here:

- Ear-specific test results are necessary for accurate hearing assessment. Information on hearing in each ear is essential for accurate diagnosis of hearing loss and for proper management of hearing loss.

- Air-conduction sounds presented at a high-intensity level to one ear may cross over to the nontest ear. Crossover of sound is most likely when hearing is poorer in one ear than in the other ear.

- Cross hearing from the test ear to the nontest ear occurs when the stimulus-intensity level exceeds interaural attenuation. Interaural attenuation is the difference between the intensity level of stimulus sound in the test ear versus the nontest ear.

- For air-conducted test sounds, interaural attenuation is at least 40 dB for supra-aural earphones and at least 60 dB for insert earphones

- In air-conduction (AC) testing, cross hearing is possible when the intensity level of the sound in the test ear (TE) minus the amount of interaural attenuation (IA) is greater than bone-conduction hearing levels in the nontest ear (BC_{NTE}). Stated as an equation: $AC_{TE} - IA \geq BC_{NTE}$. If this equation is true, cross hearing is possible.

- Interaural attenuation is 0 dB for bone-conducted sound. Presentation of bone-conduction sound to one side may produce activation of the inner ear on both sides.

- Cross hearing with bone-conduction hearing is possible at any intensity level.

- Cross hearing for bone conduction should be suspected whenever there is an air-bone gap of 10 dB or greater in the test ear before masking is used in the non-test ear.
- Clinically proven techniques exist for determining how much noise is needed to adequately mask the nontest ear during air- and bone-conduction hearing testing.

Throughout the chapter you'll learn how these rules are applied in various ways to ensure that test results reflect hearing only in the test ear.

Principles of Masking

The principles of masking are similar for pure tone hearing testing and speech audiometry. We'll first review briefly seven specific principles of masking, including (1) interaural attenuation, (2) minimum versus maximum masking, (3) effective masking, (4) over-masking, (5) air-bone gap, (6) occlusion effect, and (7) central masking. Then these principles will be incorporated into separate discussions of masking in pure tone audiometry, masking in speech audiometry, and of techniques for masking.

Interaural Attenuation

During air-conduction hearing testing with pure tones using any type of earphone, a patient's response can always be attributed to the test ear if sounds are presented at low- to moderate–intensity levels, up to about 40 dB HL. The head offers some insulation to prevent transmission of sound energy from the test ear to the nontest ear. The reduction in the amount of sound energy transmitted from one ear through or around the head to the other ear is referred to as **interaural attenuation (IA)**. The term **transcranial transmission loss** is also used to describe this phenomenon.

Air-conduction stimulation of the test ear will not cross over to the nontest ear until the stimulus is sufficiently intense to vibrate the bones of the skull or travel by air around the head to the other ear. Acoustic crossover of sound from the test ear to the nontest ear, called *cross hearing* or **transcranial hearing**, occurs when the intensity level of the sound exceeds interaural attenuation. Figure 7.1 illustrates the concept of interaural attenuation and crossover of energy from the test ear to the nontest ear during pure tone hearing testing.

Interaural Attenuation with Supra-Aural Earphones. The lowest intensity level at which cross hearing occurs or is possible differs substantially for supra-aural earphones versus insert earphones. With supra-aural earphones, it is possible for some of the sound energy to leak out of the seal between the earphones and the head and travel through the air from the test ear to the nontest ear. Bone-conducted vibrations offer a more likely route for crossover of energy from the test ear to the nontest ear. The rather firm cushions of supra-aural earphones rest on the pinna and the skin covering the skull. Air conduction stimulation with supra-aural earphones may begin to vibrate the bones of the skull at intensity levels of about 45 dB.

The actual amount of interaural attenuation with supra-aural earphones is usually greater than 45 dB, increasing to 60 dB or more for higher test frequencies ($\geq$ 2000 Hz). Figure 7.1 also depicts increased interaural attenuation for insert earphones versus supra-aural earphones. Importantly, interaural attenuation for supra-aural earphones varies from one person to the next. When the intensity level for supra-aural earphones exceeds interaural attenuation, vibrations of the skull may activate not only the cochlea on the test ear; the energy may also cross over to the nontest ear.

Interaural Attenuation with Insert Earphones. Interaural attenuation is substantially higher, and the likelihood of cross hearing of stimulation much lower, when air-conduction

FIGURE 7.1

Illustration of the interaural attenuation for air-conduction stimulation with supra-aural and insert earphones and for bone conduction pure tone stimulation. Crossover of a stimulus sound to the nontest ear occurs when the intensity of the pure tone sound exceeds interaural attenuation.

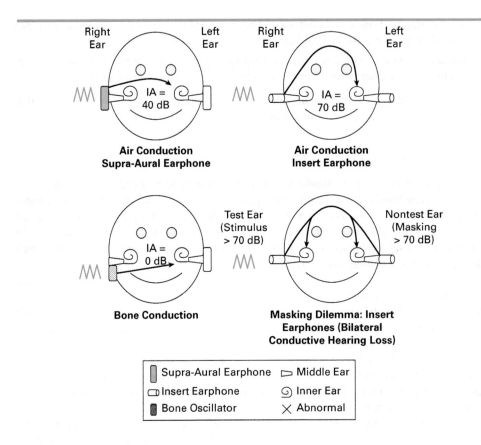

hearing testing is performed with insert earphones. With the foam insert tips properly placed in the right and left external ear canals, there is no possibility of sound escaping from one ear, traveling around the head via air, and reaching the inner ear on the opposite side.

Also, the soft foam tips used with insert earphones make contact mostly with the cartilaginous portion of the external ear canal, not the surface of the skull. Stimulus-intensity level must be at least 55 to 60 dB HL before energy begins to vibrate the skull bones (Munro & Agnew, 1999). And deeply fit insert earphones may increase interaural attenuation up to a level of 70 dB (e.g., Killion, Wilbur, & Gudmundson, 1985). Stated differently, there is no concern about cross hearing when patients with mild or moderate hearing loss are routinely tested with insert earphones. As you will soon learn when we discuss masking techniques, the lower likelihood of cross hearing associated with the greater interaural attenuation of insert earphones offers an important advantage in clinical hearing testing.

No Interaural Attenuation in Bone Conduction. With neither ear covered with an earphone and without masking of the nontest ear, a bone-conduction signal presented anywhere on the skull reaches the inner ear on each side of the head. For bone-conduction stimulation, we must assume that the head offers no insulation to the crossover of energy from one ear to the other. In other words, there is no interaural attenuation for bone conduction. Figure 7.1 also shows the concept of interaural attenuation and crossover of energy from the test ear to the nontest ear for bone-conducted pure tone sounds.

Cross hearing with bone conduction can occur at any intensity level above 0 dB HL. Placement of the bone vibrator on one mastoid certainly doesn't ensure activation of only that ear. Without adequate masking of the nontest ear, bone-conduction results are not ear specific or limited to the test ear. When bone-conduction hearing is tested with both ears uncovered, it is not possible in many cases to confidently determine whether the test ear or the opposite ear is activated or whether both ears are activated.

Too Little or Too Much Masking

We'll now discuss five related terms that are critical to understanding masking and how to apply masking in clinical audiology.

Under-Masking. **Under-masking** is inadequate and ineffective masking. Masking noise must be sufficient to eliminate the nontest ear from contributing to the patient's response to pure tone stimulation. The intensity level of masking noise can't be too low or too high. With under-masking the intensity level of masking noise is too low and the nontest ear may still contribute to the patient's response.

Minimum Masking. **Minimum masking** is the lowest level noise that just masks a pure tone or a speech signal of a certain intensity level. For example, a masking noise at 40 dB would minimally mask a tone with an intensity level of 40 dB assuming masking intensity is properly calibrated. Two practical concerns arise in determining minimum masking levels and attempting to minimally mask a nontest ear in hearing testing. Calculation of the minimum masking level is based on the assumption that interaural attenuation is accurately determined and bone-conduction hearing thresholds in the nontest ear are accurately estimated. In clinical hearing testing it is not possible to precisely determine interaural attenuation for a specific patient, and information on bone-conduction hearing is not always available when the calculations are made.

Another concern has to do with the normal variability in any measurement of hearing threshold. For example, a person's average hearing threshold for a 1000-Hz pure tone might be 40 dB if the threshold was measured repeatedly. However, the threshold might be 35 dB on some of the individual tests and 45 dB on some others. Minimum masking calculations will probably be off by 5 dB some of the time due to normal dispersion of the threshold values around the average value. This unavoidable problem is solved if a 10 dB "safety" or "correction" factor is added to the minimum masking level to ensure that masking is adequate.

Initial Masking. The phrase **initial masking** is used to describe the minimum level of masking noise necessary to produce a 5 dB-shift or increase in air-conduction thresholds in the nontest ear. Initial masking eliminates the possibility that the nontest ear is contributing to the patient's response in hearing testing.

Maximum Masking. We've already discussed the problem of a stimulus sound exceeding the interaural attenuation of an earphone and crossing over to the nontest ear. The purpose of masking is to isolate the test ear and to eliminate cross hearing as a factor in test results. **Maximum masking** is the highest level of masking noise that should be presented to the nontest ear. Too much masking noise is possible. At high-intensity levels, exceeding interaural attenuation for the earphones, masking noise can cross over from the nontest ear to the test ear.

Over-Masking. Crossover of masking noise from the nontest ear to the test ear is a problem called **over-masking**. Energy of the masking sound reaches the test ear from the nontest ear via bone conduction. The level of maximum masking and the possibility of over-masking are calculated with an equation that takes into account the effective masking (EM) level, interaural attenuation (IA) with the earphone, and bone-conduction (BC) hearing in the test ear (TE):

$$EM_{NTE} > BC_{TE} + IA$$

The level that is needed to effectively mask non-test ear must be greater than the bone conduction hearing in the test ear plus the amount of interaural attenuation. The bone-conduction threshold of the test ear is a key part of the equation. Masking levels quickly reach the point of over-masking for patients with large air-bone gaps in one or both ears. High-intensity levels of noise are required for minimum or initial masking of a nontest ear with an air-bone gap, yet maximum masking is reached at slightly higher levels of noise, creating the possibility of over-masking reaching the test ear. In short, enough masking may quickly become too much masking. We'll consider this masking challenge or "dilemma" later in the chapter, and we will identify possible solutions.

Effective Masking

Effective masking is defined as the amount of noise that definitively makes a specific signal such as a pure tone inaudible. For example, a person listening to a 30 dB pure tone will no longer hear the tone in 30 dB of effective masking. The tone would be heard if its intensity were increased to 35 dB. It is worthwhile to reiterate that the intensity level of masking noise during hearing testing cannot be too low or too high.

For most patients masking is effective over a range of intensity levels for noise extending from the level of minimum masking to the level of maximum masking. The term *plateau* is used to describe the condition in which the nontest ear is effectively masked, and further increases in masking levels do not produce a change in hearing thresholds for the test ear. Establishing the masking plateau between the minimum and maximum levels is the basis of a popular masking technique.

There is no danger or downside to regularly exceeding the minimum amount of masking so long as the maximum masking level is not exceeded. Some authors have expressed concerns about the possibility of "burdening" patients with more "unpleasant" noise than is necessary to minimally mask the nontest ear (Martin & Clark, 2012). There is no experimental or clinical evidence supporting the notion that patients experience discomfort when noise levels are increased above those minimally needed to effectively mask the nontest ear. The rationale for exceeding minimal masking levels for a given patient is consistent with the basic premise and goal of masking, that is, to assure that the nontest ear does not contribute to the patient's response.

Occlusion Effect

The occlusion effect is another factor to take into account in hearing testing. It certainly plays a role in calculations about levels of noise that are necessary for effectively masking the nontest ear. The occlusion effect can also play a role in bone-conduction hearing in the test ear. The **occlusion effect** is an enhancement or improvement in bone-conduction hearing for lower-frequency sounds. It occurs in patients with middle ear disorders and also in normal-hearing persons when an ear is covered with an earphone. Covering an ear with a supra-aural earphone produces an average occlusion effect of 30 dB for 250 Hz, 20 dB for 500 Hz, 10 dB for 1000 Hz, and 0 dB for higher frequencies (Elpern & Naunton, 1963). The occlusion effect is also recorded with insert earphones.

The occlusion effect is not a factor when larger circumaural earphones are used for masking. As the term implies, *circumaural earphones* totally surround the ear and rest on the skull, whereas supra-aural earphones rest on the pinna. As noted by Margolis (2010), with earphones that did not produce an occlusion effect "we could place the bone-conduction vibrator on the forehead, earphones over both ears, and test air conduction and bone conduction without moving the transducers. This would make manual testing more effective and make automated testing possible" (Margolis, 2010, p. 17).

Explanations for the Occlusion Effect. Two factors presumably contribute to the occlusion effect when an ear is covered or occluded by an earphone. One factor is an enhancement of osseotympanic bone conduction, one of the three mechanisms of bone conduction reviewed in Chapter 5. Some of the energy generated by osseotympanic vibration deep in the ear canal escapes from the ear canal in the uncovered test condition. In the covered condition the energy is instead added to energy that vibrates the tympanic membrane and ultimately activates the hair cells of the inner ear. Also, ambient sound in the test environment is reduced in the ears-covered condition and less likely to interfere with the perception of the bone-conduction sound. The earphones block some ambient sound from entering the ear canal and from partially masking the bone-conducted sound.

Central Masking

Central masking is an interesting phenomenon that factors into clinical hearing testing. Even a modest amount of masking noise in the nontest ear may produce a slight change in hearing thresholds in the test ear. Central masking usually results in a threshold shift or increase of 5 dB for pure tone or speech signals. It is not related to the problem of over-masking. Central masking occurs with noise levels in the nontest ear that are well below noise levels that exceed interaural attenuation for any earphone. The explanation for central masking lies in the brain, and not the ears.

If noise is sufficient to activate the cochlea in the nontest ear, there is also activation of auditory regions within central nervous system. The modest decrease in hearing thresholds is called central masking because the process takes place in the central auditory nervous system. The mechanisms for central masking are not clear. Neurons in specific regions of the brain that are activated by the masking noise may be less responsive to pure tone or speech signals. Central masking may also result from stimulation of the efferent auditory pathways that serve to inhibit and reduce cochlear activity. In any event, a slight increase in hearing threshold in the test ear is not unexpected when any amount of masking noise is presented to the nontest ear.

Masking in Pure Tone Audiometry

Air-Conduction Testing

Now that we've covered the general rules and principles of masking, we will turn our attention to the topic of masking in pure tone audiometry. We'll first consider air conduction testing and then bone conduction testing. Our discussion will address some very practical questions that arise in hearing testing, such as: When is masking needed in air-conduction testing?

Factors Affecting the Need for Masking. Three factors affect the decision about whether masking of the non-test ear is needed with air-conduction hearing testing. One is the interaural attenuation offered by the head with the earphones being used to perform air-conduction hearing testing. The concept of interaural attenuation was illustrated earlier in Figure 7.1. As you've learned, masking to prevent cross hearing must be considered whenever the stimulus-intensity level to the test ear exceeds 40 dB HL for supra-aural earphones and 60 dB HL for insert earphones.

Regular use of insert earphones in air-conduction hearing testing reduces the need for masking and also lessens the challenge of masking effectively during bone-conduction hearing testing. Because interaural attenuation is 60 dB or more with insert earphones, masking during air-conduction hearing testing is required only when measuring thresholds in a patient with hearing loss exceed 60 dB HL. In other words, with deeply placed insert earphones there is no danger of cross hearing until the intensity level exceeds 60 dB HL. Consequently, masking is never needed in air-conduction testing of persons with normal hearing or mild hearing loss, and it is rarely required even for patients with moderate hearing loss.

Another factor contributing to the decision about masking during air-conduction hearing threshold measurement is the level of bone-conduction hearing in the nontest ear. The need for masking during air-conduction hearing testing is relatively greater when bone-conduction hearing is normal in the nontest ear. The need for masking during air-conduction hearing testing decreases as bone-conduction hearing thresholds increase or are poorer in the nontest ear. This point leads directly to the third factor playing a role in the decision to mask or not to mask.

The pattern of hearing test results influences masking decisions. Masking of the nontest ear is required less often in patients with certain patterns of hearing loss, such as normal-hearing persons and patients with a similar degree of sensorineural hearing loss in each ear. On the other hand, the need for masking in the nontest ear is more likely for patients with an asymmetrical hearing loss and those with an air-bone gap in one or both ears.

Research findings and clinical experience suggest that a rather sizable proportion of patients undergoing air-conduction testing with insert earphones in a typical audiology facility do not require masking. Margolis and Saly (2008) analyzed audiogram data from over 20,000 patients seen in a medical center audiology clinic. Over one-third of the patients (33%) had normal hearing thresholds. Also, over one-half of the patients had either a mild (29%) or a moderate degree of hearing loss (28%). These findings confirm that the use of insert earphones greatly reduces the need for masking of the nontest ear during air-conduction pure tone hearing testing.

Calculating the Need for Masking. A simple equation is sometimes employed to determine whether masking of the nontest ear is needed in air-conduction hearing testing. Masking of the nontest ear is necessary when the level of sound reaching the nontest ear via crosshearing exceeds the bone-conduction hearing thresholds in the nontest ear. The relation between air-conduction (AC) hearing in the test ear (TE), interaural attenuation (IA), and bone-conduction (BC) hearing in the nontest ear (NTE) is sometimes summarized with the following expression:

$$AC_{TE} - IA > BC_{NTE}$$

If this equation is true, then masking is necessary.

Masking is required when the intensity level of sound crossing to the nontest ear via bone conduction is sufficient to be heard by the patient in the nontest ear.

Sample Masking Scenarios. Figure 7.2 shows some examples of air-conduction hearing thresholds in the test ear and bone-conduction hearing thresholds in the nontest ear. Thresholds in Figure 7.2A were measured with supra-aural earphones, whereas those in Figure 7.2B were obtained for the same levels with insert earphones. We will now take a moment to review each set of test results, as we consider when masking of the nontest ear is required and when it is not necessary.

Let's look first at thresholds for the 500-Hz pure tone frequency. The air-conduction hearing threshold is 40 dB HL and the bone-conduction threshold in the nontest ear is 5 dB HL. The difference is 35 dB ($AC_{TE} - BC_{NTE} = 35$ dB). Even a conservative estimation of the interaural attenuation for supra-aural earphones (40 dB) is greater than 35 dB. In this example there is no chance that the 500-Hz test signal presented with supra-aural earphones might cross over to the nontest ear. Masking of the nontest ear is not necessary. The same statement is true for insert earphones since interaural attenuation is even higher (60 dB), as depicted in Figure 7.2B.

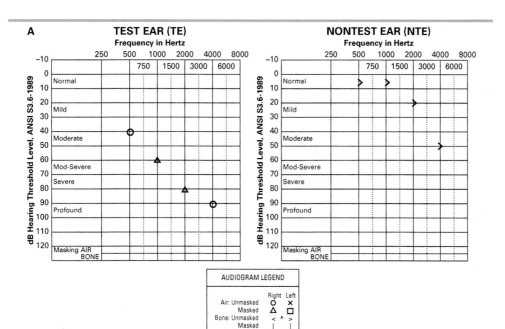

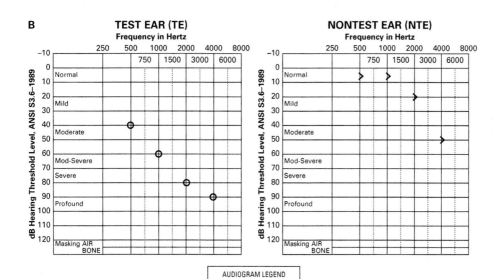

FIGURE 7.2

Audiograms for the test ear and nontest ear illustrating when masking is needed during air-conduction pure tone audiometry using **(A)** supra-aural earphones and **(B)** insert earphones. Each test frequency represents a different masking condition, that is, a different hearing threshold for unmasked bone-conduction testing. Masking for each test frequency is discussed in the text.

We'll move on to the 1000-Hz pure tone frequency shown in Figure 7.2A. The air-conduction hearing threshold is 60 dB HL and the bone-conduction threshold in the nontest ear is again 5 dB HL. The difference is 55 dB ($AC_{TE} - BC_{NTE} = 55$ dB). Since interaural attenuation for a supra-aural earphone is 40 dB, it is likely that the 1000-Hz tone will be detected in the nontest ear. You'll notice that the masked symbol is used for the air-conduction hearing threshold at the 1000-Hz test frequency. The masked symbol for air-conduction hearing threshold with the supra-aural earphone indicates that the audiologist realized the need for masking and applied adequate masking to the non-test ear. In contrast, as shown in Figure 7.2B, masking is not needed with the insert earphones since the interaural attenuation of 60 dB is greater than $AC_{TE} - BC_{NTE}$, or 55 dB.

A somewhat different combination of threshold test results is evident for the 2000-Hz frequency. You can see in Figure 7.2A that the air-conduction hearing threshold is 80 dB HL, at the upper limit of the severe range of hearing loss. This level is clearly greater than the estimated 40 dB interaural attenuation associated with supra-aural earphones. However, the bone-conduction threshold in the nontest ear is 20 dB for the 2000-Hz pure tone. Using the same equation, $AC_{TE} - BC_{NTE} = 60$ dB. Again, crossover hearing from the test ear to the nontest ear is likely for the 2000-Hz pure tone. The symbol for the air-conduction threshold for the supra-aural earphone graph indicates that masking was applied to the nontest ear. As shown in Figure 7.2B, masking was again not needed with the insert earphones since the interaural attenuation of 60 dB did not exceed interaural attenuation for insert earphones, which is also 60 dB (as $AC_{TE} - BC_{NTE} = 60$ dB).

Finally, we'll inspect the thresholds for the 4000-Hz test frequency. As shown in Figure 7.2A, the air-conduction hearing threshold decreased further to 90 dB HL. Yet it is plotted with the unmasked symbol. The explanation lies with the even greater decrease of the bone-conduction threshold in the nontest ear to 50 dB HL. The equation confirms that interaural attenuation of 40 dB for the supra-aural earphones is equivalent to but does not exceed the difference between air-conduction threshold in the test ear and the bone-conduction threshold in the nontest ear, that is $AC_{TE} - BC_{NTE} = 40$ dB. Masking is not necessary. As shown in Figure 7.2B, masking of the nontest ear again is not required with the insert earphone.

These simple scenarios highlight two important points about masking in air-conduction hearing testing. First, the need for masking depends on the combination of the air-conduction hearing threshold in the test ear and the bone-conduction hearing in the nontest ear, rather than air conduction alone. Masking of the nontest ear may be needed for patients with moderate hearing loss, as we saw above for the 1000-Hz pure tone, and not for severe-to-profound loss, as at 4000 Hz. The other point is that masking of the nontest ear is required less often when insert earphones are used for air-conduction hearing testing.

Predicting Who Needs Masking. Audiologists often have clues about the need for masking even before a patient sets foot into a sound-treated room for hearing testing. A patient history offers valuable information regarding the possible need for masking the nontest ear during air-conduction or bone conduction hearing testing. The need for masking is lower for patients who have no history of middle ear disorders and it is considerably higher for patients whose history confirms middle ear abnormalities. Objective tests of middle ear function performed before pure tone hearing testing may also guide an audiologist's decisions about whether masking is needed during pure tone audiometry or whether it is probably unnecessary. You'll learn in the next chapter about two important objective auditory tests.

A Caveat. You may have already identified one flaw with the strategy we've just reviewed for determining the need for masking in air-conduction hearing testing. The principles and formulas guiding decisions about the need for masking during air conduction testing include the bone conduction hearing threshold in the non-test ear (BC_{NTE}). However, when air-conduction hearing thresholds are being measured for one ear at the beginning of the testing process, accurate bone-conduction hearing thresholds are generally not available for the nontest ear. The rather straightforward strategy and the equation used for calculating the need for masking of the nontest ear is based on an assumption. The strategy and equation assume that the audiologist first measures air-conduction hearing thresholds in the test ear without masking and also measures bone-conduction thresholds in the nontest ear without masking. The audiologist must then repeat air-conduction testing with adequate masking of the nontest ear. This testing process is somewhat cumbersome and time consuming.

Usually Mask. There is an alternative approach for deciding when to apply adequate masking, a strategy that is simple and more clinically efficient. First of all, routinely perform air-conduction hearing testing with insert earphones unless it is not possible for some reason. Then, apply masking to the nontest ear whenever the stimulus-intensity level of the pure tone in the test ear exceeds interaural attenuation for the earphones. With insert earphones, masking of the nontest ear is not needed until air-conduction stimulation of the test ear exceeds 60 dB HL. Finally, assume that bone-conduction thresholds are 0 dB in the nontest ear.

This technique takes a conservative "worse-case scenario" approach to determining whether masking of the nontest ear is required. There is no doubt that masking will sometimes be applied unnecessarily to the nontest ear if this strategy is used. Upon completion of pure tone audiometry, it may become clear that masking was not really needed for some or all of the air-conduction hearing thresholds. Nonetheless, no harm was done. Information from patient history and from auditory tests that objectively and specifically assess middle ear function certainly contribute to decisions about masking, even before bone-conduction test results are available. Audiologists who suspect conductive hearing loss can routinely mask the nontest ear whenever air- conduction levels exceed interaural attenuation values.

An audiologist who takes this conservative and pre-emptive approach to masking the nontest ear during air-conduction hearing testing is adhering to the guideline, "I'd rather sometimes use masking when it is not really necessary than not use masking when it really is necessary."

Masking in Bone-Conduction Testing

When Should Masking Be Used in Bone-Conduction Testing? Bone-conduction testing is not always performed in clinical audiology. Authors of the study cited earlier (Margolis & Saly, 2008) reported that bone-conduction thresholds were not measured for over 42 percent of 16,818 patients in an medical center audiology clinic who underwent hearing testing of both ears. Bone-conduction testing was performed for only one ear for another 43 percent. The vast majority of patients who were not tested with bone conduction had either normal hearing (53%) or the sloping high-frequency audiogram configuration (31%) that is typically found in patients with sensorineural hearing loss.

You'll learn in the next chapter about clinical tests that provide valuable, objective, and rather specific information about middle ear function. These sensitive tests of middle ear function are often performed before a patient is taken into a sound booth for pure tone hearing testing. The results of the tests are particularly useful for differentiating patients who have normal middle ear function from those with middle ear disorders and possible conductive hearing loss. Sensitive tests of middle ear function also offer a good clue as to which patients need to be tested with bone conduction.

 WebWatch

You'll find on the Internet interactive tutorials and simulations that explain masking principles and procedures. You might begin your search at the AudSim website.

The Occlusion Effect. The test ear is not "covered" by an earphone or insert ear tip when bone conduction is performed with a bone vibrator placed on the mastoid. Figure 7.3A shows a typical arrangement for the bone vibrator on the mastoid bone of the uncovered test ear. Figure 7.3B shows an earphone covering the nontest ear (Figure 7.3B). Looking closely, you'll see the metal band for the bone vibrator underneath the band for the earphone headset.

As you've already learned, covering or occluding the test ear produces a phenomenon known as the **occlusion effect**. As a general rule, the test ear is not covered during bone conduction testing. Covering the test ear produces an occlusion effect for low frequencies that renders bone-conduction thresholds inaccurate. Calibration of bone vibrators and determination of reference levels for bone conduction testing is based on the assumption that the test ear is uncovered.

In preparing a patient for bone conduction testing an audiologist usually places a supra-aural earphone on or an insert earphone in the nontest ear, but the test ear is always left uncovered (Figure 7.3A). Some patients assume that the earphones should always be located on both ears, so it is occasionally necessary for the audiologist to specifically instruct the patient to refrain from moving an earphone onto the uncovered ear during bone conduction testing. Again, calibration of the bone vibrator assumes that testing will be conducted in the uncovered ear condition.

The decision about covering the nontest ear with an earphone rather than leaving it uncovered during bone-conduction testing depends on whether the nontest ear will be masked. Bone-conduction stimulation anywhere on the skull reaches the right cochlea and the left cochlea. There are test situations when bone conduction can be measured without masking of the nontest ear. An example situation is when a patient has air-conduction hearing thresholds that are very similar in both ears, with differences no greater than 5 or 10 dB at any test frequency between air conduction thresholds and unmasked bone conduction thresholds.

Audiometric Bing Test. Since the early 1800s, physicians have utilized tuning forks during physical examination of the ear and hearing. You learned about tuning forks in Chapter 2. Audiologists sometimes use audiometers to perform two tuning fork tests. One of the tuning fork tests is the **Bing test**. The audiometric Bing test quantifies the size of the occlusion effect. The test is named after Albert Bing, an Austrian otologist who published extensively on ear disease in the late 1800s.

FIGURE 7.3

(A) A typical set-up for bone-conduction testing. The bone vibrator is located on the mastoid of the test ear with the test ear uncovered.
(B) A typical set-up for bone-conduction testing with masking. An earphone used to present masking sound covers the nontest ear. The bone vibrator is located on the mastoid of the other ear.

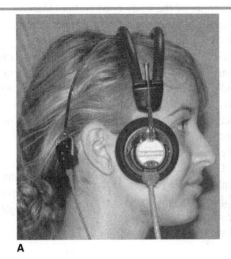
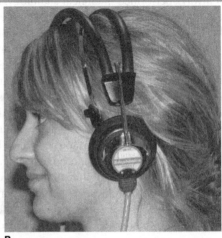

A   B

We'll review briefly now how the Bing test is performed. Bone-conduction hearing thresholds are first measured with the test ear uncovered, usually for several low test frequencies like 250 Hz or 500 Hz. Adequate masking noise is delivered to the nontest ear to assure that the bone-conduction responses reflect activation of the test ear. Then, bone-conduction thresholds are measured again for the test ear in an occluded condition. The process of measuring uncovered and occluded bone-conduction hearing is then repeated for the other ear.

Audiometric Weber Test. The audiometric **Weber test** is a measure of lateralization of sound. The occlusion effect is also the mechanism underlying the Weber test. In performing the Weber test, a bone vibrator is placed on the middle of the forehead. The ears are not covered with earphones. Figure 7.4.shows the setup for the audiometric Weber test.

The patient is instructed to report where the tones are heard, that is, toward the right side, toward the left side, or toward the middle of the head. It is sometimes easier for patients, especially children, to simply point to the location on their head where they think they are hearing the sounds. As with the Bing test, the Weber test is performed with low frequencies such as 250 Hz and 500 Hz.

Figure 7.5 illustrates some Weber test outcomes. A patient with normal hearing sensitivity bilaterally typically localizes the pure tone sound to the middle of the head. This response is labeled "A" in Figure 7.5. Bone-conduction stimulation activates each ear equally. A patient with a *symmetrical hearing loss* also gives a midline response. A symmetrical hearing loss is when there is the same degree of loss or similar hearing loss for both ears.

Figure 7.5B shows a Weber finding for a person with normal hearing sensitivity in both ears when the right ear is covered with an earphone. The bone-conducted sound is heard in the right ear because of the occlusion effect produced by the earphone.

If there is a middle ear disorder on one side only, bone-conducted sounds will lateralize to that ear. Figure 7.5C illustrates lateralization during the audiometric Weber test of bone-conducted sound to an ear with conductive hearing loss. The patient perceives stimulus sounds more loudly in the ear with conductive hearing loss due to the occlusion effect. This is the same phenomenon that explains the lateralization of sound to a normal-hearing ear when the ear is covered.

A patient will lateralize sound to the better-hearing ear on the Weber test when there is a sensorineural hearing loss one ear. The diagram labeled "D" in Figure 7.5 shows a typical finding for the audiometric Weber test in a patient with a sensorineural hearing loss in the right ear and normal hearing in the left ear.

The audiometric Bing and Weber tests are quick and simple procedures for confirming the type of hearing loss, that is, conductive versus sensory hearing loss, in one or both ears.

Masking Noises in Pure Tone Audiometry

Two types of noise are available on most clinical audiometers for masking the nontest ear in air- and bone-conduction hearing testing. *White noise* or *broadband noise (BBN)* contains approximately equal amounts of acoustic energy over a broad band of frequencies. Like white light, white noise consists of energy over a broad spectrum of frequencies. White noise is like a hissing or rushing water sound. The exact acoustic spectrum of white noise depends on the frequency response of the earphone. White noise is not ideal for masking in pure tone hearing

FIGURE 7.4

An example of the set-up for the audiometric Weber test. The bone vibrator is placed on the forehead.

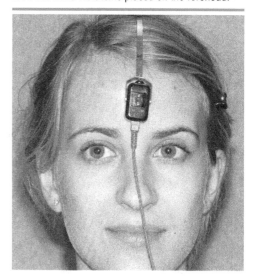

FIGURE 7.5

Weber test examples of a patient showing whether the sound is heard in the middle of the head **(A)**, to a normal-hearing ear that is covered with an earphone **(B)**, the right ear with a conductive hearing loss **(C)**, and to the left ear for a patient with a sensory hearing loss on the right ear **(D)**.

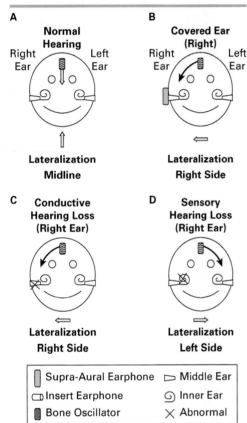

A   **Normal Hearing**
Right Ear   Left Ear

Lateralization Midline

B   **Covered Ear (Right)**
Right Ear   Left Ear

Lateralization Right Side

C   **Conductive Hearing Loss (Right Ear)**

Lateralization Right Side

D   **Sensory Hearing Loss (Right Ear)**

Lateralization Left Side

	Supra-Aural Earphone		Middle Ear
	Insert Earphone		Inner Ear
	Bone Oscillator	×	Abnormal

testing. The only components of the noise that are effective in masking are within a restricted band near the pure tone frequency.

Critical Band Concept. Early studies of masking confirmed what is known as the **critical band** concept (Fletcher & Munson, 1937). Harvey Fletcher, one of the people conducting research on critical bands, was featured in Leaders & Luminaries in Chapter 2. The sound energy within a critical band of noise that is centered at a pure tone frequency is most effective in masking the tone. Masking efficiency of noise is actually decreased as the band is widened because added frequencies in the noise increase the overall intensity without producing further change in hearing threshold for the tone. Only acoustic energy within the critical band contributes to masking efficiency. Masking efficiency is also decreased if the band of noise is narrowed to less than the critical limits.

Narrowband Noise (NBN). The most effective type of masking sound in pure tone testing is a narrow band of noise that is centered on the frequency of the test tone (Liden, Nilsson, & Anderson, 1959b; Studebaker, 1967). *Narrowband noise* on modern clinical audiometers is somewhat wider than the critical band. The relatively limited spectrum of narrowband noise in masking is focused on the frequency region of the stimulus, including a limited range of frequencies below and above the test frequency. For example, if the stimulus is a pure tone at 1000 Hz, the masking noise might consist of a band of frequencies from approximately 850 to 1150 Hz. Narrowband masking noise has superior masking efficiency.

The intensity level of masking noise produced by an audiometer must be specified and regularly calibrated, just as pure tone stimuli are calibrated. Calibration should include verification of the linearity of the intensity levels of different types of masking noise. Linearity is consistency in the intensity steps from a minimum intensity of less than 0 dB HL to the maximum intensity, often greater than 100 dB HL. The intensity level of masking noise can be defined in dB sound pressure level (SPL) or dB hearing level (HL).

Masking in Speech Audiometry

Revisiting the Advantage of Insert Earphones

Masking is as important in speech audiometry as it is in pure tone audiometry. The concepts of masking already reviewed apply in both types of hearing testing. We'll consider here one masking concept common to pure tone audiometry and speech audiometry. The clinical advantages of insert earphones already cited for pure tone audiometry are equally important for speech audiometry tests. Research findings confirm that interaural attenuation with spondee words presented via supra-aural earphones is no less than 48 dB. The minimum interaural attenuation value for supra-aural earphones with spondee words can be rounded down to 45 dB since 5-dB-intensity steps are typically used in clinical testing (Martin & Blythe, 1977; Snyder, 1973).

Insert earphones increase interaural attenuation for spondee words up to about 60 dB HL (Killion, Wilber, & Gudmundsen, 1985; Sklare & Denenberg, 1987). Insert earphones offer

L E A D E R S   A N D   L U M I N A R I E S

Mead Killion

Mead C. Killion, PhD, ScD, earned degrees in mathematics from Wabash College and the Illinois Institute of Technology. He completed his doctorate in audiology at Northwestern University. He was awarded an honorary doctor of science (Sc.D.) degree from Wabash College. Dr. Killion founded Etymotic Research in 1983 for the purpose of designing products that measure, enhance, and protect hearing. The term *etymotic* means "true-to-the-ear." Etymotic products best recognized by audiologists include ER-3A insert earphones for audiometry and ABR, Companion Mics®, QuickSIN/BKB-SIN tests, K-AMP® and Digi-K® hearing aid circuitry, ERO-SCAN and OtoRead OAE devices, directional and array microphones, and Musicians Earplugs.™ Etymotic's Consumer Division produces high-end earphones and headsets for musicians and audiophiles, ready-fit and electronic earplugs, and personal noise dosimeters. The company holds more than 100 patents.

Dr. Killion is an adjunct professor at Northwestern University. He is an accomplished choir director, violinist, and jazz pianist. Dr. Killion's current passion is flying, a hobby he started in college and had abandoned for about fifty years.

greater interaural attenuation for speech presented via air conduction and less chance of crossover of the speech to the nontest ear. Put another way, the regular use of insert earphones during air-conduction speech audiometry reduces the need to mask the nontest ear. Also, higher levels of noise can be used to mask the nontest ear with insert earphones before overmasking occurs. Masking levels of up to 60 dB HL are possible without concern that the masking noise will cross over to the test ear.

Conservative estimates for minimum interaural attenuation values during speech audiometry are 45 dB HL for supra-aural earphones and 60 dB HL for insert earphones. There is considerable variability in interaural attenuation values from one patient to the next. Consequently, the likelihood of cross hearing also varies considerably from one patient to the next. Patient differences in interaural attenuation are due to frequency characteristics of the speech stimulus and also patient factors like head size and skull thickness.

Differences between Masking during Pure Tone and Masking During Speech Audiometry

Four distinctions between masking of the nontest ear for speech audiometry and masking for pure tone audiometry are as follows: (1) Information on bone-conduction hearing from pure tone testing is already available during speech audiometry, (2) frequency characteristics of speech differ from pure tones, (3) speech stimuli are often presented at supra-threshold levels, and (4) different masking noises are required for speech than for tone signals. We now discuss briefly each of these differences.

Pure Tone Hearing Information Guides Masking in Speech Audiometry. The need for masking in speech audiometry is generally determined by the best threshold for pure tone hearing in the nontest ear. That is, masking in speech audiometry should be used if the difference between the air-conduction stimulus level for speech signals in the test ear and best pure tone bone-conduction hearing threshold for the nontest ear exceeds interaural attenuation of the earphones. Recall the simple equation for determining the need for masking, when: $AC_{TE} - IA > BC_{NTE}$.

Determination of the need for masking of the nontest ear can also be made with a calculation of the difference between the intensity level of the speech stimulus in the test ear and a speech threshold measure for the nontest ear. Masking of the nontest ear should be applied when this difference exceeds minimal interaural attenuation for the type of earphones used in testing.

Audiologists have a distinct advantage in calculating the need for masking in speech audiometry. The results of pure tone hearing testing are almost always available before speech audiometry is performed. Each of the components of the equation is known. Also, air-conduction thresholds for spondee words are measured during speech audiometry. The minimum interaural attenuation values for speech signals for supra-aural and insert earphones are well established. And, bone-conduction thresholds in the nontest ear are available from pure tone hearing testing.

Speech Threshold Testing. Masking decisions are similar for measurement of pure tone and speech thresholds. The decision about whether to mask is based on bone-conduction thresholds in the nontest ear. Speech includes energy over a broad band of frequencies. Therefore, the safest decision about when to mask is based on the best bone-conduction hearing threshold in the nontest ear for test frequencies in the region of 250 to 4000 Hz (Coles & Priede, 1970). Masking is used when there is a possibility of speech presented to the test ear crossing over to the nontest ear and exceeding the lowest or best hearing thresholds in the nontest ear.

How much masking is appropriate in speech recognition testing? Masking levels must exceed the minimum to effectively mask the nontest ear. The minimum level is conservatively determined by considering the best bone-conduction threshold in the non-test ear and also the maximum air-bone gap at any test frequency (Coles & Priede, 1970). Keep in mind that the level of masking noise presented via air-conduction to the non-test ear must exceed the air-bone gap in the non-test ear.

The intensity level of noise presented to the non-test ear in speech threshold testing can be increased up to the maximum masking level. Exceeding the maximum masking level results in crossover of the masking noise from the nontest ear to the test ear. Crossover occurs when the level of the masking noise exceeds interaural attenuation and is sufficient to reach the best bone-conduction hearing threshold in the test ear somewhere within the frequency region of 250 to 4000 Hz.

It is clear from the foregoing discussion that accurate measurement of air- and bone conduction hearing thresholds contributes importantly to decisions about masking decisions during speech audiometry. To reiterate, the final decision about whether masking is necessary in speech audiometry depends on bone-conduction levels in the nontest ear, air-bone gap, and bone-conduction levels in the test ear. The need for masking decreases when there is poor bone-conduction hearing in the nontest ear and when there is no air-bone gap. In clinical audiology, measurement of speech thresholds for patients with normal-hearing sensitivity or mild hearing loss is conducted at relatively low-intensity levels. As a result, stimulus-intensity levels for air-conduction testing are often less than the minimum interaural attenuation values, especially for insert earphones.

Word Recognition Testing. A more conservative or careful approach is recommended in determining the need for masking during word recognition testing at supra-threshold-intensity levels (Yacullo, 1998). The reason for more conservative decision making about masking has to do with the intensity level of the stimulus and also with the nature of the response.

Word recognition testing is invariably carried out at supra-threshold levels. Consequently, the need for masking is encountered more often with word recognition testing that is typically carried out at intensity levels 40 dB or more above hearing threshold in the test ear. The likelihood of exceeding interaural attenuation and of cross hearing is increased as stimulus level increases (Sanders & Hall, 1999; Studebaker, 1967).

Presentations for monosyllabic test words are usually at least 30 dB HL and may be as high as 80 or 90 dB HL. Consequently the need for masking of the nontest ear should regularly be considered before word recognition measurement begins, even in patients for whom masking was not necessary during pure tone or speech threshold testing. A simple and conservative or safe approach to masking during speech audiometry assumes an interaural attenuation of 40 dB for measurement of speech reception thresholds and word recognition testing (Yacullo, 1999).

As you learned in Chapter 6, performance is measured very differently for speech recognition threshold testing than for word recognition testing. The performance criterion in speech threshold testing is recognition of 50% of the spondee words that are presented. Let's say that the nontest ear is not adequately masked during speech threshold testing and the patient repeats some of the test words that reach the nontest ear. The speech reception threshold measurement will not be affected unless one-half of the words reaching the inadequately masked nontest ear are recognized.

How does performance criterion affect scores for word recognition testing? Let's assume inadequate masking of the nontest ear during word recognition testing. A list of twenty-five words is presented to the test ear. Let's say that the patient recognizes five of the words reaching the inadequately masked nontest ear. Let's also assume that the patient hears 40 percent of the words in the test ear and correctly recognizes them. The patient's score on the word recognition test will actually reflect combined word recognition performance for the test and the nontest ear. It is possible that the patient's overall word recognition performance could appear better than accurately measured performance with the nontest ear properly masked.

Inadequate masking of the nontest ear during word recognition testing is particularly troublesome in measurement of rollover at very high-intensity levels. Rollover or decreased word recognition performance at high-intensity levels is sometimes found in patients with neural auditory disorders. Word recognition performance, including rollover, is not valid unless the nontest ear is adequately masked.

You can now appreciate that the rules of masking apply in speech audiometry as they do in pure tone audiometry. In some cases, decisions about masking levels in word recognition testing can be simplified. An appropriate simplified approach is to select masking for the nontest ear when word recognition performance is at intensity levels 30 to 40 dB above thresholds in patients with no air-bone gap. Yacullo (1999) states: "effective masking level is equal to the presentation level of the speech signal in dB HL at the test ear minus 20 dB."

Masking Noises in Speech Audiometry. Distinctly different types of masking noise are used for speech audiometry than for pure tone audiometry. This has to do with the frequency characteristics of pure tone versus speech signals. You'll recall that the two most common types of masking sound in pure tone audiometry are narrow bands of noise centered on the pure tone frequency and broadband noise. Narrowband noise is preferable for pure tone audiometry. Speech signals consist of a wider range of frequencies than pure tones or even narrow frequency bands. The goal in masking the nontest ear during speech audiometry is to ensure that the patient does not detect any of the energy in the speech signal in the nontest ear.

Speech noise is employed most often in speech audiometry. Speech noise is a special type of masking sound. Energy in speech is relatively greater for lower frequencies and less for higher frequencies. Energy in vowels and some nasal consonants contributes considerably to the low-frequency energy in speech. Speech energy gradually decreases for higher-frequency consonant sounds. Speech noise consists of a broad band of noise with relatively greater energy in the lower frequencies. Speech noise is available on all clinical audiometers and is best suited for masking during speech audiometry.

The concept of *effective masking* reviewed for pure tone hearing testing is relevant also for speech audiometry. Masking noise must be sufficient to eliminate the nontest ear from contributing to the patient's response to speech stimulation. As in pure tone audiometry, the intensity level of masking noise during speech audiometry cannot be too low or too high. Effective masking noise for speech is defined as the amount of masking noise that produces an equivalent shift in speech threshold. A specific level of effective masking noise, like 10 dB, produces a shift in speech threshold of 10 dB. Speech spectrum noise, often simply referred to as speech noise, is the most efficient masker for speech signals.

 WebWatch

An Internet search will reveal YouTube videos illustrating the application of masking techniques during hearing testing of children and of adults.

Masking Techniques

We'll now review specific techniques for masking in clinical audiology, beginning with pure tone hearing testing. You'll apply your new knowledge of the principles of masking in the following discussion. The masking techniques described are appropriate for pure tone hearing testing and for speech audiometry. We begin with a reminder that masking is necessary whenever there is a possibility that the test sound might cross over to the nontest ear at a level sufficient to be heard by the patient. Two different strategies are available to audiologists for masking the nontest ear in bone conduction hearing testing.

Unmasked Then Masked

With one approach bone conduction hearing thresholds are first measured without masking of the nontest ear and the need for masking is then assessed. In some cases, an audiologist can determine from unmasked bone conduction testing that there is no air-bone gap in either ear. Thus, masking is not needed to verify ear-specific bone-conduction thresholds. However, in cases where review of air-conduction and unmasked bone-conduction thresholds confirms that masking is needed to verify ear-specific test results, bone-conduction testing is repeated with adequate masking of hearing in the opposite nontest ear.

Using this unmasked-plus-masked approach, bone conduction hearing testing is essentially measured twice in the same ear for some patients. Greater test time is required to complete two sets of bone-conduction measurements, that is, the unmasked and then the masked. Time is also spent reviewing the initial results obtained without masking. An audiologist also uses additional time in returning to the sound booth to replace the bone oscillator and place the earphones used for the masking sound.

Mask Immediately

An alternative approach is to routinely apply masking whenever hearing thresholds are assessed with bone-conduction stimulation. This strategy might at first appear to increase the time and effort required to complete bone conduction hearing testing. However, in clinical settings where conductive hearing loss is regularly encountered, a policy of consistently measuring masked bone-conduction hearing thresholds actually saves test time and effort.

We've discussed already how information from patient history and specific tests of middle ear function guide audiologists as to which patients are likely to require masking of the nontest ear for air- and bone-conduction testing. Routine masking the nontest ear is a reasonable test approach if information about middle ear abnormality is available before pure tone hearing testing There is no serious disadvantage to masking the nontest ear during bone-conduction testing and during air-conduction testing when the stimulus intensity exceeds interaural attenuation. For patients who require masking of the nontest ear, test time is reduced when masked thresholds are measured one time for each ear using appropriate masking of the non-test ear. Routine use of masking during bone-conduction testing and as needed during air-conduction testing is particularly efficient in clinics where patients with conductive or mixed hearing loss are regularly encountered.

Determining Effective Masking

Formula Approach. Mathematical formulae have been developed for calculating the minimum amount of noise needed to adequately mask pure tone signals at different intensity levels (Liden et al., 1959a, b; Sanders & Hall, 1999). Unfortunately, the rather complicated formulae are not easily learned and their application consumes valuable test time. The need for masking is determined frequency by frequency and then the minimum level of necessary masking is calculated. Using the formulae, masking may be applied at some test frequencies and not at others.

In fact, there is no clinical rationale for using the lowest possible or minimal-intensity level of noise to just barely mask a pure tone signal in the nontest ear. Rather, there are advantages in a clinical setting for regularly beginning bone-conduction threshold measurement with a higher level of masking noise. As noted earlier, consistent presentation of masking noise at a higher-intensity level for all test frequencies, instead of at minimum noise levels only at selected frequencies, does not pose any risk or discomfort to the patient. To the contrary, patients may adapt more readily to the constant presence of a consistent level of masking noise. A simple yet effective and clinically popular masking technique will now be described.

Plateau Method. The plateau method for determining effective masking was first reported over fifty years ago (Hood, 1960). It is widely applied clinically. Figure 7.6 shows the plateau or plateau-seeking method of masking for bone-conduction hearing measurement.

We'll now go through each step in plotting test results on the graph shown in Figure 7.6. With the example shown, bone-conduction stimulation is presented to the mastoid of a

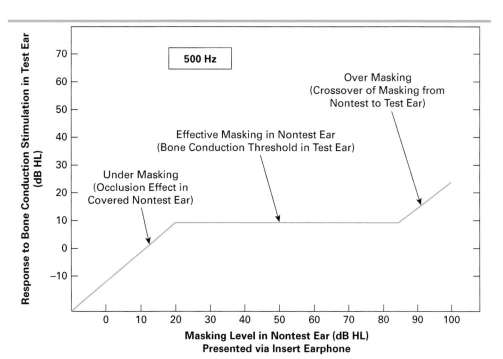

FIGURE 7.6

The Hood plateau method for masking the nontest ear in hearing testing.

normal-hearing ear. Masking is delivered with an insert earphone to the nontest ear where hearing is also normal. This general test setup was illustrated earlier in Figure 7.3.

We'll begin our review of the test results in the lower left corner of the graph. With the bone oscillator on the mastoid of the test ear and the foam tip of the insert earphone in the ear canal of the nontest ear, the patient responded to very low-intensity bone-conduction stimulation for a test frequency of 500 Hz. The patient's response was for bone-conduction sound of less than 0 dB because of the occlusion effect created by sealing the nontest ear canal with an insert earphone tip. The occlusion effect enhanced the effect of vibrations presented to the mastoid of the test ear with increased activation of the nontest cochlea.

During bone conduction testing, masking noise was presented to the nontest ear via air conduction. The intensity level of masking noise was systematically increased in 10-dB increments. At each new masking level, a new response was obtained with bone-conduction stimulation of the test ear using 5-dB-intensity increments, as shown on the graph.

When testing began, increased bone-conduction stimulus intensity was needed for the sound to be audible to the patient each time an additional 10 dB of masking was presented to the nontest ear. Repeated shifts in bone-conduction hearing thresholds associated with increases in the level of masking confirmed that these initial responses were arising from stimulation of the nontest ear and not the test ear. Masking was not yet sufficient to eliminate the nontest ear from contributing to the response. That was evidence of undermasking. The minimum effective masking level was not yet reached.

You'll notice in Figure 7.6 that a response to bone-conduction stimulation was repeatedly obtained at 10 dB HL beginning with a masking-intensity level of 20 dB. In this example, the minimum masking level is 20 dB. Progressively higher levels of masking noise over a range of masking intensities (30 dB, 40 dB, 50 dB, and so forth) had no effect on the bone-conduction response. The consistency in the intensity level producing the patient's response is the *plateau* for which the technique is named. A plateau confirms effective masking of the nontest ear. A plateau is optimally defined by consistency in the patient response level for at least three different intensity levels of masking. For our example in Figure 7.6, the plateau was considerably greater.

Finally, the right side of Figure 7.6 shows an increase in bone-conduction hearing thresholds with high-intensity levels of masking noise in the nontest ear. The final upward line on the Hood plateau graph is evidence of over-masking. The level of the masking noise exceeded interaural attenuation even for the insert earphones that are used for masking the nontest ear. Noise crossed over via bone conduction from the nontest ear to the other side where it masked the test ear. The term **cross masking** rather than cross hearing is sometimes used to describe the crossover of masking noise from the nontest ear to the test ear. If masking was delivered via a supra-aural earphone with less interaural attenuation, over-masking would probably begin at a masking level of 50 to 55 dB. The plateau is shorter when over-masking occurs at a lower-intensity level.

To summarize, there is under-masking when increases in the intensity of the masking noise are associated with increases in the bone-conduction stimulus level needed to produce a patient response. The response is still produced by activation of the nontest ear. The stimulus-intensity levels producing the plateau despite increased masking levels in the nontest ear reflect the patient's actual bone-conduction hearing threshold in the test ear. The plateau documents effective masking. Subsequent shifts in threshold at higher masking levels, if they occur, are due to over-masking.

The foregoing explanation is meant as an introduction to the concept of the plateau method for masking. Masking is not difficult for normal-hearing persons and patients with mild hearing loss in one or both ears. And, when insert earphones are used properly during air-conduction pure tone audiometry and also in masking the nontest ear during bone-conduction testing, masking challenges are largely limited to patients with moderate-to-severe hearing loss or conductive hearing loss with an air-bone gap.

Speech Audiometry

Either of the two general approaches for masking in pure tone hearing measurement, the acoustic formula approach or the plateau method, can be applied effectively in speech audiometry (Lawson & Peterson, 2011; Sanders & Hall, 1999; Studebaker, 1962, 1967; Yacullo, 1999). The plateau method is generally learned more readily and it certainly requires few calculations. There is an added advantage to the plateau method in speech audiometry. Masking can be implemented during speech threshold or word recognition measurement without first determining pure tone hearing thresholds (Lawson & Peterson, 2011).

To review briefly, masking speech noise is usually presented to the nontest ear in 10-dB increments. Masking begins at a level corresponding to the best hearing for any pure tone frequency in the nontest ear, or corresponding to the speech threshold in the nontest ear if it has already been measured. At each new masking level, additional words are presented to the patient. Repeated increases in the threshold for speech associated with increases in the level of masking confirm that the initial responses are only from the nontest ear. Masking is not yet sufficient to eliminate the nontest ear from contributing to the response. There is undermasking. The patient's speech threshold is confirmed when the threshold for speech in the test ear doesn't change even with additional masking of the nontest ear. A plateau in speech responses confirms effective masking of the nontest ear.

Masking Dilemma

Masking dilemma is one of the most interesting phrases in audiology. It refers to a troublesome practical problem in the ear-specific measurement of air- and bone-conduction hearing thresholds. The testing predicament can be succinctly defined in seven words: The masking dilemma occurs "when enough masking is too much masking." Audiologists encounter the masking dilemma most often in patients with risk factors for conductive hearing loss and air conduction test results showing a moderate or severe hearing loss in both ears. Suspicion or risk of middle ear dysfunction is based on patient history, an ear examination, or other hearing test results.

In patients presenting a masking dilemma, the audiologist is trying to determine whether there is a bilateral conductive hearing loss, a mixed hearing loss in one or both ears, or perhaps a conductive hearing loss in one ear and no hearing in the other ear. Audiologists sometimes use the slang term *dead ear* in referring to the ear with no hearing. Solving the masking dilemma is not simply a theoretical masking challenge. Information on bone-conduction hearing status in each ear plays a very important role in decisions regarding audiological and also surgical management of hearing loss.

Example of Masking Dilemma

A patient with bilateral ear malformation offers perhaps the most obvious example of the masking dilemma. You'll learn about ear malformations in Chapter 11. You may wish to take an early look at the appearance of a patient with a severe malformation in Figure 11.2A and B. With some serious malformations that are present from birth, the ear shows limited development of the pinna, absence of an external ear canal, and even malformed or absent ossicles within the middle ear. Patients with serious ear malformations usually have conductive

ClinicalConnection

Conductive hearing loss is commonly encountered in patients with a variety of etiologies for hearing loss, ranging from abnormalities present at birth to ear infections that are acquired by children or adults. Audiologists rely on behavioral and objective test procedures to detect middle ear dysfunction and describe associated conductive hearing loss. Fortunately, the masking dilemma can usually be solved with some of these procedures. You'll learn about the tests for evaluating middle ear function in Chapters 8, 9, and 10. We will review the causes of conductive hearing loss in Chapter 11.

hearing loss. In some cases air-conduction hearing threshold levels for both ears are as poor at 65 to 70 dB HL.

As you've learned, adequate masking of the nontest ear is necessary to verify which ear is responsible for a patient's responses to air- and bone-conduction stimulation. The intensity level of an effective masking noise must exceed the air-conduction threshold levels in the nontest ear. Cross masking from the nontest to the test ear is likely at the intensity levels of masking required to overcome severe conductive hearing loss in ear malformations. The absence of ear canals further complicates hearing testing of some patients with bilateral malformations. Supra-aural earphones are the only option for presenting air-conduction stimulation as the absence of an ear canal precludes the use of insert earphones.

Solving the Masking Dilemma

An audiologist can employ a handful of rather simple techniques when faced with a potential masking dilemma in air- or bone-conduction hearing testing. The techniques provide clues as to which ear is actually being activated and is producing the patient's responses. The benefits of insert earphones for pure tone audiometry have been repeatedly noted in this chapter. Audiologists use insert earphones whenever possible to substantially reduce problems with the masking dilemma. Because interaural attenuation with insert earphones exceeds 60 dB, the possibility of cross hearing associated with high levels of air-conduction stimulation or masking noise is limited to patients with severe-to-profound hearing loss.

Weber Test. For older children and adults, the audiometric Weber test offers a clue about whether a patient's response is actually due to activation of the test ear rather than the nontest ear. You'll recall that the Weber test assesses lateralization of bone-conduction stimulation. An audiologist can instruct a patient to describe where the sound is heard whenever there is a concern about which ear is producing a response. If a patient with a moderate or severe hearing loss in both ears consistently responds to one ear on the Weber test, it's likely that bone conduction hearing is better for that ear.

Sensorineural Acuity Level (SAL). Over fifty years ago, an alternative technique was introduced for estimating bone-conduction hearing thresholds (Jerger & Tillman, 1960). The **sensorineural acuity level (SAL) technique** is a clear departure from conventional bone conduction hearing measurement. The usual protocol for bone-conduction testing calls for presentation of pure tone sounds at the patient's mastoid bone via bone conduction while the nontest ear is masked via air conduction. In contrast, with the SAL technique, (1) masking noise is presented by bone conduction rather than by air conduction, (2) the bone oscillator is always located on the forehead, (3) earphones remain in place on both ears throughout the testing, and (4) the SAL technique yields an estimation of the air-bone gap instead of directly measuring bone-conduction hearing threshold levels.

Briefly, air-conduction hearing thresholds at frequencies including 500, 1000, 2000, and 4000 Hz are first measured for each ear without any masking, using insert earphones whenever possible (Hall & Mueller, 1997; Sanders & Hall, 1999). Pure tone hearing thresholds are then obtained for test frequencies of 500, 1000, 2000, and 4000 Hz while a high level of narrowband masking noise at corresponding frequencies is delivered via the bone oscillator. Noise levels presented with the bone vibrator to the forehead are usually in the range of 60 to 65 dB HL.

For patients with normal bone-conduction hearing, including normal hearers and those with conductive hearing loss, there is a shift in the air-conduction thresholds equivalent to the amount of bone-conduction masking. All of the noise presented via bone conduction is effective in masking the normal inner ears. Bone-conduction masking is less effective in persons with mild or moderate sensory hearing loss. There is no difference between air-conduction thresholds without bone-conduction masking noise and air-conduction thresholds with bone-conduction masking noise for patients with severe sensory hearing loss (greater than 60 to 65 dB). The bone-conduction masking is ineffective due to the degree of sensorineural hearing loss. The noise may not even be audible to the patient.

With the SAL test, a patient's air-bone gap is determined by calculating the patient's change in pure tone hearing thresholds produced by the bone-conducted masking noise and comparison to the typical shift in hearing levels with bone-conduction masking for persons with normal hearing. Let's consider, for example, a patient with a 50-dB air-conduction hearing loss. The patient's air-conduction thresholds increase by 50 dB when masking noise is presented via bone conduction. We can assume that all of the bone-conduction masking was effective. That finding confirms normal bone-conduction hearing thresholds. The SAL test shows that the patient has a 50-dB air-bone gap. Let's say another patient also has a 50-dB air-conduction hearing loss. This patient's air-conduction thresholds remain unchanged when masking noise is presented via bone conduction. The second patient has no air-bone gap because bone-conduction masking noise produced no shift in air-conduction hearing thresholds. The bone-conduction masking was ineffective because the patient has a sensorineural hearing loss.

WebWatch

Computer programs are now available for simulation of hearing testing. Using the programs, students can practice different procedures for hearing assessment, such as pure tone hearing testing with masking. Special software simulates the test conditions (including the masking dilemma) and findings for a variety of different patients. You can learn more about clinical simulators and even access free demonstrations of simulated hearing testing on several websites. Try searching the Internet using key words like *audiology* and *simulation* to locate them.

Concluding Comments about Masking

Understanding the Principles of Masking

In 1972 Jay W. Sanders, a well-known audiology researcher and instructor then at Vanderbilt University, made the following statement on masking: "Of all the clinical procedures used in auditory assessment, masking is probably the most often misused and the least understood. For many clinicians the approach to masking is a haphazard, hit-or-miss bit of guesswork with no basis in any set of principles" (Sanders, 1972, p. 111; Sanders & Hall, 1999, p. 86).

The purpose of the review above was to provide a basic understanding of the concepts and clinical purposes of masking. Masking is a critical skill in clinical audiology. The ability to properly use masking in clinical audiology is acquired not only by reading and studying principles and techniques. Masking is mastered through classroom lectures, laboratory sessions, computer simulations, and practice with classmates. Masking skills further develop during supervised clinical practicum experiences, as knowledge of masking principles and procedures is applied with different patient populations and patients with various types and degrees of hearing loss.

Final Advice

We'll conclude the review of masking with restatement of a general policy. In deciding when and how much to mask, it is always "better to be safe than sorry." Whenever there is a possibility of cross hearing during air- or bone-conduction audiometry, the nontest ear should be adequately masked. Recall the simple motto: "When in doubt, mask."

Audiogram Interpretation

The Art of Pattern Recognition

Audiogram analysis and interpretation is the process of distinguishing different patterns of hearing loss from the information plotted on an audiogram and relating the patterns to specific auditory disorders. You are now ready for some practice in audiogram analysis. You'll apply your knowledge of sound (Chapter 2), auditory anatomy (Chapter 3), pure tone hearing testing (Chapter 5), and even speech audiometry (Chapter 6) in the following section on audiogram review and analysis.

In the review you'll be introduced to audiogram interpretation. Audiogram interpretation focuses on how test findings are related to possible causes of hearing loss or the patient's underlying auditory dysfunction. The connection between audiogram patterns and causes of hearing loss will become clearer following a review in Chapters 11 and 12 of auditory diseases and disorders. And after reading Chapters 8, 9, and 10 you will also begin to appreciate the value of many other auditory tests in the diagnosis of hearing loss in children and adults.

We've already discussed in this chapter topics that are essential for analyzing and interpreting audiograms. The topics include measurement of air- and bone-conduction hearing thresholds, masking of the nontest ear, and symbol systems used to plot hearing thresholds. Accurate audiogram interpretation requires practice and clinical experience. Analyzing and interpreting information collected on the audiogram is clinically challenging, rewarding, and actually fun.

Pattern Recognition. Hearing test results for normal-hearing persons like most of your classmates may all look quite similar. In a clinical setting where people are scheduled for testing because they have hearing problems, almost no two audiograms are exactly the same. From one patient to the next, there are limitless possible variations in findings for different test conditions, such as air- and bone-conduction thresholds in each ear for different frequencies.

What patterns of audiogram findings are most common in a busy audiology clinic? Let's return to the study cited earlier in the chapter. Margolis and Saly (2008) reviewed 23,798 audiograms for 16,818 patients in an academic health science center audiology clinic. Findings of the study provide an interesting *evidence-based* perspective on the likelihood of different audiogram patterns, including the configuration, degree, and type of hearing loss. *Evidence-based* means based on research findings. The authors found that one-third of all records showed normal hearing in one ear and about one out of four patients had normal hearing sensitivity bilaterally.

Sloping audiogram configurations were by far the most common (40%), followed by flat hearing loss (16%), with rising configurations in less than 5 percent of the patients. Considering severity of hearing loss, about 30 percent of the total cases had a mild degree, slightly less than 30 percent had a moderate loss, 5 percent were in the severe category, and 4 percent had profound hearing loss. Finally, with air-conduction and bone-conduction testing of both ears, 21 percent showed conductive hearing loss, 34 percent sensorineural hearing loss, and 33 percent mixed hearing loss.

Experienced audiologists immediately recognize these distinct patterns of hearing loss when they are plotted on an audiogram. The information derived from the audiogram is often one of the first and most important steps in the diagnosis of hearing loss.

Practice Makes Perfect. A basic step in audiogram interpretation is familiarity with the symbols used to plot findings for different test conditions. You may want to review again the symbols summarized in Table 5.2 (Chapter 5). The most important symbols and those plotted most often on audiograms reflect pure tone hearing thresholds for the right and left ears, air conduction and bone conduction, and unmasked and masked test conditions.

With repeated exposure to a variety of audiograms, you'll begin to recognize patterns and relationships among findings for air- and bone conduction threshold measurements for each ear. To really hone skills in audiogram interpretation, there is no substitute for the knowledge gained by performing hearing assessments with many patients and manually plotting the findings on an audiogram form. All clinical audiologists during their graduate studies and clinical practicum rotations devote considerable time and effort to developing skill in audiogram analysis and interpretation.

The payoff for this investment in time and effort is considerable. Audiogram interpretation leads to a description of the degree, configuration, and type of hearing loss. Most importantly, audiogram interpretation is essential for diagnosis of auditory dysfunction and decisions about appropriate management strategies.

Audiogram Interpretation 101

You reviewed in Chapter 5 several audiograms illustrating pure tone hearing test findings. Here you'll have the opportunity to examine two additional audiograms illustrating clinically common patterns of hearing loss. A rather detailed description is provided for the first audiogram to be sure you appreciate the information necessary for proper interpretation.

After the audiogram is described, you'll be asked some questions about the essential features of the hearing loss, such as the degree, configuration, and type. Try to answer these questions on your own before reading further.

The results of hearing testing are then summarized concisely for the audiogram, much as they are in a clinical report of hearing test findings. The final interpretation of findings in an audiology report and most medical reports is often called the *impressions*.

The interpretation of an audiogram is not just a rehash of the results. Rather, the interpretation considers test findings in the context of the patient history and other findings. In addition, audiogram interpretation relates test findings to the patient's communication status.

Finally, findings displayed in the audiograms are related to concepts that you've been introduced to earlier in this chapter. Audiogram patterns for one case are displayed with the traditional format, whereas the other is shown on the separate ear audiogram format. You will have an opportunity to review other audiogram findings later in the book.

Tips for Audiogram Analysis and Interpretation. Here are five tips for approaching the analyses of an audiogram..

1. Scan the audiogram form immediately for information on
   - The patient's age
   - Earphones used during air-conduction testing, usually supra-aural or insert earphones.
   - The reliability of the patient's responses if indicated, such as good, fair, or poor.

2. Immediately inspect the audiogram to determine whether findings are entirely normal for either ear or both ears. Normal hearing threshold findings usually don't need to be reviewed further. However, other hearing test findings may still be abnormal, even for patients with normal audiograms.

3. In analyzing findings, begin with
   - The right ear, unless there is a good reason to begin with the left ear.
   - The lowest test frequency, and then progressively analyze thresholds at higher frequencies.
   - Air-conduction findings, and then proceed to bone-conduction findings for the same ear.

4. With a consistent strategy for analysis of each audiogram, you are less likely to overlook important details and more likely to minimize mistakes in your analysis. Focus only on one ear at a time, and complete your analysis for that ear before going on to the other ear.

5. Examine each symbol with a critical eye. Don't assume that every audiogram is entirely accurate and that each symbol is plotted correctly. It is particularly important to verify that masking was used whenever necessary. When masking was required, was it reported properly? If the unmasked symbol is plotted for any air- or bone-conduction threshold level, e.g., for bone-conduction testing at 500 Hz in the right ear, you should cautiously assume the nontest ear was not masked during the testing process at this test condition.

Review and Refresh. Before reading further, you might wish to review quickly the symbols used for plotting the traditional audiogram that are shown in the key within the figure. Remember, AC is an abbreviation for air conduction and BC stands for bone conduction.

In the following two summaries of test results, hearing sensitivity is sometimes described using the criteria for categories of degree of hearing loss shown earlier in Figure 5.10 (Chapter 5). The impression section for each case includes a comment about the possible impact of hearing loss on communication, specifically speech perception. This interpretation will be based in part on audibility of sound in the frequency region important for speech perception.

The patient's audiogram is discussed in the context of a count-the-dots audiogram shown previously in Figure 6.5 (Chapter 6). You'll probably need to occasionally refer back to these figures while interpreting the audiograms.

Case 1: Sensorineural Hearing Loss

Brief History. The patient was an alert and generally healthy 75-year-old female who reported a gradual onset of hearing loss over the past ten years, maybe a little longer. She complained of difficulty hearing people speak, especially understanding women's and children's voices and hearing in noisy settings.

Results. The patient's audiogram is shown in Figure 7.7. Insert earphones were used during pure tone audiometry. Hearing test reliability was very good. We'll begin with a description of results for air-conduction testing of the right ear. For frequencies of 250 through 1000 Hz, hearing thresholds were 10 to 15 dB HL and within normal limits as indicated by the category descriptions on the audiogram form. Then, hearing thresholds progressively decreased or worsened for higher test frequencies, reaching a maximum threshold level of 85 dB HL for the 8000-Hz test frequency. During air-conduction testing the patient required a greater stimulus-intensity level to detect the sound each time a higher pure tone test frequency was presented.

You'll notice that circles ("O") were used to plot air-conduction hearing thresholds for the right ear at lower frequencies where hearing thresholds were better. A triangle was used for the highest two test frequencies of 4000 and 8000 Hz because the stimulus-intensity levels of 75 and 85 dB respectively for those test frequencies exceeded the level of interaural attenuation for insert earphones. Information about bone-conduction hearing in the nontest ear was not available when the audiologist performed air-conduction pure tone audiometry. Crossover of the stimulus from the test ear to the nontest ear was possible at the highest stimulus-intensity levels, so masking was used on the nontest ear.

Figure 7.7 also shows that the pure tone average (PTA) was 20 dB for the right ear. You recall that the PTA is calculated with the formula: PTA = (threshold in dB HL at 500 Hz + 1000 Hz + 2000 Hz)/3. The PTA for each ear is in good agreement with the speech reception threshold (SRT).

Bone-conduction thresholds were measured at each of the typical test frequencies (500, 1000, 2000, and 4000 Hz) for the right ear. Looking closely at the symbols in Figure 7.7 you'll note that bone conduction testing was completed without masking. Comparison of the air- and bone-conduction hearing thresholds at each test frequency showed no evidence of an

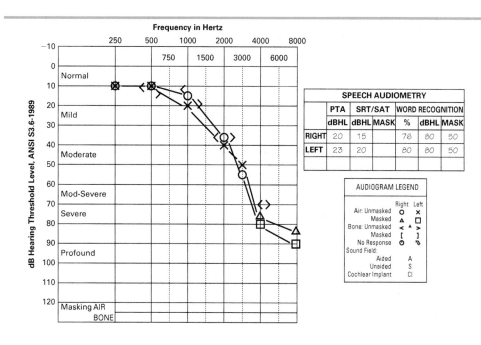

FIGURE 7.7

Audiogram for a 75-year-old female patient (Case 1) with a sensorineural hearing loss. Insert earphones were used during pure tone audiometry. Results are described and analyzed in the text.

air-bone gap. The agreement between air- and bone-conduction thresholds for the right ear was consistently within ±5 dB. Masking could have been applied to the nontest left ear but it was not necessary in this case. Recall that one rule for masking the nontest ear is an air-bone gap of 10 dB or more in the test ear. That indication for masking was not met for this patient.

Turning to results for the left ear shown in Figure 7.7, you'll see the trend for air- and bone-conduction thresholds was quite similar to the right ear findings. Hearing sensitivity was slightly better for the left versus right ear for test frequencies of 250 Hz up to 2000 Hz. For air-conduction testing, masking was only indicated at the highest two test frequencies (4000 and 8000 Hz) where the intensity level exceeded a conservative estimate of interaural attenuation for insert earphones (i.e., 60 dB).

The PTA for the left ear was 23 dB HL ([10 + 20 + 40]/3). Again, unmasked bone conduction testing revealed no evidence of an air-bone gap for the left (test) ear. The agreement between air- and bone-conduction thresholds for the left ear was consistently within ±5 dB for all test frequencies except for 4000 Hz where it was 10 dB HL.

Following completion of air- and bone-conduction hearing testing of the patient, it was clear that the audiogram was similar for each ear and there was no difference between air- and bone-conduction hearing thresholds and no air-bone gap. In retrospect, masking of the nontest ear was not needed for air-conduction or bone conduction sounds. Masking was not necessary during air-conduction testing based on the equation:

$$AC_{TE} - IA > BC_{NTE}$$

That is, the difference between air conduction hearing thresholds minus interaural attenuation (60 dB for insert earphones) did not exceed bone conduction thresholds in the nontest ear.

Subtracting the interaural attenuation value from the highest two stimulus-intensity levels used during air conduction (80 at 4000 Hz and 90 dB at 8000 Hz), we can verify that the patient didn't hear the level of stimulus sound reaching the nontest ear at either test frequency. That is, 80 dB − 60 dB = 20 dB and 90 dB − 60 dB = 30 dB. On the other hand, the use of masking for air and bone conduction posed no problem for the patient and it did not prolong air-conduction testing time. In this case the consistent use of masking added a few minutes to the test time during bone-conduction measurement, as the audiologist reentered the sound booth twice to place the bone vibrator on the test ear and the insert earphone into the ear canal of the nontest ear.

Returning again to Figure 7.7 you'll see that word recognition scores were 76% for the right ear and 80% for the left ear at an intensity level of 80 dB HL. These values represent the maximum percent correct scores for testing. Word recognition scores were lower for lower-intensity levels.

Impression. The patient has a moderate-to-severe high frequency sensorineural hearing loss bilaterally, slightly greater for the right ear. There was no evidence of significant air-bone gap in either ear. Hearing loss is likely to interfere with speech perception and communication.

Clinical Comments. The findings plotted in Figure 7.7 for Case 1 illustrate the use of symbols to indicate when masking was presented to the nontest ear to eliminate the possibility of responses due to cross hearing. Inspection of hearing thresholds for air versus bone conduction showed no evidence of an air-bone gap. Equivalent thresholds for air- and bone conduction stimulation rule out conductive hearing loss. The symmetrical high-frequency hearing loss shown in the audiogram is most likely due to inner ear dysfunction associated with aging. The term *presbycusis* is used for hearing loss related to aging. You'll learn more about presbycusis in a review of inner ear disorders in Chapter 11.

If we were to plot the patient's air-conduction hearing thresholds on a count-the-dots audiogram, it would show that much speech information for frequencies above 1000 Hz was not audible. We would predict from the patient's audiogram that she has a deficit in speech perception. This was confirmed by the patient's maximum scores of 76 percent for the right ear and 80 percent for the left ear on word recognition testing in quiet. However, these scores probably underestimate the patient's difficulties with speech perception in everyday listening situations for two major reasons.

First, scores indicate the patient's word recognition performance at a high-intensity level of 80 dB HL. The intensity level of everyday conversational speech is within the range of 20 to 50 dB HL. If the patient's audiogram were superimposed onto the count-the-dots audiogram form, speech information for just over 50 percent of the dots would be audible. In other words, the patient may miss up to 50 percent of speech information in conversations.

Second, word recognition testing was conducted without background noise in a quiet sound booth. You'll recall that the patient complained of difficulty hearing people talk in noisy settings. Ambient noise is always greatest in the low-frequency region. Based on the patient's audiogram findings, we would expect her to experience considerable difficulty with speech perception in noisy settings, such as restaurants or in crowds of people. Low-frequency ambient noise interferes with the patient's ability to utilize her relatively better hearing in the low-frequency region. The patient reported more difficulty in understanding women and children speak, in comparison to men's voices. As you learned in Chapter 2, vocal frequency is relatively higher for women than for men, and higher still for children.

In summary, findings for air-conduction hearing testing of this 75-year-old woman help to explain her complaints, specifically the problems she experiences communicating in noisy listening environments. However, hearing assessment of any patient almost always goes beyond the simple audiogram and measures of speech threshold and recognition in quiet. Comprehensive hearing assessment includes objective auditory measures to better define the extent and type of hearing loss.

Furthermore, an audiologist's role in providing services to a patient like this one usually does not end with the hearing assessment. Following the hearing assessment, an audiologist would most likely review with the patient and family members different management options, with the goal of improving the patient's communication. In upcoming chapters, you'll learn about each of these additional tests and also about options for management available to audiologists and speech pathologists.

Case 2: Conductive Hearing Loss

Brief History. The patient was a 55-year-old female patient. She reported a hearing problem in both ears for at least the past five years and maybe longer. The hearing loss seemed to be getting worse. She said her hearing in the left ear was better, but not normal. She used the left ear when talking on a telephone. Lately she'd been experiencing more difficulty hearing on the telephone and also understanding what passengers where saying when she was driving her car. She did not describe any discomfort or pain in her ears.

 ClinicalConnection

Measurement of air- and bone-conduction pure tone thresholds is just one component of the typical comprehensive hearing assessment. Diagnosis of hearing loss requires a combination of various tests, as described in the next few chapters. The diagnostic testing process, in combination with medical consultation, usually leads to an explanation for the hearing loss. You'll learn in Chapters 11 and 12 about disorders and pathologies causing auditory dysfunction, including the causes of hearing loss for the two cases reviewed here.

Results. Test results for the second case are plotted on a separate ear or "split" audiogram in Figure 7.8. Insert earphones were used during pure tone audiometry and also to present masking noise during bone conduction testing. Hearing testing began with the reportedly better-hearing left ear. Air-conduction hearing thresholds were within the mild hearing loss range, but decreased more for low pure tone frequencies. For the right ear, hearing thresholds for air-conducted sounds were generally in the moderate range and again worse for lower test frequencies. Masking of the nontest ear was not used during air-conduction testing because hearing thresholds never exceeded interaural attenuation values (60 dB) for insert earphones.

Bone-conduction thresholds were normal for both ears with the exception of the 2000-Hz test frequency for the right ear. There was a slight notching bone-conduction hearing loss at that test frequency for the right ear and a similar pattern for the left ear. Masking of the nontest ear was required for bone conduction hearing testing in order to obtain ear-specific

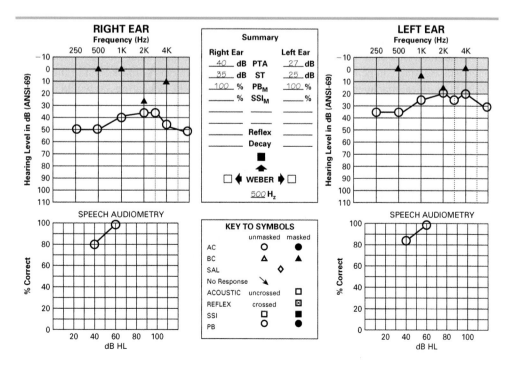

FIGURE 7.8

Audiogram findings for a 55-year-old female patient (Case 2) with a conductive hearing loss. Insert earphones were used during pure tone audiometry. Results are described and analyzed in the text.

results. Masking-noise-intensity levels up to 60 dB HL were needed to effectively mask the nontest ear due to the normal bone-conduction thresholds and the presence of a 50 dB air-bone gap at some test frequencies.

One additional test was performed with the bone vibrator. The audiometric Weber test was conducted with the bone vibrator located on the patient's forehead and with each ear uncovered (no earphones). The patient consistently heard tones of 250 and 500 Hz in the middle of her head. Finally, speech reception thresholds were in close agreement with pure tone averages. Word recognition scores were 100 in both ears at an intensity level of 60 dB HL (see center portion of the audiogram form).

Impression. The patient has a moderate conductive hearing loss in the right ear and a mild conductive hearing loss in the left ear. The midline outcome for the Weber test is consistent with a bilateral conductive hearing loss. The conductive hearing loss produces an occlusion effect in each ear.

Clinical Comments. Audiogram findings explain why the patient is experiencing difficulty with hearing and communication. Superimposing the patient's hearing thresholds on the count-the-dots audiogram form would show that she is missing important information at typical conversational levels of speech. Excellent word recognition performance at 60 dB underestimates the patient's communication problems. Test results are also in agreement with the patient's report of better hearing for the left than the right ear.

What could cause a conductive hearing loss like this and what steps should the audiologist take next? Diagnosis of auditory dysfunction cannot be made from an audiogram alone. However, this pattern of test findings in a middle-aged female suggests the possibility that a fixation or stiffening of the ossicular chain is interfering with the transmission of sound through the middle ear to the inner ear. It is possible that the stapes (the innermost ossicle) isn't moving normally due to some disease process. The progressive course of the hearing loss and the dip in bone-conduction hearing at 2000 Hz provide additional evidence of this possibility. In Chapter 11, you'll learn about fixation of the ossicular chain and disease processes associated with it. You'll also read in the next chapter about other auditory tests that provide valuable diagnostic information in cases like this.

An audiologist would refer this patient to an otologist for additional evaluation and formal diagnosis. Hearing can be restored with surgery for some patients with fixation of the ossicular chain. Surgical management is also discussed in Chapter 11. A hearing aid would probably be of considerable benefit to the patient if surgery was not an option or if she decided against surgery.

PULLING IT ALL TOGETHER

It is essential in clinical audiology to verify that a patient's response represents hearing in the test ear, not the nontest ear. Audiologists ensure ear-specific test results with proper application of masking to the nontest ear. You learned in this chapter about time-tested rules that underlie masking during air-conduction and bone conduction hearing testing. After reading the chapter, you can answer basic questions including: "What is masking?" "Why is it needed?" and "When is it needed?" You now also appreciate principles that guide the use of effective masking in patients with different types and degrees of hearing loss. These principles include interaural attenuation, the occlusion effect, and central masking. You are familiar with new terms, such as under-masking, over-masking, and effective masking.

We've also reviewed in this chapter different noises used for masking during pure tone audiometry and speech audiometry. Masking techniques have been covered, with a special emphasis on the plateau method for determining effective masking of the nontest ear. The masking dilemma was defined and tests to help resolve the dilemma were explained. Finally, you reviewed two cases to learn more about how audiologists analyze hearing test results. The review provided you with a glimpse at how audiologists use information from the audiogram to diagnose and manage hearing loss in children and adults.

READINGS

American Speech-Language-Hearing Association. (1988). Guidelines for determining the threshold for speech. *Asha, 30,* 85–89.

American Speech-Language-Hearing Association. (2005). Guidelines for manual pure-tone threshold audiometry [Guidelines]. Available from www.asha.org/policy

Lawson, G., & Peterson, M. (2011). *Speech audiometry.* San Diego: Plural Publishing.

Sanders, J. W., & Hall, J. W. III. (1999). Clinical masking. In F. E. Musiek & W. F. Rintelmann (Eds.), *Contemporary perspectives in hearing assessment.* Boston: Allyn & Bacon.

Valente, M. (2009). *Pure tone masking.* San Diego: Plural Publishing.

8

Electroacoustic Measures of Auditory Function

LEARNING OBJECTIVES

In this chapter, you will learn:

- About two procedures for evaluating the ear and other parts of the auditory system that do not require any behavioral response from the patient
- What is meant by the term *acoustic immittance measurement*
- Why acoustic immittance measurements are very useful in the diagnosis of auditory dysfunction
- The definition of tympanometry
- How to analyze tympanograms (*TIM pan o grams*), the graphs produced during tympanometry
- About the acoustic stapedial reflex and how it can be used to assess auditory function
- What is meant by the term *otoacoustic emissions* (OAEs)
- The difference between two types of otoacoustic emissions: transient-evoked otoacoustic emissions and distortion-product otoacoustic emissions
- That otoacoustic emissions are used for newborn hearing screening and diagnosis of hearing loss
- How to analyze otoacoustic emissions recordings
- Specific clinical applications of otoacoustic emissions for children and in adults

KEY TERMS

Acoustic immittance
Acoustic ohms and mhos
Acoustic reflex
Admittance
DecaPascals (daPa)
Distortion product otoacoustic
  emissions (DPOAEs)
DPgram
Electroacoustic procedures
Hermetic seal
Impedance
mm H$_2$O (millimeters of water
  pressure)
Objective auditory procedures
Otoacoustic emissions (OAEs)
Manometer
Probe tone
Spontaneous otoacoustic
  emissions (SOAEs)
Stapedius muscle
Tensor tympani muscle
Transient evoked OAEs
  (TEOAEs)
Tympanogram
Tympanometry

CHAPTER FOCUS

In previous chapters, you were introduced to two types of behavioral hearing tests, pure tone and speech audiometry. Behavioral hearing tests require an awake and alert patient who can listen to sounds and give a response an examiner can clearly observe. For very young children, the response to sound might be relatively simple and sometimes difficult to detect, such as an eye opening or head-turning movement. Older children and adults may be asked to give different responses to sound, for example, raising a hand, pressing a button, pointing to a picture, or repeating a word.

A variety of listener variables influence the accuracy of behavioral hearing testing, including the patient's developmental age, cognitive function, state of alertness, understanding of the test, attention to the sounds, and motivation to perform the task. Accurate behavioral hearing testing may not be possible for some patients, such as newborn infants and older children or adults who are developmentally delayed or very ill.

CHAPTER FOCUS *Concluded*

Given these limitations of behavioral audiometry, it is not surprising that **objective auditory procedures** play an important role in clinical hearing assessment. The term *objective* is used to describe procedures that do not require a behavioral response from the patient and do not require the tester to observe a behavioral response. With an objective auditory procedure, a stimulus produced by a device activates an automatic acoustical or physiological response from the patient. The patient doesn't need to listen to the stimulus or actively participate in the testing as the response is being measured. In fact, the patient may even be sleeping. The patient's response is detected and quantified by the measuring device. The tester may visually inspect and then analyze a graphical or numerical display of the response, or the device may automatically analyze the response.

Objective measures are essential for comprehensive and accurate diagnosis of hearing impairment. They are particularly valuable for hearing assessment of young children.

Overview of Electroacoustic Tests

Electroacoustic procedures involve the measurement of sounds within the external ear canal. An audiologist inserts a small rubber or foam-tipped probe into the external ear canal. Inside the probe assembly is a very small microphone. The probe is connected to equipment that can measure the intensity of sound in the ear canal. Some electroacoustic procedures provide information about how well the middle ear system transmits energy from the outer ear to the inner ear. Other electroacoustic procedures detect sounds in the ear canal that actually reflect energy associated with movement of outer hair cells within the cochlea. Importantly, electroacoustic auditory responses are not dependent on the patient's attention to the stimulation.

Clinical Uses of Electroacoustic Tests

How are electroacoustic auditory measures used in audiology? Any objective test permits assessment of auditory function in patients who for a variety of reasons cannot participate in behavioral hearing testing. Behavioral hearing testing is limited in young children between the ages of 6 months and 2 to 3 years and not feasible for infants under the age of 3 to 6 months. Infants are unable to respond consistently to sound due to immaturity of the nervous system. Electroacoustic procedures are very useful for assessment of auditory function of infants and young children. It is even possible with electroacoustic procedures to perform hearing screening of newborn babies, thus permitting early identification of hearing loss.

Audiologists occasionally encounter older children who are difficult or impossible to test. A difficult-to-test child may not allow an audiologist to place a probe within the ear canal or an earphone over the ear. If there are concerns about the child's hearing status, maybe because of a delay in speech and language development, an audiologist can perform an objective hearing test while the patient is sleeping. If necessary, the child can be given a sedative drug to enhance a sleep state since electroacoustic measurements are not influenced by sedation.

Also, electroacoustic procedures offer a highly sensitive tool for documenting abnormal function of the auditory system. Electroacoustic auditory findings often reveal problems in auditory function that are not evident on an audiogram. There are many examples of the diagnostic value of electroacoustic procedures in clinical audiology. Infections of the middle ear cavity are a common health problem in children. Electroacoustic tests contribute to the detection of auditory dysfunction in children at risk for middle ear infections and fluid in the middle ear space, even young children who cannot be tested with behavioral techniques. Electroacoustic procedures also identify some abnormalities in inner ear function that are not detected with simple pure tone hearing tests. Examples of this are persons at risk for cochlear damage caused by exposure to excessive levels of noise or certain medications. In some cases, electroacoustic techniques provide the first indication of cochlear dysfunction, before the audiogram shows evidence of a permanent hearing loss.

Acoustic Immittance Measures

The phrase **acoustic immittance** (im MIH tance) is really a combination of the two terms **im**pedance (im PEE dance) and **ad***mittance*. The terms *impedance* and *admittance* have related but reciprocal meanings. Measurement of acoustic impedance defines the total amount of opposition to flow of energy through the middle ear system from the eardrum to the inner ear, whereas acoustic admittance refers to the ease with which energy flows through the middle ear. So, abnormal middle ear function characterized by *high* impedance, like fluid within the middle ear cavity, is associated with *low* admittance. In years past, the term *impedance* was typically used to describe middle ear measurements. The hybrid or combination term *acoustic immittance* is now more common and will be used in this chapter.

Historical Perspective

Discovery of Immittance Technique. Although attempts to assess function of the middle ear date back to the 1800s, the earliest devices for clinical acoustic immittance measurement were not designed until the 1930s. In 1946, Otto Metz published the first systematic study of acoustic immittance findings in persons with different middle ear disorders (Metz, 1946). Metz (1903–1995) was a German otolaryngologist who relocated to Denmark just before World War II. He made aural immittance measurements with a mechanical device that included a rather scary-looking rigid rod with a probe at the end that fit within the external ear canal.

Acoustic immittance recording was cumbersome with this mechanical device and required a high level of technical ability even for assessment of cooperative adult patients. In addition, complicated mathematical calculations were required to produce clinically useful information. Josef Zwislocki, a well-known hearing scientist at Syracuse University, introduced a mechanical acoustic immittance device in the United States in the early 1960s (Zwislocki, 1963). However, technical challenges in conducting immittance measurements with the device prevented widespread clinical application of the new procedure.

Development of Clinical Equipment. In the 1950s, Danish investigators developed an electrical, rather than mechanical, device for recording acoustic immittance (Terkildsen & Nielsen, 1960; Terkildsen & Thomsen, 1959). The electroacoustic impedance device was a major breakthrough for clinical application of the technique. Within a few years, a Danish audiology equipment company, Madsen, manufactured a device for purchase by audiologists. The Madsen ZO61 electroacoustic impedance device was much easier to operate than previous mechanical instruments. Soon audiologists and otolaryngologists in Scandinavia began to measure middle ear function in clinical hearing assessment, even in children.

Introduction of Immittance Measurements in the United States. During a visit to Denmark in the early 1960s, James Jerger observed measurement of middle ear impedance with the then-new electroacoustic impedance device. You first read in Chapter 1 about James Jerger and his many contributions as "Father of Diagnostic Audiology." He's featured in Leaders & Luminaries in this chapter. Recognizing the potential clinical value of acoustic immittance measurements, Jerger acquired one of the new impedance devices for use in his busy audiology clinic at Baylor College of Medicine and Methodist Hospital in Houston, Texas.

Jerger and his colleagues promptly began to systematically collect data from a series of over 1,000 children and adults with a wide variety of confirmed ear pathologies. The technique was at that time called *impedance audiometry* rather than acoustic immittance measurement. In 1970, Jerger published the first of a series of studies of acoustic immittance using different clinical devices (Jerger, 1970; Jerger, Jerger, & Mauldin, 1972; Jerger, Anthony, Jerger, & Mauldin, 1974). Then, in 1975, he edited an entire textbook entitled *Clinical Impedance Audiometry* (Jerger, 1975). For over forty years acoustic immittance measurement has played an important role in the assessment of auditory function in adults and even more so in children.

Principles of Acoustic Immittance Measurement

A good background in mathematics and physics is useful to understand the concepts underlying acoustic immittance measurement. Technical explanations of acoustic immittance are available in articles, book chapters, and monographs. Some of the resources on acoustic immittance measurement are listed at the end of this chapter. Acoustic immittance instrumentation, calibration, terminology, and units of measurement are also thoroughly described in a set of standards published in 1987 by the American National Standards Institute (ANSI).

Here you'll be introduced to clinical acoustic immittance measurements including key terms and concepts.

Clinical Value of Acoustic Immittance Measures. Let's step back for a moment and consider why measurement of acoustic immittance is so valuable in clinical audiology. The

L E A D E R S A N D L U M I N A R I E S

James Jerger

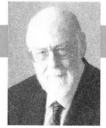

Dr. Jerger completed his PhD degree in audiology at Northwestern University in 1954. He served for seven years on the faculty of the audiology program at Northwestern. After a two-year period at Gallaudet College in Washington, DC, he moved to Houston as Director of Research at the Houston Speech and Hearing Center. In 1968 he joined the faculty of the Department of Otolaryngology and Communicative Sciences at Baylor College of Medicine at the Texas Medical Center. There he directed the audiology and speech pathology services of the Methodist Hospital of the Texas Medical Center. He also developed audiology graduate programs, including a PhD tract and the first Doctor of Audiology program in the United States. Dr. Jerger is now Distinguished Scholar-in-Residence in the School of Behavioral and Brain Sciences at the University of Texas at Dallas. He is affiliated with the program of applied cognition and neuroscience and with the program of communication sciences and disorders at the Callier Center for Communicative Disorders.

In the 1970s at Baylor College of Medicine and the Methodist Hospital Dr. Jerger conducted extensive research on acoustic immittance measurements, then called "impedance audiometry." He systematically analyzed patterns for acoustic immittance findings in large numbers of children and adults with normal and abnormal middle ear function. Results of Dr. Jerger's clinical research were published in dozens of journal articles and book chapters, as well as in several textbooks. He also traveled throughout the United States and internationally giving lectures and workshops on acoustic immittance principles and procedures. More than anyone else, Dr. Jerger contributed to the development of acoustic immittance technique as an essential part of the test battery for assessment of auditory function.

measurements allow audiologists to objectively describe and quantify how well the middle ear is working.

The outcome of acoustic immittance measurement is directly related to function of major structures within the ear. An abnormality anywhere in the series of interconnected auditory structures from the external ear canal to the inner ear may alter the measurements. There is usually a link between the type of abnormality and the pattern of acoustic immittance findings.

For example, a hole in the tympanic membrane affects acoustic immittance findings differently than fluid within the middle ear space behind the tympanic membrane. Also, the results of acoustic immittance measurement are distinctly different for a patient with a disorder that increases stiffness of the middle ear system than for a patient with a disorder producing excessive flexibility within the ossicular chain.

Our discussion of the principles of acoustic immittance measurement will address three general questions: (1) What instrumentation is used to measure acoustic immittance? (2) How is acoustic immittance measured? and (3) What components of acoustic immittance are measured? The discussion of the principles of acoustic immittance measurement will then logically lead to a review of different clinical acoustic immittance tests.

Instrumentation. A simple diagram of instrumentation used to measure acoustic immittance is depicted in Figure 8.1. One important part of the device is a miniature loudspeaker that produces a pure tone. The frequency of the pure tone is usually quite low, such as 226 Hz. The tone is referred to as a **probe tone** since it is delivered to the ear canal via a tube in a probe assembly. Some acoustic immittance devices also include the option of presenting other, higher-frequency probe tones, such as 1000 Hz.

Another component of acoustic immittance instrumentation shown in Figure 8.1 is a small microphone located within a second tube in the probe assembly. Sound in the ear canal from the probe tone that has returned from the tympanic membrane is picked up by the microphone and converted to an electrical signal. The electrical version of the probe tone signal is amplified, processed, and then sent to an analysis system for measuring the acoustic immittance of a specific patient.

The final part of the instrumentation illustrated in Figure 8.1 is an air pump for changing air pressure within the sealed external ear canal and a device called a **manometer** for quantifying air pressure within the ear canal. Air pressure is described in either **mm H$_2$O**

FIGURE 8.1

Diagram of the major components of equipment used for aural acoustic immittance measurements.

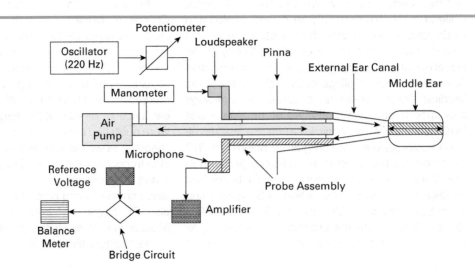

(millimeters of water pressure) or **daPa (decaPascals)**. These two units of pressure are so similar (1 mm H_2O = 0.98 daPa) that they are considered equivalent. In the following review, we'll consistently refer to air pressure in daPa. Air pressure within the external ear canal can be increased to as high as +200 daPa or decreased to as low as −300 or −400 daPa during acoustic immittance measurement.

Figure 8.2 shows an example of clinical instrumentation for aural acoustic immittance measurement. Different manufacturers market devices for measuring middle ear function. The physical appearance and specific features of the devices vary from one manufacturer to the next. However, all instrumentation includes the components diagrammed in Figure 8.1, including a probe assembly that is inserted into the ear canal.

Before beginning acoustic immittance measurement, an audiologist selects a rubber probe tip for the patient's ear based on the size of the ear canal. Figure 8.3A shows a sampling of different-sized rubber probe tips. Differences in the size of probe tips are coded with different colors. Probe tips are available in a wide array of sizes so that an airtight or **hermetic seal** can be formed between the probe assembly and an ear canal of any size. An audiologist selects an appropriate-size probe tip for the patient's ear canal. Then, an audiologist slips a new or disinfected soft rubber tip onto the probe assembly and gently but firmly inserts the probe into the patient's ear canal. Figure 8.3B shows the probe insertion technique.

The Measurement Process. Acoustic energy from a probe tone delivered to an external ear canal vibrates the patient's tympanic membrane. Much of the energy from the probe tone that vibrates the tympanic membrane flows through the middle ear system to the inner ear. However, there is some opposition to energy flow even for a normal tympanic membrane and middle ear system. A portion of the sound impinging on the tympanic membrane returns back through the ear canal to the microphone. A microphone within a probe assembly was illustrated in Figure 8.1.

As mentioned earlier, the term *acoustic impedance* is used to define opposition to energy flow through the middle ear system, whereas ease of energy flow through the middle ear system is referred to as *acoustic admittance*. The two terms are reciprocal terms. Both are used

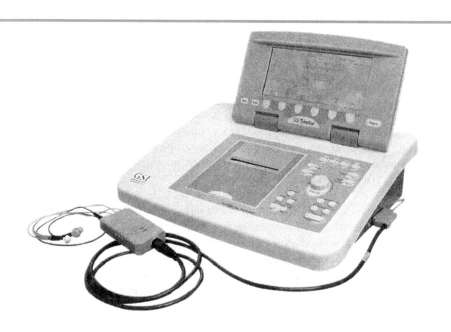

FIGURE 8.2

Clinical instrumentation for aural acoustic immittance measurement. Courtesy of Grason Stadler Inc.

FIGURE 8.3   **(A)** A sample of rubber probe tips of different sizes. Sizes of probe tips are color coded to facilitate quick selection of a tip that will fit snugly in a patient's ear canal. **(B)** An example of the technique for insertion of a soft rubber-tipped probe into the external ear canal for aural acoustic immittance measurement.

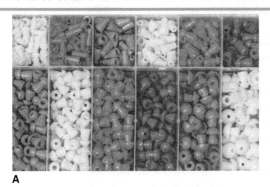
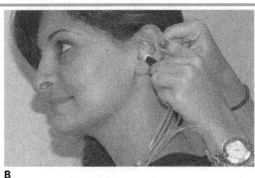

A   B

in clinical measurement of acoustic immittance. The sound pressure level that is measured at the end of the probe tip is directly proportional to acoustic immittance. In other words, higher sound pressures are recorded when acoustic impedance of the middle ear system is higher. Or, viewing the process the opposite (or reciprocal) way, lower sound pressure levels in the ear canal are associated with greater acoustic admittance and more energy flow through the middle ear system.

It is important to keep in mind that each measure of acoustic immittance—impedance and admittance—is made at the tip of the probe and not at the tympanic membrane. Clinical acoustic immittance measurements are influenced by air in the ear canal as well as characteristics of the middle ear system. The goal of clinical immittance measurement is to assess function of the middle ear system. Therefore, the external ear canal contribution needs to be removed from the measurement.

A relatively simple two-step process eliminates the ear canal as a factor in acoustic immittance measurement. The air pump in acoustic immittance instrumentation is used to develop considerable positive pressure in the external ear canal, such as +200 daPa. The tympanic membrane and middle ear system become stiffened at the high positive pressure. In the stiffened state there is almost no energy flow through the tympanic membrane and middle ear system. Acoustic impedance and opposition to energy flow is maximal, while acoustic admittance and ease of energy flow is minimal. In this condition, acoustic immittance measurement is limited to air in the external ear canal between the probe tip and the tympanic membrane. The measured acoustic immittance value is quantified as a number.

Next, acoustic immittance measurement is made with a typical neutral pressure of 0 daPa in the external ear canal. This measurement includes acoustic immittance for air in the ear canal plus the middle ear system. The contribution of the ear canal can be removed or subtracted from the overall measure to determine acoustic immittance of the middle ear system at the *plane of the tympanic membrane.*

Components of Acoustic Immittance. We've answered the first two questions: (1) What clinical instrumentation is used to measure acoustic immittance? *and* (2) How is acoustic immittance of the ear measured? Now, we're ready to answer the third question: What components of acoustic immittance are being measured?

The movement of the middle ear system in response to sound is remarkably complicated. It consists of many different components or forces that combine or interact in complex ways to produce the acoustic immittance measured at the plane of the tympanic membrane.

The major components are mass, stiffness, and friction. *Mass* is determined mostly by the tympanic membrane and the ossicles. The *stiffness* component is a product of the tympanic membrane, air in the middle ear space, muscles and ligaments attached to the ossicles, and the round window leading to the inner ear. The third component, *friction,* or resistance, is produced by middle ear structures, air within the spaces, and especially cochlear fluids.

Further complicating the measurement of acoustic immittance of the middle ear system is a lag or delay in the movement of structures to sound pressure in the ear canal. The energy driving the middle ear structures may be *in phase* or *out of phase* when the middle ear structures are set in motion by sound pressure in the ear canal. Movement of the middle ear system is in phase when it occurs simultaneously with the sound pressure, whereas out of phase movement lags behind the sound pressure.

Measurement of acoustic immittance clinically involves the sum of all of the various forces that are at work and interacting as the middle ear is set in motion. Acoustic immittance is accurately described as a ratio of the force applied to the middle ear by sound pressure in the ear canal to the velocity of the movement of middle ear structures. With some devices, it is possible to further describe whether components of acoustic immittance are in phase or out of phase.

We'll conclude the brief overview of acoustic immittance components with mention of the units of measurement used to describe findings. Two units are used to report acoustic immittance measurements. Acoustic impedance is described in **acoustic ohms**, whereas the reciprocal entity, acoustic admittance, is described in **acoustic mhos**. An ohm is a term used in physics to describe resistance. You may have noticed that the odd word *mho* is actually based on ohm spelled backward.

Stiffness Dominates Immittance Measurement. Don't be discouraged if you are a little confused after first reading about acoustic immittance. The physics underlying middle ear mechanics and measurement is quite challenging. Fortunately, modern instrumentation permits rather straightforward measurement of acoustic immittance. No mathematical computations are required.

Furthermore, acoustic immittance measurement is greatly simplified by a fact proven by vast accumulated clinical experience over the past forty years. The acoustic immittance finding commonly associated with most middle ear abnormalities is increased stiffness or reduced compliance. Compliance is a term used to describe the flexibility of the middle ear system. Although other immittance forces are certainly affected by middle ear disorders, the dominant abnormality is increased stiffness of the middle ear system.

 ClinicalConnection

The middle ear space normally is filled with air. Abnormal stiffness is recorded in certain middle disorders, including fluid behind the tympanic membrane. Infection of fluid within the middle ear fluid is the most common diagnosis made by physicians in preschool children. In Chapter 11, you will read more about ear infections and other disorders affecting the middle ear.

Analysis of acoustic immittance findings of patients in a clinical setting most commonly consists of determining whether stiffness of the middle ear system is normal versus abnormally high or low. Although instrumentation exists for recording multiple complex acoustic immittance components, such as in-phase and out-of-phase components of energy passing through the middle ear system, clinical measurement of acoustic immittance is limited almost entirely to documenting stiffness or compliance and comparing the values to normal expectations.

Performing Acoustic Immittance Measurements

Early Technique for Measuring Acoustic Immittance. Acoustic immittance recording with clinical instrumentation produces at least four different measurements: (1) equivalent volume of the ear canal, (2) static acoustic compliance of the middle ear, (3) tympanometry, and (4) acoustic reflexes.

Briefly, equivalent volume of the ear canal is an estimation of the volume of the ear canal enclosed between the probe tip and the tympanic membrane. Static acoustic compliance is a measure of the compliance or stiffness of the middle ear system at rest, that is, at atmospheric pressure or 0 daPa. Tympanometry produces a graph showing compliance of the middle ear system as pressure is changed within the external ear canal. And, the acoustic reflex is measured as an increase in middle ear stiffness associated with contraction of the stapedius muscle.

For many years after the introduction of acoustic immittance as a clinical procedure in the early 1970s, audiologists were required to perform each of these four measures manually in a systematic and step-by-step fashion. The probe assembly of a clinical immittance device was inserted into the ear canal of the patient. Then an audiologist turned a knob to change air pressure in the external ear canal, slowly increasing the pressure to +200 daPa. At that point, an audiologist would view a meter on the device to determine the initial compliance value when the tympanic membrane was immobilized and made rigid due to the high positive air pressure. That number would be written down on a recording form.

Next, an audiologist would carefully manipulate the knob to slowly and steadily reduce pressure in the ear canal until the pressure was 0 daPa. The meter was observed once more and another compliance value was also recorded on the form. Sometimes an additional reading was made for a higher or lower air pressure level where compliance was at its maximum and stiffness was minimal. This pressure value, such as −25 daPa or −150 daPa, was similarly written on the acoustic immittance sheet.

Audiologists analyzed the acoustic immittance findings for the right and the left ear by comparing each of the recorded values to published normative data printed on a sheet of paper kept near the immittance device. The early technique for acoustic immittance measurement was quite lengthy and rather tedious.

Current Technique for Measuring Acoustic Immittance. The foregoing process is greatly simplified and less time consuming with today's acoustic immittance devices. Of course, the probe must still be manually inserted into the external ear canal. Then the instrumentation automatically and systematically manipulates air pressure within the external ear canal and makes all of the necessary calculations. An audiologist can in a matter of seconds view a display of all of the important acoustic immittance data and print out the results for documentation.

In fact, most modern clinical instruments include an option for automatically initiating the acoustic immittance process as soon as an airtight seal is created between the probe and the walls of the external ear canal. This feature is especially handy for testing infants and young children as the audiologist can focus on securing an airtight seal between the probe and the external ear canal without also attempting to operate the immittance device.

Insertion of the Probe. Before beginning acoustic immittance measurement, an audiologist must carefully inspect the patient's external ear canals to rule out abnormalities or other unusual findings. Otoscopic inspection was reviewed in Chapter 4. Cerumen accumulation in the external ear canal can interfere with acoustic immittance measurements. Also, otoscopic inspection of the external ear canal in young children may unexpectedly reveal some type of foreign body, such as a pebble, a raisin, or even an insect.

After assuring that the ear canal is clear, an audiologist couples an appropriate-size probe onto the probe assembly and inserts it firmly into the external ear canal in order to create an airtight seal. A sampling of probe tips of different sizes from very small to large was illustrated earlier in Figure 8.3A. A good airtight fit between the probe tip and ear canal is essential for acoustic immittance measurement. The photograph in Figure 8.3B showed an audiologist inserting a soft-tip probe into the outer portion of the external ear canal to form an airtight (hermetic) seal.

An airtight or hermetic seal is confirmed at either positive pressure of +200 daPa in the external ear canal or negative pressure of −300 daPa. If neither positive nor negative pressure can be created in the external ear canal, the probe tip may need to be replaced with a different size and then reinserted in an attempt to adequately seal the external ear canal. Practice is required to master the technique of properly and quickly seating the probe assembly into the external ear canal so as to achieve an airtight seal. Probe insertion with a wiggly or uncooperative child is particularly challenging even for an experienced audiologist.

Clinical Acoustic Immittance Measures

We'll now go through each of the steps involved in acoustic immittance measurement with a modern clinical device. During this explanation, you'll want to refer often to the graph and the data displayed in Figure 8.4. Numbers in the figure identify acoustic immittance features and test results for steps in the measurement process. Figure 8.4 represents actual findings for a 4-month-old infant during measurement of acoustic immittance with a popular clinical device. The printout illustrates the information an audiologist analyzes following acoustic immittance measurement.

We'll focus first on the top half of Figure 8.4. The tympanogram for the left ear is on the left side of the graph, whereas right ear findings are shown on the right side. Our discussion will be limited at this time to tympanograms recorded with a rather typical low-frequency probe tone of 226 Hz identified by #1 in the figure.

FIGURE 8.4   Acoustic immittance data for a patient printed out with the clinical device shown in Figure 8.2. Information identified with each number is explained in the text. Courtesy of Grason Stadler Inc.

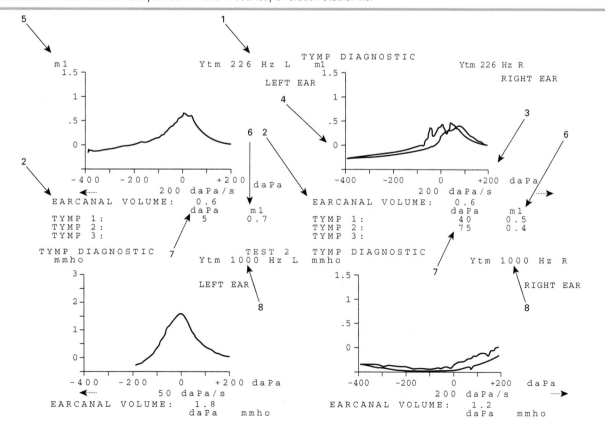

Estimation of Ear Canal Volume. Estimation of ear canal volume is a very useful clinical finding in immittance measurement. The abbreviation V_{ea} is sometimes used for volume of the external ear canal. Ear canal volume is estimated for the space enclosed between the medial edge of the probe tip and the tympanic membrane. At high ear canal pressures such as +200 daPa or low pressures in the range of −200 to −400 daPa, the middle ear is essentially eliminated from immittance measurement. Thus, the device estimates compliance of air within the enclosed external ear canal.

In Figure 8.4, the estimated ear canal volume for each ear is 0.6 ml for the 226-Hz probe tone as identified by #2. In other words, compliance of the volume of the external ear canal recorded between the probe and the tympanic membrane was equivalent to the compliance of air in a cavity of 0.6 cubic centimeters (cc) or milliliters. Here we'll use the unit milliliters (ml) for volume. Ear canal volume is normally between 0.3 and 1.0 ml for children within the age range of 3 to 10 years, and between 1.0 and 2.0 ml for adults over 18 years (Margolis & Hunter, 1999). Referring back to #2 in Figure 8.4, you can confirm that the child's ear canal volume of 0.6 ml is within the normal limits.

An acoustic immittance device measures an abnormally large ear canal volume if there is a perforation or hole in the tympanic membrane. Air passes from the external ear canal into the middle ear. Thus, volume that is measured includes the space in the external ear canal plus the middle ear space. A large volume is also recorded for patients with a ventilation tube in the tympanic membrane.

A ventilation tube is a tiny cylinder made of plastic or metal that allows air to flow in and out of the middle ear space. Otolaryngologists place ventilation tubes in the tympanic membranes of some patients with chronic ear infections. You'll learn about ear infections and ventilation tubes in Chapter 11.

During acoustic immittance measurement, air passes through an open ventilation tube much as it does through a perforation in the tympanic membrane. Acoustic immittance findings for patients with open ventilation tubes are similar to those for patients with perforation of the tympanic membrane.

Ear canal volumes are directly related to age, body size, and to a lesser extent gender. That is, ear canal volumes increase with age from infancy through adolescence and with growth in the physical dimensions of the head. Ear canal volumes are generally larger for males than for females. Also, ear canal volumes are similar or symmetrical in each ear, assuming a consistent technique is followed for inserting the probe tip in the right ear and the left ear. Meaningful interpretation of acoustic immittance findings requires knowledge of normal expectations for ear canal volume and factors influencing ear canal volume. Research studies over the years have yielded normal data for ear canal volume in subjects with different age and gender characteristics (Hall & Chandler, 1994; Margolis & Hunter, 1999).

Static Acoustic Compliance. As already noted, air pressure within the ear canal can be manipulated with an acoustic immittance device. Usually, testing begins with positive pressure of +200 daPa (see #3 in Figure 8.4) and then decreases to negative pressure of −400 daPa (see #4 in Figure 8.4). Compliance is shown on the Y-axis of the figure, labeled #5. The milliliter unit (ml) is used in the figure to describe equivalent volume, as indicated at the top of the Y-axis in each graph.

For a normal middle ear system, maximum compliance or minimum stiffness is found near 0 daPa, corresponding to atmospheric pressure. At 0 daPa there is little or no difference in air pressure from one side of the tympanic membrane to the other. The middle ear system is most flexible, or least stiff, at this neutral pressure.

Acoustic immittance recorded at a single air pressure value is referred to as *static admittance* or *compliance*. The acoustic immittance device automatically subtracts compliance of air within the external ear canal from the total compliance to calculate static admittance or compliance of the middle ear system. Since the final value takes into account or compensates for compliance of air within the external ear canal, the measure is sometimes described as *compensated static admittance* or compliance.

Static acoustic compliance values in Figure 8.4 are indicated by #6. We now need to compare the patient's static acoustic compliance values, specifically 0.07 ml for the left ear and 0.5 or 0.4 ml for the right ear, to normal expectations. Normal data for acoustic immittance measures are published in research articles and book chapters and typically supplied by the manufacturers of equipment used to make the measurements (Hall, 1987; Hall & Chandler, 1994; Jerger, Jerger, & Mauldin, 1972; Van Camp et al., 1986). Normal limits for static compliance extend from 0.30 to 1.50 ml. The patient's static acoustic immittance values shown in Figure 8.4 fall well within this normal range.

Let's inspect the information identified by #7 in Figure 8.4. The patient's maximum static compliance was recorded at an air pressure of +5 daPa for the left ear and at slightly higher-pressure values of +40 and +75 daPa for the two tracings made from the right ear. Maximum static compliance is recorded at slightly different air pressures in different patients with normal middle ear function but the values fall within a normal range. The conventional lower limit for normal negative pressure is −100 (Jerger, 1970). A more negative cutoff of −150 is also used in clinical acoustic immittance measurement (Hall, 1987; Hall & Chandler, 1994).

Tympanometry. We'll begin this section with a brief description of how **tympanometry** is performed. Then analysis of tympanometry findings will be described. Tympanometry is the most commonly recorded acoustic immittance test. It is a fundamental and essential procedure for detection of middle ear dysfunction.

Tympanometry yields a graph called a **tympanogram**, as shown in Figure 8.4. The tympanogram is generally recorded as a plot showing compliance or flexibility of the middle ear system as air pressure is changed within the ear canal. Air pressure in the external ear canal is typically decreased from a positive to a negative extreme. Compliance in ml is depicted in Figure 8.4 on the Y-axis and identified as number 5. Again, air pressure in daPa is depicted on the X-axis and identified as #3.

Tympanometry provides a graphic representation of changes in stiffness or compliance of the tympanic membrane as air pressure is manipulated within the external ear canal. Tympanometry quickly, objectively, and noninvasively yields clinically valuable information on the functional status of the tympanic membrane and the middle ear system. Middle ear disorders are almost always detected by simple analysis of the results of tympanometry. Analysis of tympanograms often permits differentiation among different types of middle ear abnormalities.

Tympanometry begins after insertion of a probe assembly into the external ear canal and verification of an airtight seal. To reiterate, air pressure in the ear canal is first increased to +200 daPa and then decreased to atmospheric pressure (0 daPa) and on to −300 daPa or even −400 daPa. Patients need to remain reasonably still during tympanometry, but a modest amount of bodily movement doesn't affect test results.

Tympanometry may need to be repeated when it is performed with a crying or uncooperative child. Figure 8.4 included an example of the effect of crying on tympanometry. The bumpy tympanogram for the right ear shown in the upper right corner of the figure was recorded while the child was crying. The smoother tympanogram in the same part in the figure was recorded after the child stopped crying. Young children are sometimes uncooperative during tympanometry, but older preschool and school age children almost always tolerate the procedure very well.

Tympanometry should be explained before insertion of the probe with older children and adult patients. Otherwise patients may be startled by the rather loud probe tone sound or by pressure changes in the ear canal they experience during the test. The procedure should also be explained in advance to parents of young children. Cooperation with young children is often enhanced if the child sits on the parent's lap and an audiologist or assistant distracts the child with a toy, a stuffed animal, or a distraction like soap bubbles. It is often helpful to encourage young children to touch the probe tip to see that it is soft and sometimes to actually demonstrate with a parent how tympanometry is performed before the procedure is performed on the child.

We will now review how tympanograms are analyzed and categorized as normal or abnormal. Figure 8.5 shows a simple approach for analysis of tympanogram findings, first introduced in 1970. This analytic approach remains clinically popular even today (Jerger, 1970). By convention, changes in air pressure are shown on the X-axis and the resulting admittance or compliance of the middle ear system is displayed on the Y-axis.

The shaded box indicates the normal region for tympanometry. The normal region is defined in the horizontal direction as the pressure region where the peak of the tympanogram should appear. The vertical dimension of the box defines the low and high limits for normal middle ear compliance.

The three general categories for tympanograms are called simply Type A, Type B, and Type C. There are also several variations of these tympanogram types. A *Type A* tympanogram

FIGURE 8.5   Different types of tympanograms are shown as categorized according to a popular system first described in the 1970s (Jerger, 1970). Characteristics of each tympanogram type are explained in the text.

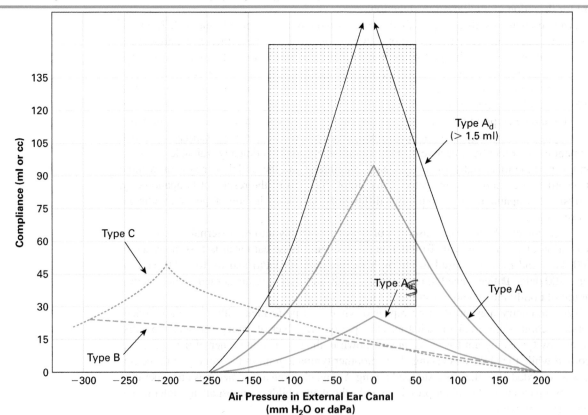

reflects normal outcome for tympanometry. In recording a type A tympanogram middle ear compliance systematically increases as air pressure in the ear canal is decreased from +200 daPa to atmospheric pressure of 0 daPa. As shown in Figure 8.5, a normal type A tympanogram has maximum or peak compliance between 0.30 and 1.50 ml. The tympanogram peak falls somewhere within the pressure region of +50 daPa to −150 daPa. Then, as air pressure in the ear canal decreases into the negative region, there is a reduction of middle ear compliance. The minimum value for tympanogram compliance is usually recorded at a negative pressure of > −200 daPa.

Occasionally a tympanogram peak is observed at a positive air pressure rather than at 0 mmH$_2$O (daPa) or in the negative pressure region. The tympanograms shown earlier for the right ear in the upper right corner of Figure 8.4 were good examples of positive peak pressure. The peak for one tympanogram was at +40 daPa and the other was at +75 daPa, labeled as #7.

There is a logical explanation for the slightly positive middle ear pressure. Air was forced up from the nasopharynx through the Eustachian tube into the middle ear space as the child cried during testing. A positive pressure peak of more than +50 daPa is also sometimes observed in patients after they vigorously blow their nose.

The *Type A$_s$* tympanogram is a variation of the Type A pattern. The "s" refers to *shallow* or *stiffness*. A Type A$_s$ tympanogram indicates a restriction in the flexibility or an increase in stiffness of the middle ear system. The pattern may be associated with a fixation of the ossicles connecting the tympanic membrane to the inner ear. The third and innermost ossicle, the stapes, is the most likely to be immobilized.

At the other extreme, a very deep *Type A$_d$* tympanogram suggests a highly compliant middle ear system or tympanic membrane. A Type A$_d$ tympanogram finding may reflect a tympanic membrane that is flaccid, or highly flexible. There are two likely explanations for a highly flexible tympanogram. One is a tympanic membrane that has healed following a perforation. Another less likely explanation is a discontinuity or break in the ossicular chain.

Consideration of pure tone hearing test findings in combination with tympanometry clearly distinguishes between these two possibilities. A Type A$_d$ tympanogram in a patient with normal pure tone hearing thresholds is most consistent with a tympanic membrane abnormality. Despite the slight abnormality in function of the tympanic membrane, sound is conducted reasonably well through the middle ear to the inner ear. In contrast, a discontinuity in the ossicular chain must be suspected for a patient with a Type A$_d$ tympanogram and a substantial hearing loss on pure tone audiometry. A break between any two ossicles will almost always produce a conductive hearing loss.

Figure 8.5 also shows abnormal tympanogram types. With an abnormal *Type B* tympanogram there is no clear peak as air pressure is varied across the range of +200 daPa to −300 daPa. The Type B tympanogram sometimes appears rounded, but it may also look like a flat line. The finding of a Type B tympanogram usually indicates severely restricted mobility of the middle ear system. One possible explanation for a Type B tympanogram is fluid in the middle ear space immediately behind the tympanic membrane. However, other disorders requiring immediate medical attention may also be associated with a Type B tympanogram.

Figure 8.5 also shows an abnormal *Type C* tympanogram that consists of a peak only when negative pressure is created in the ear canal. The peak occurs when the negative pressure in the ear canal is beyond −100 or −150 daPa. A Type C tympanogram most often indicates Eustachian tube dysfunction. You'll recall from Chapter 3 that the Eustachian tube connects the middle ear space to the nasopharynx toward the back of the mouth. Blockage of the Eustachian tube often

🎧 **Clinical**Connection

Tympanometry is very useful for identifying middle ear disorders in children and adults. Tympanogram types contribute importantly to the diagnosis of ear abnormalities, especially when the findings are analyzed in combination with findings for other auditory measures, like air- and bone conduction hearing thresholds. You read in Chapter 5 about the diagnostic value of pure tone audiometry. In Chapter 11, you'll learn about diseases and disorders affecting the middle ear.

contributes to inadequate ventilation of the middle ear space. In turn, insufficient aeration of the middle ear space may be associated with the collection of fluid there, and sometimes development of an infection.

An audiologist will occasionally encounter patients who appear to have a Type B tympanomgram. On close inspection the tympanogram is not flat but, rather, compliance appears to increase consistently as pressure is decreased in the negative direction. The tympanogram has no peak within the typical limit for negative pressure of −200 or −350 daPa. However, a peak is apparent at more extreme pressures. A tympanogram with a peak at high negative pressure is not a Type B tympanogram. The presence of a peak somewhere in the negative pressure range confirms a Type C versus Type B tympanogram. The finding probably indicates severe Eustachian tube dysfunction rather than fluid within the middle ear space.

Ruling Out Technical Problems in Tympanometry. Before linking a Type B tympanogram to middle ear abnormalities, an audiologist must first rule out technical problems and external ear canal explanations. Sometimes debris or cerumen in the external ear canal plugs up one or more of the small tubes in the probe assembly. The result can be an apparent but invalid Type B tympanogram. The problem is solved by removing the probe assembly from the acoustic immittance device and reaming out the probe tubes with a thin wire.

Excessive cerumen occluding the external ear canal also produces what appears to be a Type B tympanogram. Cerumen that completely blocks the ear canal prevents the probe tone from reaching the tympanic membrane and the middle ear system. A valid tympanogram reflects variation in middle ear compliance with changes in air pressure at the tympanic membrane. A Type B tympanogram due to ear canal blockage is not valid. Changes in air pressure in the space enclosed between the probe tip and the cerumen don't reach the tympanic membrane and don't produce the expected variation in middle ear compliance.

Cerumen occupying much of the external ear canal results in an abnormally small estimated ear canal volume. Accumulation of excessive cerumen within the external ear canal is identified with otoscopic inspection of the ear and verified with an unusually small ear canal volume measurement.

While we're discussing technical aspects of middle ear measurement, it is important to re-emphasize that tympanometry can be conducted only after an airtight or hermetic seal is obtained between the probe tip and the external ear canal walls. If a hermetic seal cannot be established or if high positive or negative air pressure cannot be developed in the ear canal because of a hole in the tympanic membrane, then it is not possible to perform tympanometry. The first requirement for tympanometry, manipulation of air pressure in the external ear canal, is not met. Modern acoustic immittance devices produce a display warning about an inadequate seal or a leak in the probe fit whenever air pressure cannot be developed in the external ear canal.

Low- and High-Frequency Probe Tones. Up to this point, we've considered acoustic immittance measurements only with a low-frequency 226-Hz probe tone. American National Standards Institute (ANSI-1987) standards for acoustic immittance devices are based on a low-frequency probe tone. The conventional low-frequency probe tone is quite effective for detecting stiffness-related middle ear abnormalities in older children and adults.

The use of both a high-frequency probe tone of 1000 Hz and a low-frequency probe tone is required for tympanometry in infants up to the age of at least 4 months. Normal acoustic immittance characteristics differ substantially between infants and older children and adults (Holte & Margolis, 1987; Holte, Margolis, & Cavanaugh, 1991; Hunter & Margolis, 1992; Kei et al., 2007). Indeed, tympanogram patterns in normal newborn infants vary greatly and unpredictably (Holte, Margolis, & Cavanaugh, 1991). The explanation for the age-related variability in tympanometry involves some of the principles we have already reviewed, including the effects of stiffness, mass, and middle ear resonance.

Longstanding published reports have repeatedly described normal-appearing tympano-grams in infants with documented middle ear pathology when tympanometry is performed with a low-frequency probe tone (Hunter & Margolis, 1992; Margolis & Popelka, 1977). A number of factors help to explain these findings, including birth substances within the middle ear space, immature status of the middle ear system, and increased compliance of the ear canal walls in young infants. A probe tone frequency of 1000 Hz is recommended for middle ear measurement in neonates up to the age of six months (Joint Committee on Infant Hearing, 2007). However, estimation of ear canal volume with acoustic immittance measurement in these infants should always be conducted with a low-frequency probe tone (Kei et al., 2007).

The importance of recording tympanograms with low- and high-frequency probe tones in infants is well illustrated by the acoustic immittance findings shown earlier in Figure 8.4. Recall that the patient was a 4-month-old infant. A normal Type A tympanogram was recorded in each ear with a 226-Hz probe tone. Tympanograms recorded with a high-frequency 1000-Hz probe tone were shown in the lower half of Figure 8.4 and labeled with #8.

For the left ear, the tympanogram was normal for the high-frequency 1000-Hz probe tone and also for the low-frequency probe tone. In contrast, tympanometry findings for the right ear were different for the low- and high-frequency probe tones. Results with the low-frequency probe tone (Type A tympanogram) suggested normal middle ear function, but tympanometry with the higher-frequency probe tone revealed a clear abnormality. In this child, tympanom-etry with a low-frequency probe tone was invalid for the right ear. Although the results sug-gested normal middle ear function, repeating tympanometry with the higher-frequency probe tone confirmed an abnormality.

Clinical Applications of Tympanometry. Tympanometry is a sensitive indicator of middle ear functioning. Indeed, tympanograms sometime reveal evidence of abnormalities that are not clearly visible upon examination of the ear. Clinical advantages of tympanometry have contributed to widespread use of the technique by audiologists and other healthcare profes-sionals, including nurses and physicians. Tympanometry is highly sensitive to middle ear dys-function, a quick and objective test, and feasible for patients of any age.

The value of tympanometry in audiology is well established by extensive research and many years of clinical experience (Hall, 1987; Van Camp, Margolis, Wilson, Creten, & Shanks, 1986). However, it is important to keep in mind several limitations of the technique.

A tympanogram provides diagnostically useful information on the status of the middle ear system, but tympanometry alone does not permit the diagnosis of ear pathology. Also, tympanometry is *not* a valid measure of hearing. Normal tympanograms may be recorded in children with sensory hearing loss affecting speech and language development, including severe to profound hearing impairment. Conversely, abnormal tympanometry findings are not always associated with communicative or clinically significant deficits in hearing sensitivity.

Wideband Reflectance Measurement

Wideband middle ear power reflectance measurement is an innovative and recently developed approach to middle ear assessment (Hunter & Shahnaz, 2013). The word *wideband* is used because middle ear function is evaluated with a wide range of frequencies.

As wideband reflectance stimuli are delivered into the external ear canal, some of the energy is reflected back from the tympanic membrane. Figure 8.6 shows a format for display-ing wideband reflectance findings recorded with a clinical device. Reflectance is displayed on the Y-axis and stimulus frequency is on the X-axis. High reflectance, such as 90 percent,

FIGURE 8.6

A graph showing wide-band middle ear power reflectance for a child with otitis media (ear infection) in comparison to a normal region.

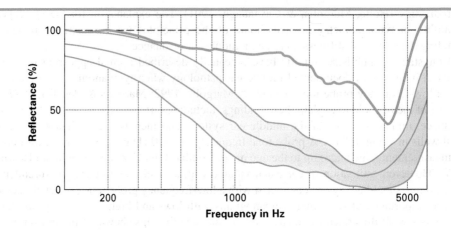

ClinicalConnection

In Chapter 11, you'll learn about diseases and disorders affecting the middle ear that are associated with abnormal findings on acoustic immittance and wideband reflectance testing. Both of these electroacoustic measures quickly provide information on middle ear functioning in children and adults that is not available from physical examination of the ear.

indicates that most of the stimulus is returning from the tympanic membrane, whereas low reflectance, like 10 percent, indicates that the middle ear system is absorbing most of the stimulus power.

Wideband middle ear power reflectance offers three potential advantages over conventional tympanometry, particularly for detection of pathology in neonates and young children (Hunter et al., 2010; Feeney, Grant, & Marryott, 2003). First, wideband middle ear power reflectance is measured at ambient pressure or with induced ear canal pressure. A hermetic airtight seal between the probe tip and the ear canal wall is not required. Second, the technique quickly provides information on middle ear function across a wide frequency region, rather than one or two frequencies, such as 226 Hz and 1000 Hz. Finally, rather distinctive wideband reflectance patterns seem to be associated with normal middle ear function and different types of middle ear dysfunction.

Acoustic Reflex Measures

Acoustic reflexes are *sonomotor responses*. The response is a contraction of muscles upon sound stimulation. In years past, acoustic reflexes were referred to as middle ear muscle contractions or intra-aural muscle reflexes (Djupesland, 1975). Acoustic reflexes fall into the same general category as other sonomotor responses, such as the eye blink reflex to loud sounds, involving muscles around the eyes, and the startle response to loud sounds that involves many large muscles in the body.

Two small muscles and associated tendons are attached to the first and third ossicles within the middle ear space. You learned about middle ear muscles in the review of auditory system anatomy in Chapter 3. The **tensor tympani muscle** is connected to the malleus and innervated by the fifth or trigeminal cranial nerve. The **stapedius muscle** is connected to the neck of the stapes and innervated by the seventh or facial cranial nerve.

Extensive research in the 1960s and 1970s confirmed that high intensity sound stimulation typically activates the stapedius muscle alone, without involvement of the tensor tympani muscle (Djupesland, 1975). In contrast, the tensor tympani muscle contracts along with other muscles in the head and neck region as part of a startle or defensive response to very high-intensity sounds.

The stapedius muscle normally contracts in response to a high-intensity sound exceeding about 70 dB HL. When one normal ear is stimulated with sound, the stapedius muscles in both ears contract. Contraction of the muscles stiffens the middle ear systems and compliance of both middle ear systems decreases. This is detected in acoustic immittance measurement. This phenomenon is called the **acoustic reflex** or the acoustic stapedial reflex.

The acoustic reflex is activated and recorded with four combinations of measurement conditions. The sound stimulus in an ipsilateral condition is presented to one ear and the change in middle compliance is recorded in the same ear. In the contralateral condition, the activating sound stimulus is presented to the ear opposite the ear with the probe assembly that is recording changes in middle ear compliance. There are four measurement conditions, since each ear can be used for stimulus presentation and each can be used for recording changes in middle ear compliance.

Acoustic Reflex Pathways. Figure 8.7 shows the major pathways involved in the acoustic reflex, often called the *acoustic reflex arc*. We will now review the acoustic reflex pathways while referring to the diagram in Figure 8.7. The ascending and afferent pathway takes information from the ear to the brain. Afferent structures consist of the cochlea and the auditory portion of the eighth cranial nerve. The cochlear nuclei in the brainstem contribute to the acoustic reflex arc in the ipsilateral and contralateral measurement conditions.

Additional neurons in the trapezoid body and medial superior olivary complex contribute to the acoustic reflex pathways in the contralateral measurement condition. In the contralateral

ClinicalConnection

Audiologists often evaluate patients who complain about hearing annoying sounds in the ears. The term *tinnitus* is used to describe the perception of sounds in the ears even in very quiet settings. A very small proportion of patients with tinnitus describe intermittent sounds like clicking rather than the more typical ringing type of sound. Research suggests that one source of intermittent sound in the ear is associated with rapid contraction of the tensor tympani muscle. The likelihood of tensor tympani activity may be increased when a patient is anxious or concerned about hearing loud sounds.

F I G U R E 8 . 7   Acoustic reflex pathways include the auditory nerve, brainstem neurons, and the facial nerve. Abbreviations: CN = cranial nerve, VCN = ventral cochlear nucleus, DCN = dorsal cochlear nucleus, SOC = superior olivary complex, MSO = medial superior olive, TB = trapezoid body, 7th N Nuc = nucleus of the 7th cranial nerve.

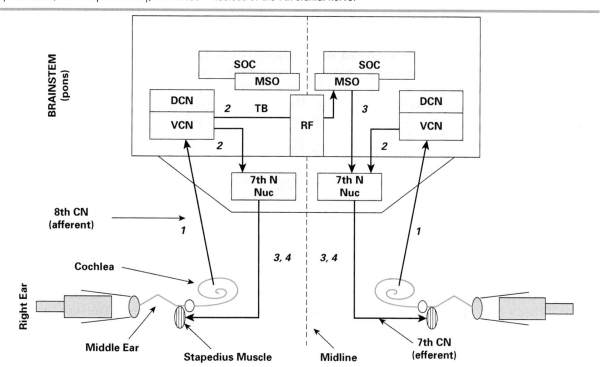

condition, a stimulus is presented to one ear and measurement of stapedius muscle contraction is made on the opposite side.

A descending efferent pathway passes from the brainstem back to the ear. The descending pathway includes motor fibers within the seventh (facial) cranial nerve. The facial nerve includes a small branch that innervates the stapedius muscle.

Ipsilateral acoustic reflex pathways remain on one side of the body. Ipsilateral pathways appear on each side of the dashed line in Figure 8.7. Since the pathways do not cross the midline, the ipsilateral acoustic reflex is sometimes described as an *uncrossed acoustic reflex*.

The trapezoid body (TB) is one of multiple sets of pathways crossing from one side of the brainstem to the other. For this reason, acoustic reflexes involving contralateral pathways and the trapezoid body are often described as *crossed acoustic reflexes*. The contralateral or crossed pathways include neurons within the reticular formation, sometimes called the reticular activating system. The reticular formation (RF) is a complex set of pathways in the mid-region of the brainstem (Hall, 1982, 1985).

Careful analysis of acoustic reflexes recorded under the four measurement conditions provides valuable information on the auditory function of children and adults. It is important to emphasize here that the presence of acoustic reflexes is highly dependent on status of the ear and particularly dependent on normal middle ear function. Most middle ear abnormalities obscure confident detection of acoustic reflexes. In fact, acoustic reflexes may absent in patients with even relatively subtle middle ear dysfunction as indicated by a modest 5- to 10-dB gap between air- and bone-conduction pure tone thresholds (Jerger, Anthony, Jerger, & Mauldin, 1974).

Recording the Acoustic Reflex. Acoustic reflex measurement with the probe in one ear is recorded immediately after tympanometry has been completed, with the probe assembly still sealed in the ear. Acoustic reflexes are recorded at external ear canal air pressure where there is a tympanogram peak and where compliance reaches its maximum value. Modern acoustic immittance devices automatically find and maintain this measurement condition. Acoustic immittance devices include a range of stimuli that can be used to activate the acoustic reflex. Stimulus options include pure tones of 500, 1000, 2000, and 4000 Hz and noise signals like broadband noise (BBN).

As already mentioned, stimuli in acoustic reflex measurement can be presented to an ear via the probe assembly in the ipsilateral condition or in a contralateral condition via stimulation through an earphone on the ear opposite to the probe. The ear that is stimulated is used in describing the test condition. The stimulus ear is also the probe ear in the ipsilateral measurement condition. So, the right ipsilateral acoustic reflex is recorded with the probe and the stimulus in the right ear. The left ipsilateral reflex is recorded with the probe and the stimulus in the left ear. In the contralateral condition, the right ear acoustic reflexes are activated with stimulation of the right ear even though the probe is in the left ear.

Acoustic Reflex Threshold. Acoustic reflex recording begins with presentation of a stimulus at a moderate-to-high-intensity level of around 70 to 80 dB HL. Stimulation is typically presented manually by pressing a stimulus button for about 1 second. As the stimulus is presented acoustic immittance is monitored with either a meter or a digital display. A decrease in compliance or an increase in stiffness immediately following stimulus presentation indicates an acoustic reflex.

If a change in compliance is observed indicating the activation of an acoustic reflex, stimulus intensity is decreased10 dB and a stimulus is presented again. The stimulus intensity level is increased 5 dB if there is no change in compliance and the stimulus is presented again.

The goal of the threshold-seeking process is to find the minimum stimulus-intensity level that activates the acoustic reflex, commonly referred to as the *acoustic reflex threshold (ART)*.

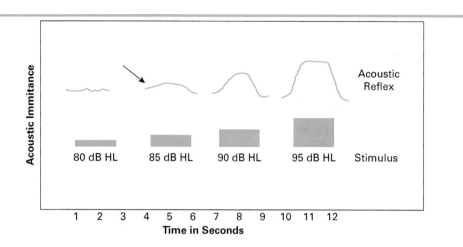

FIGURE 8.8

Examples of acoustic reflexes recorded at different intensity levels confirming the threshold level of 85 dB HL. The arrow indicates acoustic reflex threshold.

The efficient process of estimating acoustic reflex threshold may be more clearly appreciated with a simple example. Figure 8.8 shows graphic displays of tracings during acoustic reflex measurement at an intensity level that is too soft to elicit an acoustic reflex, at the acoustic reflex threshold (see arrow in the figure), and then at intensity levels above acoustic reflex threshold.

Let's say an audiologist delivers a 1000-Hz tone stimulus to a patient at an intensity level of 80 dB HL but does not detect any change in middle ear immittance (or compliance). An acoustic reflex is not present. Next, the audiologist delivers the same stimulus 5 dB higher, at 85 dB HL, and detects a small change on the immittance device meter. The acoustic reflex threshold is 85 dB HL. The same process is carried out at higher intensity levels to verify a response if there is any doubt about the presence of an acoustic reflex threshold.

Acoustic reflex thresholds for pure tone stimulation are rarely observed for pure tone stimulus levels less than 75 to 80 dB HL. For pure tone stimulation, the normal upper limit for intensity level required to elicit an acoustic reflex is 95 dB HL (Gelfand, Schwander, & Silman, 1990). For a broadband-noise (BBN) signal, in contrast, the acoustic reflex may occur for intensity levels as low as 60 dB (Jerger, Burney, Mauldin, & Crump, 1974). Acoustic immittance devices are usually capable of generating very high stimulus-intensity levels, up to 125 dB HL. However, intensity levels exceeding about 110 to 115 dB are avoided to minimize discomfort to the patient and the risk of sound-related damage to the ear.

The general testing technique used in estimating acoustic reflex threshold should be familiar to you. The sequence of decreasing intensity level by 10 dB and increasing stimulus-intensity level by 5 dB in a search for threshold is fundamental to hearing testing with pure tone and speech sounds. However, the acoustic reflex testing process differs in at least two important ways from pure tone and speech audiometry.

First of all, the patient does not need to pay attention or listen to the sounds. In fact, patients should be told just before acoustic reflex measurement begins that they will hear some sounds, but they don't need to pay attention to the sounds or indicate when a sound is presented. Indeed, the patient should not vocalize during testing. Patient talking interferes with accurate detection of acoustic reflexes.

There is another important difference between acoustic reflex measurement and behavioral audiometry. For any given stimulus condition, the acoustic reflex threshold estimation process is done only once. Threshold estimation in pure tone audiometry, in contrast, requires repeated presentation of descending and ascending intensity levels. Acoustic reflex threshold estimation is completed more efficiently than threshold estimation for pure tone audiometry because measurement involves an automatic electroacoustic response, a reflex, rather than a behavioral response.

Hearing Loss Estimation with Acoustic Reflexes. The use of acoustic reflex thresholds for estimation of hearing loss was first reported in the early 1970s (Jerger et al., 1974; Niemeyer & Sesterhenn, 1974). Assuming the middle ear is functioning normally, the acoustic reflex threshold for several different stimuli can help to distinguish normal-hearing ears from ears with sensory hearing loss. Acoustic reflex thresholds for pure tone signals generally remain constant at about 80 to 85 dB for patients with normal-hearing thresholds and hearing loss up to 50 or 60 dB HL. Recall that the upper limit for normal acoustic reflex thresholds with pure tone stimulation is 95 dB HL (Gelfand, Schwander, & Silman, 1990). For greater degrees of hearing loss, higher stimulus-intensity levels are needed to elicit an acoustic reflex.

In contrast, there is a more direct relation between hearing loss and the acoustic reflex thresholds elicited with noise stimulation. In particular, the acoustic reflex threshold for broadband noise (BBN) increases rather systematically with hearing thresholds. The differences in acoustic reflex thresholds for pure tone from those for noise stimuli in patients with hearing loss underlie a technique called Sensitivity Prediction by the Acoustic Reflex (SPAR), introduced by Jerger and colleagues in 1974 (Hall, Berry, & Olson, 1982; Jerger et al., 1974b).

Figure 8.9 illustrates the differential effect of sensory hearing loss on acoustic reflex thresholds elicited with tonal versus BBN signals. Hearing level in dB HL is on the X-axis, whereas acoustic reflex threshold in dB HL is on the Y-axis. You can readily see a clear difference between the lines representing tonal and noise-stimulation acoustic reflex thresholds, with a rather predictable relation between hearing loss and the reflex threshold for noise stimulation.

According to research findings in an adult population, patients with normal hearing usually have an acoustic reflex threshold of better than 90 dB for a BBN stimulus. In contrast, patients with a pure tone average worse than 35 dB HL rarely have acoustic reflex thresholds for BBN at noise-intensity levels less than 85 dB SPL (Hall, Berry, & Olson, 1982).

Acoustic reflex measurement for a BBN stimulus, applied in combination with other objective tests of auditory function, provides a readily available, quick, and objective method for ear-specific identification of hearing loss in infants and young children.

Acoustic Reflex Decay. In a normal ear, the acoustic reflex response will continue for as long as 10 seconds if the activating sound is present for that length of time. That is, the stapedius muscle contraction persists and compliance remains decreased throughout the stimulus presentation. Prolonging the stimulus sound for as much as 10 seconds is done in a test called the *acoustic reflex decay test.* Figure 8.10 shows a normal response for the acoustic reflex decay test.

In the early years of clinical acoustic immittance measurement, researchers discovered that the normal ongoing acoustic reflex activity during stimulation was not always observed in certain types of hearing losses (Jerger, Harford, Clemis, & Alford, 1974; Jerger & Jerger (1974); Klockhoff, 1961). Instead, the amount of acoustic reflex activity recorded with ongoing stimulation in some patients did not persist. Acoustic reflex activity decreased or decayed over a 10-second period in patients with certain types of auditory dysfunction. The observation led to the clinical application of the acoustic reflex decay test.

Here's how the acoustic reflex decay test is performed. First, the acoustic reflex threshold is determined

FIGURE 8.9

The differential effect of hearing loss on acoustic reflex thresholds for pure tone signals versus broadband-noise (BBN) signals.

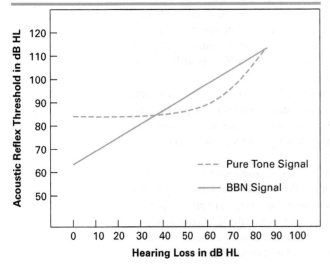

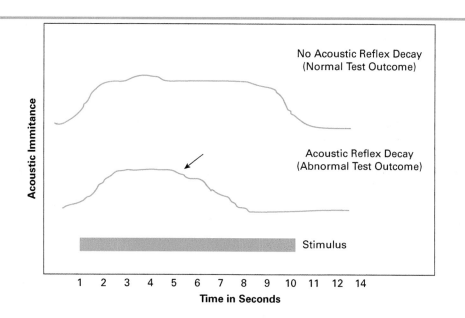

FIGURE 8.10

Examples of acoustic reflex decay tests show-ing normal outcome (no acoustic reflex decay) and an abnormal outcome (evidence of acoustic reflex decay). The arrow indicates acoustic reflex decay.

for one ear with a stimulus, like a 1000-Hz tone. Then, the same stimulus is presented continu-ally for 10 seconds at an intensity level 10 dB higher than the threshold. Most clinical acoustic immittance devices have an option for a timed 10-second stimulus presentation. Abnormal acoustic reflex decay is defined as a decrease of 50 percent or more in the amplitude of middle ear compliance during the 10-second time period.

Figure 8.10 shows an example of normal acoustic reflex activity over a 10-second period and an example of abnormal acoustic reflex decay. Acoustic reflex decay is a sign of auditory dysfunction involving the auditory nerve or the auditory brainstem, rather than the inner ear (Hall, 1985; Jerger & Jerger, 1977). Patients with this test outcome are promptly referred to a medical specialist like an otolaryngologist for further evaluation. Acoustic reflex abnormali-ties are sometimes recorded in combination with other abnormal auditory findings.

Diagnostic Value of Acoustic Reflex Patterns. Now that you're familiar with acoustic reflex pathways and acoustic reflex measurement, we'll conclude this section of the chapter with a brief discussion of how reflexes can be used in the diagnosis of hearing loss. Close analysis of the patterns of acoustic reflex findings in the four measurement conditions (ipsilateral and contralateral for the right and left ear) is useful for distinguishing persons with normal auditory function from those with various types of hearing loss. In other words, acoustic reflex findings are useful not only for predicting whether a patient has a hearing loss but also for determining type of hearing loss. The diagnostic information from acoustic reflexes is greatly increased when the findings of pure tone audiometry and tympanometry are also included in the analysis. Indeed, diagnosis of hearing loss is never based on acoustic reflex findings alone.

Combinations or patterns of findings for pure tone audiometry, tympanometry, and acous-tic reflex recordings are often linked to certain clinical etiologies or diagnoses. You'll now be introduced to some common patterns of findings for these three major groups of auditory tests. A systematic, step-by-step approach to analysis of the combined findings for the three tests helps to minimize diagnostic errors. Results of pure tone hearing testing, tympanometry, and acoustic immittance measurements can be described with brief phrases in a narrative format or summarized as numbers in a table. However, patterns of findings are more read-ily and clearly recognized when displayed in graphic formats, such as the audiogram and tympanogram. Even acoustic reflex findings can be shown in a graphic figure rather than described verbally.

Case Studies: Audiogram and Acoustic Immittance Findings

We will conclude the discussion of acoustic immittance measurement with a presentation of findings for two patients with different types of hearing loss. You will have the opportunity to examine findings for each procedure and the relations among the findings. Although it is tempting and natural to focus first on the audiogram, you'll discover that efficiency and accuracy in analysis of test findings is enhanced if you first examine the results of tympanometry. Try to ask the questions posed about each case. You'll find a complete description of the cases and a review of the findings at the end of the chapter.

Case 1

An audiogram and acoustic immittance findings for a 6-year-old boy are displayed in Figure 8.11. Look closely at the findings for each ear on tympanometry, acoustic reflexes, and then the audiogram, in that sequence. Be sure to compare hearing thresholds for air- and bone-conduction pure tone testing. How would you describe the findings? Does the patient have evidence of an abnormality in auditory function? If results are not normal, can you suggest a possible disorder that would explain the findings in Figure 8.11?

ClinicalConnection

The cases in this section of the chapter represent only two of the many types of abnormalities and hearing test patterns that are encountered in an audiology clinic. Disorders and diseases associated with the hearing problems for these cases are described in Chapter 11.

Case 2

Figure 8.12 shows findings for a 4-year-old girl. After inspecting the tympanograms, the acoustic reflex pattern, and the audiogram, how would you describe the findings? Does the patient have an evidence of an abnormality in auditory function? Are test results normal? If not, how would you describe the patient's hearing?

FIGURE 8.11

Audiogram and acoustic immittance findings for a 6-year old boy with a mild unilateral conductive hearing loss in the right ear (Case 1).

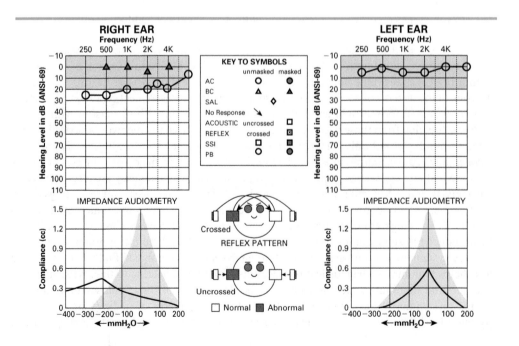

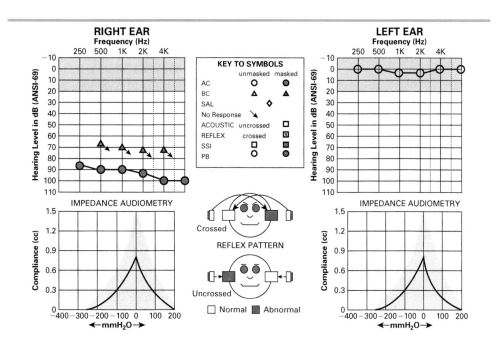

FIGURE 8.12

Audiogram and acoustic immittance findings for a 4-year-old girl with a unilateral severe-profound cochlear hearing loss (Case 2).

Otoacoustic Emissions (OAEs)

What Are Otoacoustic Emissions (OAEs)?

Otoacoustic emissions (OAEs) are sounds measured in the external ear canal that are associated with activity of the outer hair cells. You learned in Chapter 3 about outer hair cells and how they are activated during sound stimulation. The term *motility* is often used to describe rapid changes in the shape of the outer hair cells in response to sound. Mechanical energy produced by outer hair cell motility serves as an amplifier within the cochlea, contributing to better hearing. Indeed, normally functioning outer hair cells are essential for perfectly normal auditory function.

Outer hair cell motility clearly plays an important role in the production of OAEs. However, ongoing investigations for the past thirty years have yielded varying theories, even some controversy, as to the precise mechanisms underlying OAEs (Dhar & Hall, 2012).

The OAE measurement process begins with insertion of a probe into the external ear canal. The probe device is used to present stimulus sounds to the ear and to detect very faint sounds produced by the ear. OAE sounds represent energy associated with outer hair cell motility that makes its way from the cochlea through the middle ear, finally propagating outward into the external ear canal. The sound energy reaching the ear canal and recorded as OAEs is relatively modest. A sizable portion of the cochlear energy produced by outer hair cell motility is lost as it moves outward through the middle ear system. The amplitude of OAEs recorded in the ear canal is normally in the range of 0 to 15 dB SPL.

Types of OAEs. There are different categories of OAEs, distinguished by whether or not a sound used to stimulate the ear and by other characteristics. **Spontaneous otoacoustic emissions (SOAEs)** are not evoked or elicited with a stimulus. SOAEs are tones at one or more frequencies that are, as the term suggests, recorded in the external ear canal without sound stimulation. They are spontaneously generated by the cochlea and usually indicate outer hair cell integrity. SOAEs are absent in some normal-hearing persons. SOAEs can be recorded in only about 70 percent of normal ears and more often in females than males. SOAEs are not

WebWatch

You can quickly and easily get a sense of the remarkably large and diverse literature on otoacoustic emissions by conducting a PubMed search via the National Library of Medicine website (www.nlm.nih.gov). Simply select the link for Health Care Professionals, and then enter the key words "otoacoustic emissions." Be prepared for a response of over 3,000 peer-reviewed articles published in scientific journals, including some papers reviewing current research on how OAEs are produced by the ear and applied in different patient populations.

useful clinically because their presence or absence has limited value in distinguishing between normal and abnormal cochlear function.

We'll focus here on two types of OAEs that are elicited or evoked by sound stimulation. **Transient evoked OAEs (TEOAEs)** are elicited with very transient or brief sounds such as clicks or tone bursts that are usually presented at an intensity level of 80 dB SPL. TEOAEs are normally detected within the frequency range of 500 to about 4000 Hz.

Distortion product otoacoustic emissions (DPOAEs) are elicited with pairs of two pure tones labeled f_2 and f_1, rather than a single transient stimulus. Two stimulus frequencies are closely spaced together and presented simultaneously at moderate intensity levels usually in the range of 55 to 65 dB SPL. DPOAEs can be recorded across a frequency region of 500 to 8000 Hz and sometimes even for higher test frequencies.

Historical Overview

Discovery. In the 1970s, David Kemp first discovered sounds in the external ear canal produced by activity within the inner ear (Kemp, 1978, 1980). The discovery had a dramatic impact on theories and understanding of cochlear function. Within a decade, other hearing scientists proved unequivocally that acoustic stimulation of the ear resulted in movement of outer hair cells (e.g., Brownell, Bader, Bertrand, & Ribaupierre, 1985). When activated by a stimulus, outer hair cells rapidly and repeatedly changed in shape from tall and skinny to short and fat.

The rather revolutionary discovery of outer hair cell motility suggested an anatomical and physiological explanation for the generation of otoacoustic emissions. The discovery of outer hair cell motility also opened up an exciting new avenue in the study of cochlear function. Outer hair cell activity clearly plays an important role in the production of OAEs. Over the past thirty years, investigations have yielded varying theories and controversy as to the precise mechanisms underlying of OAEs and their origin (Dhar & Hall, 2012).

LEADERS AND LUMINARIES

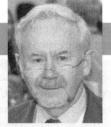

David Kemp

David Kemp is a Professor at the University College London who founded the Ear Institute. Dr. Kemp is known for his discovery and scientific exploration of otoacoustic emissions (OAEs) as well as his invention of practical technologies for their application in screening and diagnosis. A physicist by training, Dr. Kemp gained experience in electronics and audio-frequency signals at London University England in the 1960s while researching extremely low-frequency radio waves. He found his acute hearing useful in analyzing signals and diagnosing instrument faults. Moving into audiology Kemp studied low-level auditory perceptual aberrations experienced by normally hearing subjects, concluding they were due to reflections and distortions inside the cochlea. His findings were totally at variance with contemporary auditory theories but his observations predicted acoustic emissions. Dr. Kemp subsequently recorded otoacoustic emissions. The discovery led to the identification the cochlear amplifier, nonlinear compression, a new clinical tool, and indeed a new industry. You can learn more about Dr. Kemp and this very important test technique by downloading the Story of Otoacoustic Emissions from the Otodynamics website.

Early Clinical Applications. TEOAEs were applied almost exclusively in clinical settings from their discovery in 1978 until the mid-1990s (Hall, 2000). During that period, a clinical device based on laboratory equipment used by Kemp in his initial research was utilized by small groups of clinical audiologists around the world. Early clinical studies of OAEs certainly confirmed their value in varied patient populations. Unfortunately, audiologists had few options for purchase of clinical devices and the available devices only permitted measurement of TEOAEs and DPOAEs.

Increased Application of OAEs in Clinical Audiology. In the mid-1990s, three major developments contributed to substantially increased and widespread clinical application of OAEs (Dhar & Hall, 2012). First, different manufacturers developed and marketed a variety of clinical OAE devices, including instrumentation for recording DPOAEs. Also, two billing codes were approved that allowed healthcare professionals in the United States to charge for OAEs testing. The combination of readily available clinical devices and a means to bill for OAEs services naturally contributed to a rapid increase in the clinical application of the procedure.

The third factor responsible for the widespread use of OAEs, particularly in children, was a direct outgrowth of the increased availability of the technique. Clinical reports soon appeared in the literature documenting the value of OAEs for hearing screening and in the diagnosis of auditory dysfunction in a wide variety of patient populations (Dhar & Hall, 2012; Hall, 2000). OAEs are now firmly entrenched as an evidence-based procedure within the audiology test battery. And, OAEs are an essential tool in hearing assessment of infants and young children (JCIH, 2007).

Current Clinical Applications. OAEs are now an indispensable part of the hearing test battery. They are regularly applied in hearing screening of newborn infants. OAE measurement permits early detection of inner ear abnormalities associated with a wide variety of causes, including hearing loss related to noise exposure, to certain medications that affect cochlear hair cells, and to aging. Sometimes early detection of cochlear changes with OAEs contributes to prevention of hearing loss and its impact on communication and quality of life.

In combination with other test findings, abnormal OAE findings may also indicate a middle ear disorder that can be treated with surgical or medical management. With proper identification and diagnosis of hearing impairment, medical and nonmedical treatment options often lead to effective management.

Anatomy and Physiology

Clinical audiology practice requires an understanding of auditory system anatomy and physiology. This point is particularly relevant for the clinical application of OAEs. A clear understanding of how OAEs are generated within the cochlea is essential for recording OAEs and analyzing findings in varied patient populations.

Four general regions of auditory system anatomy are involved in OAE measurement. Each region is illustrated very simply in Figure 8.13. We will now discuss the role of each of the four regions in the stimulation and generation of OAE activity, and the influence of abnormal function of each of the regions on OAE recordings. You may wish to review information in Chapter 3 on structure and function for each of the four regions of the auditory system.

External Ear Canal. The external ear canal plays two critical roles in the measurement of OAEs. The stimulus and recording roles of the external ear canal are illustrated in Figure 8.13. Recording of OAEs is performed with a probe inserted in the external ear canal. Stimuli used to evoke OAEs are presented via the probe. Within the probe are one or two tiny tubes for presenting

FIGURE 8.13

Simple diagram of four regions of the auditory system involved in measurement and generation of otoacoustic emissions (OAEs).

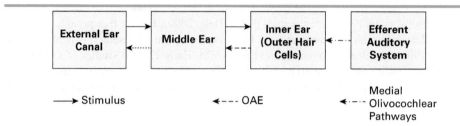

FIGURE 8.13

Simple diagram of four regions of the auditory system involved in measurement and generation of otoacoustic emissions (OAEs).

stimuli and another tube leading to a microphone for detection of OAE-related sound in the external ear canal. The effectiveness of stimulation may be reduced by debris or cerumen in the external ear canal. Debris or cerumen can occlude the external ear canal between the probe and the tympanic membrane. Debris or cerumen can also block one or more of the tubes in the probe.

Normal resonance and acoustics in the external ear canal may also influence stimulation during OAE measurement. In particular, interactions between the stimulus sounds, OAE sounds, and ear canal resonance may affect calibration of the stimulus used to elicit DPOAEs (Dhar & Hall, 2012).

The same nonpathologic conditions found in the external canal (like excessive cerumen) that can disrupt stimulation of the cochlea may also interfere with propagation of energy outward from the cochlea to the microphone located in the probe within the external ear canal. Outgoing OAE energy is markedly decreased by external ear canal blockage, preventing the detection of any OAE-related activity.

Middle Ear. The middle ear system plays a critical role in OAE measurement. Figure 8.13 depicts how stimuli used to elicit hair cell activity during clinical OAE measurement are transmitted to the cochlea via the middle ear. The arrows in Figure 8.13 indicate the direction of the stimulus inward to the cochlea and propagation of OAE energy outward from the cochlea to the ear canal.

OAEs are reduced in amplitude and often cannot be detected in the external ear canal in patients with middle ear abnormalities. It is important to assess function of the middle ear system whenever OAEs are reduced in amplitude or not present. You learned earlier in this chapter about how acoustic immittance procedures are used to evaluate the middle ear system. Middle ear dysfunction should be ruled out before OAE abnormalities can be attributed to cochlear auditory dysfunction.

Inner Ear. Multiple structures in the cochlea are important in the generation of OAEs. Each of the structures was reviewed in the sections of Chapter 3 on cochlear anatomy and physiology. Functional integrity of outer hair cells is essential for generation of OAEs. Outer hair cells change shape in response to sound stimulation. The up-and-down changes in hair cell shape amplify movement of the basilar membrane. The increased basilar membrane movement associated with outer hair cell motility contributes importantly to cochlear function, hearing sensitivity, and the ability to hear small differences in frequency, known as frequency selectivity.

Another cochlear structure, the stria vascularis, also plays a crucial role in the generation of energy that contributes to outer hair cell movement and the production of OAEs. Inner hair cells are not involved in the generation or measurement of OAEs.

Efferent Auditory System. Referring again to Figure 8.13, you'll see that the efferent auditory system is the fourth and final anatomic region involved in the measurement of OAEs. The efferent system is not essential for the generation or the clinical application of OAEs.

However, OAEs are influenced by efferent auditory activity. As you'll recall from Chapter 3, the efferent auditory system descends from the cerebral cortex, passing through the brainstem and then downward to hair cells in the inner ear. Efferent pathways primarily exert an inhibitory influence on cochlear activity. Stimulation of the efferent pathways, particularly those that course from the lower brainstem to the outer hair cells, suppresses outer hair cell activity and reduces OAE amplitude.

How Are Otoacoustic Emissions Recorded?

Probe Insertion. OAE recording is noninvasive, technically rather simple to perform, and quick. Usually OAE recording requires only a few minutes of test time for both ears. No behavioral response from the patient is required in OAE recording. In other words, the procedure is not affected by a patient's motivation, attention, or cognitive status. Before OAE recording, a soft disposable tip is secured to the end of a probe, as with acoustic immittance measurement. The probe is then gently inserted into the outer portion of the external ear canal.

In contrast to acoustic immittance measurement, a hermetic or airtight seal between the probe tip and the ear canal is not necessary when recording OAEs. One or two miniature loudspeakers within the inserted probe assembly generate sound stimuli at a moderate intensity level in the external ear canal. Stimuli in DPOAEs recording are usually at intensity levels of 55 to 65 dB SPL and 80 dB SPL for TEOAEs.

Stimulus Calibration. Immediately after the probe is inserted and just before OAE recording starts, the measurement device automatically calibrates stimulus-intensity levels within the patient's ear canal. Audiologists select the specific intensity level that an OAE device produces in the patient's external canal, such as 65 dB SPL. A miniature microphone in the probe of the OAE device detects the stimulus and the correct or target intensity level before testing begins.

Stimuli in Measurement of TEOAEs and DPOAEs. The types of stimuli are quite different for TEOAE and DPOAE measurement. The stimuli in TEOAE recording are very brief 0.1- or 0.2-millisecond clicking sounds. As you'll recall from Chapter 2, clicks contain a broad spectrum of frequencies. Click stimuli in TEOAE measurement almost instantaneously activate a wide frequency region in the cochlea. Some of the TEOAE energy related to outer hair cell movement in response to click stimulation returns from the cochlea through the middle ear to the ear canal.

In contrast, DPOAE activation follows simultaneous presentation of two different pure tone stimuli. The two pure tones are similar in frequency. The ratio of the higher-frequency tone to the lower-frequency tone is slightly higher than 1.0, usually about 1.22. For example, if the higher frequency is 2000 Hz then the lower frequency would be 1639 Hz, producing a ratio of 1.22.

The two stimulus tones in DPOAEs measurement activate a very limited region of the cochlea. Energy in the cochlea with activation of outer hair cells in the cochlea occurs at the two stimulus frequencies and also at other additional frequencies. The additional activity in the cochlea produced by the two closely spaced stimulus frequencies is called *distortion products*. The distortion products travel from the cochlea back through the middle ear to the external ear canal where they are detected with the probe connected to the OAE device.

Detection of OAEs. The miniature microphone within the probe assembly detects OAE-related sound as well as any other sound in the ear canal during the recording. OAE activity must be distinguished from other noise in the external ear canal. Specialized computer-based programs in the OAE device are designed to distinguish the OAE activity from background noise.

Noise is always present in the external ear canal during OAE measurement. Ambient acoustical noise from the test environment enters the external ear canal even with a probe securely in place. Sources of ambient noise include test equipment, people talking, noise from room ventilation systems, and so forth. Physiological noise also enters the external ear canal. Physiological noise arises from patient sources, such as breathing sounds and bodily movement. An audiologist can usually minimize excessive noise levels in the ear canal during OAE measurement by controlling sources of ambient noise and taking steps to quiet the patient.

Display of OAE Findings. At the completion of OAE recording, results are displayed on a computer screen or in another display format. Some modern OAE devices also include software for automated data analysis, including the calculation of amplitude values and noise-floor levels and statistical confirmation of the presence or absence of OAEs. Automated OAE devices designed for operation by nonaudiologists are generally used for hearing screening of children and adults. On the other hand, audiologists usually visually inspect amplitudes and noise levels when OAEs are included as part of a diagnostic test battery. Then the audiologist analyzes the patient's OAE amplitude values in comparison to normative amplitude data for the device.

TEOAE and DPOAE techniques are both used in clinical audiology. There are similarities and also differences in the way each type of OAE is recorded. We'll now review in a little more detail how TEOAEs and DPOAEs are measured.

Transient Evoked Otoacoustic Emissions (TEOAEs)

Information on a TEOAE Display. In recording any type of OAE, response amplitude in dB is plotted across a stimulus-frequency region. Figure 8.14 shows a display from the screen of a clinical TEOAE device. Information on the screen allows an audiologist to verify characteristics of the stimulus, such as the intensity level, and to analyze the response. An audiologist using a TEOAE device views all of this information to assure that the ongoing stimulus and noise conditions are adequate for OAE measurement and to determine whether a response is present.

We'll focus for a moment on some of the information displayed in Figure 8.14. The TEOAE temporal waveforms for each ear are identified at the top of the figure. The waveforms reflect the actual OAE sound produced by the cochlea as recorded within the external ear canal. If you look closely you'll see two separate waveforms that look quite similar. The size of the waveforms reflects the amplitude of the TEOAEs generated by the ear. OAE activity from the high-frequency base region of the cochlea is toward the left in the waveforms, with lower-frequency activity toward the right side.

Just below the waveforms is a display of TEOAE amplitude and also noise in dB SPL across a frequency region of 0 to 5000 Hz identified as TEOAE Spectrum in Figure 8.14. The jagged lighter-shaded area represents OAE amplitude at different frequencies evoked by the click stimulus as it activated the outer hair cells. The darker shaded area below the TEOAE amplitude labeled Background Noise Spectrum depicts noise in the external ear canal during the recording. As already noted, noise is always present during OAE recording. However, you can easily see that the TEOAE rises well above the noise floor.

Finally, below this spectral display of OAE and noise you'll see numbers in the portion labeled Response Data Summary that summarize the overall size of the TEOAE response in dB SPL and the noise during recording, also in dB SPL. Also shown in this section are the intensity level in dB SPL and presentation rate of the stimulus, 19 per second in this example. Displays of TEOAE findings include other details, but the information just described is most important for analyzing test results.

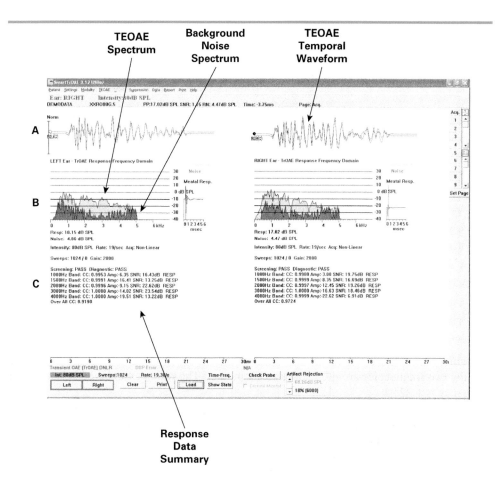

TEOAE Spectrum

Background Noise Spectrum

TEOAE Temporal Waveform

Response Data Summary

FIGURE 8.14

Transient evoked otoacoustic emissions (TEOAE) test conditions and findings displayed on the screen of a clinical device. The information labeled in the figure is described in the text. Courtesy of Intelligent Hearing Systems.

TEOAE Analysis. How is TEOAE information analyzed? First, the audiologist verifies that the stimulus-intensity level is appropriate and noise conditions are adequate during measurement. Then, attention is focused on the actual TEOAE findings. The TEOAEs displayed in Figure 8.14 are clearly present, as indicated by the robust waveform. In addition, there is a substantial difference between the TEOAE amplitude and the noise floor in the recording.

You can see in Figure 8.14 that signal-to-noise ratio (SNR) differences summarized in the printout below the graph are within the range of 13 to 19 dB for different bands of frequencies. If the patient were an infant undergoing hearing screening with TEOAEs, the outcome would definitely be a "Pass." In other words, the presence of TEOAE activity well above the noise floor is not consistent with hearing loss.

Distortion-Product Otoacoustic Emissions (DPOAEs)

Information on a DPOAE Display. The graph in Figure 8.15 shows information about DPOAE stimulation and DPOAE recordings. The display of DPOAE stimulus and response information is quite different from what we've just reviewed for TEOAEs. The graph shown in Figure 8.15 is the screen for a clinical DPOAE device.

Two stimuli are used to activate the cochlea in DPOAE measurement, shown on the right side of the display. Each frequency is shown as a spike in the displays, with amplitude indicated by the height of the spike. The higher-frequency stimulus (on the right) is referred to as f_2 and the lower-frequency stimulus (on the left) is f_1. You'll see that the

FIGURE 8.15

Distortion product
otoacoustic emissions
(DPOAE) stimuli and
findings displayed on
the screen of a clinical
device. Image courtesy
of Natus Medical Incor-
porated.

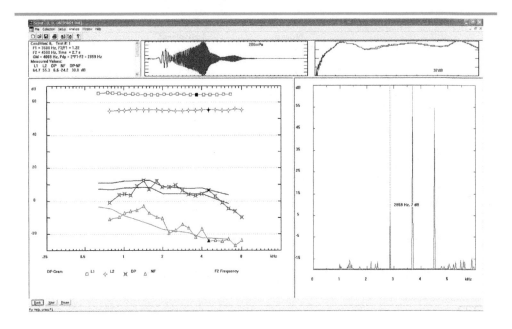

f_1 stimulus is at an intensity level of 65 dB SPL and the f_2 stimulus is at 55 dB SPL. Notice that the two frequencies are quite close to each other. The ratio of the higher to the lower frequency is 1.22.

The frequency range in the display extends from about 500 Hz on the left side to 8000 Hz on the right side. Different numbers of test stimuli are presented within each octave, depending on the goal of DPOAE measurement. When the goal is to simply screen for hearing loss, as few as three or four test frequencies may be presented within a relatively limited frequency region, for example, from 2000 to 4000 Hz. On the other hand, DPOAE recordings that are made along with other hearing tests in the diagnosis of hearing loss may include as many as five to eight test frequencies within the same frequency region and other similar frequency ranges from 500 to 8000 Hz.

The distortion-product (DP) activity generated in the cochlea by the two closely spaced stimuli (f_1 and f_2) is shown at a slightly lower frequency just to the left of the stimulus spikes in Figure 8.15. The DP is represented as a short spike at a frequency just below 3000 Hz. The distortion product in clinical DPOAEs measurement is almost always measured at a frequency of $2f_1 - f_2$. This frequency is defined as two times the lower of the stimulus frequencies (f_1) minus the higher stimulus frequency (f_2). The symbols on a graph of DPOAEs findings in the left portion of the figure indicate the amplitude or size of the DP at the frequency of $2f_1 - f_2$.

DPOAEs Analysis.   The graph in Figure 8.16 reflects the typical format for plotting DPOAE results with clinical devices. Results for the right ear are usually indicated by Os (circles), whereas left ear findings are shown as Xs. The plot of DP amplitude as a function of the stimulus (f_2) frequency is known as a **DPgram**. DP amplitude may be shown for a limited frequency region like 2000 to 4000 Hz, or across a much wider range such as 500 to 8000 or 10,000 Hz. Noise in the external canal during the DPOAE recording is shown below the DP amplitude symbols.

Looking closely at the figure, you'll notice that noise levels are highest in the lower-frequency region and that noise levels decrease for higher frequencies. Noise levels are usually diminished for frequencies above 2000 Hz, as shown in the figure.

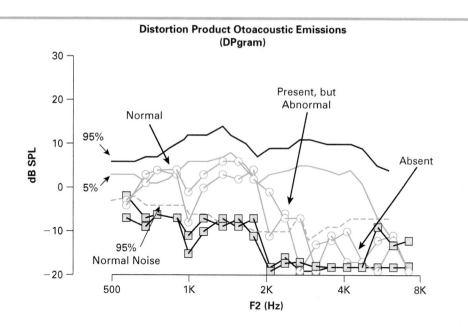

FIGURE 8.16

Analysis of distortion product otoacoustic emissions (DPOAE) findings, including documentation of noise levels, DP amplitude, and differentiation of findings into three categories: (1) normal, (2) present but abnormal, or (3) absent or no response.

Even a quick inspection of the graph in Figure 8.16 confirms that DP amplitude is well above the noise floor for most of the test frequencies. The minimum criterion for confirmation of the presence of an OAE is a 6 dB difference between the DP amplitude and noise at the same frequency. Some patients have large and clear DPOAEs at some frequencies, but small amplitude or even absent DPOAEs at other frequencies. Absence of DPOAEs is indicated by minimal or no difference (<6 dB) between the amplitude of the DP and that of the noise floor.

Analysis of OAE Findings

There are three general steps in the analysis of OAE findings. We will focus here on the analysis of DPOAE findings since they are applied more often in clinical audiology in the United States than TEOAEs. However, the principles of analysis are similar for each type of OAE.

Measurement Conditions. The first step in OAE analysis is to verify that measurement conditions are adequate. Specifically, noise levels in the ear canal during OAE recording must be sufficiently low to permit confident detection of OAE activity. Noise levels lower than -10 dB SPL are desirable, but sometimes slightly higher levels are unavoidable with young children who move about during testing.

Noise in the external canal during DPOAE recording shown earlier in Figure 8.15 is displayed with more detail in Figure 8.16. Let's take a moment to get oriented to the slightly different DPgram format shown in Figure 8.16. Sound levels recorded in the external ear canal are depicted on the vertical (Y) axis in dB SPL, to the left. One of the stimulus frequencies, specifically the f_2 frequency, is shown on the horizontal (X) axis that extends from 500 to 8000 Hz.

The upper limit for normal noise is shown as a dashed line, the lowest of three lines within the graph. The noise level line indicates that 95 percent of a group of normal adult subjects had lower noise levels during DPOAE measurement with the same device. The square symbols indicate noise levels in the external ear canal during DPOAE recording for the patient with this device at each of the test frequencies. Comparing the square symbols to the lowest solid line in the figure confirms that noise levels were adequately low for this patient.

Are OAEs Present? The next step in data analysis is to determine whether any OAE response was recorded. Let's again refer to the DPOAE findings in Figure 8.16. The presence of a DPOAE response at any test frequency is verified when OAE amplitude in dB SPL exceeds the noise level by 6 dB or more. If you look closely at Figure 8.16, particularly the frequency region of 500 Hz up to about 1500 Hz, you'll see that the circle symbols for DP amplitude are more than 6 dB above the square symbols for noise. A DPOAE response is present for these test frequencies. In contrast, DPOAEs are not consistently present at higher test frequencies.

Are OAEs Normal? Finally, once we've confirmed that the difference between OAE amplitude and noise floor ≥ 6 dB SPL, we can analyze DPOAE amplitudes with respect to an appropriate normal region. The DP normal region in Figure 8.16 is enclosed by the set of two solid lines that are in the range of approximately 0 to 10 dB. The normal region was developed from DPOAE data collected from a group of normal-hearing persons, using the same clinical device. If you compare the DP amplitude values to the normal region for the lower test frequencies, you'll notice that there is very little difference. That is, DPOAE amplitude is either within the two solid lines, at the lower end of normal, or just below normal limits.

Also, the two sets of circles confirm that DPOAE amplitudes for this patient were consistent or repeatable for two consecutive recordings. Now examine data for stimulus frequencies of 2000 Hz and higher. DPOAE amplitude clearly falls below normal limits. In fact, as noted already, there is really no difference between DPs and the noise floor for higher test frequencies. DPs are not detected for higher test frequencies.

 ClinicalConnection

Increased clinical application of OAEs in the mid-1990s contributed importantly to recognition of a new type of hearing problem called auditory neuropathy spectrum disorder (ANSD). Audiologists who began to apply OAEs in children were surprised when normal findings were encountered in patients with evidence of severe to profound hearing loss on other tests. You'll learn about the identification and diagnosis of ANSD in Chapter 12 and management strategies for ANSD in Chapter 16.

OAEs and Auditory Function

What do these DPOAE findings tell us about the auditory function of this patient? The nearly normal DPOAE amplitudes for lower test frequencies provide evidence that outer hair cells for that portion of the cochlea are intact. Also, given the clear and repeatable DPOAE responses within the lower-frequency region, it is likely that the patient's middle ear is functioning normally. Remember, measurement of OAE sounds in the external ear canal is dependent on the propagation of the OAE energy from the cochlea outward through the middle ear. The expectation of normal middle ear function could be easily confirmed by conducting acoustic immittance measurements.

The decreased DPOAE amplitude for higher frequencies and the absence of detectable DPs for test frequencies above 3000 Hz are evidence of cochlear dysfunction involving outer hair cells. The possibility of a hearing loss would be further evaluated with pure tone and speech audiometry.

OAEs and the Audiogram

Introduction. OAE findings sometimes agree closely with the audiogram. Patients with normal hearing sensitivity often have entirely normal OAEs and, conversely, abnormal hearing sensitivity is often associated with abnormal or absent OAEs. However, clinical experience has repeatedly revealed the possibility of discrepancies between the pure tone audiogram and OAE findings. For example, some patients with normal audiograms have abnormal OAE findings. Also, some patients with hearing loss as documented by pure tone audiometry have entirely normal OAE findings.

There are a variety of possible explanations for discrepancies between pure tone audiometry and OAE findings. It would be reasonable to question whether disagreement between findings on pure tone hearing testing and OAE findings reflects a problem with OAE measurement.

Actually, just the opposite is true. OAEs have remarkable diagnostic value in clinical audiology *because* they provide information on auditory function that is not available from pure tone audiometry. This important clinical principle will become quite clear in later chapters as we review the findings of many different test procedures for patients with various types of auditory dysfunction and hearing loss.

We'll now compare findings for pure tone audiometry versus distortion product otoacoustic emissions for a patient with a sensorineural hearing loss.

Case: High-Frequency Hearing Loss. Figure 8.17 shows findings for a person with a mild high-frequency hearing loss. Pure tone hearing thresholds begin to decrease at 3000 Hz even though they are still within normal limits, and then further decrease to about 30 dB HL at 8000 Hz. Bone-conduction hearing thresholds are the same as air-conduction thresholds, and there is no air-bone gap.

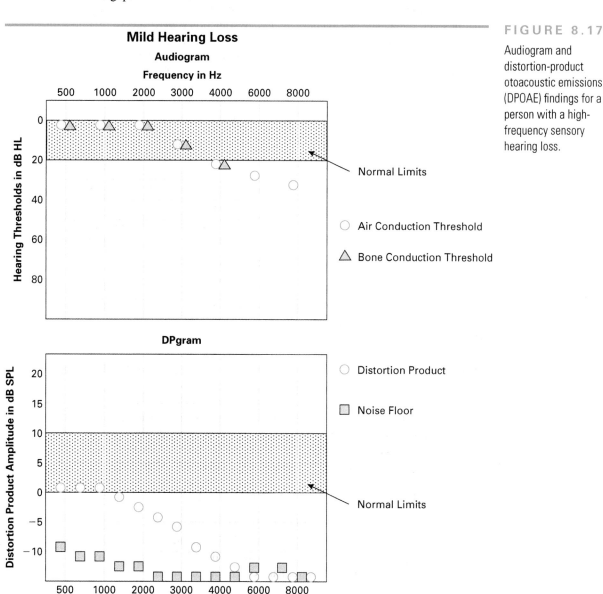

FIGURE 8.17

Audiogram and distortion-product otoacoustic emissions (DPOAE) findings for a person with a high-frequency sensory hearing loss.

In the lower portion of the figure, the pattern of amplitudes for DPOAEs appears to mirror pure tone thresholds. Looking closely, however, you'll notice that DPOAE amplitudes fall out of the normal region not only for frequencies of 3000 Hz and higher, but also for frequencies between 1500 and 3000 Hz. Abnormal DPOAE findings provide evidence of cochlear dysfunction involving outer hair cells even at test frequencies where pure tone hearing thresholds are normal.

Clinical Applications of Otoacoustic Emissions

OAEs contribute importantly and in a truly unique way to the diagnosis of auditory dysfunction, yet they have essentially no value in defining the degree of hearing loss. This apparent paradox in no way minimizes or detracts from the role of OAEs in clinical audiology today. In terms of anatomic site sensitivity and specificity, that is, detection and verification of outer hair cell dysfunction, OAEs have no rival in the audiological test battery. Because most permanent hearing loss in children, including newborn infants, is caused by cochlear abnormalities and outer hair cell damage and/or dysfunction, OAEs are well suited for hearing screening of infants, preschool and school-age children, and even adults.

OAEs are also an attractive screening option because the technique is relatively inexpensive and simple. OAE measurement just requires insertion of a disposable or reusable probe into the ear, without the need for electrode application. Given their sensitivity to cochlear dysfunction and the clinical advantages just cited, it is not surprising that OAEs are useful in auditory assessment of diverse patient populations.

Common Clinical Applications. Some of the more common clinical applications of OAEs include:

- Hearing screening of infants, pre-school children, and school age children
- Diagnosis of auditory dysfunction in children and adults
- Monitoring cochlear (outer hair cell) auditory function in patients receiving drugs that potentially damage the ear
- Early detection of false or exaggerated hearing loss
- Early detection of ear damage due to exposure to excessive levels of noise

One of the most common applications of OAEs is hearing screening of persons at risk for hearing impairment. OAE screening outcome is generally described as either *Pass* or *Refer*. A *Pass* outcome is reported when OAEs are present as defined by amplitudes ≥ 6 dB above the noise floor for the majority of test frequencies. Although the presence of OAEs does not always indicate normal hearing sensitivity, a Pass outcome rules out serious degrees of hearing loss.

A *Refer* OAE screening outcome indicates a clear risk for hearing loss that could affect communication. Patients who yield a Refer outcome for OAE screening should be referred for diagnostic hearing assessment and possible audiological or medical management.

OAEs also contribute to determination of sites of auditory dysfunction and can help to distinguish between cochlear and neural auditory abnormalities. Along with other test procedures, OAEs can play a role in the diagnosis of a variety of diseases and disorders causing hearing loss or some form of auditory dysfunction. The scientific literature contains hundreds of publications reporting evidence in support of OAE measurement in children and adults (Dhar & Hall, 2012).

Combined Acoustic Immittance and OAE Devices

In recent years, manufacturers have introduced instrumentation that can be used to record both OAEs and acoustic immittance measures. Clinical devices for simple and integrated measurement of OAEs and tympanometry contribute substantially to improved accuracy of newborn hearing screening. We have reviewed the critical role of the middle ear in OAE measurement. The middle ear is the link between activation of the cochlea and the stimulus presented to the ear and also in the outward propagation of OAE-related energy from the cochlea to the external ear canal. A device that combines OAE and tympanometry technology permits quick and effective description of middle ear and cochlear functioning.

Figure 8.18 shows an example of a combined acoustic immittance/OAE device. The device is small and easily handheld. It includes a lightweight probe designed for use with infants and young children. The device permits TEOAE and DPOAE measurement and also tympanometry with low or high probe tone frequencies.

The device can also be simply programmed to perform any combination of these three procedures in any sequence. The results are displayed for instant analysis on a small screen. Figure 8.18 also shows that test results for tympanometry and OAE recordings can be printed for later analysis and recordkeeping.

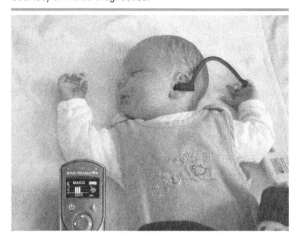

FIGURE 8.18 A portable device for recording both acoustic immittance measures and otoacoustic emissions. Courtesy of Maico Diagnostics.

PULLING IT ALL TOGETHER

The two categories of electroacoustic procedures, acoustic immittance measures and otoacoustic emissions, are valuable in describing auditory function. Tympanometry, an acoustic immittance test commonly applied by audiologists and other healthcare professionals, provides information on middle ear function and on the integrity of the tympanic membrane. Another acoustic immittance procedure, measurement of the acoustic reflex, also provides information on middle ear status. In addition, acoustic reflex findings are useful in assessing the functional integrity of the cochlea, the auditory (eighth cranial) nerve, parts of the brainstem, and even a portion of the seventh cranial nerve.

Otoacoustic emissions are a highly sensitive measure of cochlear function, specifically outer hair cell functioning. Many etiologies for hearing loss involve outer hair cell damage or dysfunction. For these reasons, otoacoustic emissions testing is now relied on for hearing screening and also, along with other auditory tests, for diagnosis of auditory function in children and adults. Otoacoustic emissions findings do not always agree pure tone audiometry. A discrepancy in findings between the two tests often leads to further diagnostic testing, more accurate diagnosis of auditory function, and more effective intervention for patients with hearing loss.

The clinical value of these electroacoustic procedures is enhanced by their objectivity, that is, their independence from behavioral test factors. As a result of their objective nature, acoustic immittance measures and otoacoustic emissions provide accurate information on auditory function in infants and young children, as well as uncooperative adult patients.

CASE 1

The patient is a 6-year-old boy. Case history revealed that the patient has allergies and often has upper respiratory congestion during the winter months. In the bottom portion of Figure 8.11, tympanograms are different for the two ears. The left ear tympanogram is normal (Type A), whereas the right ear tympanogram is abnormal. It is a type C tympanogram with a peak at about −200 mm H20 (daPa). The diagram between the two tympanograms indicates that acoustic reflexes are normal with the probe in the left ear but abnormal, perhaps absent, with the probe in the right ear. Consistent with the tympanometry findings, hearing thresholds are normal for the left ear and abnormal for the right ear.

Specifically, there is evidence of a conductive hearing loss in the right ear. There is a rising configuration on the audiogram. Air-conduction hearing thresholds are decreased for the lower frequencies and improve at higher frequencies. In contrast, bone-conduction thresholds are normal at all frequencies. There is a 25-dB air-bone gap at 250 and 500 Hz. The patient clearly has evidence of abnormal auditory function.

The findings in Figure 8.11 document abnormal middle ear function on the right side. The most likely explanation for the findings is Eustachian tube dysfunction that has resulted in decreased air pressure in the middle ear. You'll learn more about Eustachian tube dysfunction and ear infections in Chapter 11.

CASE 2

The patient is a 4-year-old girl. According to history, mother and preschool teachers noticed that the girl does not consistently respond to sounds that she hears from the right side. The patient also seems to have difficulty understanding what people are saying in noisy settings, like the preschool classroom. The tympanograms in the lower part of Figure 8.12 are normal, but the acoustic reflex pattern is definitely abnormal. Acoustic reflexes are not observed whenever the stimulus sound is presented to the right ear, yet they are entirely normal when sound is presented to the right ear. This particular pattern for acoustic reflexes raises the suspicion of a severe hearing loss in the right ear.

Even a quick glance at the patient's audiogram confirms the suspicion of a severe hearing loss in the right ear. Pure tone hearing thresholds are within the range of 90 to 100 dB HL for all test frequencies. As you learned in Chapter 7, stimulus sounds presented at high-intensity levels to one ear might cross over to the other nontest ear. With this audiogram format, adequate masking of the nontest ear is indicated by filled-in (black) symbols for air-conduction and bone-conduction pure tone audiometry. We can assume in this case that hearing thresholds plotted for the right ear actually reflect right ear hearing, and not a crossover response from the left ear.

What is the cause of the patient's unilateral hearing loss? That important question will not be answered with hearing tests alone. The question might be answered with additional information from medical tests. The audiologist who performed the hearing test will refer the patient to an otolaryngologist for additional evaluation. A more detailed history also might yield clues about the cause of the hearing loss. For example, the results of newborn hearing screening would be helpful in determining whether a hearing loss was present from birth. A family history of unilateral hearing loss would suggest a genetic explanation for the hearing loss.

READINGS

Dhar, S., & Hall, J. W. III. (2011). *Otoacoustic emissions: Principles, procedures, and protocols.* San Diego: Plural Publishing.

Gelfand, S. A. (2009). *Essentials of audiology.* New York: Thieme.

Hall, J. W. III. (1987). Contemporary tympanometry. *Seminars in Hearing, 8, 321.*

Hall, J. W. III. (2000). *Handbook of otoacoustic emissions.* San Diego: Singular Publishing.

Hall, J. W. III, & Chandler, D. (1994). Tympanometry in clinical audiology. In J. Katz (Ed.), *Handbook of clinical audiology* (4th ed., pp. 283–299). Baltimore: Williams & Wilkins.

Jerger, J. (Ed.). (1975). *Handbook of clinical impedance audiometry*. Dobbs Ferry, NY: American Electromedics Corporation.

Hunter, L., & Shahnaz, N. (2013). *Acoustic immittance measures: Basic and advanced principles*. San Diego: Plural Publishing.

Hunter, L. L., Feeney, M. P., Lapsley Miller, J. A., Jeng, P. S., & Bohning, S. (2010). Wideband reflectance in newborns: Normative regions and relationship to hearing screening results. *Ear & Hearing, 31,* 599–610.

Lilly, D. J. (1972). Acoustic impedance at the tympanic membrane. In J. Katz (Ed.), *Handbook of clinical audiology* (pp. 434–439). Baltimore: Williams & Wilkins.

Margolis, R. H., & Hunter, L L. (1999). Tympanometry: Basic principles and clinical applications. In F. E. Musiek & W. F. Rintelmann (Eds.), *Contemporary perspectives in hearing assessment* (pp. 89–130). Boston: Allyn & Bacon.

Otoacoustic Emissions Portal Zone. www.otoemissions.org

Robinette, M. S., & Glattke, T. J. (Eds.), *Otoacoustic emissions: Clinical applications* (3rd ed.). New York: Thieme Publishers.

Van Camp, K. J., Margolis, R. H., Wilson, R.H., Creten, W. L., & Shanks, J. E. (1986). Principles of tympanometry. *ASHA Monograph,* 24.

Wilson, R. H., & Margolis, R. H. (1999). Acoustic-reflex measurements. In F. E. Musiek & W. F. Rintelmann (Eds.), *Contemporary perspectives in hearing assessment* (pp. 131–165). Boston: Allyn & Bacon.

9 Special Speech Audiometry Tests and Auditory Evoked Responses

KEY TERMS

Auditory brain stem response (ABR)

Auditory evoked responses

Auditory processing disorders (APD)

Binaural integration

Binaural separation

Competing message

Contralateral pathways

Dichotic listening task

Distorted speech tests

Electrodes

Filtered word test

Hearing in Noise Test (HINT)

Ipsilateral pathways

Monaural frequency distorted speech tests

Performance-intensity (PI) function

PI-PB function

Retrocochlear disorder

Right ear advantage (REA)

Rollover

Signal-to-noise ratio (SNR)

Special speech audiometry

Speech-in-noise tests

Test battery

Test reliability

Test validity

Tone bursts

LEARNING OBJECTIVES

In this chapter, you will learn:

- New terms used by audiologists who assess and diagnose auditory disorders
- About additional procedures for evaluating how well a person perceives speech
- The difference between traditional speech audiometry tests, like speech recognition threshold and word recognition, and special speech audiometry tests used to evaluate central auditory nervous system function
- How special speech perception tests are useful in evaluating auditory processing and diagnosing auditory processing disorders
- What is meant by the term "auditory brain stem response," abbreviated ABR
- How ABR is recorded in children and in adults
- How audiologists analyze ABR recordings
- Different applications of ABR for children and adults
- How audiologists can evaluate an infant's hearing with ABR
- About other responses from the ear, auditory nerve, and brain that are stimulated by sound

CHAPTER FOCUS

The chapter begins with a review of some *special speech audiometry* procedures used to evaluate patients who have hearing problems that are not detected or adequately described with pure tone audiometry or conventional speech threshold and recognition procedures. Dozens of special speech audiometry tests have been developed over the past sixty years. Some of the test approaches are rather simple.

One example is the measurement of word recognition performance in slightly different test conditions, such as high-intensity levels as well as lower, more comfortable levels. Another example is measurement of speech perception in the presence of background noise or with some frequencies in the speech filtered out. Other speech procedures are more clever and sophisticated. With one common speech test for assessment of central auditory functioning, a patient is required to repeat a word presented to the right ear and also another different word that is presented to the left ear at exactly the same time.

Special speech tests are particularly valuable in evaluating patients with abnormalities affecting the central auditory nervous system. You were

CHAPTER FOCUS *Concluded*

introduced to the central auditory nervous system in Chapter 3. In this chapter and in a later chapter on disorders affecting the central auditory nervous system pathways and centers, we will emphasize an important concept: *We hear with our brain.* Auditory and language areas in the central nervous system are critically important for hearing, listening, and communication. Some hearing problems related to dysfunction in the central nervous system are called *auditory processing disorders.* You'll learn more about auditory processing disorders in later chapters.

You'll also be introduced in this chapter to objective test procedures called *auditory evoked responses.* You've already learned about some objective auditory procedures that do not require a behavioral response from the patient or observation of the response by a tester. In the previous chapter, we discussed two objective auditory tests that are commonly applied in clinical audiology. You'll recall that aural immittance measurement provides information about how well the middle ear system conveys energy from the external ear to the inner ear, and otoacoustic emissions are a sensitive measure of the function of the outer hair cells within the inner ear.

Auditory evoked responses are objective tests used to detect bioelectrical activity in all regions of the auditory system, from the cochlea and the hearing nerve to the highest levels in the brain. Brain activity is elicited or evoked by very brief sounds presented via earphones or bone vibrators. Auditory evoked responses are detected with special electrodes and wires attached to skin on the head and near the ear. Auditory evoked responses are sometimes referred to as electrophysiological measures.

Auditory evoked responses play an important role in clinical audiology. They are used along with special diagnostic speech tests for the assessment of patients at risk for central auditory nervous system dysfunction, including auditory processing disorders. Auditory evoked responses are especially valuable for the evaluation of auditory function in infants, young children, and other persons who cannot or will not participate in behavioral hearing testing.

Hearing testing with auditory evoked responses is also well within the audiologist's scope of practice. According to the American Academy of Audiology, "Assessment of hearing includes the administration and interpretation of behavioral, physioacoustic, and electrophysiologic measures of the peripheral and central auditory systems (American Academy of Audiology, 2004).

Rationale for Special Testing

Going beyond Simple Testing

You learned in Chapters 4, 5, and 6 that a patient undergoing behavioral hearing testing must be alert. The patient is required to listen for stimulus sounds and then the patient gives a response that an audiologist can observe. Pure tone and simple speech audiometry play an essential role in the assessment of hearing. In fact, these two types of procedures are routinely used during hearing testing of older children and adults.

The results of pure tone audiometry are useful in confirming a hearing loss for most patients who complain of hearing problems. Patients with a hearing loss may also demonstrate difficulty on speech audiometry tests such as decreased speech recognition thresholds and lower than normal scores on word recognition. When a patient's hearing and listening complaints are confirmed by abnormal performance on pure tone and/or simple speech audiometry, there is usually no need for further hearing assessment. That is, initial test results provide the information an audiologist needs to describe the hearing loss and to develop a management plan for the patient.

Audiologists sometimes encounter patients who complain of difficulty in hearing, yet the complaints are not confirmed by pure tone audiometry or even by performance on tests of word recognition. This important point will now be illustrated with three different patients.

Three Case Examples

Let's consider as an example an older adult male patient who reports daily problems in communicating. He particularly notes a problem in understanding what his wife is saying when they converse in a noisy setting like a restaurant or while driving in their car. Understandably, the elderly couple is very discouraged and frustrated by their communication struggles.

An audiologist conducts a hearing assessment of the elderly patient, expecting to discover at least a moderate hearing loss. However, pure tone audiometry for the patient reveals reasonably good hearing sensitivity with only a mild hearing loss limited to the highest test frequencies. And, word recognition scores of 88 to 92% for the right and left ears are quite good. Findings on special speech audiometry tests for this case would probably document abnormal performance of speech perception in background noise.

Based on the additional diagnostic test results, the audiologist could develop an effective management plan to help this older gentleman communicate effectively in the real world. Appropriate management planning would not be possible based only on the patient's audiogram and or the results of simple speech audiometry.

Let's consider a second example. A mother schedules her 8-year-old son for a hearing assessment at the beginning of a school year. This is the third year in a row the child has undergone a simple hearing assessment with pure tone audiometry. Mother remains convinced that her child has a hearing loss. At the start of each school year, teachers report to the mother that the boy seems to have problems listening in the classroom. The third-grade student is a struggling reader and is not doing well academically. However, year after year the child's audiogram is entirely within normal limits, with word recognition scores of 100% in each ear.

It is likely that comprehensive hearing assessment with special speech measures would reveal evidence of deficits in auditory information processing, even though hearing sensitivity and simple word recognition scores are normal. The diagnostic test results would lead to effective intervention strategies for enhancing communication in the classroom, improving academic performance, and perhaps even strengthening the boy's reading skills.

A different and final example is a 24-year-old male graduate student who complains of difficulty hearing with the left ear when talking on his cell phone, especially in noisy settings. An ear examination by his primary care physician showed no signs of ear disease. The report of follow-up testing at a local audiology clinic indicated that the young man's audiogram and speech recognition thresholds were "within normal limits" and word recognition scores were "good" at a comfortable intensity level. Up to this point, all test findings have been normal.

What outcome might we expect if this patient underwent further additional speech audiometry testing and perhaps assessment with the auditory brain stem response? There is a good chance that diagnostic testing would reveal abnormal findings for the left ear. Based on the unilateral left-sided auditory test abnormalities, an audiologist would almost certainly refer the patient directly to an otolaryngologist or otologist to further investigate the possibility of a disease or pathology affecting the left auditory nerve.

The ear specialist would likely schedule the patient for a brain imaging study to determine whether the auditory problems were due to a tumor involving the left auditory nerve. If this concern were confirmed, management options would probably include surgical removal of the tumor. An otologist and perhaps a brain surgeon would perform the operation. However, an audiologist might also be in the operating room to measure auditory and facial nerve function and help minimize the chance of damage to the nerves during surgery.

Why Special Tests Are Important

These three cases illustrate that pure tone and simple speech tests are not always adequate measures of hearing status. Some patients who experience serious difficulties with hearing have no problem detecting soft pure tone sounds or repeating single-syllable words in a quiet setting. Why is it important to detect auditory problems in patients who have little or no problem hearing faint pure tone signals or recognizing words? Detection of all auditory problems in all patients is important for two reasons.

First, the patient's auditory problems are likely to contribute to ineffective and inefficient communication in real-world listening environments like the classroom or the workplace. Detection of auditory problems usually leads to effective nonmedical intervention, implemented by an audiologist, sometimes in collaboration with a speech pathologist. Almost all patients with auditory problems can be helped with appropriate rehabilitation and assistive listening technology. The first two cases just reviewed highlight the clinical value of further testing for hearing and listening problems that are not explained by basic auditory assessment.

Second, findings from diagnostic assessment may contribute to identification of hearing problems or auditory dysfunction resulting from pathology or disease. Patients with abnormal findings on special diagnostic hearing tests are almost always referred to one or more medical specialists for further diagnostic evaluation and additional testing, such as laboratory tests and brain scans. In some patients, referral to a physician results in medical management with drugs or even surgical intervention like an operation to remove a tumor. The third case was an example of auditory dysfunction caused by pathology that was not apparent on basic hearing assessment.

Special Speech Audiometry Procedures

What Are Special Speech Audiometry Tests?

Speech audiometry test procedures are used mainly to estimate threshold for speech and to assess recognition of simple speech signals in a quiet test condition. It is true that even simple speech audiometry procedures contribute to the diagnosis of hearing loss. However, the main goal of simple speech tests is to determine the impact of a hearing loss on ability to perceive speech under ideal listening conditions. In contrast, **special speech audiometry** procedures are more challenging tasks that are more sensitive to the detection of auditory dysfunction and more useful in distinguishing among different categories of auditory dysfunction.

James Jerger and Deborah Hayes explain the importance of special speech audiometry, also known as diagnostic speech audiometry, in a 1977 publication entitled simply "Diagnostic Speech Audiometry." They state,

> The diagnostic value of traditional speech audiometry is extremely limited. If measurement is confined to the usual combination of spondee threshold and "PB max" at a single suprathreshold level, the performance variation within distinct diagnostic categories is so great that there is a real problem of overlapping ranges. (Jerger & Hayes, 1977, p. 216)

Historical Origins in the 1950s

The application of special speech audiometry in clinical evaluation of auditory function can be traced back over sixty years. In 1954, four Italian otolaryngologists published a paper entitled "Testing 'cortical' hearing in temporal lobe tumours" (Bocca, Calearo, Cassinari, &

L E A D E R S   A N D   L U M I N A R I E S

Deborah Hayes

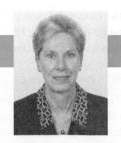

Deborah Hayes received her bachelor's and master's degrees from Northwestern University and her PhD in audiology from Baylor College of Medicine in Houston, Texas. Dr. Hayes began her career in the 1970s as an audiologist and supervisor in the audiology clinic at the Methodist Hospital in Houston Texas. There she collaborated with James Jerger in conducting large-scale clinical studies of various diagnostic procedures for hearing assessment of children and adults. Together they published now-classic papers, including "The Cross-Check Principle in Pediatric Audiology" in 1976 and "Diagnostic Speech Audiometry" in 1977.

Since 1983, Dr. Hayes has served as Chair of Audiology, Speech Pathology, and Learning Services at Children's Hospital Colorado (Denver) and professor in the Department of Physical Medicine and Rehabilitation and the Department of Pediatrics at the University of Colorado School of Medicine. She has held numerous leadership positions in professional organizations, including serving as president of the American Academy of Audiology and the American Auditory Society. In recent years, Dr. Hayes organized an international consensus meeting on the identification and management of children with auditory neuropathy that resulted in evidence-based clinical guidelines for its identification, diagnosis, and management.

Migliavacca, 1954). The subjects in the study were eighteen adult patients who had normal hearing thresholds and also normal word recognition scores. However, each of the patients complained about extreme difficulty understanding speech. The Italian physicians made a special tape recording of two-syllable words with higher-frequency information filtered out. Energy was removed from the words beginning at the frequency of 500 Hz, with no energy in the words above the frequency of 2000 Hz. This is described as *low pass filtering* words, since only the low frequencies are allowed to pass through the filter. When words are filtered in this way, they sound fuzzy or unclear even to a listener with normal hearing.

The **filtered word test** was first administered to a group of normal-hearing subjects who had no hearing complaints and who were recruited specifically for the study. Test scores for the normal subjects were consistently within the 60 to 80% range and scores were similar for each ear. In contrast, the scores of the eighteen patients were much poorer for one ear than the other. Medical diagnostic tests confirmed that each of the patients had a tumor or lesion in the auditory region of the brain, specifically the temporal lobe in the cerebrum. A *lesion* (pronounced LEE shun) is a region of damaged or diseased tissue, in this case brain tissue. In the words of the authors, "The result of the test has been nearly constant in all cases and has demonstrated that the discrimination of distorted voice is poorer in the ear contralateral to the cortical lesion. In nearly all cases normal tone and speech audiometry failed to reveal any deviation from normal in both ears" (Bocca, Calearo, Cassinari, & Migliavacca, 1954, p. 302).

Inspired by the exciting findings of this study, groups of hearing researchers around the world began to use filtered word tests to assess auditory problems not detected on the simpler hearing tests (Hall, 1991; Konkle & Rintelmann, 1983). One early variation on filtered word testing was a binaural version of the filtered speech test in which low frequencies were removed from words presented to one ear and high frequencies were removed from words presented to the other ear. Persons with normal auditory function automatically combined the information from each ear and had no difficulty repeating the filtered words. In contrast, patients with auditory processing disorders performed poorly on the test (Matzker, 1959).

Auditory researchers also began to develop other very different types of diagnostic speech audiometry procedures for the assessment of central auditory function and auditory processing (e.g., Jerger, 1960a; Kimura, 1961; Milner, Taylor, & Sperry, 1968; Pinheiro & Tobin, 1969; Sanchez-Longo, Forster, & Auth, 1957; Speaks & Jerger, 1965). In 1954 a well-known British psychologist named Donald Broadbent described a very different strategy for evaluating auditory abilities (Broadbent, 1954). Broadbent developed what came to be called the **dichotic listening task**. The word *dichotic* is pronounced "die KAH tick." A dichotic listening task involves binaural hearing. Specifically, during a dichotic listening test different sounds are presented to each ear at the same time.

Commonly, in a dichotic listening test different speech signals such as words, numbers, or sentences are presented simultaneously to each ear. The speech signals are usually in the same category; for example, a word is presented to the right ear while another word is presented to the left ear or a sentence is presented to the right ear while another sentence is presented to the left ear. The person being tested is asked to repeat what is heard in each ear.

As a cognitive psychologist, Broadbent was not interested in developing a new clinical test for audiology. Rather, he was studying very specific auditory skills of normal-hearing people, namely a person's ability to remember auditory information for a brief time in auditory memory and to selectively attend to a certain sound when many other sounds were also present. In fact, Broadbent's research began during World War II when he was attempting to determine how air traffic control workers could focus their attention on radio communications from one airplane when at the same time pilots of many other airplanes were also communicating with the control tower. It was not long, however, before dichotic listening tests were developed to clinically evaluate auditory function in patients who were suspected of having brain dysfunction.

Toward the end of the 1950s, a student named Sinha reported in an unpublished master's thesis what was probably one of the first clinical applications of a speech-in-noise test (Sinha, 1959). Early speech-in-noise tests measured the patient's recognition of speech while noise was presented in the background to the same ear. The noise typically consisted of either broadband noise or noise with frequencies in the same range as the speech signal. The speech signal was higher in intensity than the background noise, resulting in a signal-to-noise ratio (SNR) in the range of 1 to 10 dB. Sinha used one of these early speech-in-noise tests to study a small group of patients with confirmed brain tumors. He reported that the patients had depressed performance for speech recognition in background noise when words were presented to the ear on the side opposite to a tumor in the auditory cortex part of the temporal lobe of the brain.

Coincidentally, another event in 1954 contributed to growing interest in diagnostic speech tests in clinical audiology. Helmer Myklebust published a textbook entitled *Auditory Disorders in Children: A Manual for Differential Diagnosis* (Myklebust, 1954). Myklebust was a psychologist by training who had a strong clinical and research interest in hearing and auditory learning. He emphasized in his teaching and writings the importance of special speech audiometry for the detection and description of auditory function of the central nervous system, as well as function of the ear. As a faculty member at Northwestern University for over twenty years, Myklebust introduced many generations of audiologists, speech pathologists, and learning disability specialists to the clinical importance of evaluating how the brain processes speech.

Clinical Applications in the 1960s

The Canadian research psychologist Doreen Kimura first applied the dichotic listening procedure to evaluation of patients with known neurological disorders (Kimura, 1961). Using speech signals consisting only of numbers, she found that even normal hearers yielded slightly

FIGURE 9.1

Photographs of persons who made important early contributions to special speech audiometry and audiology in general: **A.** Jack Katz and **B.** Robert Keith.

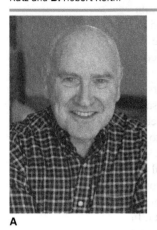 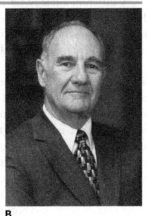

A   **B**

better scores for the right ear than the left ear on dichotic listening tasks. In contrast, patients with neurological abnormalities involving the auditory cortex or the corpus callosum, the pathway connecting the right and left hemispheres of the brain, typically showed remarkably poor scores for words presented to the left ear.

A few years after Kimura's report on dichotic listening in patients with neurological disorders, audiologist Jack Katz (1962) (Figure 9.1A) developed a version of the dichotic technique that soon become quite popular among audiologists. The *Staggered Spondaic Word (SSW) Test* is still used today. Indeed, dichotic listening tests in general are among the most commonly applied special speech procedures. We'll soon review hearing processes involved in dichotic listening and several dichotic listening tests currently used regularly by audiologists in clinical assessment of children and adults who have hearing complaints yet normal audiograms.

In the 1960s the diagnostic audiology test battery continued to expand beyond dichotic listening tests (Hall, 1983, 1991). It grew to include other tests, such as tests involving tones rather than speech. Tests were developed to evaluate fundamental processes, such as auditory adaptation or decay and also the just-noticeable-difference intensity of sound. You learned about these auditory processes in Chapter 2. The primary focus of diagnostic audiology in the 1960s and early 1970s was the detection of retrocochlear auditory dysfunction in patients with unilateral hearing loss. The term **retrocochlear disorder** at that time referred to patients with a tumor involving the auditory nerve.

Measurement of word recognition performance was also a regular part of the traditional diagnostic test battery. Exceptionally poor word recognition scores are a characteristic feature of retrocochlear auditory dysfunction. Clinical experience and research involving patients with confirmed auditory nerve tumors revealed that word recognition test performance often became poor at very high-intensity levels when compared to performance at a comfortable listening level (Jerger & Jerger, 1971; Schuknecht & Woellner, 1955). Speech recognition testing at different intensity levels soon grew popular in diagnostic hearing testing.

Today audiologists typically use a group of speech audiometry tests to evaluate auditory function. A group of such tests is called a **test battery**. Currently the typical test battery includes procedures that are sensitive to different auditory processes and to abnormalities in the auditory system. An audiologist often selects a collection of tests specific tailored to assess a particular patient.

Clinical Value of Special Speech Tests

By the mid-1970s, a clinically proven battery of special speech audiometry procedures was available to audiologists (e.g., Jerger & Jerger, 1975a). Clinical evidence from research studies showed that patients with confirmed pathologies or disorders affecting the auditory system had abnormal findings when evaluated with procedures in the test battery. During the same time period, a well-known audiologist named Robert Keith (Figure 9.1B) published a textbook devoted exclusively to the use of speech tests to assess auditory processing in persons with central nervous system dysfunction (Keith, 1977). With these developments, hearing testing was extended beyond the audiogram to include diagnostic assessment of the central auditory nervous system and auditory processing.

Dozens of other speech audiometry procedures were later developed for the diagnosis of auditory dysfunction. Not all of the procedures have stood the test of time. Some are not used clinically. The various speech audiometry procedures are generally categorized according to their characteristics, such as word tests versus sentence tests, monosyllabic versus multisyllabic tests, or monaural versus binaural tests.

Test Reliability and Validity

Early clinical studies of diagnostic testing in patients with confirmed pathology and disease produced valuable information on **test reliability** and **test validity**. You may not be familiar with these terms. *Reliability* indicates that the results of a test are repeatable from one test session to the next. A reliable test yields equivalent results each time it is carried out on the same person. For example, a patient with a score of 88% on the test today will produce a similar score on the test tomorrow or next week. The term *validity* means the test actually measures what it was designed to measure. A valid test accurately describes a specific auditory dysfunction for a specific patient. Establishment of the reliability and validity of hearing tests has led to the clinical test batteries used in audiology.

Development of a clinical test procedure should include studies to document its reliability and validity with a sizable number of normal-hearing persons and persons with well-defined auditory dysfunction. Unfortunately, this scientific process is not always adequately followed for newly developed speech audiometry procedures or other auditory tests. Procedures are generally not included in an audiological test battery unless there is research evidence confirming clinical performance, such as reliability and validity.

 WebWatch

You can locate on the Internet published clinical guidelines for assessment and management of persons with hearing impairment and related problems like tinnitus and balance disorders. Clinical guidelines are usually developed by professional organizations, such as the American Academy of Audiology, the American Speech-Language-Hearing Association, and multidisciplinary professional groups.

Evidence-Based Tests

We will now review selected speech tests, with an emphasis on those currently used by audiologists in the diagnosis of auditory dysfunction. The discussion will focus mostly on tests that are evidence based. The meaning of the phrase *evidence based* is directly related to our discussion of clinical studies of auditory test batteries and the concepts of test reliability and validity. Evidence or findings from research should guide clinical practice. Research findings for evidence-based tests are published in the *peer-reviewed literature*. Peer-reviewed literature includes scientific articles published only after close review by multiple experts to verify that proper research methods have been followed and that analysis of the results is appropriate.

Performance-Intensity (PI) Functions for Phonetically Balanced (PB) Words

In the 1960s, James and Susan Jerger first described a simple diagnostic speech audiometry procedure involving phonetically balanced words (Jerger & Jerger, 1967). You were introduced in Chapter 6 to phonetically balanced (PB) words and to the PI-PB word recognition technique. PB word lists consist of a series of twenty-five or fifty words with a distribution of speech sounds or phonemes in each list corresponding to the likelihood of the sounds in everyday speech. That is, the lists are constructed so that the frequency with which each speech sound, like /s/, /t/, /i/, or /o/, occurs in a list approximates its frequency in conversational speech.

Jerger and Jerger used the phrase **performance-intensity (PI) function** for PB words, abbreviated **PI-PB function**, to refer to a graph showing word recognition scores for word lists as the testing is conducted at different intensity levels (Jerger & Jerger, 1971). In performing the PI-PB function test, an audiologist first measures word recognition at a moderate intensity level that the patient considers comfortable. The words are presented through the audiometer via a tape recorder or some other device such as an MP3 player. An audiologist can say the words using a microphone and the monitored live voice technique. (You may remember from Chapter 6 that the use of recorded speech materials rather than the monitored live voice technique is strongly recommended for multiple reasons.)

Normal PI-PB Functions. Word recognition scores normally increase as the intensity level increases. That is, scores are lowest when a list of words is presented at an intensity level slighter higher than a patient's hearing threshold. Recall that hearing threshold may be defined by the patient's pure tone average (PTA) or speech reception threshold (SRT).

Let's say the first word list is delivered to the patient's right ear at an intensity level of 40 dB HL, and the patient repeats back correctly 23 of the 25 words in the list. The audiologist records the patient's percent correct score of 92% and then another list of words is presented at a higher-intensity level. This process may be followed at two or more different intensity levels until the audiologist has verified the patient's optimal or maximum (max) word recognition score. The score in percent (%) correct at each intensity level is usually plotted on a graph, as shown in Figure 9.2. Word recognition performance often improves steadily as the intensity of word lists is increased up to a high-intensity level. The line labeled "A" in Figure 9.2 shows a typical PI-PB function for a person with normal hearing.

Rollover of the PI-PB Function. In some patients, word recognition performance atypically and paradoxically worsens for the highest presentation levels. Jerger and Jerger coined the term **rollover** to describe the *decrease* in word recognition scores as intensity level *increases*.

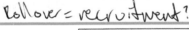

FIGURE 9.2

Performance-intensity (PI) functions for phonetically balanced (PB) words. The PI-PB function is a graph of word recognition performance, a score described as the percentage of correct responses for a word list, at different intensity levels. Decreased performance at the highest intensity level, quantified as the rollover index, is indicated for three separate PI-PB functions. The different PI-PB functions are described in the text.

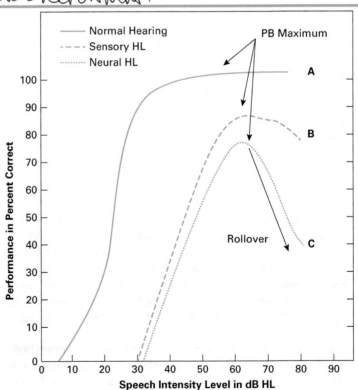

The concept of rollover in word recognition performance is also illustrated in Figure 9.2. PI-PB functions for two patients with sensorineural hearing loss are shown in Figure 9.2. One patient, represented by line "B," with a sensory hearing loss due to cochlear auditory dysfunction, shows a modest amount of rollover. Rollover is noticeably greater for a third patient (line "C") with a retrocochlear disorder. A retrocochlear disorder is a neural hearing loss often due to a tumor affecting the auditory portion of the eighth cranial nerve. You'll learn more about neural diseases and pathologies in Chapter 12.

Rollover Index. How much rollover is considered abnormal? Audiologists sometimes define significant rollover as a decrease in word recognition scores of 20% or greater from the maximum score to the score at the highest-intensity level. Rollover can also be quantified by a value called the *rollover index* that is calculated by the size of the decrease in performance in comparison to the maximum score.

The rollover index (RI) is defined by the expression:

$$RI = \frac{(PBmax - PBmin)}{PBmax}$$

when PB = phonetically balanced, max = maximum score, and min = minimum score at an intensity level above the maximum score.

PI-PB functions are rightfully considered in a discussion of special speech audiometry because the amount of rollover contributes to the differentiation or diagnosis of different types of auditory dysfunction. The diagnostic value of rollover was illustrated with the examples of patients in Figure 9.2. Persons with normal auditory function show little or no rollover. A modest degree of rollover is expected in persons with sensory hearing impairment due to cochlear auditory dysfunction. In contrast, excessive rollover is a characteristic feature of retrocochlear abnormality.

Let's take a moment to calculate the rollover index (RI) for each of the examples in Figure 9.2 using the equation above. The rollover index for patient A = (100 − 100)/100, or 0/100, or 0. For patient B, RI = (85 − 80)/85 = 5/85 = 0.06. And, for patient C the RI = (75 − 40)/75 = 35/75 = 0.47. Research data show that an RI of 0.45 separates patients with cochlear from patients with retrocochlear auditory dysfunction. That is, patients with cochlear hearing loss have an RI of less than 0.45 whereas patients with confirmed auditory nerve pathology have an RI of 0.45 or more (Dirks et al., 1977; Jerger & Jerger, 1971). Thus, PI-PB findings are consistent with cochlear hearing loss for patient B and retrocochlear hearing loss for patient C.

Explanation for PI-PB Rollover. You might be curious to know why findings for PI-PB function tests are normal in persons without auditory dysfunction and abnormal in most patients with dysfunction affecting the auditory cranial nerve or auditory regions of the brain stem. It is always reasonable to ask "what" and "why" questions about auditory tests. That is, *what* are the mechanisms or functional explanations for auditory test abnormalities? *Why* are test results normal in some patients and abnormal in others?

Unfortunately, "what" and "why" questions were not regularly asked and perhaps couldn't be answered in the 1950s and 1960s when most special speech audiometry tests were first developed. As you learned in reading Chapter 3, our understanding of the structure and function of the auditory system has increased considerably within the past twenty years. Most remarkable is the dramatic increase of information about how the brain processes sound. As a result, answers are now available to many longstanding questions about auditory function and dysfunction.

The explanation for rollover in patients with neural auditory dysfunction is related at least partly to how sound intensity is coded in the auditory system. Recall again the material on the anatomy and physiology of the auditory and vestibular systems covered in Chapter 3. Briefly, increased acoustic stimulus intensity level is coded or represented in the auditory nervous system by increased firing rate of neurons and probably also by the number of neurons activated.

One group of neurons is primarily responsive to increases in stimulus intensity at lower or softer levels. At progressively higher stimulus intensity levels another group of neurons is activated and fires more rapidly as stimulus intensity level increases. Presumably, poorer word recognition at high stimulus intensity levels is associated with the inability of abnormally functioning neurons to respond or fire at a high rate.

Also, performance on PB word tests is to a large extent dependent on accurate perception of high-frequency consonant sounds. If retrocochlear auditory pathology is due to a tumor pressing on the auditory nerve, dysfunction is most pronounced for fibers toward the outer portion of the nerve. You'll recall from Chapter 3 that nerve fibers from the low-frequency or apical portion of the cochlea are located toward the center of the auditory nerve, whereas high-frequency fibers are toward the outer portion. Organization of frequency information is maintained in the auditory system from the cochlea through the auditory nerve to the central nervous system.

Clinical Use of PI-PB Functions. Surveys of audiologists suggest that measurement of performance-intensity functions for PB words is applied more than other special speech audiometry procedures (Martin, Champlin, & Chambers, 1998). Can we assume that the test is evidence based? The answer to this question is "yes." The initial article by Jerger and Jerger (1971) reported that all study patients with confirmed eighth cranial nerve disorders and one-half of the patients with brain stem auditory disorders showed abnormal rollover on PI-PB functions. In contrast, most patients with cochlear disorder showed little or no rollover.

Within the next decade, over a dozen papers published in the peer-reviewed literature confirmed the diagnostic value of the PI-PB function test in differentiating persons with normal hearing from those with sensory or cochlear hearing loss and from those with neural auditory dysfunction (Hall, 1983, 1991).

Although it deserves a place in the diagnostic audiology test battery, the PI-PB function test, like other auditory procedures, is not perfect. Not all patients with neural auditory dysfunction show marked rollover at high-intensity levels. Also, even though the rollover index would seem to be a reliable measure of word recognition at different intensity levels, it is influenced by a variety of factors, including the specific words used to assess word recognition, the patient's age, the degree of hearing loss, and the highest intensity level included in the PI function. For a patient with an auditory nerve tumor, rollover is also influenced by the type, size, and specific location of the tumor.

Distorted Speech Tests

As you've already learned, **distorted speech tests** like the filtered word test were among the very first diagnostic speech audiometry procedures. Measurement of "auditory performance with degraded acoustic signals" (ASHA, 2005) remains important in audiology today. Distortion speech tests fall into the larger category of procedures referred to as "tests of monaural low-redundancy speech perception" (AAA, 2010).

The phrase refers to tests in which some kind of speech material like a list of words is presented to one ear after removal or reduction of some of the information typically in the speech. Redundancy of information in speech can be lowered in different ways, including filtering out some frequencies, compressing the timing of the speech, or presenting speech in the presence of background noise or additional speech.

All of us at times struggle to understand distorted or low-redundancy speech. A common example is listening to a cell phone conversation when the signal is poor or when the talker's voice is breaking up. A conversation under such conditions requires considerable effort and concentration, and the experience is frustrating. Still, by putting together bits and pieces of the speech signal we're usually able to recognize the message and to understand what is being said. Most speech is redundant. Speech contains more information than is absolutely necessary for correct recognition. The normal human brain is capable of effectively utilizing whatever portions of the speech signal are available and then essentially filling in the gaps of missing information.

Demands on the auditory pathways and centers of the brain are similarly increased when information in speech is artificially removed by filtering out selected frequencies or when the information in speech is compressed into a briefer time period. Patients with auditory dysfunction are more likely to have difficulty accurately recognizing speech signals like words or sentences when redundancy is reduced. The difficulty is reflected in abnormally low scores on distorted speech tests.

Many procedures are included in the category of distorted or low-redundancy speech tests. Distortion speech tests can be further subdivided based on how the speech is distorted or modified. With one group of distorted speech tests, single-syllable words are modified by removal of frequency information while the duration characteristics of the words remain unchanged. Another group consists of words that are altered by compressing or shortening the duration or by removal of brief segments of the words. In either case, the goal in modifying or degrading the speech is to reduce the amount of information available to the patient.

Monaural Frequency Distorted Speech Tests. As stated earlier, removal of selected frequencies from words was among the earliest approaches to reducing redundancy in speech. This technique is used to make a *frequency distorted speech test*. Usually these tests are administered to one ear at a time so they are called **monaural frequency distorted speech tests**. Not long after the studies by the Italian physicians in the 1950s (Bocca et al., 1954), other hearing researchers confirmed the diagnostic value of filtered speech tests in detecting and describing auditory dysfunction in persons with confirmed pathology in the hearing region of the temporal lobe of the brain (e.g., Jerger, 1960a; Lynn & Gilroy, 1972).

Low-pass filtering in distorted speech tests removes the high frequencies and preserves or passes low frequencies of speech. Figure 9.3 shows a count-the-dots audiogram form illustrating removal of high-frequency speech information with low-pass filtering at two different cutoff frequencies. You learned about the count-the-dots audiogram form in the discussion of speech audiometry in Chapter 6. There are 100 dots on the form. Each dot represents 1% of the information in speech across the audiogram frequency region. Greater concentrations of dots reflect a frequency region that is more important for speech audibility, whereas fewer dots reflect less importance for speech audibility.

In examining Figure 9.3, you'll notice that filtering out high frequencies reduces audibility for multiple speech sounds, especially consonant sounds that are important for recognizing words. Filtering of frequencies only above 1700 Hz preserves reasonably good word recognition since some consonant energy remains. In contrast, filtering out frequencies above 1000 Hz progressively reduces frequency information available for word recognition as much of the consonant energy is removed. For a person with normal hearing, words are perceived as muffled and unclear when much of the consonant energy is removed.

Binaural Frequency Distorted Speech Tests. Up to this point, we've talked about monaural filtered speech tests. That is, tests consisting of filtered words presented to one ear at a time. Also within the category of distorted speech procedures are binaural versions of filtered

FIGURE 9.3

The filtered speech technique is illustrated with count-the-dots audiogram form showing removal of high-frequency speech sound energy for cut-off frequencies of 1000 Hz and 1700 Hz. The effect of filtering on word recognition scores can be estimated by counting the dots in the audiogram for frequencies below the cut-off frequency.

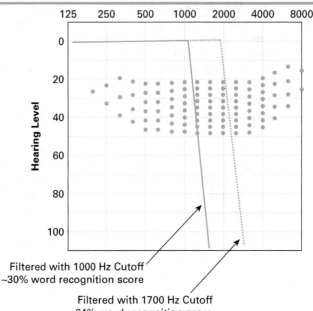

Filtered with 1000 Hz Cutoff
~30% word recognition score

Filtered with 1700 Hz Cutoff
~64% word recognition score

word tests. The category includes *binaural fusion tests*. In binaural fusion tests, a word with certain frequencies filtered out is presented to one ear and the same word with other frequencies filtered out is presented to the other ear. Because critical frequency information is removed by filtering, neither word would be recognized when presented to one ear alone. However, in the binaural test mode the auditory regions of the brain fuse incomplete speech frequency information in the word presented to one ear with incomplete speech frequency information in the word presented to the other ear.

For normal-hearing persons the synthesis of information from both ears results in accurate word recognition. In contrast, some patients with auditory dysfunction of the central nervous system experience difficulty performing binaural fusion tests. Abnormal test scores are most often recorded for patients with auditory abnormalities of the brain stem, where information arriving simultaneously from both ears is processed. Binaural fusion tests for two-syllable spondee words are available for clinical use.

Temporal Distortion Speech Tests. Various approaches are used to modify or degrade the temporal or timing characteristics of speech in diagnostic tests. As already noted, the overall goal of all distorted speech procedures is to reduce the redundancy of speech by removing information. Developers of early tests either recorded a speaker who talked faster than normal or played back to the patient at a very fast rate speech that was recorded at a normal rate.

In creating any distorted speech test, it is important to modify only one characteristic of speech. In the frequency distorted tests just described, temporal information like the duration of speech sounds and the gaps between speech sounds remained intact. Only the frequency characteristic of speech was altered. Creating temporal distortion tests is challenging. Simply speeding up a recording of speech produces considerable frequency distortion. If you've ever listened to music of the recording group The Chipmunks and their popular holiday records, you know exactly what rapid speech sounds like. Special instrumentation is used to electronically modify and compress the timing of speech without altering frequency characteristics. Properly recorded time-compressed speech tests do not have frequency distortion.

Time-compressed speech materials have been available to audiologists since the 1970s (e.g., Beasley, Schwimmer, & Rintelmann, 1972). Different versions of the tests are now available in digital format. The most common tests consist of lists of words that are compressed in time by 30%, 40%, or 60%. With 60% compression, the duration of the words in the test is less than half the normal duration. Evidence from many studies over the course of thirty years confirms the diagnostic value of time-compressed speech in detection of auditory dysfunction, especially at the level of the auditory cortex (Hall, 1983; Hall & Mueller, 1997; Konkle & Rintelmann, 1983).

Characteristics of Distorted Speech Tests. The various distorted speech tests just reviewed share at least four clinical disadvantages as diagnostic procedures. First, scores vary widely for normal subjects. For some of the filtered speech tests using single-syllable words, the range of normal performance extends from below 50% all the way up to 100%. The wide range of normal performance limits the sensitivity of the tests in detection of abnormal auditory dysfunction. Second, performance on monosyllabic word tests may be affected by dysfunction involving different regions of the auditory system. For example, abnormal findings on disordered speech tests can be recorded in persons with sensory hearing loss due to cochlear dysfunction, neural hearing loss due to auditory nerve dysfunction, or dysfunction of the central auditory nervous pathways.

Third, there is considerable variation in design among different distorted speech tests. For example, filtered word tests differ according to the specific words that are included in the lists and in exactly how the certain frequencies are filtered out of the words. More than fifty years after initial development of test materials, there remains little consistency or standardization of distorted speech tests. Finally, evidence on test reliability and test validity from formal clinical investigations is lacking.

Despite these limitations, distorted speech tests are sometimes included in test batteries for the evaluation of specific types of auditory dysfunction. Distorted speech tests can contribute to the description of auditory skills and accurate diagnosis of auditory dysfunction. We'll return to distorted speech tests later in this chapter in a review of the assessment of **auditory processing disorders** (APD). Auditory processing disorders are difficulties some patients experience in processing auditory information even when the audiogram is normal. Given the limitations just cited, audiologists do not rely only on distorted speech tests in the diagnosis of auditory dysfunction.

Tests of Speech Perception in Noise

Speech-in-Noise Tests. Many **speech-in-noise tests** are now available to assess speech recognition with some type of background sound or acoustic competition. Tests involving speech perception in noise evaluate "auditory performance in the presence of competing acoustic signals" (ASHA, 2005).

It makes sense to include tests of speech perception in background noise in diagnostic auditory assessment because problems recognizing and understanding speech in noisy listening conditions are common complaints of persons with hearing loss. Background sound reduces redundancy of speech.

Clinical experience also confirms that speech-in-noise tests are useful in detecting auditory dysfunction associated with brain disorders (Hall, 1983). Despite these arguments for inclusion of speech-in-noise procedures in the diagnostic test battery, the majority of audiologists do not routinely use them. Instead, audiologists continue to rely almost entirely on the assessment of word recognition in a quiet condition (Martin, Champlin, & Chambers, 1998; Wilson, McArdle, & Smith, 2007).

Features of Speech-in-Noise Tests. All speech-in-noise tests have three distinct features: (1) the type of speech used in the test, (2) the type of sound or noise in the background during the test, and (3) the intensity difference or ratio between the speech signal and the other sound, commonly called the **signal-to-noise ratio (SNR)**.

We'll now consider briefly each of these three features of speech-in-noise tests. The type of speech signal used in the test is most often either single-syllable words or sentences.

The second feature, the type of background sound, requires a little explanation. Some speech-in-noise tests were aptly named because the background sound was actually noise. Typical types of noise include broadband noise or noise filtered to resemble the spectrum of frequencies found in speech. However, the phrase "speech-in-noise test" is not always accurate because the background sound may also consist of speech. There are also different types of background speech sound such as unintelligible multi-talker speech versus babble like *cafeteria noise* versus *cocktail party noise*. Multi-talker babble is unintelligible background sound consisting of more than one person talking at the same time, whereas cafeteria noise is an unintelligible mixture of many talkers plus environmental noise. Cocktail party noise consists of multiple speakers. With considerable effort it's possible to occasionally understand some of the words spoken.

Background sound may also consist of real everyday sentences or an ongoing meaningful story. The term **competing message** is sometimes used to describe speech that is intelligible and meaningful and that competes with the speech signal for the listener's attention. The difficulty of speech-in-noise tests and the specific auditory functions or processes assessed vary considerably depending on the nature of the background sound.

The final feature, the *signal-to-noise ratio (SNR),* is an important factor in the difficulty of the test and affects its sensitivity to auditory dysfunction. For all diagnostic speech audiometry procedures, the term *signal* refers to the speech that a patient is instructed to listen to. Any other sound that the patient hears during the test can be considered noise. Difficulty of a speech-in-noise test is inversely related to the SNR. In other words, the bigger the difference in the intensity level between the speech signal and the background noise, the easier the task. An SNR is increased if the intensity level of the speech is increased or if the noise level is decreased, or both.

Recognition of speech is relatively easy with large signal-to-noise ratios such as +10 or +12 dB, even for some persons with hearing problems. In contrast, speech recognition with an SNR of 0 dB, with no difference between the intensity of the speech and background sound, or a negative SNR such as −5 dB, is very challenging even for normal hearers.

Patient Factors Affecting Speech-in-Noise Tests. In addition to the three test factors just noted, that is, type of speech material, the type of background sound, and the SNR, a variety of patient or listener factors affect performance on speech-in-noise tests. These factors include

- Age
- Cognitive factors like attention
- Degree of hearing loss affecting audibility of the signal
- Auditory processing abilities
- Whether the patient is a native speaker of the test language

Noisy Listening Settings Are Common. Learning more about the magnitude of noise levels in common communication settings like restaurants might help you better appreciate the relation between SNR and listening difficulty. The average level for conversational speech is 65 dB SPL. This is equivalent to the level of your speech during a conversation with a friend in a quiet place. Formal studies show that sound levels in restaurants typically range from 59 to 80 dBA, with an average of 71 dBA (Lebo et al., 1994). On the average, then, the difference between the level of speech and the levels of background noise in restaurants ranges from +6 dB (65 dB – 59 dB) to –15 dB (65 dB – 80 dB).

Let's briefly consider the relations between speech perception performance and the level background noise in a noisy setting. A 6-dB difference between the intensity of speech and background sound (a signal-to-noise ratio of 6 dB) is generally needed for a normal-hearing person to understand speech. A hearing-impaired person requires for speech understanding a more favorable ratio of +12 dB between the level of speech and background noise (Wilson, McArdle, & Smith, 2007).

These calculations confirm the negative impact of background noise on communication. Background noise in some restaurants makes conversation very difficult for normal-hearing persons and impossible for persons with hearing impairment (Lebo et al., 1994). One objective in performing diagnostic speech audiometry as part of hearing assessment is to identify persons who are likely to experience serious communication problems in noisy listening settings like restaurants.

 ClinicalConnection

Persons seeking help from an audiologist often describe difficulty hearing in background noise. One of the most common complaints among this patient population is: "I can hear people talking, but I can't understand what they are saying." When prompted to further explain this complaint, a patient often offers a statement like: "I can hear okay if I'm in a quiet place close to the speaker. I can hear you just fine in this quiet room, but I can't understand a thing in a noisy place like a busy restaurant."

Word Tests. Multiple tests are available to audiologists for assessing recognition of single-syllable words in the presence of some type of background sound. Many of the word lists used on speech-in-noise tests were developed years ago for word recognition (as reviewed in Chapter 6). The words are simply presented with multi-talker babble or cafeteria noise, rather than in quiet.

Speech-in-noise tests are sometimes pre-recorded at a specific SNR such as +6 dB. It is also possible to purchase digital versions of the tests that allow an audiologist to manipulate the SNR by changing intensity level of the words and the background sound. For example, words in speech-in-noise tests might be first presented at an intensity level of 50 dB HL while multi-talker babble or cafeteria noise is presented in the same ear at 45 dB HL for an SNR of +5 dB. Then, another list of words could be presented at the same level of 50 dB HL with the multi-talker babble or cafeteria noise also at 50 dB HL, producing an SNR of 0 dB.

Two other speech-in-noise tests involving single-syllable words deserve mention. Each was developed within the past fifteen years. The *Speech Recognition in Noise Test,* abbreviated *SPRINT* (Cord, Walden, & Atack, 1992; Wilson & Cates, 2008), is a test of word recognition in noise developed by the U.S. Army for evaluation of communication abilities in military personnel at risk for hearing impairment and determination of the serviceman's or servicewoman's fitness for duty. As you can imagine, the ability to communicate in background sound is a critical skill for military personnel, especially in combat settings. The SPRINT consists of a specific collection of single syllable words presented to both ears at the same time at an intensity level of 50 dB HL and in multi-talker babble at a fixed SNR of +9 dB. The words are called NU-6 words. They are drawn from six lists of fifty words each that were developed at Northwestern University (NU) in the 1960s (Tillman & Carhart, 1966).)

The *Words-in-Noise (WIN) Test* takes a different approach to evaluating word recognition in the presence of background sound.

 ClinicalConnection

As noted in Chapter 1, hundreds of audiologists serve as officers in the U.S. Army, Navy, and Air Force, where their responsibilities include coordinating hearing conservation programs to protect hearing from the damaging effects of noise, assessing hearing abilities for fitness of military duty, and, in recent years, diagnosing auditory dysfunction following combat-related trauma.

Audiology researchers in the Veterans Administration Hospital System developed the WIN test (Wilson, 2003; Wilson, McArdle, & Smith, 2007). Like other tests of speech perception in noise, the WIN test consists of monosyllabic NU-6 words presented in multi-talker babble. However, rather than assessing performance at a fixed SNR, the WIN test is administered at seven different SNRs ranging in 4-dB increments from 0 dB to 24 dB. A score in percent correct is obtained at each SNR.

The WIN test illustrates a new direction in describing word recognition abilities in patients with hearing loss. The traditional testing approach, followed for over fifty years, relied on assessment of word recognition performance with a fixed intensity difference between the words and the background sound. That is, scores were reported in percent correct either in quiet or at only one signal-to-noise ratio, such as 9 dB or 6 dB. Scores for hearing-impaired subjects varied widely, often from a low of 40% to a high of 80%.

When a test like the WIN test is administered over a range of different SNRs, it is possible to estimate what signal-to-noise ratio an individual patient requires to yield word recognition performance in background sound equivalent to that of a normal-hearing subject. You'll soon learn that expressing performance as an SNR rather than as a score in percent correct is also a trend for speech-in-noise procedures utilizing sentences.

Sentence Tests. Over thirty years ago, James Jerger stated eloquently, "We are, at the moment, becalmed in a windless sea of monosyllables. We can sail further only on the fresh winds of imagination" (Jerger, 1980). Diagnostic speech audiometry tests utilizing sentences were first developed in the 1960s. However, audiologists until recently relied mostly on single-syllable word tests to evaluate speech perception. Now there is a trend in clinical audiology toward greater use of sentence tests in the assessment of hearing, perhaps because several sentence-based procedures designed specifically for better assessment of speech perception in background sound are now available.

Everyday conversational speech generally consists of sentences that are often heard in the presence of background sound. Also, during a conversation the listener has some idea what he or she might hear. Traditional monosyllabic word tests are not very realistic. That is, we don't in a typical conversation hear single-syllable words in a quiet setting. Also, word recognition with most tests is assessed using an open set format. You may recall from Chapter 6 the difference between closed and open set speech test materials. In an open set test, the patient has no advance notice about which items he or she is about to hear. The test items could be any words, perhaps including words not in the patient's vocabulary. Listeners can take advantage of a variety of auditory and nonauditory clues in perception of conversational speech.

In an attempt to overcome the limitations of single-syllable open set word tests administered in quiet, Jerger and his colleagues in the late 1960s developed a test known as *synthetic sentence identification with ipsilateral competing message,* abbreviated *SSI-ICM* (Jerger, Speaks, & Trammell, 1968: Speaks & Jerger, 1965). The SSI-ICM test was a departure from most other speech audiometry procedures available at that time. The test materials were sentences, not words. To minimize the influence of language abilities on test performance, the SSI-ICM consists of "synthetic" or nonsense sentences rather than grammatically correct sentences.

Sentences in the SSI test are each composed of seven real words, but not in a typical order with proper syntax. The words are selected from an accepted listing of the 1,000 most familiar words. Three examples of the synthetic sentences are: "Go change your car color is red," "Small boat with a picture has become," and "Battle cry and be better than ever." The sentences are printed out on a sheet of paper and numbered 1 through 10. The patient identifies the sentence heard by either pointing to it or by saying the number of the sentence.

The developers of the test recognized that listening to sentences in quiet would be a very easy task and not representative of typical conversation. Therefore, sentence identification is performed in the presence of a competing message in the same ear, referred to as an ipsilateral competing message or ICM. In the English language version of the SSI-ICM, the competing message is an ongoing story about Davy Crockett. In administering the SSI-ICM, the intensity difference between the sentences and the competing message is varied from one list of ten sentences to the next.

The SSI-ICM test offers at least four advantages for speech perception assessment. First, the patient gives a simple verbal response, such as identifying the number of a sentence, or a nonverbal response like pointing to the printed sentence. The simple response mode is an advantage for patients with speech or voice disorders and for nonverbal patients. Second, because the SSI-ICM includes a meaningful competing message, rather than simple background noise, the test may provide a more "real-world" measure of the patient's performance in a difficult listening setting. Third, clinical experience suggests that the SSI-ICM test can provide a useful and valid measure of auditory processing even in patients with significant high-frequency hearing loss. Finally, the SSI-ICM test has been adapted to non-English languages, such as Spanish, French, German, and Arabic.

The **Hearing in Noise Test (HINT)** was developed for assessment of speech perception in persons with normal hearing or peripheral hearing loss (Nillson, Soli, & Sullivan, 1994). The HINT requires a patient to repeat sentences that are presented in quiet or in the presence of background noise. Difficulty of the listening task during the HINT is increased or decreased with manipulation of the level of the background noise, and thus the SNR.

The sentences are presented at a consistent level of 65-dB SPL, a typical level for conversational speech. The background noise is called speech spectrum noise. It consists of frequencies represented in speech. An example of a HINT sentence is: "A/The girl ran along a/the fence." Either the word "a" or "the" would be scored as correct. The HINT is usually administered binaurally with the sentences coming from one loudspeaker in front of the patient and noise delivered via multiple additional loudspeakers. Notably, there are versions of the HINT for more than a dozen non-English languages (Soli, 2008).

Among the new generation of special speech audiometry procedures are two versions of another sentence-type speech-in-noise test called the *Speech in Noise (SIN) Test* and a shortened version called the *QuickSIN test* (Killion, Niquette, Gudmundsen, Revit, & Banerjee, 2004). You have probably noticed that catchy acronyms for test procedures are very common in the field of audiology. Despite any alternative meaning the acronym might imply, the SIN test is a good test. The SIN test consists of a series of sentences delivered at 53 dB SPL and also at 83 dB SPL in the presence of multi-talker background speech noise consisting of one male and three female speakers. Examples of sentences are: "Rice is often served in round bowls," and "The juice of lemons makes fine punch."

Performance on the SIN test is evaluated for five or ten sentences presented at four signal-to-noise ratios: +15, +10, +5, and 0 dB. SNRs are fixed on a digital recording of the test. Within each sentence are five key words. The audiologist scores the sentences by tallying up how many of key words the patient repeats correctly. As with the HINT, scores on the SIN and QuickSIN tests are reported as the SNR required for the patient to hear in background noise. This is sometimes known as the "SNR loss."

Up to this point we've discussed tests in which the main variable is the difference in intensity level between speech and noise. However, the ability to hear in background noise is determined not only by the level of the noise, but also by differences in the sources or locations of the speech signal and the background noise. For example, you've no doubt experienced how much easier it is to follow a conversation in a crowded room when the speaker is in front of you rather than off to one side. Information utilized by a listener about the location of the signal or the speaker and the source of the background noise is referred as a *spatial cue*. Recognizing where the signal is coming from in space helps to reduce the negative impact of background noise and enhances effective communication.

Appreciating the impact of spatial cues on the ability to hear in noise, an Australian research group developed a clever clinical measure of this ability called the *Listening in Spatialized Noise with Sentences (LISN-S) Test* (Cameron & Dillon, 2007; Cameron, Dillon, & Newall, 2006). The LISN-S test is conducted with earphones using software that creates "a three-dimensional auditory environment" (Cameron & Dillon, 2007, p. 380). The LISN-S evaluates perception of target sentences with background speech coming from directly in front of the listener, from the right side, and from the left side. Unlike other speech perception tests, the LISN-S test also assesses speech recognition performance in background speech when the vocal quality of the speaker is the same as the background speech and when it is different from the background speech.

Listening is easiest and listener scores highest for conditions that distinguish the target sentences from the background speech. The biggest listening advantage occurs when (1) there is a difference between the locations of the sentences and the background speech, and (2) when two different speakers' voices are used, one for the sentences and one for background speech, providing a vocal quality cue. The LISN-S is the first clinical test available for assessment of the use of spatial and vocal cues while listening in the presence of background noise. The LISN-S test is now available for clinical assessment of rather complex speech recognition skills in children and adults.

Dichotic Listening Tests

You have already learned that dichotic listening tests were first developed over sixty years ago. Dichotic procedures are still a valuable and clinically popular tool for identification and description of auditory function in persons at risk for auditory dysfunction involving the central nervous system, especially persons with normal hearing sensitivity. There are hundreds of published papers describing findings for a variety of different dichotic listening tests, as well as numerous book chapters and even several books on the topic (e.g., Hall, 1983; Baran & Musiek, 1999; Chermak & Musiek, 1997; Hugdahl, 1988; Keith & Anderson, 2007).

We will now review the dichotic listening task and the hearing processes involved in dichotic listening. Then you will be introduced to some of the dichotic speech procedures commonly applied in clinical audiology.

Pathways in Dichotic Listening. The key feature of the dichotic listening task is simultaneous presentation of two different items separately, one to each ear. Examples of dichotic procedures and how patients respond during testing will help to clarify the concept of dichotic tests. Dichotic tests are conducted with one earphone on each ear. One word might be presented to the right ear at the same time another word is presented to the left ear. Or, two numbers (digits) might be presented to one ear at the same time two different numbers are presented to the other ear. Items are presented to both ears at the same intensity level. Dichotic testing creates a challenging auditory task. To accurately perform the task, the auditory regions of the listener's brain must quickly and efficiently process different information simultaneously arriving in each ear.

The dichotic listening mode puts great demands on the auditory system. In usual everyday listening the same information is heard with both ears. For example, a word like "hello" is heard in each ear and the information travels up through the central nervous system via pathways on the right and the left side. In contrast, in the dichotic listening condition information that enters each ear travels up the auditory nerve and then the information takes pathways that cross over to the other side of the brain.

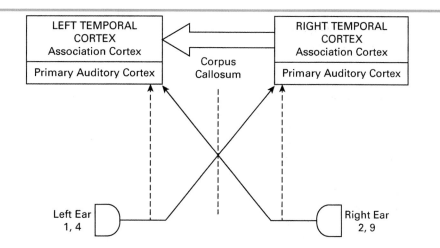

F I G U R E   9 . 4

Dichotic listening paradigm with digit pairs (two sets of numbers) presented to each ear. Suppression of ipsilateral pathways is indicated with dashed lines, whereas solid lines show the dominance of contralateral pathways.

Figure 9.4 shows the general pathways and centers involved in dichotic listening tests. In humans, pathways that lead from one ear to the central auditory system on the opposite side are dominant and more plentiful than pathways carrying information from the ear to higher structures on the same side. Pathways that cross over from one side to the other are called **contralateral pathways**, whereas those that remain on one side are called **ipsilateral pathways**. Under typical binaural listening conditions information can travel from the ears to the auditory cortex via ipsilateral pathways (shown as dashed lines in Figure 9.4) or contralateral pathways (shown as solid lines in Figure 9.4).

In the dichotic listening condition, information from each ear reaches the auditory cortex only via the contralateral or crossing pathways. Activity is suppressed in ipsilateral pathways during dichotic listening. Returning to Figure 9.4, you'll notice that crossing pathways in the lower part of the brain stem are indicated with solid lines. So, the contralateral pathways carry auditory information from the right ear to the left side of the brain while information from the left ear crosses over to right side of the brain. Pathways of the central auditory nervous system were reviewed in Chapter 3. We'll now review in a little more detail the steps in the journey of auditory information from the cochlea to the cortex during a dichotic listening test.

Let's look at the route of auditory information from each inner ear to the cortex during a dichotic listening test in which the listener hears two numbers in each ear. As shown in Figure 9.4, right ear information has a relatively direct route along major pathways leading to the left primary auditory cortex in the temporal lobe, and then associated auditory cortical regions also on the left side. For almost everyone, including most left-handed people, the left hemisphere is dominant for speech and language. In other words, the left cerebral hemisphere rather than the right hemisphere specializes in processing verbal information.

As a result, in a dichotic listening test the words or numbers presented to the right ear enjoy a clear advantage as they travel along dominant auditory pathways to the cerebral hemisphere dominant for language processing. The numbers 2 and 9 enclosed in the box representing the left hemisphere indicate prompt processing of information that arrives from the right ear.

Information presented to the left ear takes a less direct and more complicated journey to the left hemisphere. Speech information from the left ear reaches the auditory cortex in the right temporal lobe by traveling along the prominent contralateral pathways. However, since the right cerebral hemisphere does not specialize in processing verbal information, the neural representation of the speech signals must leave the right cerebral hemisphere and pass within the *corpus callosum* to the left hemisphere. You learned in Chapter 3 that the corpus callosum consists of multiple thick bands of nerve fibers connecting and permitting communication between the two hemispheres. Information from the left ear is processed only after it reaches the left hemisphere via the corpus callosum.

Principles of Dichotic Listening Tests. There are seven principles underlying dichotic listening tests: (1) Test materials must be presented to each ear simultaneously or with a time difference of only several milliseconds; (2) test materials presented to each ear must be different, but within the same category (examples of categories are consonant-vowel syllables, one-syllable words, digits, two-syllable words, and sentences); (3) test materials must be presented to each ear at the same intensity level; (4) hearing thresholds must be symmetrical or very similar for both ears; (5) persons with normal auditory function typically show higher scores for the right ear than the left ear, a phenomenon known as the **right ear advantage (REA)**; (6) there is a clear effect of maturation on dichotic test performance up to the age of approximately 12 years (the right ear advantage or left ear deficit is more pronounced for younger children, and with maturation score differences are less pronounced); and (7) a listener repeats or in some other way identifies what is heard in each ear.

Response Modes in Dichotic Listening Tests. During a dichotic listening test, the listener's task is to repeat back or to identify in another way the CV syllables, words, or sentences heard in each ear. Scores on dichotic tests, however, vary depending on the instructions given to the listener. In the most common dichotic test response mode, known as *free recall* or *divided attention,* the listener is simply told to repeat back what is heard in each ear. The term **binaural integration** is used to describe this listening task, as the listener is required to combine or integrate information from each ear.

A variation of this approach, called *divided attention with pre-cued direction,* requires the listener to repeat what is heard in both ears, but to first say what was heard in either the right or the left ear. Typical instructions are "repeat back both words but say the word you hear in your left ear first." Scores on dichotic tests usually increase for the ear that the listener to focuses on first. The typical right ear advantage may actually disappear when the listener is given this pre-cued instruction for the left ear.

Another dichotic test response mode, called *directed attention,* requires the patient to focus on information in one ear, the pre-cued ear, while ignoring information in the other ear. The term for this task is **binaural separation**. There is no question that the results for dichotic listening tests and the difficulty of dichotic tests are influenced by the listener instructions.

Consonant-Vowel Dichotic Tests. Studies of dichotic listening tests utilizing consonant-vowel (CV) syllables such as /ba/ and /da/ date back over forty years (Berlin, Lowe-Bell, Jannetta, & Kline, 1972; Hugdahl, 1988). Nonetheless, dichotic tests with CV syllables are rarely applied in clinical audiology. Two factors probably contribute to the infrequent clinical application of CV dichotic tests.

First, peripheral hearing loss influences performance on CV tests more than for other dichotic procedures. Commonly encountered high-frequency hearing loss interferes with the perception of high-frequency consonant sounds required for recognition of CV syllables. Also, the precise intensity level of words presented to each ear seems to be more critical for CV test materials than for other types of dichotic tests. In other words, it's hard to determine whether deficits on dichotic tasks with CV words are due to ear problems causing hearing loss or auditory dysfunction within the brain.

Staggered Spondaic Word (SSW) Test. The staggered spondaic word (SSW) test is one of the oldest clinical dichotic listening tests, and it is still used in clinical audiology today

(Katz, 1962). It was developed by Jack Katz, shown earlier in Figure 9.1A. As the name implies, the SSW test consists of two-syllable spondee words presented separately to the right and left ear in the dichotic mode. Each syllable is a word itself. The name of the test also indicates that the two words are not presented to each ear at exactly the same time but, rather, presentation time between ears is delayed slightly or staggered.

Let's briefly go through the SSW test sequence for these two words in chronological order. You may wish to refer back to Figure 9.4, substituting spondee words *baseball* and *cowboy* for the numbers 2, 9 and 1, 4 shown for the right and left ear in the figure. The word *base* is heard in the first ear. Then, the rest of the word (*ball*) is heard in the same ear at the same time that the first part of word *cowboy* is presented to the second ear. The overlapping words are called the competing test condition. Finally, the last part of *cowboy* is presented to the second ear. The ear that receives the first word is called the leading ear, whereas the other ear receiving the second ear is the lagging ear. The listener's task is to repeat both words (*baseball* and *cowboy*) starting with the word presented to the leading ear.

The full SSW test includes forty sets of spondee words. Twenty words are presented with the first word leading to the right ear and the other twenty words are presented with the first word leading to the left ear. The listener's task is to repeat back both words after both have been presented. A separate percent correct score is kept for each of the four test conditions: (1) right leading and non-competing, (2) right competing, (3) left competing, and (4) left lagging and non-competing. There is also a screening version of the SSW test consisting of only twenty sets of words.

The longstanding popularity of the SSW test as a clinical procedure can probably be attributed to at least five factors. The spondee words are well known to clinical audiologists and are not seriously influenced by high-frequency hearing loss. Administration of the test is rather quick and easy, making the SSW test feasible even for children as young as kindergarten age. Normative reference data used in SSW analysis are available for a wide age range, from 5-year-old children to 70-year-old adults. Also, over the years many published papers have confirmed sensitivity of the SSW in detecting auditory disorders in various patient populations (Keith & Anderson, 2007). Finally, for over fifty years generations of students and practicing audiologists have been systematically instructed on SSW test administration and scoring.

Dichotic Digits Test. The dichotic digits test is applied in the assessment of children and adults. Here the term "digits" refers to numbers. Considerable research in patients with confirmed pathology of the central nervous system documents the clinical value of dichotic digits testing in diagnostic hearing assessment (Musiek, 1983; Musiek, Wilson & Pinheiro, 1979; Musiek & Chermak, 2007).

The test can be performed with one, two, or three digits presented to each ear. The digits include the numbers 1 through 10, excluding 7 because it has two syllables. Early studies with the test utilized three digits per ear (Kimura, 1961), but the triple-digit version is rather difficult even for persons with normal auditory function. The single-digit version of the test, on the other hand, is too easy for older children and adults. The two-digit or double pairs version of the test, consisting of two numbers presented to each ear, is typically used in the clinic to assess auditory processing.

During administration of the dichotic digits test, an audiologist usually instructs the listener to wait until all four numbers are presented and then to repeat back in any order each number that is heard. This is the free recall or divided attention response mode you learned about in the preceding general discussion of dichotic listening. Listeners may also be instructed to respond in other ways to digits presented in dichotic fashion.

The full version of the dichotic digits test consists of fifty sets of two numbers per ear or a total of 100 numbers. Upon completion of the test, the audiologist calculates the percent correct score separately for the right and left ears. Normal hearers yield a modest advantage in correct scores for the right ear, usually about 2 to 6%. Patients with central auditory nervous system dysfunction, including auditory processing disorders, often show marked deficits for the left ear on dichotic digits testing.

The dichotic digits test offers multiple advantages for clinical use. Numbers are highly familiar and often-used vocabulary words for native English speakers, even school-age children. The closed set test format enhances listener recognition of the materials and simplifies scoring for the tester. The dichotic digits test is described as a closed set response procedure because the same nine numbers are presented in random order throughout the test. Perception of digits is not seriously influenced by hearing loss. Administration of the dichotic digits test is quite time efficient.

Clinical investigations have confirmed the sensitivity of the dichotic digits test to disorders in the auditory brain stem and cerebral cortex (Musiek & Chermak, 2007). For these reasons, the dichotic digits test is recommended by current evidence-based clinical guidelines as a screening test and also as a diagnostic procedure for disorders of the central auditory nervous system (American Academy of Audiology, 2010).

> 🎧 **Clinical**Connection
>
> Special speech audiometry is an important tool for the assessment of children and adults who are referred to an audiologist for possible auditory processing disorders. Auditory processing disorders are hearing problems that involve the central nervous system, rather than only the ear. You'll learn more about them in Chapter 12.

The SCAN Test Battery

We'll conclude the discussion of special speech audiometry tests with review of a measure designed to screen for central auditory nervous system abnormalities. The *SCAN* is a brief test battery consisting of four separate subtests. Robert Keith (shown earlier in Figure 9.1B) developed the SCAN test battery (Keith, 1994). There are now several versions of the SCAN. The original SCAN consists of four speech procedures like those we've reviewed in this chapter: (1) the Filtered Words subtest, which is a distorted speech test with high frequencies removed; (2) the Auditory-Figure Ground subtest, which is a words-in-noise test with an SNR of +6 dB; (3) the Competing Words subtest, which is a dichotic test consisting of words; and (4) the Competing Sentences subtest, which is a dichotic sentence test.

There are two versions of the original SCAN test battery, one for younger children (SCAN-C) and another for children over age 11 and adults (SCAN-A). There is also a more recent and expanded edition of the SCAN test battery. The SCAN is used not only by audiologists but also by speech pathologists interested in identifying children who might have auditory problems related to language impairment (Lovett & Johnson, 2009).

Auditory Brain Stem Response (ABR)

We will now briefly review the discovery of the auditory brain stem response (ABR). Then you will learn about the anatomical generators of the ABR within the auditory system and how the response is recorded and analyzed. We will also discuss current applications of the ABR in children and adults, and also future directions in ABR technology. Our discussion will only scratch the surface of the topic. The ABR is thoroughly explained in thousands of published articles, dozens of book chapters, and textbooks devoted entirely to the topic. Readings with detailed information on the ABR and other auditory evoked responses are listed at the end of this chapter.

Discovery of Auditory Brain Stem Response

Discovery of the **auditory brain stem response (ABR)** in 1970 forever changed pediatric audiology. Don Jewett and several colleagues published classic papers describing how brain activity was consistently and noninvasively recorded in humans in response to sounds (Jewett,

Romano, & Williston, 1970; Jewett & Williston, 1971). The stimulus sounds were very brief or transient sounds like clicking sounds and short portions of tones. The responses were detected with tiny metal discs connected to wires that were attached to the scalp on the top of the head or on the forehead and also on the earlobes or the mastoid region.

The observation of brain activity evoked or elicited by sound was not new. As early as the 1930s, other investigators had demonstrated that it was possible to detect **auditory evoked responses** from cooperative and awake subjects (Davis, Davis, Loomis, Harvey, & Hobart, 1939; Weaver & Bray, 1930). However, some of these auditory evoked responses could not be consistently recorded in infants and young children who were active and moving about. They also could not be detected in children or other persons who were sleeping (Hall, 2007).

Jewett's discovery in the early 1970s was particularly noteworthy for at least four reasons. First, auditory brain stem response recordings were highly consistent and almost identical from one person to the next. Second, the response could be activated by sounds that were presented very rapidly, more than fifty times per second, so the ABR could be recorded quickly. Third, the ABR was clearly visible when elicited with different types of stimulation, including clicking sounds and short bursts of tones. Finally, sleep, sedation, or anesthesia had no effect on the ABR, so babies did not need to be awake during testing. Muscle activity associated with movement in babies who are awake generally interferes with the detection of tiny electrical brain responses evoked by auditory stimulation from the brain. Sedation anesthesia or natural sleep solves the problem of movement in babies undergoing ABR testing.

Early Clinical Applications of ABR

Pediatric Applications. A few years after the first report of ABR, Robert Galambos confirmed that the new response could be consistently recorded in infants and young children (Hecox & Galambos, 1974; Kileny & Seewald, 2011). Naturally, the description of ABR recording in humans immediately caught the attention of audiologists who had been seeking a technique for hearing screening and diagnostic assessment of infants and young children.

LEADERS AND LUMINARIES

Don Jewett

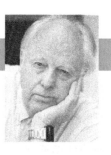

Don Jewett earned his Doctor of Philosophy degree from Oxford University in England. In the 1960s he completed a research position at Yale University under the direction of the well-known auditory physiologist Robert Galambos. The laboratory investigations focused on auditory responses from cats, mostly electrophysiological responses arising from high levels of central nervous system function. The two researchers inadvertently recorded some earlier activity at the brain stem level.

Within a few years, Dr. Jewett moved on to his first faculty appointment at the University of California in San Francisco, where he began to seriously study the early auditory responses in human subjects. The research led quickly to the discovery of the auditory brain stem response (ABR). Results were initially published in the prestigious journal *Science* and then fully described in a classic paper in the journal *Brain*. News of the discovery soon spread throughout the audiology and hearing science world. Dr. Jewett's discovery of the ABR truly revolutionized auditory assessment of young children and led directly to early identification and diagnosis of infant hearing loss. Dr. Jewett now conducts innovative research beyond the boundaries of hearing science. His latest grant is for the WebCompendia Project, which includes the ForwardLink-Protocol and the Hash-Algorithm Against Plagiarism.

FIGURE 9.5

Clinical device for recording auditory brainstem (ABR) response known as the Nicolet CA-1000 that contributed in the 1980s to the application of ABR in pediatric and adult populations. The abbreviation CA referred to "clinical averager."

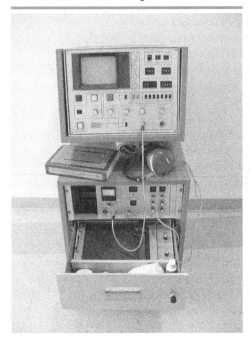

 ClinicalConnection

The ABR is a valuable tool for hearing assessment in children with a wide assortment of diseases and disorders affecting the auditory system, from the ear to the brain. In Chapters 11 and 12, you'll learn about many etiologies of childhood hearing impairment. ABR findings play a critical role in the management of children with hearing impairment. You will read about management strategies and approaches used with children in Chapters 13 through 16.

Galambos and his colleagues went on to publish a series of papers describing the feasibility of newborn hearing screening with ABR, even screening of infants born prematurely.

By the early 1980s audiologists at major medical centers were beginning to acquire instrumentation allowing them to record the auditory brain stem response for pediatric hearing assessment and to screen newborn infants for hearing loss. An early auditory brain stem response recording device manufactured during this era is shown in Figure 9.5. Audiologists tested pediatric and adult patients in the clinic with these devices and also rolled the bulky devices from the clinic to the nursery for infant hearing screenings or to hospital rooms to test children who could not be transported to the clinic. Before long the ABR was an indispensable part of the pediatric test battery.

Adult Applications. Availability of equipment for recording ABR in the clinic contributed to exploration of various uses for this new technique in adult populations as well as in children. In the late 1970s, investigators from around the world demonstrated that the new technique was valuable for assessment of patients with various serious neurological disorders (Starr & Achor, 1975; Stockard & Rossiter, 1977).

ABR measurement during the same period was also applied in the early detection of tumors affecting the auditory nerve (Selters & Brackmann, 1977; Thomsen, Terkildsen, & Osterhammel, 1978). Brain scanning techniques like computed tomography (CT) or magnetic resonance imaging (MRI) were not yet available. Clinical experience and research confirmed that the ABR was useful in identification of acoustic tumors prior to the development of serious neurological complications. In subsequent years, hundreds of papers confirming other clinical applications of the auditory brain stem response also appeared in the scientific literature (see Hall, 1992, 2007).

Anatomy and Physiology

The ABR reflects the activity of many auditory nerve fibers and of pathways within the auditory brain stem. You'll recall from our review of the anatomy and physiology of the auditory system in Chapter 3 that vibrations from sound are converted to electrical energy by the hair cells in the inner ear. The hair cells transmit the energy to auditory nerve fibers. Very brief sounds produce a time-locked synchronous response from many nerve fibers. The term *synchronous* here means that many hundreds of activated nerve fibers fire at precisely the same time.

The summed or combined electrical activity from a sizable group of nerve fibers firing together is picked up with detectors located as far away as the scalp on the forehead and near the ear. The detectors are called **electrodes** consisting of small metal pieces or sticky band-aid type pieces that attach to the skin and connect to the ABR system with wires. Figure 9.6 shows a patient set up for ABR recording with electrodes attached to the forehead and earlobes and insert earphones in place.

Electrical responses to sound in the auditory nerve fibers and in the brain stem must pass through brain tissue and the skull to reach the electrodes on the skin. Electrical responses to sound stimulation originate deep within the brain, so only an extremely small amount of ABR energy is detected by electrodes on the scalp.

Knowledge of the different auditory structures contributing to the ABR is very important for audiologists and other persons who use the technique to diagnose hearing loss. Information on generators of the ABR in the auditory system was gathered from a variety of different studies conducted over thirty years ago (Hall, 2007). The ABR consists of a series of peaks and valleys. Taken together, the peaks or waves are referred to as the ABR waveform. Each of the waves represents activity in one or more regions of the auditory system and is labeled with a Roman numeral. The major ABR waves are wave I, wave III, and wave V.

Generators of ABR Waves. Figure 9.7 depicts the auditory pathways contributing to these three main waves in the ABR. The first component in the ABR is called *wave I.* Wave I arises from activity in auditory nerve fibers, particularly fibers in the distal end of the auditory nerve near the cochlea. Of course, with air-conduction ABR measurement sound stimulation from the ear canal must first be transmitted through the middle ear to activate hair cells in the cochlea before a response is produced by the auditory nerve fibers.

The next major ABR component, *wave III,* is produced by activity in multiple pathways in the auditory system. As illustrated in Figure 9.7, generators of wave III are located in the pons portion of the brain stem. ABR wave III actually reflects combined activity from two or three pathways in the lower part of the brain stem.

Wave V is the final major ABR component and is the most prominent wave. It is generated in the rostral midbrain portion of the auditory brain stem. Figure 9.7 shows that the major source of wave V consists of fibers within the lateral lemniscus, the primary pathway carrying information upward through the auditory brain stem.

FIGURE 9.6

An adult prepared for auditory brainstem response (ABR) recording with insert earphones and electrodes in position. ABR measurement is described in the text.

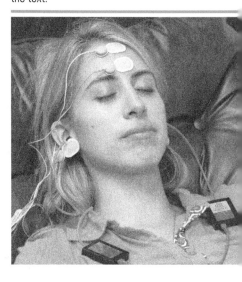

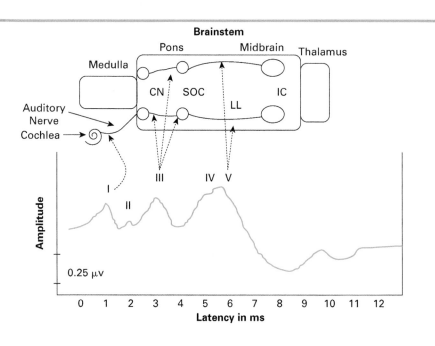

FIGURE 9.7

Anatomical generators of the auditory brainstem response (ABR). The relation between ABR components and auditory structures is described in the text.

Abbreviations are as follows:

CN = cochlear nucleus

SOC = superior olivary complex

LL = lateral lemniscus

IC = inferior colliculus

ABR Measurement

Stimulation. Figure 9.8 highlights the important steps in ABR measurement. Sounds are usually presented with insert earphones for ABR measurement in infants and young children. Stimuli used most commonly in clinical ABR measurement are either clicking sounds or very brief tones called **tone bursts**, presented at frequencies such as 500, 1000, 2000, and 4000 Hz. A tone burst consists of only four or five cycles of a pure tone sound, with a total duration of less than 10 ms.

A single ABR waveform is recorded when hundreds or even thousands of stimuli are presented very rapidly, at rates like 37 stimuli per second, at a single intensity level, such as 80 dB or 20 dB. When testing children, a series of ABR waveforms are usually recorded with stimulation presented at different high-level intensities. The goal is to record a clear ABR at intensity levels close to the patient's hearing threshold. Click and tone burst stimuli used to elicit the ABR are delivered with the types of transducers you learned about earlier in the book, including insert earphones, supra-aural earphones, and bone vibrators.

Detection. The actual auditory response produced by the stimuli is detected with electrodes located on the scalp and the ears as illustrated in Figure 9.8. The setup for recording an ABR was also shown earlier in Figure 9.6. The electrodes on the scalp detect only a tiny amount of electrical activity from the auditory regions of the brain. The amplitude of the brain activity is increased with an amplifier connected to the equipment. Non-response frequency information in the brain activity is filtered out. Then, the patient's brain activity, including the auditory response, is conveyed to a computer within the ABR system, as depicted in Figure 9.8.

As testing is conducted an ABR waveform appears on a computer screen as shown in the right side of Figure 9.8, assuming the test protocol is appropriate and the stimuli are effective in producing a response from the patient's auditory system. Using cursors on the computer keyboard, an audiologist marks different points on the ABR waveforms and performs calculations to analyze test results.

ABR Analysis and Interpretation

Latency Analysis. Two calculations made most often during ABR analysis are determination of the latency and amplitude of the waves. These terms will need to be explained. *Latency* of a wave is the time interval from the presentation of the stimulus to the occurrence of a

FIGURE 9.8   Diagram of major steps in measurement of the auditory brainstem response (ABR) including the types of stimuli, transducers used to present the stimuli, location of electrodes on the scalp and ears, subject factors influencing the ABR, and other components of an ABR system. An ABR waveform is shown on the right side of the figure.

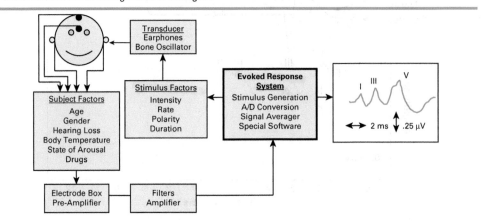

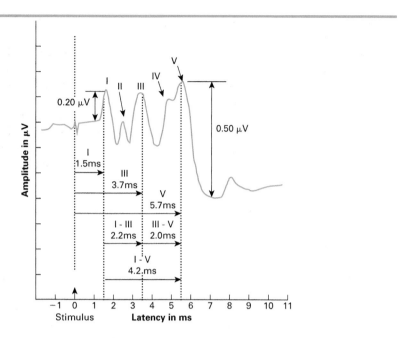

FIGURE 9.9

Calculations made in analysis of the auditory brain stem response, including latency and amplitude of wave I, wave III, wave V, and inter-wave latency values. An explanation of ABR analysis is provided in the text.

wave. Using a cursor or mouse, an audiologist marks the peaks for each of the ABR waves. The ABR system then determines the latencies for each of the waves in milliseconds (ms) and also the time differences in milliseconds between the waves.

Figure 9.9 shows latency calculations for a typical normal-appearing ABR waveform. Published normal data are available for the latencies of different ABR waves (Hall, 2007). An audiologist compares a patient's latency values to normal values to determine whether the response is normal or abnormal. Most forms of auditory dysfunction result in longer-than-normal ABR latency values.

Other patient factors must also be taken into account in the analysis of ABR latencies. For example, due to neurological immaturity, ABR latencies are longer for infants from birth to 18 months than they are for older children and adults. An audiologist accounts for maturational delays in latency before analyzing ABR findings in infants. Lower-than-normal body temperature also prolongs a patient's ABR latency values.

Amplitude Analysis. Wave *amplitude* is another calculation made in ABR analysis. Amplitude is depicted with vertical double-ended arrows in Figure 9.9. Amplitude is calculated as the size of the wave in microvolts (μv) from its peak to the valley that occurs before or after the peak. In marking ABR waves, an audiologist places one cursor on the peak and a second cursor in the valley. The computer software then calculates the size or amplitude of the wave and displays the value in microvolts.

Amplitude of ABR waves is remarkably small, even in normal-hearing persons. One microvolt (μv) is only one-millionth of one volt. The biggest ABR component is wave V but it is only 0.5 μv. Normal data are available for the amplitudes of each major ABR wave, allowing the audiologist to determine whether the response is normal or abnormally reduced in amplitude.

Objective Hearing Testing in Infants and Young Children
Early Identification and Diagnosis of Hearing Loss in Infants. Approximately 4 to 5 out of every 1000 children (about 0.4 to 0.5%) are born with some degree of hearing loss that may interfere with their speech and language development (JCIH, 2007). By school age

the proportion of children with hearing impairment increases to over 2%, or 20 per 1000 (Fortnum, Summerfield, Marshall, Davis, & Bamford, 2001).

The importance of detecting and defining hearing loss in early childhood was recognized in the earliest years of audiology. Now there is unquestionable and compelling evidence that early identification, diagnosis, and intervention of hearing loss in infants and young children is very important for development of the auditory regions of the brain and for adequate acquisition of speech and language skills (JCIH, 2007; Yoshinaga-Itano, Sedley, Coulter, & Mehl, 1998).

How is the word "early" defined? Research clearly confirms that early intervention means the initiation of appropriate management within the first six months after a child with hearing impairment is born. A newborn infant is surrounded and stimulated by sound immediately after birth. A normal-hearing child's exposure to and immersion in the speech and language of family members and others provides stimulation that is critical for development of the auditory regions of the brain. Early and adequate auditory stimulation is also essential for acquisition of verbal communication, particularly speech and language development.

Unfortunately, before the 1970s there were limited options for testing hearing in children under the age of 2 to 3 years. Behavioral audiometric techniques like pure tone testing successfully identified hearing loss in older preschool and school-age children. Pure tone and word recognition testing also permitted diagnosis of hearing loss for those children who did not pass the screening procedure. However, accurate and widespread hearing screening of infants and children under the age of 2 to 3 years is not possible using behavioral test techniques, even when performed by experts in pediatric audiology. Newborn infants with immature neurological status do not respond consistently and reliably to sounds that they actually can hear.

Diagnostic behavioral hearing testing of infants and young children is not accurate. Based on false test results, children who actually have normal hearing may be suspected of hearing loss. An even more serious error occurs when inaccurate test results suggest normal hearing in a child who really has a hearing loss that will affect speech and language acquisition.

Older children with developmental delays and emotional problems may also be difficult or impossible to test using behavioral tests. So, before the 1970s audiologists were faced with a major dilemma. There was a demand to identify, diagnose, and manage hearing loss in young children in order to maximize speech and language development. However, no accurate or clinically feasible technique was available.

Estimating Auditory Thresholds with ABR. For approximately forty years, ABR has played a vital role in the early detection and diagnosis of hearing loss in infants and young children (Hecox & Galambos, 1974). Now evidence-based test protocols permit accurate estimation of hearing thresholds for different audiometric test frequencies, even in infants within days after birth (Hall, 2007; Hall & Swanepoel, 2010). Audiologists have access to equipment specifically designed for recording the ABR of infants and young children in different settings, such as an audiology clinic or even a newborn nursery or operating room in a hospital.

ABR test results in this young patient population provide information that is critical for early diagnosis of hearing loss and for prompt management with hearing aids or other devices. Following a comprehensive assessment of auditory function with ABR, it is possible to describe hearing loss with remarkable detail, even for infants who are only a month old.

Although assessment with pure tone audiometry is always performed later, the diagnostic ABR testing of an infant initially confirms the presence of abnormal auditory function. Initial ABR findings also allow an audiologist to estimate the degree and configuration of hearing loss. ABR also permits differentiation among types of hearing loss, including conductive, sensory, mixed or neural forms of auditory dysfunction.

To objectively estimate auditory thresholds in infants and young children, the ABR is repeatedly recorded at progressively lower stimulus intensity levels for click stimuli and for tone burst stimuli at different frequencies. Testing begins at a high-intensity level to confirm the presence of a response and concludes at a lower-intensity level that fails to produce a response. Figure 9.10 shows normal ABR waveforms at different intensity levels for click stimulation and frequency-specific tone burst stimulation at 4000 Hz.

Looking closely at the waveforms in Figure 9.10 you'll notice three major changes in the waveforms as stimulus intensity level is decreased. First, the latency of the waves increases as the stimulus intensity level decreases. The longer latencies for wave V at lower stimulus intensity levels are tracked with the dotted line in Figure 9.10. The line connecting the wave V peaks at each intensity level slopes to the right or outward on the latency scale (the X-axis).

Second, amplitude of the waves decreases as the intensity level decreases. The gradually smaller amplitude of ABR waves as intensity decreases is indicated by the amplitude markings on the Y-axis in the figure. Finally, as intensity level is progressively decreased, only wave V remains. Wave I and wave III disappear at the lower-intensity levels.

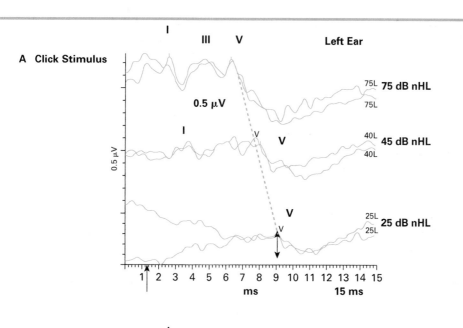

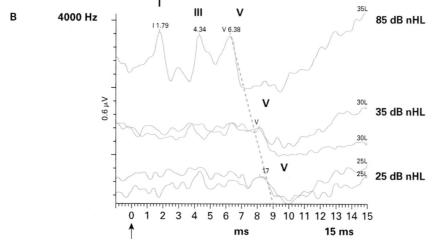

FIGURE 9.10

Auditory brain stem response (ABR) waveforms at decreasing intensity levels for click stimulation **(A)** and stimulation with 4000 Hz tone bursts **(B)** in the estimation of auditory threshold.

The patient's auditory threshold corresponds to the intensity level where ABR wave V disappears. Research has demonstrated a relation between the first appearance of the wave V component of ABR and behavioral estimation of hearing threshold (Hall & Swanepoel, 2010; Stapells, 2000). As a rule hearing threshold assessed by behavioral testing is about 10 dB lower than the minimum intensity level producing an ABR wave V.

Invaluable but Not a Test of Hearing. To meaningfully apply ABR in the clinic, audiologists must appreciate four facts about the generation of the ABR within the auditory system. First, ABR does not reflect activity of all of the neurons in the auditory system. Auditory system neurons differ remarkably in their structure and function and in their specific response to sound stimulation. As you learned in the review of the auditory system in Chapter 3, there are at least seven or eight different structural and functional types of neurons in the auditory system. Presumably, activity of each of the different types of neurons contributes to normal hearing functions, from detection of simple sounds to perception of complex speech sounds in demanding listening conditions. Research shows that the ABR reflects activity of only one of these different types of neurons, the *onset neurons.* Onset neurons fire only at the very beginning of a stimulus, not during the remainder of the stimulus. The ABR provides no information on other neurons of the auditory system, even though these other neurons are essential for hearing (Hall, 2007).

Second, the ABR primarily reflects activity of nerve fibers and not the many complex nuclei or collections of nerve cell bodies within the auditory system. Processing of information in the auditory system during communication takes place in the major nuclei mentioned in Chapter 3, such as the superior olivary complex and the inferior colliculus. Although these complex neural centers are very important for hearing, they apparently play a minor role in generating ABR.

Third, there is not a one-to-one relation between a single auditory structure and a single ABR wave, with one exception. Wave I is the exception, as it is generated only by sound-evoked activity in the auditory nerve. Later waves, such as wave III and wave V, represent a combination of activities from more than one pathway or center in the auditory brain stem. It is not possible to determine exactly which part of the auditory system is or is not contributing to these waves. And finally, ABR provides no information on the function of auditory structures above the level of the brain stem. Major regions of the central auditory nervous system such as the thalamus and the cerebral cortex contribute importantly to hearing function, but they are not involved in the generation of ABR.

Taken together, these rather complex facts about the anatomical underpinnings of ABR lead to a simple conclusion. Even though it is a valuable clinical tool, *the ABR is not a test of hearing.* The ABR may be abnormal or even undetectable in a person who seems to communicate quite well. Or, conversely, the ABR may be normal in persons with serious communication problems. In fact, a perfectly normal ABR may even be recorded in persons who are unconscious or in a deep coma. These observations do not minimize the considerable value of ABR in audiology, particularly the objective estimation of auditory thresholds in infants and young children. However, ABR alone is not a complete measure of hearing.

Why Is ABR Important in Hearing Assessment of Children? In conducting hearing assessment of infants and young children between the ages of birth and 6 months, audiologists follow guidelines developed by the Joint Committee on Infant Hearing (JCIH, 2007). The JCIH is further described in the next chapter. Briefly, the JCIH is a multidisciplinary group consisting of representatives from various professions involved in the hearing healthcare of children and specifically the identification, diagnosis, and management of pediatric hearing loss.

The JCIH periodically publishes peer-reviewed and evidence-based clinical guidelines that describe proven techniques for infant hearing screening, for confirming hearing loss in

LEADERS AND LUMINARIES

Nina Kraus

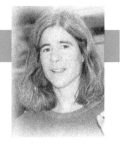

Nina Kraus earned her bachelor's degree at Swarthmore College and her PhD at Northwestern University. She currently holds an appointment as Hugh Knowles Professor in the Departments of Communication Sciences, Neurobiology and Physiology, and Otolaryngology at Northwestern University, where she also directs the Auditory Neuroscience Laboratory and mentors numerous doctoral and postdoctoral students. In the 1980s, Dr. Kraus published dozens of articles on the application of the auditory brain stem response in diagnosis of hearing in young children and on the anatomical origins of the auditory middle latency response. She now investigates biological bases of speech and music with techniques such as the speech-evoked auditory brain stem response. Dr. Kraus investigates learning-associated brain plasticity throughout the lifetime in normal, expert listeners (like musicians) and in clinical populations with various disorders, including dyslexia (reading disorder), autism, and hearing loss. In addition to being a pioneering thinker who bridges the multiple disciplines of aging, development, literacy, music, and learning, Dr. Kraus is a technological innovator who roots her research in translational science (that is, research that leads to clinical applications). You can learn more about Dr. Kraus and her work at the website www.brainvolts.northwestern.edu.

children, and for management of or intervention with children when a hearing loss is confirmed. JCIH guidelines strongly recommend reliance on three objective techniques for hearing assessment of infants and young children from birth to 6 months. You have already been introduced to two of these objective techniques, acoustic immittance measurements and otoacoustic emissions. The ABR is the third objective technique and the most important for describing both degree and type of hearing loss.

Recent Advances in ABR Technology and Techniques

Equipment for ABR measurement has become steadily more sophisticated over the past forty years. Figure 9.11 shows two modern devices for recording the ABR including a hand-held screening device (Figure 9.11A) and a diagnostic system (Figure 9.11B). To a large extent,

FIGURE 9.11 **A.** A handheld combination device for recording automated auditory brainstem response (ABR) and otoacoustic emissions. **B.** A diagnostic system for recording the ABR, the auditory steady state response (ASSR), and other auditory evoked responses. Images Courtesy of Grason Stadler, Inc.

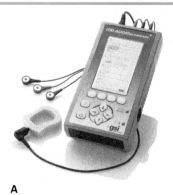

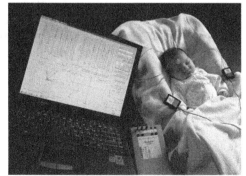

A   B

development of ABR instrumentation has paralleled and benefited from advances in computer technology. Four major advances have included (1) *automated ABR technology* that allows a technician or another nonaudiologist to initiate automatic recording and analysis of ABR findings using statistical processing computer software; (2) *combined OAE/ABR technology* permitting measurement of either otoacoustic emissions and/or ABR with the same device; (3) instrumentation for ABR measurement, without sedation or anesthesia, in young children whose movement would disrupt ABR recording with conventional ABR systems; (4) equipment for recording and analyzing ABRs elicited by speech stimuli like /da/, rather than simple click or tone burst sounds. *Speech-evoked ABR* measurement can be performed during clinical evaluation of auditory processing, even with young children who cannot participate in behavioral speech audiometry; and (5) the *auditory steady state response (ASSR)* that can be used to estimate auditory thresholds even in patients with severe-to-profound hearing loss who cannot be adequately tested with conventional ABR techniques.

The ASSR is generated in the same general auditory regions as the ABR and recorded with instrumentation that is also used for ABR measurement (Hall, 2007; Hall & Swanepoel, 2011). However, the ASSR is not elicited or activated by very brief sounds like the ABR but, rather, by longer-duration pure tone sounds. The longer-duration pure tone stimulation of ASSR measurement can be presented at much higher-intensity levels than the short-duration ABR stimulation.

 ClinicalConnection

Auditory steady state response (ASSR) plays an important role in the estimation of auditory thresholds in infants and young children with severe and profound hearing impairment. ASSR findings lead directly to prompt management of such children, including consideration of cochlear implantation as a treatment option. You'll learn about the management of children with severe hearing loss in Chapters 13 through 16.

Other Auditory Evoked Responses (AERs)

We'll conclude the chapter with a brief review of five other auditory evoked responses. These auditory evoked responses are available to clinical audiologists for objective evaluation of auditory function from the cochlea to the highest levels of the cortex. Audiologists rely mostly on the ABR for objective hearing assessment of infants and young children. The other auditory evoked responses are not routinely recorded clinically. However, each of the responses has an important place in the diagnostic audiology test battery.

Electrocochleography (ECochG)

Electrocochleography (abbreviated ECochG) was first described back in 1930 (Hall, 2007). ECochG provides information on activity in the cochlea and the auditory nerve. Figure 9.12 shows a typical ECochG waveform with a summating potential (SP) and action potential (AP) component. The response occurs within several milliseconds after the presentation of stimuli. ECochG is recorded very much like the ABR. The key difference in ECochG recording is that one of the electrodes is located as close as possible to the inner ear. Various clinical applications of ECochG discovered over the years include diagnosis of inner ear disease, monitoring of auditory function during surgical procedures involving the ear, and diagnosis of abnormalities affecting the auditory nerve and auditory regions in the brain stem (Hall, 2007).

 ClinicalConnection

Electrocochleography (ECochG) techniques are valuable in the diagnostic assessment of a wide range of auditory problems, from disorders of the ear such as Ménière's disease to neural auditory dysfunction, including auditory neuropathy spectrum disorder. These and many other etiologies for hearing loss are reviewed in Chapters 11 and 12.

Cortical Auditory Evoked Responses

Multiple auditory evoked responses arise from regions of the central nervous system above the level of the brain stem. Audiologists sometimes apply them in the assessment of central auditory nervous system function and auditory processing disorders. As illustrated in Figure 9.12, the *auditory middle latency response (AMLR)* is

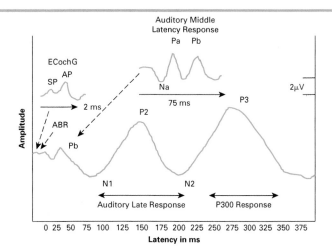

FIGURE 9.12

Waveforms for auditory responses in addition to the auditory brain stem response (ABR), including electrocochleography (ECochG), auditory middle latency response (AMLR), and auditory late response (ALR) and P300 response waveforms. You will note that the time frames and the amplitude scales are different for each response.

recorded after earlier responses such as ECochG and ABR yet before even later responses (Hall, 2007). AMLR measurement is made with the same equipment used to record ABR, with modification of some of the test settings. The AMLR is detected with electrodes located on the side of the head, over the auditory regions within the cerebral cortex. The AMLR includes anatomical contributions from the thalamus and the primary auditory cortex, two auditory regions that are essential for normal hearing.

As shown in Figure 9.12, the *auditory late response (ALR)* is recorded even later in time than the ABR or AMLR. Major ALR waves occur with a latency of 100 to 300 ms after the stimulus is presented. The structures in the cerebral cortex giving rise to the ALR are vital not only for hearing but also for language functioning. ALR is effectively elicited with speech sounds as well as pure tone stimuli. Recent studies confirm that ALR can be used for objective confirmation of speech sound processing in young children who are unable to participate in behavioral hearing assessment (Hall, 2007).

The *auditory P300 response* is another cortical response recorded by some audiologists. As you see in Figure 9.12, the P300 response consists of a relatively large wave that occurs 300 ms after the stimulus. Unlike the other responses we've discussed, the P300 response is recorded with two different sets of sounds presented at the same time. As an example, one set of sounds might consist of 2000-Hz tones presented steadily and frequently and the other sound might be a lower-frequency 500-Hz tone presented infrequently, such as 20% of the time, and in no predictable pattern. The latter rare stimulus elicits a very large wave that appears at about 300 ms. The P300 response is sometimes referred to as a "cognitive response" since it appears to measure more complex processing of sound by the auditory system (Hall, 2007).

 ClinicalConnection

The cortical auditory evoked responses mentioned here, including the auditory middle latency response, the auditory late response, and the P300 response, are useful for documenting the presence and extent of central auditory nervous system dysfunction. Etiologies for auditory abnormalities involving the brain are reviewed in Chapter 12.

Electrical Auditory Evoked Responses

Up to this point, we've discussed the recording of electrical responses from the auditory system that are elicited with different types of *sound*. We will conclude the chapter with mention of responses that arise following electrical stimulation to the auditory system. Measurement of electrically evoked auditory responses is not possible or necessary with most patients, yet the technique is valuable for some patients with profound hearing loss. Patients with very little hearing who cannot receive any benefit from hearing aids may be candidates for surgically implanted electrical devices that are designed to directly stimulate the auditory nerve. You'll learn about these devices in Chapter 13. Electrically evoked responses provide verification before the implantation surgery that auditory nerve fibers are intact and can be stimulated. Electrically evoked responses can also be used after implantation surgery to make sure the electrical device is working adequately, especially in young children who cannot be tested using behavioral audiometry techniques.

PULLING IT ALL TOGETHER

You learned in this chapter about a wide variety of speech audiometry procedures that go beyond simple speech recognition threshold and word recognition. Some of the tests utilize words whereas others consist of sentence-length speech items. Performance on each of the procedures is challenging for even normal-hearing persons because speech information is distorted, missing, presented simultaneously with other speech signals, or embedded within noise or a competing meaningful message. The special speech audiometry tests are highly sensitive in detecting abnormalities in persons with dysfunction in the neural regions of the auditory system. Findings are also valuable as audiologists develop management plans for children and adults who have serious auditory dysfunction despite normal hearing sensitivity.

Auditory evoked responses arising from the ear and different pathways within the central nervous system provide audiologists with a means to identify and define hearing loss in patients of all ages, even newborn infants. ABR, the most clinically applied auditory evoked response, is the technique of choice for estimating hearing thresholds in young children who cannot be tested behaviorally. ABR results permit early and accurate audiological management of infants with hearing loss in the first few months after birth. Other responses evoked by sound identify dysfunction anywhere in the auditory system, from the cochlea to the cortex.

READINGS

Chermak, G. D., & Musiek, F. E. (1997). *Central auditory processing disorders: New perspectives*. San Diego: Plural Publishing.

Hall, J. W. III. (1992). *Handbook of auditory evoked responses*. Boston: Allyn & Bacon.

Hall, J. W. III. (2007). *New handbook of auditory evoked responses*. Boston: Allyn & Bacon.

Hall, J. W. III, & Swanepoel, D. (2011). *Objective assessment of hearing*. San Diego: Plural Publishing.

Hugdahl, K. (1988). *Handbook of dichotic listening: Theory, methods, and research*. Chichester, England: John Wiley & Sons.

Konkle, D. F., & Rintelmann, W. F. (Eds.). (1983). *Principles of speech audiometry*. Baltimore: University Park Press.

Musiek, F. E., & Rintelmann, W. F. (Eds.). (1999). Contemporary perspectives in hearing assessment (pp. 375–413). Boston: Allyn & Bacon.

10

Differential Diagnosis of Auditory and Vestibular Disorders

LEARNING OBJECTIVES

In this chapter, you will learn:

- About early identification of hearing loss and why it is important
- Risk factors for hearing loss in infants and young children
- How clinical guidelines developed by the Joint Committee on Infant Hearing (JCIH) contribute to early hearing loss detection and intervention (EHDI)
- New terms used by audiologists in the diagnosis of auditory disorders
- How an audiologist uses information from a patient history and test findings to narrow down possible explanations for hearing or vestibular disorders to a handful of the most likely diagnoses
- When patients should be referred by an audiologist to other healthcare personnel for consultation, evaluation, and possible management
- The difference between *hearing loss* and *hearing handicap*
- About procedures in the traditional diagnostic site-of-lesion test battery, the persons who developed the procedures, and why the site-of-lesion tests are no longer important in modern audiology
- The meaning of *best practices, evidence-based practice,* and *standard of care*
- About special equipment used to measure vestibular function
- About procedures of a current test battery used for the assessment of vestibular and balance functioning

CHAPTER FOCUS

This chapter covers the rationale and methods for identification and diagnosis of auditory and vestibular disorders. You will first be introduced to hearing screening principles and procedures, with an emphasis on widely accepted multidisciplinary guidelines from the Joint Committee on Infant Hearing (JCIH). Techniques for diagnostic assessment of the auditory system have evolved considerably over the years. The chapter includes a historical overview of early diagnostic tests and a discussion of clinical guidelines and current strategies for hearing evaluation.

In this chapter you will apply knowledge acquired earlier in the book. An appreciation of the diagnostic process in clinical audiology requires knowledge of auditory system anatomy and physiology, topics we covered in Chapter 3. The diagnostic process is also dependent on the application of different procedures available for evaluating auditory function, as reviewed in Chapters 4 through 9.

KEY TERMS

Alternate binaural loudness balance (ABLB)
Best practices
Chief complaint
Cognitive variables
Differential diagnosis
Early hearing detection and intervention (EHDI)
Electronystagmography (ENG)
Frenzel goggles
Loudness recruitment
Medical home
Nystagmus
Otolaryngology
Otologist
Presbycusis
Quality of life
Rule out
Site-of-lesion
Standard of care
Universal newborn hearing screening (UNHS)
Vertigo
Vestibular evoked myogenic potential (VEMP)
Video-nystagmography (VNG)

> **CHAPTER FOCUS** *Concluded*
>
> Diagnosis of auditory and vestibular disorders is possible for patients of all ages, from newborn infants to older adults. Prompt and accurate diagnosis of hearing loss and related disorders like tinnitus and vestibular impairment is a very important step toward effective management. Understanding the diagnostic process in audiology is central to understanding what audiologists do and how they think clinically.

The Diagnostic Process

Importance of Accurate Diagnosis

Accurate diagnosis of hearing impairment and vestibular disorders contributes importantly to effective nonmedical and medical management. Misdiagnosis of auditory dysfunction may lead to inappropriate and ineffective management. The consequence of misdiagnosis or delayed diagnosis of auditory dysfunction may be suboptimal outcome, unnecessary risk, or even harm to the patient. Early and accurate diagnosis makes possible early and effective intervention and contributes to the best possible outcome.

How Patient History Contributes to Diagnosis

The process of diagnosing disorders involving the auditory or vestibular system begins with a good patient history. Information gleaned from the patient history and other patient-related factors guides an audiologist in selecting specific test procedures that are then administered under well-defined test conditions. Some important patient-related factors are chronologic age, developmental age, and cognitive level.

Patient age is an important factor in the decision to perform or not perform certain procedures in the assessment of hearing, especially in the pediatric patient population.

A single test procedure might be adequate for hearing screening of a patient at any age, from newborn infants to older adults. However, diagnostic hearing assessment beyond simple screening requires multiple test procedures that are usually grouped into a test battery. A skilled and experienced audiologist takes into account patient age in selecting the most appropriate procedures to include in the test battery.

Basic information from the history plays an important role in decisions about the hearing assessment approach that's most appropriate for a specific patient. A history often begins with questions about the patient's **chief complaint**. The chief complaint is the reason the patient is seeking a hearing assessment. For example, a chief complaint might be difficulty hearing or, more specifically, difficulty hearing people speak when there is background noise. If the patient's chief complaint is imbalance and occasional vertigo, then vestibular testing is appropriate in addition to a basic hearing assessment.

Often in a medical practice setting such as a hospital or physician's office, an audiologist's decisions about how to evaluate a patient are influenced or even dictated by a very specific aspect of the patient's history. Based on the patient's history and suspected diagnosis, a referring physician may even make a formal request or an "order" for a single test procedure.

Let's consider an example of a very specific procedure performed in response to a physician's order. A patient involved in a motor vehicle accident is admitted to a trauma hospital with a skull fracture that results in weakness of the facial nerve. An audiologist is asked to perform a test of facial nerve function at the patient's bedside in an intensive care unit. In this example, the approach taken in assessing the patient was determined entirely by one feature of the history— the trauma-related facial nerve dysfunction. Sometime later, if the patient recovers and is discharged from the hospital, an audiologist may perform a full hearing assessment. Fracture of the temporal bone within the skull often damages the ear or auditory nerve and is associated with hearing loss.

Standard of Care

You've already learned about behavioral, electroacoustic, and electrophysiological tests for assessment of children and adults. The number of available clinical tests of auditory function has increased for over sixty years. Audiologists can utilize one or more of these procedures in hearing assessment. As newer, quicker, and more accurate procedures are developed, some older tests fall out of use.

Now, in the era of healthcare cost containment, there is a financial incentive for limiting the tests administered in a hearing assessment to those that are most likely to contribute to diagnosis and improved outcome of patients with hearing impairment. Professional organizations such as the American Academy of Audiology and the American Speech-Language-Hearing Association have developed guidelines and protocols for how to conduct hearing assessments in specific patient populations.

Once all of the procedures selected for a specific patient are performed and the results are analyzed, an audiologist must interpret the findings for the test battery. That is, an audiologist takes into consideration all of the test findings and examines them for patterns or trends that suggest a likely diagnosis. A patient's history is taken into consideration in the interpretation of the hearing test findings. The assumption is that interpretation of test findings contributes directly to decisions regarding management. Proper interpretation of hearing test findings in the context of the patient's history and findings on other procedures is one of the most challenging yet rewarding aspects of clinical audiology.

The Fascinating Diagnostic Process

Most audiologists enjoy the intellectual stimulation of the diagnostic process and take satisfaction from making an accurate diagnosis of auditory or vestibular dysfunction. Indeed, many audiologists will readily admit that the challenge of performing test procedures, precisely quantifying disorders of auditory function with calibrated instrumentation, and then putting all of the information together to reach the correct diagnosis is to a large extent what attracted them to the profession. Particularly appealing and ultimately satisfying to the clinical audiologist is the daily opportunity to develop an effective management plan based on the diagnostic information, with the goal of providing clear and quantifiable benefit to a person with a hearing or vestibular disorder.

At the beginning of the diagnostic process, an audiologist may know very little about a patient. An hour or so later, after reviewing the patient history, administering an appropriate test battery, carefully analyzing test findings, and thoughtfully interpreting all of the information gathered, an audiologist can develop and begin to implement a logical treatment plan. In some cases, a patient may leave the clinic after a single visit quite satisfied and no longer concerned about or impaired by his or her auditory or vestibular problem.

We'll now review in more detail each major step in the process of **differential diagnosis**, beginning with hearing screening and the patient history. The phrase *differential diagnosis* is borrowed from medicine. It refers to the process of determining a patient's diagnosis from among two or more different disorders that have similar characteristics or symptoms. Our discussion assumes that you've already carefully reviewed information on the anatomy and physiology of the auditory and vestibular systems (Chapter 3). The discussion of the diagnostic process here bridges the gap between the information on hearing tests in the previous chapters to, in the next chapters, a summary of different patient populations and a review of management options available to audiologists.

Hearing Screening Protocols in Children and Adults

Identification of hearing loss comes before diagnosis. Early identification of auditory dysfunction is always desirable. For the newborn infant, the goal is to identify hearing loss within one month, to complete the diagnostic process within the first three months after birth, and to initiate appropriate intervention no later than six months after birth. The sequence is now sometimes referred to as the "1-3-6" strategy of early intervention for infant hearing impairment.

Early identification of hearing loss for all children is consistently achieved only with **universal newborn hearing screening (UNHS)**. Universal newborn hearing screening means that all babies undergo hearing screening within the first three months after birth to identify those who are likely to have a hearing loss. In the United States, hearing screening is almost always completed in the nursery within a day or two after birth and before discharge from the hospital. Then, diagnostic hearing assessment is performed for children who do not pass the hearing screening.

Audiologists strive to identify hearing loss of all patients as soon as possible, even in older children and adults. The major goal of early identification is to develop and implement an appropriate and effective management plan in a timely fashion. Outcome in management of hearing loss and related disorders is usually enhanced with early identification and intervention. Furthermore, early identification generally leads to improved quality of life and reduction of the psychosocial impact of hearing loss.

Infant Hearing Screening

Joint Committee on Infant Hearing. Universal newborn hearing screening (UNHS) is now a reality in the United States and most other developed countries in the world. The first efforts to identify hearing loss in infants date back to the 1960s when Marion Downs in the United States, W. G. Alex and Irene R. Ewing in the United Kingdom, and Lillian Tell in Israel published papers describing rudimentary programs for identifying hearing loss among newborn infants. In the late 1960s Marion Downs was instrumental in the development of the first Joint Committee on Infant Hearing, or JCIH (Downs & Sterritt, 1967). Marion Downs was featured in Leaders & Luminaries in Chapter 1.

The JCIH is a multidisciplinary group consisting of representatives from various professions with an interest in infant and childhood hearing impairment. During the past thirty years, different incarnations of the Joint Committee on Infant Hearing have published position statements. Each JCIH publication consists of up-to-date and evidence-based guidelines for newborn hearing screening, follow-up of infants who do not pass the initial screening, diagnosis of infant hearing loss, and intervention for infants with confirmed hearing loss (JCIH, 1994, 2007).

Risk Indicators for Hearing Loss. Early Joint Committee reports specified indicators associated with infant hearing loss that could be used to identify children who were at risk for permanent hearing loss and who required diagnostic assessment. Over the years, as evidence accumulated from clinical research and appeared in peer-reviewed scientific journals, the list of risk indicators for hearing loss grew longer.

Current risk factors or indicators for hearing loss are listed in Table 10.1. Children with one or more of the risk factors are more likely to have hearing impairment than healthy babies without risk factors. Most infants with risk factors are admitted soon after birth to the intensive care nursery, sometimes called the neonatal intensive care unit. Recent research clearly shows that childhood hearing loss is not always present at birth. The prevalence of hearing loss is

- Caregiver concern regarding hearing, speech, language, or developmental delay
- Family history of permanent childhood hearing loss
- Neonatal intensive care unit (NICU) stay of > 5 days or
  - Extracorporeal membrane oxygenation (ECMO)
  - Assisted ventilation
  - Exposure to ototoxic medicines
  - Hyperbilirubinemia requiring exchange transfusion
- In utero infections, e.g.,
  - Cytomegalovirus (CMV)
  - Herpes
  - Rubella
  - Syphilis
  - Toxoplasmosis
- Craniofacial anomalies, including involvement of the
  - Pinna
  - Ear canals
  - Ear tags and pits
  - Temporal bone
- Physical findings associated with a syndrome, e.g.,
  - White forelock
- Syndromes associated with hearing loss, e.g.,
  - Neurofibromatosis
  - Osteopetrosis
  - Usher
  - Waardenburg
  - Alport
  - Pendred
  - Jervell
  - Lange-Nielsen
- Neurodegenerative disorders, e.g.,
  - Hunter syndrome
  - Sensorimotor neuropathies
  - Friedreich ataxia
  - Charcot-Marie-Tooth syndrome
- Culture-positive postnatal infections associated with sensorineural hearing loss, e.g.
  - Confirmed bacterial or viral meningitis
- Head trauma requiring hospitalization
- Chemotherapy

Adapted from Joint Committee on Infant Hearing, 2007.

TABLE 10.1
Risk factors for hearing loss according to the Joint Committee on Infant Hearing, including factors associated with progressive and delayed onset hearing loss.

considerably higher for school-age children than in newborn infants (Fortnum, Summerfield, Marshall, Davis, & Bamford, 2001).

The rather lengthy list in Table 10.1 includes factors associated with hearing loss that progresses during early childhood or hearing loss that has an onset sometime after birth. Children with any of these risk factors in their medical history, even those who pass newborn hearing screening, should be followed closely for the possible development of hearing loss.

Emergence of Universal Newborn Hearing Screening. Gradually, collective clinical experience with screening of infants at risk for hearing loss confirmed that only about 50% of all babies with hearing impairment have a risk factor for hearing impairment. That is, about one-half of all young children with confirmed hearing loss are graduates of well baby

LEADERS AND LUMINARIES

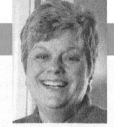

Judy Gravel

Judith Gravel (1948–2008) earned her Bachelor's degree (Phi Beta Kappa) and Master's in Audiology in 1971 from the University of Massachusetts at Amherst. She completed her PhD at Vanderbilt University in 1985. Dr. Gravel held an adjunct faculty position at Vanderbilt University and academic positions at Columbia University, Albert Einstein College of Medicine, the City University of New York, and the University of Pennsylvania. At the time of her death, Dr. Gravel was the Director of the Center for Childhood Communication at the Children's Hospital of Philadelphia.

Dr. Gravel enjoyed a worldwide reputation for her expertise and scholarship in pediatric audiology. She published extensively on a variety of topics related to children and hearing, from influential studies on communication disorders following otitis media to auditory neuropathy spectrum disorder.

She also generously served her profession as Chair of the Joint Committee on Infant Hearing (2003–2005) and on many other boards, task forces, and committees for professional organizations and the National Institutes of Health (NIH). Dr. Gravel received many awards in recognition of her work in childhood hearing including the American Academy of Audiology Distinguished Achievement Award. You are encouraged to reach some of Dr. Gravel's important publications and an online version of a published tribute to her many accomplishments.

nurseries and are not be identified with a high-risk register approach. It became clear during the 1980s that focusing hearing screening efforts exclusively on at risk children in the neonatal intensive care nursery was not adequate for early identification of all children with hearing loss. Another strategy was required.

Universal Newborn Hearing Screening. Recognizing limitations of the risk factor approach for early identification of all babies with hearing loss, the 1994 JCIH recommended universal newborn hearing screening (Joint Committee on Infant Hearing, 1994). Again, universal newborn hearing screening means that all babies undergo hearing screening within the first three months after birth, and almost always in the nursery a day or two before discharge from the hospital. This recommendation appeared about the same time as a National Institutes of Health (NIH) Consensus Statement that recommended hearing screening of all infants in the neonatal intensive care unit (NICU) and all other babies within the first three months after birth (National Institutes of Health, 1993).

Five years later the American Academy of Pediatrics similarly endorsed universal newborn hearing screening (American Academy of Pediatrics, 1999). Pediatricians represent the physician specialty that serves as "gatekeeper," or the **medical home** for healthcare of children. The American Academy of Pediatrics decision was based largely on evidence published in peer-reviewed journals confirming the feasibility of hearing screening of all infants with newly developed automated technology and supporting the benefits of early identification and intervention for hearing loss on speech and language development (Stewart, Mehl, Hall, Carroll, & Bramlett, 2000; Yoshinaga-Itano, 2003; Yoshinaga-Itano, Sedey, Coulter, & Mehl, 1998).

The advent of automated screening devices was an essential factor in the decision to endorse universal newborn hearing screening. Automated devices are designed so that non-audiology personnel can successfully conduct hearing screenings (Dhar & Hall, 2012; Hall, 2007b; Stewart et al., 2000). Screening personnel include appropriately trained technicians, nurses, and volunteers. In the United States alone approximately 4 million babies are born each year. It would be impossible to complete hearing screenings of such a large number of newborn infants without automated technology.

Early hearing detection and intervention (EHDI) programs have rapidly expanded throughout the United States since about 2000. EHDI programs are also widespread in Europe and most developed countries in the world. Serious efforts are now underway to implement EHDI programs in other countries, including South Africa (Friderichs, Swanepoel, & Hall, 2012; Swanepoel, Storbeck, & Friedland, 2009).

Current Joint Committee on Infant Hearing Recommendations. A full review of the 2007 JCIH recommendations is far beyond the scope of this chapter or this book. Interested readers can easily access the 2007 JCIH Position Statement online. You have already learned about risk factors for hearing loss established by the 2007 JCIH, including the factors used for identification of children with progressive or delayed onset hearing loss. The JCIH also offers very clear guidelines for when and how newborn hearing screening should be conducted, and also for the test protocol that should be followed in the diagnosis of hearing loss in infants and young children.

The two objective techniques JCIH endorses for newborn hearing screening are auditory brain stem response (ABR) and otoacoustic emissions (OAEs). Figure 10.1A shows a baby undergoing hearing screening with an automated handheld ABR device. Infant hearing screening using automated ABR technology dates back to the mid-1980s (Hall, 2007b). The JCIH specifically recommends the ABR technique for hearing screening of children in the neonatal intensive care unit to facilitate early detection of neural hearing loss as well as cochlear hearing loss (Joint Committee on Infant Hearing, 2007).

Figure 10.1B shows a 2-week-old infant undergoing hearing screening with the OAE technique. Hearing screening with OAEs alone, with ABR alone, or with a combination of

WebWatch

A wealth of information on EHDI programs and the topic of early identification of hearing loss in general is available from the following websites: American Academy of Audiology; Early Hearing Detection & Intervention Meeting; National Center for Hearing Assessment and Management, Utah State University; National Institute on Deafness and Other Communication Disorders (NIDCD); and the National Institutes of Health, National Institute on Deafness and Other Communication Disorders. Many states in the United States also have a special EHDI website.

FIGURE 10.1 **A.** Infant undergoing hearing screening with auditory auditory brain stem response (AABR). Photo A Courtesy of Maico Diagnostics. **B.** Two-week-old infant undergoing hearing screening with otoacoustic emissions (OAEs). Photo B Courtesy of Austin Charles Hall and Grason Stadler Inc.

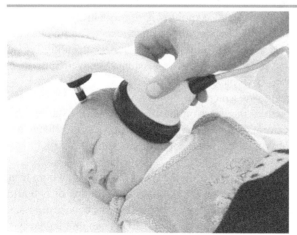
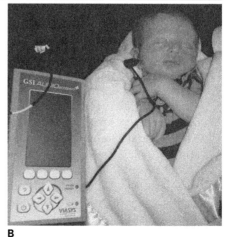

A   B

Child and Family History

Required Audiologic Procedures

- Otoacoustic emissions (OAEs)
- Auditory brain stem response (ABR) with frequency-specific stimuli during the initial evaluation to confirm type, degree, and configuration of hearing loss
- Acoustic immittance measures (using a 1000-Hz probe tone)

Supplemental Audiologic Procedures*

- Auditory steady state response (ASSR)
- Acoustic middle ear reflexes for infants older than 4 months
- Broadband reflectance measures of middle ear function

Behavioral Response Audiometry (if feasible)

- Visual reinforcement audiometry (VRA) or conditioned play audiometry
- Speech detection and recognition

Parental Report of Auditory and Visual Behaviors

Screening of Infant's Communication Milestones

*The Joint Committee on Infant Hearing concluded that there is insufficient evidence to use any of these procedures as the only test of infant hearing.

OAEs and ABR is appropriate for screening hearing in the well baby nursery setting (Joint Committee on Infant Hearing, 2007). Essentially all hearing loss is targeted in infant screening, including congenital permanent unilateral or bilateral sensory hearing loss, permanent conductive hearing loss, and also neural hearing loss. These and other types of hearing loss are reviewed in the next two chapters.

Table 10.2 summarizes the test battery recommended by the 2007 JCIH Committee for confirmation of hearing loss in infants from birth to 6 months. You are now familiar with the names of the auditory tests that are included in the table. Children scheduled for follow-up diagnostic hearing assessment include infants who do not pass hearing screening and also those have risk factors for a progressive hearing loss or a delayed onset hearing loss. Diagnostic assessment is also recommended when parents are concerned about their child's hearing or a delay in speech and language acquisition.

Confirmation of hearing loss between birth and 6 months is dependent almost entirely on the findings of three objective techniques: (1) auditory brain stem response with click and frequency-specific tone burst stimulation, (2) aural immittance measures, including tympanometry and sometimes acoustic reflexes, and (3) otoacoustic emissions. You were introduced to each of these techniques in the previous two chapters.

Valid and complete behavioral hearing assessment of infants under the age of 6 months is not feasible or likely to contribute much to the description of hearing status. Neurological immaturity of young infants affects performance on behavioral hearing testing. Behavioral hearing testing takes on a more important role for assessment of older children.

Infant Hearing Loss: Identification to Intervention. In the era of universal newborn hearing screening, an infant is screened for hearing loss in the hospital within a day or two after birth. Automated auditory brain stem response (AABR) or otoacoustic emissions testing may be used for hearing screening (Joint Committee on Infant Hearing, 2007). An infant who does not pass the hearing screening in the hospital nursery is usually scheduled to return within one to two months to an audiology clinic for follow-up hearing screening. Re-screening often includes more than one technology, such as otoacoustic emissions testing plus automated ABR recording. If the infant again does not pass the hearing screening, a full diagnostic hearing assessment is scheduled to occur within the next few months, or additional testing is carried out immediately.

Table 10.2 included JCIH recommended components of the assessment. The minimum goal of diagnostic hearing assessment is to describe the degree, configuration, and type of hearing loss for each ear. This is the information required to make timely and appropriate decisions regarding management. Based on the findings for diagnostic assessment, management of a confirmed hearing loss often begins without delay. The parents are counseled regarding the findings and also about different options for management of the hearing impairment. Then the infant is scheduled to return to the clinic within a few weeks for a hearing aid fitting. In other words, a clear program for habilitation of the hearing loss is initiated as soon as possible.

If the diagnostic process unfolds according to JCIH guidelines, an infant will begin to benefit from hearing aid use within six months after birth in order to enhance the likelihood of optimal outcome, or normal speech and language acquisition. Remember the ideal 1-3-6 schedule for identification, diagnosis, and intervention for infant hearing loss. In the real world there are different variations of this scenario, depending on the diagnostic findings and a host of health-related and other factors. The sequence of events is often different for infants who pass hearing screening at birth and then develop a progressive hearing loss or a hearing loss of delayed onset. The timing of diagnosis and intervention is also quite different for older children whose hearing loss is identified beyond the age of 6 months. However, the overall course remains the same. Early and accurate diagnosis makes possible early and effective intervention and the best possible outcome.

Hearing Screening of Preschool and Young School-Age Children

Hearing screening of children is often carried out at some time during preschool years and then every year or every two years after a child begins school. Hearing screening may be conducted by nurses, trained volunteers, or other qualified personnel. Children in certain preschool settings like Head Start Programs are required by federal regulations to undergo hearing screening at the beginning of each school year.

The purpose of the screenings is to detect hearing loss that develops after birth, including hearing loss related to ear infections. In past years, hearing screening of preschool and young school-age children was performed with a pure tone technique. Recent research confirms the value of otoacoustic emissions in combination with tympanometry for hearing screening of preschool and young school-age children (Dhar & Hall, 2012; Hall & Swanepoel, 2010).

Pure Tone Screening. The screening process for preschool and school-age children typically begins with an otoscopic inspection of the external ear canal and tympanic membrane. Most children readily accept the momentary insertion of an otoscope speculum into the ear canal for this procedure.

The conventional approach for hearing screening of preschool or school-age children utilizes pure tone audiometry. Guidelines for pure tone hearing screening of young children are available from professional organizations (American Academy of Audiology, 2011; American Speech-Language-Hearing Association, 1997). Preschool children ages 3 to 5 years are screened with pure tone signals of 20 dB HL for octave frequencies of 1000, 2000, and 4000 Hz. Children are first instructed about the task and how to respond to the stimulus sounds. According to guidelines, pure tone screening can be supplemented with tympanometry.

Preschool hearing screening programs that use the pure tone approach are hampered by at least four practical and often serious limitations. As already noted, some children are incapable of understanding the task required for pure tone hearing screening. These children do not give valid responses for a variety of reasons, including reduced cognitive function, attention deficits, or developmental delay. The number of 3-year-old children who are unable to be screened is up to thirty-three times higher than school-age children who cannot be tested (Halloran, Wall, Evans, Hardin, & Woolley, 2005). Head Start programs include children aged from 6 months to 4 years, so a sizable number are too young to screen with the pure tone technique.

Second, hearing screening of preschool children with conditioned play or visual reinforcement behavioral techniques requires skilled personnel, preferably an audiologist. However, most preschool hearing screening programs rely on volunteers, teachers, school nurses, or other nonaudiology personnel with no formal education or training in hearing testing. At the least, audiologists must oversee hearing screening with the pure tone technique.

> ### 🎧 Clinical Connection
>
> Audiologists or speech pathologists employed in public school settings are usually responsible for conducting hearing screening of children or overseeing hearing screening by other school personnel. Audiologists and speech pathologists with heavy caseloads and often limited financial resources are motivated to utilize efficient and quick screening techniques.

Third, the child's consistent detection of a low-intensity pure tone signal while wearing earphones requires a relatively quiet test environment. Unfortunately, an appropriately sound-treated room is not available in most elementary school and preschool settings. Screening is, therefore, conducted in a suboptimal environment with excessive extraneous and ambient sound.

Finally, the behavioral hearing screening technique, including instruction of the child, is time consuming, usually requiring at least three to four minutes per child, and in some cases considerably longer.

Otoacoustic Emissions. Otoacoustic emissions offer an attractive alternative to pure tone hearing screening (Dhar & Hall, 2012). A handheld device contains a computer program that controls delivery of stimuli and detection of OAE activity amidst background noise within the ear canal. The device also determines whether the screening outcome is a "pass" or a "refer."

Nonaudiology personnel can easily, quickly, and consistently record OAEs, as shown in Figure 10.2. Ambient noise in the test environment rarely precludes hearing screening with

FIGURE 10.2

Photograph of a preschool child in a Head Start Program undergoing hearing screening with distortion product otoacoustic emissions. Trained Head Start personnel shown on the right side is performing the hearing screening. Courtesy of Terry Foust of the National Center for Hearing Assessment and Management (NCHAM).

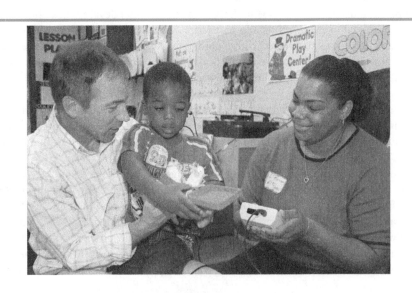

test frequencies of 2000 Hz and higher because the ear is sealed up with a sound-attenuating probe and special computer software is designed to detect OAE activity within background noise.

Brief test time is another major advantage of preschool and school-age hearing screening with OAE technology. With an appropriate OAE protocol, screening for a sample of test frequencies within the range of 2000 to 5000 Hz typically requires only 20 to 30 seconds. Therefore, it is possible to complete hearing screening of a substantial number of students within a brief period of time. Essentially, the same OAE technology and technique used with newborn hearing screening is applied with hearing screening of preschool and school-age children.

OAEs are an objective measure, not influenced by the listener variables such as development age, cognitive function, and attention that affect pure tone hearing testing. As a result, successful hearing screening of all children is almost always possible with OAEs (Dhar & Hall, 2012; Lyons, Kei, & Driscoll, 2004). Recent clinical evidence suggests that screening outcome using the DPOAE technique, supplemented by tympanometry as needed, is equivalent to conventional pure tone hearing screening. The advantages just cited make a compelling case for reliance on an objective DPOAE approach for hearing screening of preschool and early school-age children.

Tympanometry. OAE screening can be supplemented with tympanometry. Combining tympanometry with otoacoustic emissions techniques in hearing screening increases detection of middle ear dysfunction. Middle ear abnormalities are a common finding in preschool and young school-age children. You read in the previous chapter about the technique for performing tympanometry. To review briefly, testing requires insertion of a rubber probe tip into the external ear canal, forming a hermetic or airtight seal. As soon as a seal is created, the screening device automatically records middle ear compliance as a function of changes in air pressure within the external ear canal.

Clinical experience in Head Start programs with children in the age range of less than 1 to 4 years of age confirms the feasibility of performing hearing screening quickly and efficiently with a combination of otoscopy, DPOAEs, and tympanometry as needed. Average screening test time is often less than two minutes for both ears (Dhar & Hall, 2012; Lyons, Kei, & Driscoll, 2004).

Hearing Screening in Adult Populations

Hearing screening in adult populations is reserved mostly for persons at risk for noise-induced hearing loss. Two major groups are military personnel and persons employed in industries that involve noise, such as factories, mining, and heavy machinery. In the United States, Occupational Safety and Health Administration (OSHA) guidelines are followed for hearing screening of adults who work in noisy environments. The goal of a hearing conservation program is to prevent workers at risk for occupational noise exposure from developing a permanent hearing loss.

Toward this goal, employers are required by OSHA regulations to educate employees about noise exposure and possible damage to hearing and to monitor an employee's hearing at least once every year. A baseline audiogram is recorded when an employee is hired or no later than six months after the first day of work. Any employee exposed to sound intensity levels of 85 dBA or higher for a typical eight-hour work day then undergoes annual monitoring by a trained technician, under the supervision of a licensed audiologist. All audiometric testing is done with a calibrated audiometer in a quiet room with background noise not exceeding specified levels.

(i) Web Watch

You can quickly search the published literature on any topic at the website for the National Library of Medicine in Bethesda Maryland (www.nlm .nih.gov). Once you reach the website, go to the link "PubMed/MEDLINE." Then enter key words, like "OAEs" and "noise" or "OAEs" and "hearing screening" in the search field and prepare yourself for the large number of published papers you'll find.

The applicability of otoacoustic emissions in hearing conservation and screening programs has mirrored their use in newborn and preschool hearing screening. Numerous investigators have provided evidence in support of OAEs as a feasible technique for early detection of noise-induced cochlear dysfunction (reviewed in Dhar & Hall, 2012).

The advantages of OAEs already cited for hearing screening of children also hold true for adult hearing conservation programs. Test time is short, screening does not require an audiologist, devices perform automated data analysis, and OAEs are highly sensitive to cochlear dysfunction. Adherence to existing OSHA and other government regulations is still important. However, OAE screening can be used to supplement pure tone hearing screening for early detection of cochlear dysfunction in adults who are at risk for noise-induced damage, before a permanent sensory hearing loss develops.

The Concept of Differential Diagnosis

The goal of differential diagnosis is to efficiently narrow down to a "short list" possible etiologies or causes for the patient's signs and symptoms. An experienced clinical audiologist with appropriate information from the patient history and a well-selected test battery can quickly rule out most of the myriad causes of hearing loss. Then the audiologist can focus on the small number of etiologies that might explain the patient's hearing complaints.

The task can at first seem daunting. Imagine an audiologist in a busy clinical setting seeing dozens of patients each week, maybe a dozen in a single day, who have the chief complaint of "hearing loss." The majority of these patients may share the same general symptoms and auditory characteristics. How can the audiologist in a reasonable amount of time sort out the underlying auditory disorders for a series of patients who appear, at first glance, to be so similar? For a well-trained and experienced audiologist, the differential diagnostic process can proceed remarkably fast and appear almost effortless.

Patient History in Differential Diagnosis

The patient history represents the oldest and most traditional approach for diagnosing any health problem, including auditory and vestibular disorders. You were introduced in Chapter 4 to the process of acquiring a patient history. Far before the advent of the instrumentation and technology used by modern-day audiologists and hundreds of years before audiology developed as a profession, physicians relied to a large extent on careful and systematic exploration of the health history to reach a diagnosis. Often, the diagnosis was made almost entirely from information gleaned from the patient history.

A complete patient history is certainly "low tech," yet it remains one of the most important tools available to an audiologist. Most healthcare professionals, including audiologists, begin the diagnostic process by obtaining a detailed patient history. Then, as test findings accumulate during the diagnostic process, the patient is often asked additional and more focused questions. The patient history contributes importantly to a quick and accurate diagnosis and also guides an audiologist to the most appropriate diagnostic test strategy.

Questions asked in a patient history vary considerably depending on characteristics of patients, such as their age and their chief complaint. The format and content of a patient history also vary depending on whether the audiologist is the entry point for hearing healthcare or the patient is referred to the audiologist by another healthcare professional.

Some people seeking professional consultation for a hearing problem literally walk from the street into an audiology clinic. Parents with concerns about their child's hearing may also directly seek the services of an audiologist. An audiologist who is in the role of a primary healthcare professional is likely to use a general patient history format designed to gather diverse information that might be relevant to hearing or vestibular function.

Audiologists are more likely to use a patient history form designed for a specific type of auditory disorder or a vestibular disorder when a specialist like an otolaryngologist refers the patient. Most of the patient history questions pertain to the problem that is of most concern to the patient. Audiologists utilize special history forms for patients who are referred for diagnosis of problems such as imbalance, dizziness, and/or vertigo. Special history forms are also used for patients scheduled for evaluation of tinnitus or auditory processing disorders, or for those referred as candidates for a specific form of intervention.

The Diagnostic Game

Imagine that a patient with a commonly encountered diagnosis or etiology for a hearing loss arrives at the clinic. At that point, you don't know the diagnosis or anything about the patient's hearing or vestibular status. How can you discover the patient's diagnosis? Some simple facts from the patient's history will immediately help you to **rule out** many causes for the hearing loss, that is, you may scratch them off your list. "How old is the patient?" "What is the patient's gender?" These are always logical questions to ask at the beginning of a patient history. If the patient is an adult female, then you might ask: "Is the patient a young, middle-aged, or older adult?" If the patient is an elderly adult, then you can immediately eliminate from consideration or rule out dozens of possible etiologies for hearing loss that only affect children or young adults. Similarly, if the patient is a child, you will not even consider certain etiologies that rarely or never affect children.

You might continue the diagnostic process by seeking answers to multiple questions from either the history that the patient gives you or from the diagnostic hearing assessment. For example: "Did the onset of the hearing loss develop slowly over many years?" "Is the hearing loss due to inner ear dysfunction?" "Is the hearing loss greater in the high-frequency region, with a sloping audiogram configuration?" "Is the hearing loss *symmetrical* and about the same for both ears?" If the answer is "yes" to all of these questions, you might want to ask a few more questions regarding other signs and symptoms as you begin to consider a tentative etiology, questions like: "Does the patient experience dizziness or vertigo?" "Has the patient ever been exposed to loud sounds?" "Does the patient have any serious health problems?" "Is the patient under the care of a physician or receiving medical treatment for any health problem?" We'll assume for this hypothetical patient that the answer is "no" to all of these questions.

Let's try to reach a tentative diagnosis for this elderly female who is generally healthy. Testing shows a symmetrical high-frequency sensory hearing loss. She reports no history of noise exposure and no problems with dizziness or vertigo. Most audiologists could readily offer a logical explanation for the etiology or cause of the patient's hearing loss. Consider the information you have just gathered about the patient. Do you have in mind a probable etiology or diagnosis?

Naturally, you wouldn't be expected to confidently identify the most likely etiology without clinical experience and a thorough knowledge of audiology, including etiologies for hearing loss. Most clinical audiologists would arrive at the same tentative etiology for the patient's hearing loss, even with the rather cursory forgoing synopsis of the history and test findings. The most logical initial diagnosis for the patient is hearing loss associated with aging, a disorder called **presbycusis**. "Presby" means elder, and "acusis" means hearing loss.

Classification of Hearing Loss

You learned in Chapters 5 through 9 about types of hearing loss and how they're differentiated based on results of different hearing tests. With each patient, audiologists strive to classify auditory function by five or six general categories: (1) normal hearing, (2) conductive hearing loss, (3) sensory hearing loss, (4) mixed hearing loss, (5) neural hearing loss and, sometimes, (6) central auditory nervous system dysfunction or auditory processing disorder. Within each of these categories are many specific diagnoses. In Chapters 11 and 12, you'll learn about common diseases and disorders associated with each category of hearing loss.

What is the next step for audiologists, after they establish the diagnosis for a hearing problem? When most people think about diagnosis of a physical problem, they probably think the next step would be some form of medical or surgical treatment for the problem. Audiologists do not prescribe medications or perform surgery in the management of ear disease or hearing loss. Instead, audiologists take care of patients who have auditory or vestibular disorders that cannot be effectively treated with medicine or surgery.

You might be surprised to learn that most hearing loss is not medically or surgically treatable, particularly in adult populations. Indeed, for every 100 adult patients with hearing loss fewer than twenty are likely to benefit from medications or from a surgical procedure (Hall, Freeman, & Bratt, 1994; Zapala et al., 2010). The majority of persons that audiologists or physicians evaluate have a sensory hearing impairment due to inner ear dysfunction. The sensory hearing loss is most often the result of noise exposure, associated with aging, and/ or related to hereditary and genetic factors. The hypothetical patient with presbycusis cited above is a good example of this point. The majority of patients who seek healthcare services for hearing concerns are evaluated and ultimately managed by an audiologist rather than a physician.

When in Doubt, Refer Out

Audiologists must remain mindful that some patients in each category of hearing loss have medically or surgically treatable disorders or diseases. Following completion of diagnostic hearing testing, audiologists often refer patients to one or more physicians for consultation. Specific reasons for referral vary from one patient to the next, but the common reason is concern about a medical cause for the hearing loss. The physician usually conducts a physical examination and a medical workup that may include laboratory and radiological studies. Depending on the diagnosis, the physician may also begin some type of medical management such as administration of drugs or a surgical procedure. The patient may return to the audiologist for nonmedical management of permanent hearing impairment. Hearing aids are the most common form of nonmedical management of hearing loss.

Education and clinical training of audiologists includes repeated exposure to information on the signs and symptoms of serious ear disease that require prompt medical attention (Hall & Mueller, 1997; Steiger, 2005). Referrals of patients with possible ear disease or pathology are often made to an ear specialist called an **otologist**. Otology is a subspecialty of the ear, nose, and throat (ENT) specialty known as **otolaryngology**. Otolaryngologists are trained as surgeons. Thus, they can manage patients with operative procedures. Surgeries range from relatively simple surgeries performed in a day-surgery facility to complicated procedures performed with other specialists like brain surgeons. You'll learn in Chapter 11 about some surgical treatments for ear problems.

The American Academy of Otolaryngology—Head & Neck Surgery has identified ten criteria for medical referral of patients. Known as "Red Flags—Warning of Ear Disease," they include:

- Hearing loss with a positive history of any of a variety of diseases associated with hearing loss, a family history of hearing loss, or head trauma. Most of the diseases are reviewed in the next chapter.
- History of pain, active drainage, or bleeding from an ear.
- Hearing loss of sudden onset or rapidly progressing.

- Dizziness.
- Congenital or traumatic deformity of the ear.
- Appearance of blood, pus, cerumen plug, or foreign body in the ear canal.
- Conductive hearing loss or abnormal tympanogram.
- Unilateral or asymmetric hearing loss or bilateral hearing loss >80 dB.
- Unilateral or pulsing tinnitus (ringing or other sound in the ear).
- Unilateral or asymmetric poor speech discrimination (word recognition) scores.

Indeed, audiologists are bound by their scope of practice and ethical guidelines to refer to physicians any patients who have these findings by either history or hearing tests. Audiologists interact with different types of physicians in reaching hearing and vestibular disorder diagnoses.

To a large extent, referral of a patient to a specialist for a medical consultation or management is based on the pattern of auditory findings and suspicions about possible diseases or disorders. For example, if auditory findings point toward a disorder or disease affecting the ear, the patient will be referred to an otolaryngologist or perhaps a subspecialist like an otologist or a pediatric otolaryngologist.

Patients with auditory findings associated with central nervous system disorders or diseases or other findings suggesting possible neurological concerns might be referred to a neurologist or a psychiatrist for further evaluation. With regard to decisions about whether to consider referral to a physician, audiologists are wise to adhere to the clinical adage *"When in doubt, refer out!"*

 WebWatch

Documents detailing the scope of practice for audiology are available for review on the websites of the American Academy of Audiology and the American Speech-Language-Hearing Association. Additional information on the criteria for medical referral, called "Red Flags—Warning of Ear Disease" is available at the website for the American Academy of Otolaryngology—Head & Neck Surgery.

Hearing Loss and Hearing Handicap

The diagnostic process that audiologists follow goes beyond describing the type of hearing loss. The process also extends past referral of a patient to a medical specialist for diagnosis of the specific etiology of the hearing loss and possible medical management. A full and proper evaluation of a person with hearing impairment yields information about how the hearing loss affects communication. The assessment may also document how communication problems related to the hearing loss impact the patient's *psychosocial status* and **quality of life.**

These new terms need some explanation. Psychosocial behaviors and problems often associated with hearing loss include anxiety, irritability, social stress, withdrawal and isolation, loneliness, and even depression. Hearing loss can clearly have a negative impact on quality of life and also on the person's perception of his or her health. Quality of life refers to general well-being and the degree to which a person can enjoy life and pursue their personal interests and goals.

 ClinicalConnection

Paper-and-pencil inventory forms completed by a patient in an audiology clinic help to describe the impact of hearing loss on daily communication and quality of life. Inventories are also useful in identifying psychosocial effects of hearing loss, such as irritability, frustration, isolation, and depression. In Chapter 14, you will learn more about psychosocial problems in persons with hearing loss and how patients are helped with counseling.

Recognition of the difference between hearing and listening has been appreciated since antiquity. Put simply, we hear with our ears, but we listen with our brain. To use hearing for meaningful communication, we must not only passively perceive sounds like speech, we must also attend to what we are hearing and actively process auditory information. A complete diagnostic hearing assessment, therefore, must gather information on how hearing loss affects day-to-day communication in different listening environments or conditions. For children, the major concern is the influence of the hearing loss on speech and language acquisition.

For older children, it is also important to evaluate the effect of hearing loss on academic performance.

Findings on typical hearing tests in adult patients, such as the degree of hearing loss or word recognition scores, do not predict very accurately the extent of a person's actual hearing handicap. Two patients with the same audiogram patterns may report very different communicative experiences and very different degrees of difficulty in daily communication. One person might communicate effectively and perceive no hearing handicap, whereas the other might have serious complaints and concerns about his or her ability to communicate and might perceive a marked communicative disorder.

Factors that help to explain the discrepancy between hearing loss as documented with the audiogram and hearing handicap in everyday communication include **cognitive variables** like memory and processing time, personality characteristics, typical listening environments, and daily listening demands.

Diagnostic Site-of-Lesion Tests in Audiology: A Historical Perspective

Gradenigo (1893) is generally credited with first applying an auditory test in the differential diagnosis of sensorineural hearing impairment. The phrase **site-of-lesion** was often used because the goal was to find the location of pathology. The word *lesion* means pathology or injury. Major advances in the development of diagnostic audiology procedures for site-of-lesion assessment are summarized chronologically in Table 10.3. Traditional tests used in the past for diagnosis of different types of hearing loss will now be reviewed. The procedures are only mentioned briefly because all of them are outdated and rarely applied these days in hearing assessment of children or adults. However, valuable lessons have been learned from clinical experience with the classic diagnostic tests. This knowledge can be applied today in the description and differentiation of dysfunction anywhere in the auditory system.

Alternate Binaural Loudness Balance (ABLB) Test

The concept of differentiating cochlear and retrocochlear auditory dysfunction with clinical procedures was revived in 1936. The Englishman E. P. Fowler observed that in patients with unilateral sensory hearing impairment due to cochlear auditory dysfunction, an increase in intensity presented to both ears resulted in an unusually rapid growth of loudness in the impaired ear. Fowler coined the term **loudness recruitment** to describe this phenomenon and developed the **alternate binaural loudness balance (ABLB)** test to assess it.

The ABLB test compares loudness growth in an impaired ear versus a normal-hearing ear. The typical outcome found in patients with unilateral cochlear impairment is an abnormally rapid growth of loudness as pure tone stimulus intensity is increased above threshold in the impaired ear. The amount that intensity must be increased above threshold to create the sensation of equal loudness, called inter-aural loudness balance, is much less for the impaired ear than for the normal ear. There must be hearing loss in only one ear to perform the ABLB. The test is not appropriate for patients with similar hearing loss in both ears. Also, hearing thresholds must be normal (25 dB HL or better) in the noninvolved ear.

Dix, Hallpike, and Hood, working in England in 1948, reported on the clinical application of ABLB testing for differential diagnosis of cochlear versus eighth nerve disorders. The appearance of this publication for all practical purposes marked the beginning of traditional

TABLE 10.3   Chronological summary of major advances in classic diagnostic audiology procedures for site-of-lesion assessment.

Year	Procedure	Author (Year of Publication)
1935	Monaural loudness balance	Reger (1935)
1936	Alternate binaural loudness balance (ABLB)	Fowler (1936)
1946	Impedance audiometry	Metz (1952)
1947	Békésy audiometer	Békésy (1947)
1948	ABLB in site-of-lesion evaluation	Dix, Hallpike, & Hood (1949)
1948	Difference limen for intensity	Lüscher & Zwislocki (1951)
1957	Tone decay	Carhart (1957)
1959	Short increment sensitivity index (SISI)	Jerger, Shedd, & Harford (1958)
1960	Békésy threshold types	Jerger (1960)
1969	Acoustic reflex decay	Anderson, Barr, & Wedenberg (1970)
1971	Auditory brain stem response (ABR)	Jewett & Williston (1971)
1971	Performance-intensity functions for PB words	Jerger & Jerger (1974)
1972	Békésy forward-backward	Jerger, Jerger, & Mauldin (1972)
1974	Tone decay	Olsen & Noffsinger (1974)
1974b	Békésy comfortable loudness (BCL)	Jerger & Jerger (1974)
1975	Supra-threshold adaptation test (STAT)	Jerger & Jerger (1975)
1977–79	ABR in eighth nerve pathology	Selters & Brackmann (1977) Clemis & McGee (1979) Thomsen, Terkildsen, & Osterhammel (1978) Rosenhamer, 1977

diagnostic audiology. Soon, many other papers were published on the clinical application of the ABLB in patients with cochlear and retrocochlear auditory dysfunction.

Short Increment Sensitivity Index (SISI) Test

In the early 1950s James Jerger conducted research that led to the development of a diagnostic audiology procedure based on the difference limen for intensity. You're now quite familiar with a number of Jerger's important contributions to audiology. The procedure was called the *short increment sensitivity index test,* with the clever acronym SISI (Jerger, Shedd, & Harford, 1959). Just-noticeable differences or difference limens for intensity were described in Chapter 2. Briefly, *difference limen* is defined as "an increment in the physical intensity of a sound that a subject perceives as a change in loudness just 50 percent of the time" (Jerger, 1952, p. 1317).

In the conventional SISI test protocol, a patient hears a continuous tone at a test frequency such as 500 or 1000 Hz. The tone is 20 dB above the patient's hearing threshold at that frequency. The patient's task is to listen for brief, 200-ms presentations of the same pure tone frequency at an intensity increment that is 1 dB higher than the continuous tone. The intensity increment is superimposed on the continuous tone. The increments are presented periodically, such as every 5 seconds. Normal-hearing subjects and patients with neural auditory dysfunction cannot perceive the 1-dB increments, but patients with cochlear dysfunction hear them clearly.

Tone Decay Tests

Tone decay tests were common in the classic site-of-lesion test battery. In 1955 another Englishman, J. Derrick Hood, described decreased perception of a continuously presented tone in patients with neural auditory abnormalities. Hood collaborated at the time with Dix and Hallpike at the National Hospital for Nervous Diseases in London. A few years later, Raymond Carhart at Northwestern University popularized a clinical test for evaluating abnormal auditory adaptation that came to be known as the Carhart threshold tone decay test (Carhart, 1957). Numerous other investigators then applied the original tone decay test or developed and applied modified versions for differentiating cochlear from retrocochlear auditory dysfunction (Hall, 1991).

Tone decay is the phrase commonly used for a phenomenon formally known as *auditory adaptation*. With all tone decay tests, an audiologist presents a continuous tone to the patient and determines whether the patient's threshold for the tone changes or becomes poorer over time. A least a dozen different tests for tone decay were developed in the site-of-lesion diagnostic era (Hall, 1991). Each version of tone decay test was distinguished by a variation in measurement technique.

Tone decay is not an exclusive feature of auditory nerve pathology and abnormal auditory nerve function. Normal auditory nerve fibers show some degree of adaptation. Tone decay is also found in patients with presumed pure cochlear impairment. Excessive tone decay leading to loss of audibility has been reported in patients with a variety of peripheral auditory disorders, in addition to eighth nerve tumors and some CNS diseases (Hall, 1991). The specific site for adaptation in auditory function is not known. The chemical synapse between hair cells and auditory nerve fibers is one possible site. Even now, however, there is no definitive physiological explanation for the clinical phenomenon of tone decay.

Békésy Audiometry

In the late 1940s, Georg von Békésy described an automatic recording audiometer and a technique for assessing hearing threshold (von Békésy, 1947). You read about von Békésy in Chapter 1 in an overview of the scientific foundation of audiology. The so-called Békésy device was initially built expressly for von Békésy for the purpose of research at the Psycho-Acoustic Laboratory at Harvard University. A well-preserved Békésy audiometer manufactured in 1950 was shown earlier in Figure 5.1 (Chapter 5). Audiologists and otolaryngologists purchased Békésy audiometers for special diagnostic testing in the clinical setting. Indeed, Békésy audiometric findings were reported for a patient with a neural or retrocochlear tumor in the early 1950s (Reger & Kos, 1952).

The clinical role of Békésy audiometry was established with Jerger's systematic delineation in 1960 of four distinct Békésy tracing classifications among 434 patients diagnosed with normal hearing or conductive, cochlear, or eighth nerve pathology (Jerger, 1960). One of the Békésy tracing patterns was consistent with normal hearing or conductive hearing loss, one with sensory (cochlear) hearing loss, and two with neural auditory dysfunction. Over the next decade, Jerger and others confirmed the diagnostic value of variations of the Békésy audiometry techniques that differed based on whether the stimulus sound changed from low to high frequencies or whether the test was conducted near the patient's threshold or at higher-intensity levels (Jerger, Jerger, & Mauldin, 1972).

Second Generation Traditional Diagnostic Tests

Throughout the 1960s and into the mid-1970s, a second generation of these classic site-of-lesion procedures emerged. The newer versions of the tests were distinguished from their earlier counterparts by a single common feature. The newer tests were administered at supra-threshold intensities well above hearing threshold level (Hall, 1991). The supra-threshold testing approach offered two clinical advantages. At higher-intensity levels test time was shortened and the tests were more sensitive to auditory nerve dysfunction. There were supra-threshold versions of all major diagnostic procedures, including a modified SISI test, a high-intensity tone decay test like the supra-threshold adaptation test or STAT (Jerger & Jerger, 1975), and the Békésy Comfortable Loudness (BCL) test (Jerger & Jerger, 1974).

ClinicalConnection

The traditional diagnostic hearing tests are no longer applied in clinical hearing assessment in the United States and many other countries. Audiologists in locations or facilities where equipment for recording the auditory brain stem response is not available can turn to the old procedures for diagnostic hearing assessment of certain patients. Some testing for neural auditory dysfunction is helpful, particularly if brain-imaging technology is not readily available.

The End of an Era

The era of diagnostic audiometry with traditional behavioral tests drew to a rather unceremonious conclusion in the 1970s with increased clinical use of acoustic reflex recordings and independent international publications of clinical experience with the application of ABR for identification of neural or retrocochlear pathology (Clemis & McGee, 1979; Selters & Brackman, 1977; Terkildsen, Huis in't Veld, & Osterhammel, 1977). There were various reasons for the clinical preference of ABR over classic site-of-lesion tests, but the relatively high accuracy of ABR in identification of auditory nerve dysfunction predominated.

Advantages of Acoustic Reflex Recording. Measurement of acoustic stapedial reflex threshold and reflex decay offered multiple clinical advantages over the traditional behavioral diagnostic tests. Acoustic reflex measurement was objective, quick, and relatively sensitive for differentiation of cochlear from retrocochlear pathology (Anderson, Barr, & Wedenberg, 1970; Metz, 1952). In addition, acoustic reflex measurement in the suspected retrocochlear ear was not constrained by the hearing status of the opposite ear as it was for the ABLB test (Jerger, Harford, Clemis, & Alford, 1974).

Neurodiagnosis with Auditory Brain Stem Response. Diagnostic audiology changed dramatically within the decade following description by Jewett and Williston of a scalp-recorded auditory brain stem response (Jewett, Romano, & Williston, 1970; Jewett & Williston, 1971). Ironically, primitive instrumentation for measurement of sensory evoked responses was described initially in 1947 by the Englishman Dawson just as his British compatriots Dix, Hallpike, and Hood (1948) were investigating abnormal growth of loudness and difference limen for intensity in sensorineural hearing impairment.

Advent of Brain Imaging Techniques. The development of computerized tomography (CT) in the mid-1970s was also a major factor in the decline of site-of-lesion testing. Computerized tomography offered physicians a far more sensitive and specific means of acquiring structural evidence of tumors affecting the eighth nerve. With the introduction of magnetic resonance imaging (MRI) in the 1980s, physicians had access to even greater precision for anatomical imaging of tumors. Figure 10.3 shows an MRI image for a patient with a tumor affecting the auditory nerve.

FIGURE 10.3

Magnetic resonance image (MRI) of the brain showing a tumor in the region of the right cerebello-pontine angle and affecting the auditory (8th cranial) nerve. The tumor is indicated with an arrow.

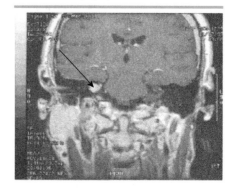

Modern MRI scanning permits identification and confident verification of location and size of even small acoustic tumors less than 1 mm in width. The classic test battery became progressively less important as CT and MRI became readily available in most large hospitals. In the 1990s MRI technology even began to replace ABR for timely detection of tumors affecting the retrocochlear auditory pathways.

Current Diagnostic Hearing Testing

No "standard" hearing test battery is used consistently with all patients. However, a series of selected procedures are almost always performed for hearing assessment with alert and cooperative adult patients. You've already learned about all of these procedures in previous chapters. Traditionally, audiologists relied heavily on three rather basic procedures for hearing assessment of adult patients and most older children, namely, (1) air-conduction pure tone audiometry, (2) bone-conduction audiometry, and (3) simple speech audiometry, like word recognition in quiet.

Audiologists now also incorporate additional procedures into the diagnostic test battery. Otoacoustic emissions (OAEs) have greater sensitivity to cochlear dysfunction than the pure tone audiogram. Special speech audiometry procedures are more sensitive to disorders of auditory processing and central auditory nervous system function than simple word recognition scores. In short, traditional tests of hearing sensitivity using simple non-speech sounds like pure tones and assessment of word recognition in quiet are often inadequate for complete description of hearing.

Selection of Diagnostic Procedures

Step-by-Step Diagnostic Process. As you've learned already, decisions regarding which procedures to perform in hearing assessment are highly dependent on information revealed in the patient history or identified by the referral source. The basic hearing test battery is similar for most adult patients, but more detailed and diverse diagnostic assessment is sometimes appropriate, depending on a specific patient's major complaint or concern. For example, a more conventional test battery is usually administered to an elderly patient whose hearing loss appears to be age related. In contrast, distinctly different test batteries are used for assessment of a patient whose chief complaint is vertigo or imbalance or a patient who comes to the clinic seeking help for troublesome tinnitus.

Effective diagnostic assessment of patients is usually an adaptive process. That is, auditory or vestibular function is repeatedly probed and tested with various procedures. Decisions about what procedure is applied next are based largely on the findings for the previous procedure or procedures. In this way, the diagnostic test battery is not static but, rather, quite dynamic. A common format for illustrating the dynamic flow of the decision-making process is called a decision-making tree or a flowchart.

Assessment of Older Children and Adults. Figure 10.4 shows a flowchart for the straightforward hearing assessment of a normal-hearing older child or adult. Following review of the patient history, the first formal step in almost all hearing assessments is otoscopic inspection of the external ear canal. It is important to verify that the ear canal is free of excessive cerumen or foreign bodies before inserting probes for auditory tests.

Excessive cerumen may interfere with valid measurement of hearing or even pose a risk to the patient upon insertion of a probe. Surprisingly diverse foreign bodies may be discovered in the ear canal, especially among children. Common foreign bodies include small pebbles and sticks, bits of food, and various species of insects. Qualified healthcare personnel, such as

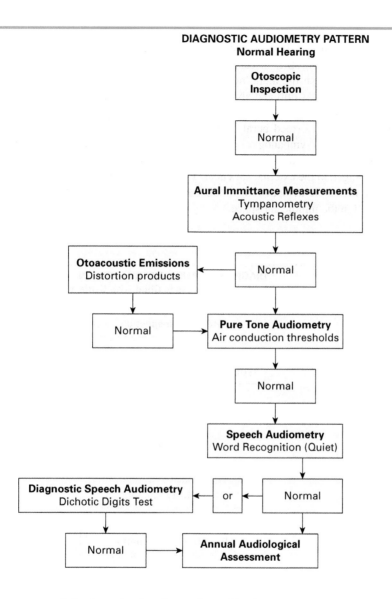

FIGURE 10.4

Flowchart of major procedures in a basic hearing test battery for an older child or adult with normal hearing sensitivity. Steps in the testing are described in the text.

a physician or an audiologist trained and experienced in the process, must remove excessive cerumen or foreign bodies before a hearing test can be completed.

Figure 10.4 and similar flowcharts in this chapter and elsewhere in the book reveal that the diagnostic hearing testing process is really a series of "if" and "then" decisions. In other words, if test A produces finding X, then test B will be performed. If test A produces finding Y, then test C will be performed. If test C produces finding Z, then test D will be performed and so forth. Certain auditory disorders are systematically ruled out or eliminated from consideration with repetitions of this adaptive step-by-step process. Other auditory disorders are considered as possibilities and then further evaluated. For the normal-hearing example, each test yielding normal findings simply leads to the next procedure in the test battery. The patient presumably came to the clinic with hearing-related complaints. Therefore, at the conclusion of a typical test battery yielding entirely normal findings it is reasonable to continue evaluation with administration of a screening measure of auditory processing, as depicted by the dichotic digits test in the lower left portion of Figure 10.4.

Assessment of a Young Child. Figure 10.5 illustrates the diagnostic process for a young school-age child with the diagnosis of a middle ear infection. You will learn in Chapter 11 about ear infections and other diseases or disorders affecting the ear. The initial remarkable finding was noted when the audiologist conducted an otoscopic inspection of the ear. The tympanic membrane was dull and abnormal in appearance. This was the first clue or sign of possible middle ear disorder and associated conductive hearing loss.

An audiologist performed aural immittance measurement a few minutes later. Testing showed a flat (type B) tympanogram. You'll recall from Chapter 8 that tympanometry measures the flexibility or compliance of the tympanic membrane and middle ear system as air pressure is changed in the external ear canal. The finding of a type B tympanogram confirmed the abnormal otoscopic evidence of middle ear dysfunction. The finding suggested the possibility of fluid in the middle ear space.

FIGURE 10.5

Flowchart of major procedures in a basic hearing test battery for a child with an ear infection. Steps in the testing are described in the text.

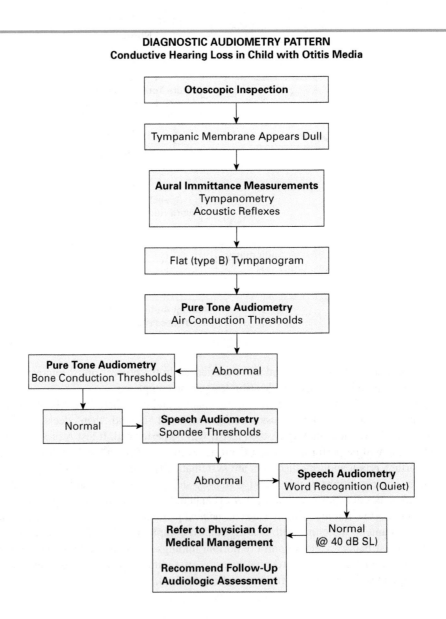

Next, it was reasonable to wonder whether the middle ear disorder was associated with hearing loss. Pure tone audiometry with air-conduction stimulation confirmed a hearing loss, yet hearing thresholds were normal for bone-conduction testing. Hearing sensitivity was worse when sounds were presented to the ear with an earphone rather than a bone vibrator. You've already learned that an air-bone gap is a typical finding in conductive hearing loss. The abnormal hearing thresholds for air-conduction pure tone audiometry were confirmed by an elevation in the speech reception threshold measured with spondee words.

Word recognition performance was then assessed for lists of single-syllable words appropriate for the limited vocabulary of a young child. The monosyllabic words were presented at an intensity level 40 dB above pure tone thresholds and speech reception thresholds. Word recognition scores were excellent for each ear (100%). This finding was also compatible with a conductive hearing loss. The child, with normal inner ear function, had no problem with the perception of speech at a high intensity level.

Selection of Procedures for a Test Battery. To summarize, results for early tests in the battery influenced the audiologist's decisions about which tests to administer next. The audiologist selected subsequent tests that were likely to contribute or add value to the diagnostic process and to the accurate diagnosis of auditory dysfunction. The pattern of findings for the test battery led the audiologist to a confident decision to refer the child to a physician for possible medical management of the middle ear disorder, as indicated in the lower portion of Figure 10.5. A follow-up assessment was scheduled to confirm improvement of hearing following medical management.

An optimal hearing test battery consists of procedures with proven sensitivity and specificity to various types and anatomical locations of hearing impairment. An effective test battery includes procedures that are likely to detect the patient's auditory abnormality or abnormalities. This is referred to as test sensitivity. An effective test battery also consists of one or more procedures that have test specificity. In other words, results of the test help to determine whether a patient has a specific disorder. Selection of tests is also dependent on a patient's main concerns or complaints and findings of other prior test procedures. In addition, selection of each procedure in the test battery is based on certain patient characteristics like age and cognitive status.

Importantly, procedures included within a test battery should add value to the diagnosis of an auditory disorder and ultimately to patient outcome. For adult and pediatric patient populations, guidelines established by national professional organizations like the American Academy of Audiology (AAA) and the American Speech-Language-Hearing Association (ASHA) and multidisciplinary committees like the Joint Committee on Infant Hearing assist audiologists in making appropriate decisions regarding the test battery. Guidelines for best practices in hearing testing of children and adults are reviewed next.

Best Practices in Audiology Today: Clinical Guidelines

Best practices are evidence-based clinical procedures and techniques for diagnosis and management of hearing, vestibular, and related disorders. The term *evidence-based clinical practice* is now used commonly in audiology, speech pathology, and health professions in general. *Evidence-based* means that test and treatment procedures and protocols are founded on research findings. An audiologist or speech pathologist following evidence-based guidelines for best practices is providing standard of care. **Standard of care** is a phrase used to define specific clinical services and quality of services that are consistent with the standards for the professions of audiology and speech pathology.

In providing standard of care, an audiologist or speech pathologist adheres to guidelines established by nationally recognized committees, agencies, or professional organizations. There has been a strong move in recent years toward evidence-based clinical practice in audiology and speech pathology. What is the proof of effective clinical services? The best proof is evidence from research that meets certain criteria or grades for quality.

Grades of Evidence

There are different strengths of research evidence based on how the evidence is obtained. The strongest evidence is generated in well-designed studies meeting certain requirements for good research. Some research studies focus on documenting the validity of diagnostic test procedures, whereas others investigate the efficacy of a specific treatment.

Grade I Evidence. Grade I evidence is strong and is usually obtained from randomized controlled trials or well-designed clinical studies. In a randomized clinical trial in audiology, for example, one group of subjects might be evaluated using a new clinical procedure or managed with a new technique. The subjects who are being evaluated are sometimes called the *experimental group*. Then the results are compared to those for a *control group*. The control group consists of subjects evaluated or managed using an existing or conventional approach or perhaps subjects receiving no treatment at all. In auditory research the control group often is a group of people with normal hearing.

Control subjects are carefully selected to be very similar to the experimental group, for example of the same age, gender, and medical history, differing only in the variable or property that is being studied. In truth, few studies published in the audiology literature report Grade I evidence in support of specific techniques for clinical assessment of hearing or vestibular function, or in support of specific management approaches for hearing or related disorders. Randomized clinical trials are often difficult to conduct for a variety of scientific reasons, and they usually require considerable research funding.

Grade II Evidence. Grade II evidence is not as strong as Grade I evidence. Grade II evidence is generated from clinical studies that are based on retrospective data analysis. Test findings are gathered and reviewed at some point after the subject visited an audiology clinic. A study that looks back at clinic data already collected is called a retrospective study. Grade II evidence also results from clinical studies in which subjects are not randomized or there is not a control group of subjects.

Grade II audiology research evidence is often reported in peer-reviewed published papers. You'll recall that a peer-reviewed paper undergoes a rigorous evaluation by experts on the topic before it is published. Unfortunately, without data for a control group of untreated subjects it is often difficult to be sure that the benefit is really due to the treatment.

Grade III Evidence. Grade III evidence is the weakest form of evidence. It is not obtained in a formal study. Grade III evidence is based on current or longstanding clinical practice and not on research findings. Unfortunately, clinical practice in audiology and speech pathology is often based on Grade III evidence.

Demand for Evidence-Based Practice

Increasingly, within the past twenty years, third-party payers like health insurance companies covering the costs of healthcare have expected audiologists and speech pathologists to provide evidence-based clinical services. Regulatory agencies and groups that oversee healthcare practices and healthcare organizations also emphasize the importance of evidence-based clinical practice. And, organizations representing healthcare professionals, including audiology and speech pathology, are now firmly behind the effort to develop and implement evidence-based clinical practices.

Clinical Guidelines: Good News and Bad News

Goals for Clinical Guidelines. As described earlier, clinical guidelines are formal recommendations developed by well-respected representatives of a task force or committee within a national organization, a multidisciplinary group, or a regulatory board or body. The Joint Committee on Infant Hearing, described in the section above on hearing screening, is a good example of such a group. The 2007 JCIH Position Statement is an example of clinical guidelines pertaining to pediatric audiology practice (JCIH, 2007).

The main goals of clinical guidelines are to

WebWatch

You can locate dozens of evidence-based guidelines for various audiology and speech pathology services and patient populations on the websites of the two main organizations representing the professions, the American Academy of Audiology or AAA and the American Speech-Language-Hearing Association or ASHA.

- Improve quality of patient care.
- Improve consistency in care. That is, guidelines should lead to greater consistency in the procedures administered to patients presenting with the same clinical problem.
- Empower patients. Guidelines help patients know what to expect of healthcare.
- Educate patients. Armed with knowledge gained from published guidelines combined with resources available on the Internet, patients sometimes are able to educate healthcare providers on appropriate care and treatment options.

Clinical guidelines can positively influence public policy and reimbursement trends. In addition, clinical guidelines may reassure healthcare providers who are uncertain about the appropriateness of their diagnosis or treatment for a patient.

Drawbacks of Clinical Guidelines. Guidelines are not without disadvantages, including unintended or unanticipated problems arising with the clinical implementation of the guidelines. For example, clinical guidelines may have unintended legal consequences when an audiologist or speech pathologist inadvertently or unknowingly does not follow guidelines and is later challenged legally. Conflicts may arise between national consensus guidelines and community practice of audiology or speech pathology. In other words, experts may recommend clinical procedures or protocols that are not consistent with or feasible for widespread clinical practice.

For a variety of reasons, there is general agreement in the medical community that guidelines are not a "magic pill" for correcting problems of inferior healthcare. Clinical guidelines play an important positive role in the clinical practice of audiology and speech pathology, but the limitations and possible negative effects of clinical guidelines must be recognized.

The Vestibular Test Battery

Assessment and management of vestibular and balance disorders is within the audiology scope of practice. Audiologists are trained to complete comprehensive diagnostic assessment of persons with various complaints that might be related to the vestibular system. The vestibular system consists of structures within the ear, nerves that connect these structures with the brain, and then vestibular centers in the brainstem. Complaints of patients with abnormal vestibular function include lightheadedness, dizziness, imbalance, unsteadiness, or **vertigo**. Patients with vertigo complain that the world seems to spin around them. Often physicians refer patients with balance and vestibular complaints to audiologists for the diagnostic assessment. Due to connections between the vestibular system and systems that control eye movements, audiologists can utilize precise measurement of eye movements to diagnose vestibular disorders.

Doctor of Audiology programs include coursework and supervised clinical experience in the diagnosis and management of vestibular disorders. Some audiologists specialize in this aspect of the profession. We'll conclude the chapter with a brief review of a test battery for evaluation of vestibular function.

Similarities and Differences in Auditory and Vestibular Systems

You learned toward the end of Chapter 3 that the auditory and vestibular systems share much in common. If it has been awhile since you read Chapter 3, this would be a good time to return for a quick review. Despite the similarities in structure and function, there are also distinct differences between these two related systems. To a large extent, anatomical and physiological differences between the two systems explain the divergent approaches audiologists take in the clinical assessment of patients with auditory and vestibular complaints and disorders.

Procedures for Vestibular Assessment

Clinical Examination with Frenzel Goggles. Vestibular assessment is usually conducted with highly sophisticated equipment in a clinical laboratory, with computer-assisted analysis of test results. However, it is possible to perform relatively simple maneuvers to activate the peripheral vestibular apparatus and to monitor eye movements using specially designed goggles in a typical clinical examination room. Figure 10.6 shows how **Frenzel goggles** permit clear visualization of eye movements during two steps of a vestibular procedure known as the *Dix Hallpike maneuver.*

The lenses of the Frenzel goggles magnify the patient's eyes, making it easier for an audiologist to visually detect and monitor eye movements under different test conditions. Frenzel goggles also help reduce the likelihood that the patient will visually fixate on an object during a procedure. The ocular response to vestibular stimulation is altered and suppressed when a patient fixes his or her gaze on an object rather than simply staring forward during testing.

Measuring Nystagmus. **Nystagmus** is movement of the eyes either horizontally, vertically, or in a clockwise or counterclockwise direction (Jacobson & Shepard, 2007). In some cases, eye movements in nystagmus are in multiple directions. Nystagmus has a slow phase

FIGURE 10.6

A patient wearing Frenzel goggles during two steps of the Dix Hallpike vestibular procedure performed by an audiologist in a clinic. Courtesy of Devin McCaslin at Vanderbilt University.

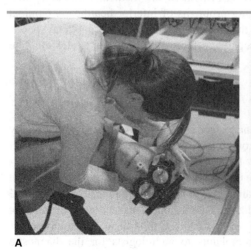
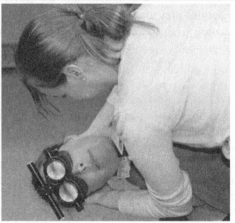

A   **B**

or movement, and a fast phase in the opposite direction. Repetitive fast eye movements in the same direction are often referred to as *beating*. So, nystagmus may be described as right beating or left beating. By convention, horizontal eye movements to the right side are plotted upward when printed out or displayed on a computer screen, whereas eye movements to the left side are displayed going downward. For vertical nystagmus, eye movements in an upward direction are shown upward on the graph and eye movements in a downward direction are plotted downward.

The types of nystagmus and the conditions under which nystagmus is observed or recorded have diagnostic significance. Nystagmus may be spontaneous and observed or recorded with the patient in an immobile sitting position with the eyes viewing a target in front of the patient. *Spontaneous nystagmus* usually is a sign of an imbalance or asymmetry in the peripheral vestibular system, with less or greater activity on one side than the other.

Nystagmus may also be produced by various maneuvers with patients like rapid head shaking from side to side or placement of the patient's head into a different position. The procedure known as the Dix Hallpike maneuver involves movement of the head in a specific way to elicit a vestibular response, as shown in Figure 10.6. Nystagmus is also effectively elicited with irrigation of the external ear canal with *caloric stimulation,* consisting of warm (44°C) and cool (30°C) water or air.

The ENG/VNG Test Battery. A common clinical approach for assessing the vestibular system is referred to as **electronystagmography (ENG)** or **video-nystagmography (VNG)**. These long words simply describe techniques for recording electrical changes associated with eye movements during vestibular testing. Nystagmus during ENG testing is detected as tiny changes in electrical activity, using electrodes placed at the outside and above the eyes. Figure 10.7 shows a patient prepared for VNG detection of eye movements during caloric stimulation and other test procedures. It is important to use calibrated equipment to record valid ENG/VNG measurements. Also, a patient is not allowed to take certain medication prior to measurement of ENG/VNG, particularly medications that suppress or otherwise alter the vestibular response.

Additional Vestibular Procedures. Additional procedures are often included in a comprehensive vestibular test battery, although most patients do not undergo all procedures. *Rotational testing* is performed with the patient in a special chair that can be programmed by a computer to turn precisely to the left or the right. Some patients who are about to undergo rotational testing in a rotary chair mistakenly think that it will spin them quickly like a ride at an amusement park. However, the speed of the angular acceleration and the velocity of the rotary movement produced by the rotary chair are relatively slow. For example, the chair may turn 100° (a little less than one-third of the way around) in about one second.

During rotational testing, the head is secured and stationary while eye positions are recorded as they are during ENG/VNG. The results of rotational testing include: (1) phase, or timing, of eye movement compared to chair movement; (2) gain, or amount of eye movement compared to chair

FIGURE 10.7

Photograph of patient prepared to under go video-nystagmography (VNG) during caloric stimulation. An enlarged view of the eyes is shown on the monitor in the left portion of the figure. Equipment for caloric stimulation with warm and cool air is shown in lower right portion of the photograph (see arrow). Courtesy of Benigno Sierra-Irizarry, AuD (Colonel, USAF, Ret).

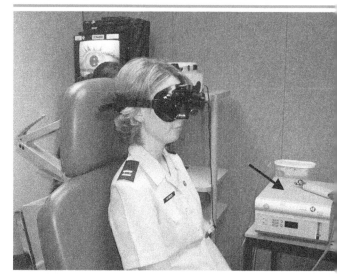

LEADERS AND LUMINARIES

Richard Gans

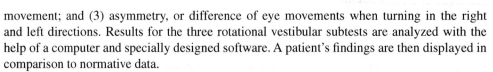

Richard Gans received his PhD from The Ohio State University in Auditory and Vestibular Physiology. He's now an adjunct professor at the University of South Florida, Nova Southeastern University, and the University of Pittsburgh. Dr. Gans served as President of the American Academy of Audiology from 2004 until 2005.

Dr. Gans is a leader in the development of vestibular evaluation and rehabilitation techniques. He utilizes the techniques in his clinical practice. Dr. Gans also gives continuing education workshops and seminars on vestibular techniques to audiologists and physicians worldwide.

Dr. Gans is the author of many journal articles as well as the book *Vestibular Rehabilitation: Protocols and Programs*. He's the founder and executive director of The American Institute of Balance (AIB) in Largo, Florida, one of the country's largest treatment centers for balance disorders.

movement; and (3) asymmetry, or difference of eye movements when turning in the right and left directions. Results for the three rotational vestibular subtests are analyzed with the help of a computer and specially designed software. A patient's findings are then displayed in comparison to normative data.

Computerized dynamic posturography is performed to evaluate balance or the ability of a person to remain in a vertical position over the body's center of gravity (Jacobson & Shepard, 2007). Balance is maintained by the coordination of information from three different senses and systems: (1) the somatosensory sense that detects the surface that the person is standing on and includes information from touch, joints between bones, and muscles; (2) the visual sense that provides information on the position of the head in comparison to objects around the person; and (3) the vestibular sense that provides information on gravitation and movement of the head in linear or angular directions.

FIGURE 10.8

Photograph of patient undergoing computerized dynamic posturography. Courtesy of Benigno Sierra-Irizarry, AuD (Colonel, USAF, Ret).

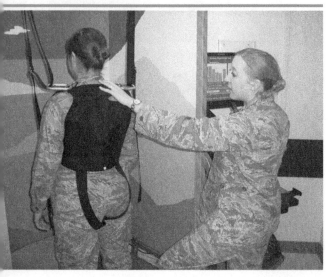

Figure 10.8 shows equipment used in computerized dynamic posturography. Specialized instrumentation is used to minimize visual and somatosensory information. Testing systematically evaluates the vestibular component and these two additional components of balance in an attempt to identify the pattern of balance abnormality. You will notice in Figure 10.8 that the patient is secured with a harness during testing to prevent a fall-related injury.

A third and relatively recent addition to the comprehensive vestibular test battery is the **vestibular evoked myogenic potential**, or **VEMP**. The VEMP has gained popularity as a clinical procedure because it provides information on the function of structures and pathways not assessed with other vestibular procedures, such as ENG/VNG. The VEMP depends on activation of the saccule. You may recall from Chapter 3 that the saccule leads to the inferior vestibular nerve and vestibular pathways in the brain stem and spinal cord.

A VEMP is recorded with the same type of instrumentation used to record the auditory brain stem response (ABR), so many audiologists are prepared to include the VEMP in their test battery without the need for purchase of additional equipment (Hall, 2007). The VEMP is recorded by stimulating the ear with a very high intensity sound as changes in tension of the sternocleidomastoid muscle or ocular muscles are detected with an electrode placed on the muscle or electrodes placed under the eyes (Hall, 2007). The sterno-cleidomastoid is a large neck muscle that is important in controlling position of the head. During VEMP measurement high-intensity sound is presented to the patient via earphones or via a bone vibrator using auditory evoked response equipment.

The comprehensive vestibular test battery just described is administered in most large medical centers and other clinics providing services to patients with balance or vestibular disturbances. The results of a vestibular test battery are analyzed and interpreted within the context of information gleaned from a specialized patient history and often information from a physical examination and review of medications, radiological studies, and laboratory tests. With the review, analysis, and interpretation of all available information, it is almost always possible to differentiate among dizziness, imbalance, and vertigo— three problems that are often confused and misunderstood.

 WebWatch

You can view dozens of videos showing a variety of vestibular tests and maneuvers on YouTube with a search using key words like "vestibular testing."

 ClinicalConnection

Diseases and disorders causing vestibular and balance disorders are reviewed briefly in Chapters 11 and 12. Then you'll learn in Chapter 16 how audiologists can successfully treat patients with specific vestibular and balance abnormalities using maneuvers and therapy performed in the clinic.

PULLING IT ALL TOGETHER

Early and accurate diagnosis of hearing impairment and vestibular disorders is an important goal for clinical audiologists. Infants offer perhaps the best example of the importance of diagnostic hearing assessment. Identification of hearing loss begins optimally within the first day or two after birth, diagnostic auditory assessment is completed a month or two later, and intervention begins by the sixth month. Accurate diagnosis of any hearing or vestibular disorder is a critical step toward management in persons of all ages. The diagnostic process begins with a completed and focused patient history. Then, using a variety of auditory procedures (as reviewed in earlier chapters), from traditional behavioral measures like pure tone audiometry to the latest electroacoustic and electrophysiological techniques, the audiologist differentiates among types of auditory and vestibular dysfunction, defines the amount of hearing loss, and then develops a strategy for management that is most likely to lead to a good outcome and patient satisfaction.

You are now prepared to learn about different patient populations and specific disorders involving peripheral auditory and vestibular structures, primarily the ear and the central nervous system regions involved in hearing loss, vestibular dysfunction, and related disorders.

READINGS

Desmond, A. (2004). *Vestibular function: Evaluation and treatment.* New York: Thieme.

Hall, J. W. III, & Mueller, H. G. III. (1997). *Audiologists' desk reference: Volume I. Diagnostic audiology, principles, procedures, and practices.* San Diego: Singular Publishing.

Herdman, S. (2007). *Vestibular rehabilitation* (3rd ed.). Philadelphia: F. A. Davis.

Jacobson, G. P., & Shepard, N. T. (2007). *Balance function assessment and management.* San Diego: Plural Publishing.

Jerger, S., & Jerger, J. (1981). *Auditory disorders: A manual for clinical evaluation.* Boston: Little, Brown and Company.

Mueller, H. G. III, & Hal,l J. W. III. (1998). *Audiologists' desk reference: Volume II. Audiologic management, rehabilitation and terminology.* San Diego: Singular Publishing.

Musiek, F. E., & Baran, J. A. (2007) *The auditory system: Anatomy, physiology, and clinical correlates.* Boston: Allyn & Bacon.

PART III

11 Outer Ear, Middle Ear, and Inner Ear Disorders

LEARNING OBJECTIVES

In this chapter, you will learn:

- Why an understanding of diseases and disorders affecting the ear is important for health care and educational professionals working with children and adults
- About the prevalence of types of hearing loss, that is, how common they are
- That factors in the prevalence of hearing loss include patient age, gender, and family history of hearing loss
- About disorders affecting the outer ear, ranging from normal variations like cerumen (ear wax) in the ear canal to serious pathology such as cancerous growths on the pinna
- About a variety of disorders affecting the middle ear, including middle ear infection, the most common health problem in children prompting a visit to a physician
- That hereditary hearing impairment accounts for about 50% of all hearing impairment present at birth
- That more than 100 genes for hearing loss have been discovered to date
- About syndromes that are associated with hearing loss and vestibular dysfunction
- That the most common causes of inner ear dysfunction in adult patients are excessive noise exposure or advancing age
- About cochlear pathologies that require prompt medical management
- That some drugs used to treat patients with health problems cause hearing loss

KEY TERMS

Aural atresia
Cholesteatoma
Craniofacial abnormalities or anomalies
Cytomegalovirus (CMV)
Foreign body
Hyperacusis
Malignant
Ménière's disease
Meningitis
Microtia
Myringotomy
Neoplasm
Otitis externa
Otitis media
Otosclerosis
Ototoxic
Perforation
Preauricular pits and tags
Prebycusis
Pseudohypacusis
Sensorineural
Stenosis
Syndromes
Tinnitus

CHAPTER FOCUS

An understanding of disorders affecting the outer ear, the middle ear, and/or the inner ear is important for professionals working with children and adults with hearing loss and with other communication disorders. The combined inclusion of the two words "and/or" here is important as some hearing loss may be due to dysfunction or abnormalities in more than one part of the ear. Audiologists, speech-language pathologists, educators of the hearing impaired, classroom teachers, and other professionals responsible for providing services to persons with hearing impairment will regularly encounter many of the disorders reviewed in this chapter.

In this chapter, you'll be introduced to the most common etiologies of hearing loss in children and adults. The review of outer ear, middle ear, and inner ear diseases and disorders may at first seem rather detailed and

> **CHAPTER FOCUS** *Concluded*
>
> technical. However, the information in this chapter is in fact a superficial overview of a sample of the diseases that can affect hearing. There are many hundreds of scientific articles, book chapters, and even entire textbooks devoted to some of the topics that are covered briefly in this chapter. Our focus is on the information most important for nonmedical professionals who are responsible for evaluating hearing loss and providing rehabilitation and therapy services for persons with hearing impairment.
>
> The chapter begins with a refresher on the concept of diagnosis and the importance of the diagnostic test battery in hearing assessment. Then, we'll review diseases and auditory disorders following an anatomical sequence from the outer ear to the inner ear. You'll first learn about causes of hearing loss that involve the pinna and external ear canal. Next we'll highlight some of the middle ear disorders that produce hearing loss. Middle ear disease is a very common cause of hearing loss, particularly in children. We'll conclude with a review of inner ear abnormalities and their impact on auditory function and hearing. Inner ear diseases and disorders account for highest proportion of patients with permanent hearing loss.
>
> Those are the topics included in this chapter. It is appropriate to note here several disorders that were left out of the chapter. One disorder is false or exaggerated hearing loss. The technical term for false or exaggerated hearing loss is **pseudohypacusis**. Pseudohypacusis is excluded because it is not an abnormality involving the outer, middle, or inner ear. In fact, many patients with the initial diagnosis of pseudohypacusis actually have entirely normal auditory function. Diagnosis and management of pseudohypacusis is reviewed in Chapter 15.
>
> **Tinnitus** and **hyperacusis** are two other disorders that are not covered here. Tinnitus is sound like ringing, buzzing, or roaring heard by a patient even in the absence of an external sound stimulus. Tinnitus is a symptom of many of the inner ear diseases reviewed in this chapter, but it is not a disease itself. Hyperacusis is intolerance to loud sound. It too is a symptom, rather than a disease. Most patients with hyperacusis actually have entirely normal hearing sensitivity. Assessment and management of tinnitus and hyperacusis are also discussed in Chapter 15.

Why Knowledge of Ear Disorders Is Important

Some audiologists and speech pathologists provide services exclusively to infants and young children. Audiologists involved in newborn hearing screening and the diagnosis of infant hearing loss must be familiar with the many risk factors for infant hearing loss, genetic factors in hearing impairment, and syndromes that include hearing loss as a component. It's also important for audiologists to be aware of the wide variety of diseases associated with hearing loss at or soon after birth. Speech pathologists who deliver early intervention services to the birth to 3 years population need to have a good appreciation and understanding of middle ear disease and how it affects hearing. The same statement is true for audiologists and speech pathologists involved in hearing screening of preschool children.

Audiologists and speech-language pathologists who interact with older children and adults encounter a diverse collection of different causes for hearing loss. For example, exposure to excessive and potentially harmful levels of sound, either noise or music, is one of the most common causes of hearing loss in older children and adults. Early recognition of sound-induced auditory dysfunction and awareness of appropriate steps to reduce risk may prevent permanent serious hearing impairment. Medical referral of patients who might have a disease or pathology is almost always important for accurate diagnosis and the most effective management. Immediate referral to an otolaryngologist or otologist is required for adult patients with certain test findings, such as evidence of middle ear dysfunction or the rapid onset of a sensorineural hearing loss.

Hearing loss is a very common health problem among the elderly. Audiologists and speech pathologists providing services to older adults can play a valuable role in identification, diagnosis, and management of age-related auditory dysfunction. Appropriate intervention for hearing loss in the elderly can substantially improve communication, cognitive functioning, quality of life, and even general health status.

You are now well prepared to learn about the many disorders or diseases that affect the auditory system, and their impact on hearing function. In Chapter 3 you learned about functional anatomy of the peripheral auditory system and the central auditory nervous system. The peripheral auditory system consists of the outer ear, middle ear, inner ear, and auditory nerve, whereas the central auditory nervous system begins at the lower portion of the brainstem and ends with the auditory cerebral cortex.

In Chapters 4 through 8 you studied a variety of procedures used to evaluate auditory function. You read about behavioral tests such as pure tone and speech audiometry. You also were introduced to objective measures of auditory function, such as acoustic immittance procedures, otoacoustic emissions, and auditory evoked responses. Audiologists select certain tests to efficiently and effectively evaluate auditory function of each patient.

Differential Diagnosis Revisited

The concept of differential diagnosis was reviewed in the previous chapter. You were introduced there to specific strategies that apply clinical test procedures in the diagnosis of auditory and vestibular dysfunction. Remember that the goal of differential diagnosis is to efficiently narrow down the likely etiologies or causes for the patient's signs and symptoms. The term *etiology* is generally used in medicine and audiology when referring to the cause of a disease or disorder.

Now, we'll systematically discuss many of the etiologies of hearing loss and vestibular abnormalities in children and adults. In this chapter we'll focus on etiologies for auditory dysfunction involving the outer ear, the middle ear, and the inner ear. Etiologies for retrocochlear auditory dysfunction and abnormalities involving the central auditory nervous system are covered in the following chapter.

Prevalence of Hearing Loss and Vestibular Disorders

Some causes for hearing loss are more common than others. Prevalence of an etiology for hearing loss is an estimate of how common the hearing loss occurs in a population during a certain time period, like a year. The prevalence of different causes of hearing loss varies greatly. Some causes of hearing loss are very rare, while others may affect the majority of people in a certain population. Also, prevalence for a specific type of hearing loss may be very different for males and females or for children and adults.

Table 11.1 illustrates the widely varying prevalence values for different causes of hearing loss. Some of the etiologies listed in the table are often encountered in clinical practice. The two most common causes of hearing loss are exposure to high-intensity noise and age-related hearing loss, or *presbycusis*. Noise-induced hearing loss and presbycusis are good examples of etiologies for cochlear dysfunction not associated with pathology and not treatable medically. Management of patients with these disorders is mainly the responsibility of audiologists. Other causes for hearing loss are far less common, but they are associated with diseases

TABLE 11.1
Prevalence of hearing loss in a general population.

Etiology	Estimated Prevalence
Presbycusis	25%
65 to 74 years	30–35%
>74 years	40–50%
Noise-induced hearing loss	15%
Chronic otitis media	4.5%
Ménière's disease	0.15%
Otosclerosis	0.06%
Sudden SNHL	0.02%
Cholesteatoma	0.01%
Multiple sclerosis	0.01%
Labyrinthitis	0.004%
Vestibular schwannoma	0.002%

Adapted from Zapala, D. A., et al. (2010). Safety of audiology direct access for Medicare patients complaining of hearing impairment. *Journal of the American Academy of Audiology, 21,* 367.

 WebWatch

You can quickly locate published papers about etiologies of hearing loss at the website for the National Library of Medicine in Bethesda, Maryland (www.nlm.nih.gov). Once you reach the website, go to the link "PubMed/MEDLINE." Then enter key words like "hearing" and "Ménière's disease" or some other disorder or disease in the search field. Add the key word "review" for an article that summarizes what is known about the topic.

or pathologies that must be identified promptly to facilitate effective medical and audiological management. You'll learn about each of these diseases and disorders later in the chapter.

Age is an important factor in the prevalence of different types of hearing loss. For example, diagnosis of presbycusis clearly is not possible in children. Some of the serious diseases requiring medical treatment are rarely or never found in children. On the other hand, some etiologies for hearing loss in children, like middle ear infections, are encountered far less often in adult patients.

We'll review in this chapter a variety of etiologies for hearing loss. For each disease or disorder information is provided on age, gender, and family history factors. Our review of ear disorders and diseases will follow the customary anatomic sequence, beginning with the outer ear and ending with the inner ear. Within each of the anatomic regions the discussion will generally progress from the most common or prevalent etiologies to those encountered infrequently in clinical practice.

Outer Ear Disorders

Audiologists have many opportunities to observe the outermost portion of a patient's ear, the pinna. The pinna is examined formally during inspection of the ear prior to the beginning of hearing assessment. The pinna is also viewed each time earphones are placed on the patient. Some deviations in the anatomy of the pinna are quite minor, easily overlooked, and inconsequential in terms of both health and hearing. At the other extreme, major malformations are immediately obvious even with a casual glance at the ear and can result in severe hearing loss. Between these two extremes are growths and tumors that vary in their appearance, but always warrant speedy referral to a physician because of the risk of serious disease, including cancer.

Audiologists routinely perform otoscopic inspection before beginning hearing assessment. Otoscopic inspection is important to verify that the external ear canal is clear before insertion of insert earphones or probes used in various auditory tests. A wide assortment of diseases may affect the outer or middle ear, including cancerous growths and other pathologies that pose a serious health concern (Lucente & Hanson, 2009; Shockley & Stucker, 1987).

Audiologists have a professional responsibility to recognize possible disease or pathology during inspection of the ear. When audiologists suspect disease or pathology, they refer patients to a physician for a medical diagnosis. Often a patient is referred to an otolaryngologist who specializes in diseases of the ear. A sizable proportion of people with hearing loss may initially seek hearing healthcare with an audiologist. An audiologist can play an important role in the early detection of ear disease and pathology.

We'll now review a small sampling of disorders involving the outer ear.

Collapsing Ear Canals

Examination of the outer ear may suggest to an audiologist the possibility of collapsing ear canals. The term *prolapsing* ear canals is sometimes used instead of collapsing ear canals. Patients with very small or slit-shaped external auditory canals are at risk for ear canal collapse. Collapsing ear canals are most common in infants and in elderly adults. Ear canal collapse occurs when pressure from a supra-aural earphone resting on the pinna deforms the relatively flexible cartilage within the ear canal walls. An audiologist sometimes pushes on the tragus of a patient to determine whether there is a likelihood of a collapsing ear canal. Collapsing ear canals are more likely if pressure on the tragus causes the external ear canal to become narrow. In years past, before the introduction of insert earphones, ear canal collapse was prevented by the insertion of an otoscope speculum into the ear canal before placement of supra-aural earphones. The problem of collapsing ear canals is usually resolved with the use of insert earphones.

The possibility of collapsing ear canals should always be considered for patients with mild high-frequency conductive hearing loss, particularly if middle ear dysfunction is not suspected based on history or other test findings. The solution for collapsing ear canals is the use of insert earphones rather than supra-aural earphones for air-conduction hearing testing.

Malignant Disease of the Outer Ear

Malignant growths or tumors are a very important category of outer ear abnormalities. The term **malignant** is from the Latin word for "bad kind." The term **neoplasm** is often used instead of tumor. The word *neoplasm* is derived from the Greek words *neo* for "new" and *plasm* for "thing." Malignant diseases, particularly cancerous growths, can develop on the pinna and in the external ear canal.

Figure 11.1 shows an example of a cancerous growth arising from skin on the pinna. Such growths are found mostly in older patients and are often related to prolonged exposure to sun. In contrast, cancer disease in the external ear canal often affects younger patients without a history of sun exposure (Lucente & Hanson, 2009; Shockley & Stucker, 1987). Patients with any unusual or suspicious growths on the pinna or in the external ear canal should be referred immediately to a physician or to a medical specialist like an otolaryngologist.

Congenital Malformations

Craniofacial Anomalies. Malformations of the outer ear range from mild variations in anatomy to the total absence of a pinna and external ear canal. A congenital malformation is present at birth. The word *congenital* means literally

FIGURE 11.1

Photograph of a very visible squamous cell cancerous growth on the pinna of an adult patient (see arrow). Patients with suspicious growths involving the outer ear or the external ear canal should be referred immediately to a physician. Reproduced with permission from Otolaryngology Houston. www.ghorayeb.com

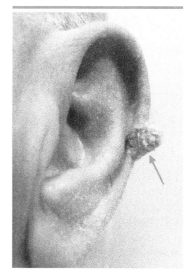

"from the beginning." Congenital malformations involving the ear fall within a larger grouping of disorders in newborn children known as **craniofacial abnormalities** or **anomalies**. Craniofacial anomalies are malformations involving the face and head. They are well-appreciated risk factors for infant hearing loss. Conductive hearing loss is most often associated with anomalies of the external or middle ear structures (Hall & Ghorayeb, 1991; Jahrsdoerfer & Hall, 1986).

Craniofacial abnormalities have long been recognized as a possible cause of hearing impairment (Joint Committee on Infant Hearing, 2007). You may recall from reading the previous chapter that the 2007 Joint Committee on Infant Hearing cite craniofacial abnormalities as risk factors or indicators for infant hearing loss.

Preauricular Pits and Tags. Preauricular pits and tags are relatively common congenital malformations. A **preauricular pit** is a small depression in the skin in front of the tragus of the outer ear. Auricular is derived from auricle, another term for the ear. Children with auricular pits or tags sometimes have a family history of ear malformations. A preauricular pit may become infected, leading to drainage of infected pus. In some cases, a preauricular pit is one feature in a complex or syndrome of physical problems originating during embryological development known as *branchio-oto-renal (BOR) syndrome* (Fraser, Sproule & Halal, 1980; Lucente & Hanson, 2009). The syndrome includes multiple defects in the neck and throat region, plus ear anomalies and kidney abnormalities. Hearing impairment is often associated with this syndrome (Fraser, Sproule, & Halal, 1980).

Preauricular tags consist of one or more small stalks of skin and tissue located directly in front of the earlobe. Since the presence of either preauricular pits or tags poses a potential risk for hearing impairment, children with either type of malformation should undergo hearing screening or assessment (Lucente & Hanson, 2009). They should also be referred to an otolaryngologist for further evaluation.

FIGURE 11.2

A. Photograph of microtia illustrating a moderate abnormality of the outer ear for a child. Courtesy of Patrick J. Antonelli, MD.
B. Photograph of microtia illustrating a more severe abnormality for an adult. Reproduced with permission from Otolaryngology Houston. www.ghorayeb.com

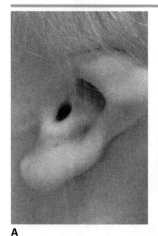
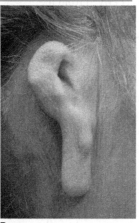

A   B

Microtia and Atresia. **Microtia** is a word meaning "small ear." It is a term used for more pronounced malformations of the ear that range from absence of portions of the pinna to total absence of the pinna and even the external ear canal (Lambert, 2001). Figure 11.2A and Figure 11.2B show two examples of microtia. Microtia is sometimes associated with conductive hearing loss.

Absence of an outer ear with perhaps only small remnants of skin and tissue is generally referred to as **aural atresia**. *Atresia* means undeveloped and *aural* refers to the ear. Aural atresia with the absence of an external ear canal is invariably associated with hearing loss. Depending on the extent of the structural abnormality, the hearing loss may be mild to severe (Hall & Ghorayeb, 1991; Jahrsdoerfer & Hall, 1986; Jahrsdoerfer, Yeakley, Hall, Robbins, & Gray, 1985).

Approximately two-thirds of children with aural atresia have no other physical abnormalities (Lambert, 2001). Microtia or aural atresia is one of multiple physical defects for the remaining one-third. About 10% of children with aural atresia are diagnosed with a syndrome consisting of a group of malformations (Smith, Kochhar, & Friedman, 2009), including craniofacial anomalies that result in a distinctive appearance. Two examples are *Treacher-Collins syndrome* and *Goldenhar syndrome.* Patients with these syndromes have substantial structural defects involving the outer ear and middle ear structure that usually result in severe bilateral conductive hearing loss (Jahrsdoerfer, Yeakley, Hall, Robbins, & Gray, 1985).

Ear Canal Disorders and Abnormalities

Cerumen. The presence of some cerumen or earwax in the external ear canal is normal. Cerumen contributes to protection of the ear canal and tympanic membrane. Normally moist and sticky, cerumen repels water, while catching dust, dirt, and pollen. The unpleasant smell and taste of cerumen is mostly due to its acidic content. The acidic nature and antibiotic property of cerumen minimizes the growth and survival of bacteria, fungus, and even small insects within the ear canal. For these reasons, a moderate amount of moist cerumen in the ear canal is healthy and beneficial.

Cerumen secreted from glands within the ear canal walls normally migrates slowly in an outward direction. Some persons produce too little cerumen or too much, whereas others have cerumen that is dry and flaky. The amount and type of cerumen observed in the external ear canals of a given patient is sometimes related to aging or genetic factors. Patients with less-than-normal cerumen or very dry cerumen often complain of constant itching in the ear canal. The itching may be relieved by application of a small amount of lightweight "baby" oil near the opening of the ear canal.

Excessive cerumen within the external ear canal is a problem commonly encountered in an audiology clinic. It often interferes with or prevents the insertion of probe tips used for different test procedures. Even if a probe tip can be safely inserted, cerumen may block the tiny tubes in the probes that carry sound into or out of the ear. Occlusion of the external ear canal with excessive cerumen blocks the passage of sound from earphones to the tympanic membrane.

A variety of techniques are available for removal of excessive cerumen. Audiologists with proper training, experience, and instrumentation often remove modest amounts of cerumen from the ear canals of cooperative adult patients. Adult patients with excessive cerumen tightly packed or impacted deep within the ear canal are generally referred to physicians, usually otolaryngologists.

Physicians remove cerumen with the aid of a microscope and special equipment like suction devices and surgical tools. Physicians usually take on the responsibility for cerumen removal in young children. Patients should never attempt to remove cerumen with cotton-tipped swabs or other approaches because of the risk of injury to the ear canal wall or the tympanic membrane.

 ClinicalConnection

Findings from objective auditory test procedures like the auditory brainstem response (ABR) contribute importantly to the diagnosis and medical management of children with craniofacial defects. As reviewed earlier in Chapter 9, ABR measurement permits hearing assessment of infants and young children, including accurate determination of auditory thresholds for air and bone conduction. Information from auditory assessment contributes importantly to medical and surgical management of children with craniofacial abnormalities.

 ClinicalConnection

An audiologist or any other healthcare professional should only attempt cerumen removal if he or she has adequate training and experience and proper instrumentation. Referral to an otolaryngologist is advisable whenever cerumen cannot be clearly visualized or if there is suspicion of additional ear pathology. Remember the adage "When in doubt, refer out!"

Debris and Foreign Bodies. Otoscopic inspection of the ear canal may reveal small flakes of skin or bits of dirt. The phrase **foreign body** is used for an object that should not be in the external ear canal. Examples of foreign bodies most often discovered in the external ear canals of children include beads, raisins, pebbles, and even insects. A physician with access to necessary instruments generally performs removal of foreign bodies from the ear canal. The removal of foreign bodies often requires the availability of local anesthesia to minimize discomfort and a capacity to deal with complications associated with the procedure, such as bleeding. An audiologist who detects an unsuspected foreign body in the external ear canal usually refers the patient to a physician for management.

Inflammation and Infections. Otoscopic inspection may also reveal evidence of ear canal inflammation or infection. The general term **otitis externa**, meaning inflammation of the outer ear, encompasses a number of diseases of the external ear canal, including *bacterial, viral,* and *fungal infections* (Rosenfeld, Brown, Cannon, et al., 2006).

Most cases of *inflammation* and *infection* affecting the external ear canal pose a health problem rather than a concern for loss of hearing (Lucente & Hanson, 2009). Prompt referral of patients with infections to a physician who can medically treat the disease is necessary to prevent spread of the infection and to minimize health risk to the patient.

A remarkably diverse collection of diseases may involve the external ear canal. External ear infections are certainly not uncommon. The likelihood and etiology of some of them is related to systemic diseases like diabetes, which are usually reported during the patient history. All patients with external ear infections require a referral to a physician. Medical management options include close monitoring, antibiotic drugs delivered as eardrops, thorough cleaning, or even surgery (Rosenfeld, Brown, Cannon, et al., 2006).

In some cases, inflammation and infection result in abnormal constriction of the canal, which prevents the passage of sound to the tympanic membrane. The technical term for a constriction or narrowing of the external ear canal is **stenosis**. Consistent production and accumulation of skin and debris in the narrow ear canal, causing total stenosis, can result in a conductive hearing loss. Hearing by air conduction is affected by blockage to sound caused by the stenosis, whereas stimulation of the cochlea directly by bone conduction yields normal hearing thresholds.

ClinicalConnection

Acoustic immittance measurement is used to determine whether a stenotic ear canal is completely blocked. Tympanometry is performed if narrowing of the ear canal does not interfere with placement of the immittance probe. A normal (type A) tympanogram indicates that changes in air pressure reach the tympanic membrane and the stenosis is incomplete. On the other hand, a flat tympanogram and measurement of an abnormally small ear canal volume suggests complete stenosis and total blockage of the ear canal. Stenosis of the ear canal prevents tympanometry air-pressure changes from reaching and moving the tympanic membrane.

Bony Abnormalities. Bone growths in the external ear canal walls are quite obvious upon otoscopic inspection. In fact, the extension of bony abnormalities into the opening of the external ear canal complicates inspection of the ear (Lucente & Hanson, 2009). Bony growths interfere with the insertion of the otoscope speculum. Two common bony abnormalities of the external ear canal are *osteomas* and *exostosis* (Rosenfeld, Brown, Cannon, et al., 2006). Like many medical terms, these two are meaningful when their Latin or Greek origins are appreciated.

Osteoma is derived from the Greek words for "bone" and "tumor." Osteomas are growths projecting into the ear canal on a stalk. They are usually found in the outer portion of one ear canal. The term *exostosis* (plural, *exostoses*) is derived from the Greek words for "out" and "bone." Exostoses are hard growths with a broad base that project outward from the ear canal wall, deep in the ear canal close to the tympanic membrane (Lucente & Hanson, 2009). They are usually found in both ears. The development of exostoses is often linked to exposure of the delicate ear canal lining to cold water. Referral of patients with osteomas or exostoses to a physician is always recommended. In fact, medical management of osteomas and exostoses is sometimes necessary before patients can be fitted with hearing aids that require insertion in the external ear canal.

ClinicalConnection

Prompt referral to a physician is appropriate for patients with any abnormality of the outer ear. Medical referral from an audiologist is particularly important when there is the possibility of a malignant disease of the external ear. Other indications for medical referral that were cited in Chapter 10 bear repeating here. These indications include evidence of drainage from the ear and patient complaints of ear fullness, discomfort, or pain.

Middle Ear Disorders

Middle ear disorders involve the tympanic membrane, the three ossicles connecting the tympanic membrane to the inner ear, the middle ear space where the ossicles are located, and spaces nearby that are continuous with the middle ear. If it has been awhile since you read about anatomy and physiology of the auditory system in Chapter 3, this might be a good time for you to briefly review information pertaining to middle ear structure and function.

The following review emphasizes middle ear disorders commonly encountered by audiologists in the clinic and those most often associated with hearing loss. Abnormalities posing a risk to the patient's health and requiring medical attention will be clearly identified even if they do not cause a hearing loss.

Eustachian Tube Dysfunction

Children. The Eustachian tube provides communication between the space in the back of the mouth and the middle ear space. The Eustachian tube is the only pathway connecting the middle ear with the outside environment. Therefore, it plays a vital role in ventilation of the middle ear space by allowing a fresh supply of air to reach the middle ear.

Young children are prone to Eustachian tube dysfunction because their craniofacial anatomy is not yet fully developed (Poe & Gopen, 2009). Eustachian tubes in infants and young children have a very small diameter and an especially small opening at the end near the middle ear. Also, Eustachian tubes in young children are oriented horizontally rather than in a more vertical direction. Upper respiratory congestion is sometimes associated with swelling of the mucous membranes lining the Eustachian tube. Swelling of the Eustachian tube walls interferes with normal opening of the tube that ventilates the middle ear space (Poe & Gopen, 2009).

Fortunately, during childhood the Eustachian tube increases in size and gradually shifts to a more vertical 45-degree orientation. Changes in Eustachian tube size and orientation are associated with overall physical growth of the body. As a result, Eustachian tube dysfunction and associated ear problems decrease as children grow older.

Adults. Eustachian tube dysfunction is commonly found in children, but it is sometimes a problem in the adult patient population. You may have experienced difficulty in clearing your ears during airplane travel, particularly when descending and landing. As the airplane ascends after takeoff, air pressure in the cabin decreases slightly. Pressure of air in the middle ear space is still equivalent to the atmospheric pressure on the ground and slightly greater than the cabin pressure. As you swallow and perhaps yawn, the relatively greater air pressure in the middle ear escapes through the Eustachian tube. You often hear a popping, squealing, or crunching sound as the air makes its way out of the middle ear.

The pressure difference between air in the airplane and air in the middle ear space is reversed as the airplane descends. Pressure in the airplane progressively increases in comparison to middle ear pressure. For some people, the Eustachian tube does not open as readily when pressure is exerted from the outside as when pressure is escaping from the middle ear. Swallowing repeatedly, chewing gum, or yawning activates the muscles that open the Eustachian tube. After the airplane lands, there may still be less pressure in your middle ear space than outside. The negative middle ear pressure may produce some discomfort and muffled hearing. Activities that utilize the Eustachian tube muscles, like yawning and swallowing, eventually help to equalize pressure between the middle ear and outside environment.

Patent Eustachian Tube. Inability to periodically open the Eustachian tube is by far the most common type of Eustachian tube dysfunction (Poe & Gopen, 2009). Occasionally, however, audiologists evaluate patients with just the opposite problem. In these patients, the Eustachian tube remains open or, to use a technical term, the Eustachian tube is *patent*. Persons with recent weight loss sometimes report problems with patent Eustachian tubes. These patients often complain about hearing whooshing sounds, produced by air rushing in and out of the

FIGURE 11.3

An example of a tympanic membrane perforation of the right ear. Courtesy of Science Photo Library/Custom Medical Stock Photo.

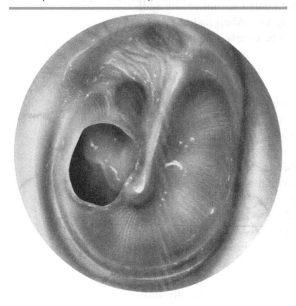

middle ear space via the always-open Eustachian tube. An audiologist suspecting a patent Eustachian tube in a patient typically refers the patient to an otolaryngologist.

Perforation of the Tympanic Membrane

Causes of Perforations. Tympanic membrane **perforation** is the technical term for a hole in the eardrum. Figure 11.3 shows a perforation of the tympanic membrane. In a clinical setting, perforations of the tympanic membrane are generally associated with trauma, middle ear disease, or a surgical procedure. Trauma producing a perforation may be caused by puncture of the tympanic membrane with an object like a cotton-tipped swab or a pen (Welling & Packer, 2009). A perforation may also result from a sharp blow to the outer ear, such as when the side of the head strikes water during a dive or an ear is slapped with the palm of a hand. Ear trauma is a common health problem in military combat explosions.

Blasts and explosions produce a variety of serious injuries (DePalma, Burris, Champion, & Hodgdon, 2005). Military personnel exposed to high-intensity blast explosions in combat with resulting physical injuries often suffer perforation of the tympanic membrane. Tympanic membrane damage is caused by the sudden and large increase in pressure from the blast explosion. Peak sound pressure levels from blast explosions reach a level of 185 dB. In fact, tympanic membrane perforation is the most common injury resulting from exposure to blast explosions during combat in the conflicts in Iraq and Afghanistan (Ritenour et al., 2009).

The majority of patients with blast injury perforations have hearing loss, and one-half of these patients have tinnitus. Speech pathologists also serve on the team that evaluates and treats persons with blast injuries, as a large proportion of the patients have cognitive, language, swallowing, or voice disorders (Newman, 2005).

Perforations of the tympanic membrane may also result from acute ear infection (Post & Kerschner, 2009). Infection and inflammation in the middle ear space during an ear infection often produces outward pressure on the tympanic membrane.

Upon examination of the ear with otoscopy, the tympanic membrane of a patient with acute ear infection is red and bulging in appearance. With excessive inflammation and increase of pressure in the middle ear space, the tympanic membrane may spontaneously rupture, releasing some of the infected pus into the external ear canal. Dry and crusted debris visible in the outer portion of the ear canal is evidence of tympanic membrane rupture and discharge of infected fluid. Dried debris will often be found on the pillow if a tympanic membrane ruptures at night while a patient with acute ear infection is sleeping.

Creation of a hole in the tympanic membrane may also be done on purpose for medical treatment of ear disease. Using a specialized miniature knife and viewing the ear through a microscope, an otolaryngologist makes a small incision or slit in the tympanic membrane. The technical term for this surgical procedure is **myringotomy**. A myringotomy is performed to relieve the excessive pressure in the middle ear and to remove with suctioning infected fluid from the middle ear space (Post & Kerschner, 2009). Hearing is often temporarily improved following the procedure. The tympanic membrane generally heals within a week or two following a myringotomy.

You may recall from the discussion about the tympanic membrane in Chapter 3 that the outer layer of skin is constantly being "shed" and migrates outward through external ear canal. This renewal process contributes to the rapid healing of the tympanic membrane following a perforation.

Hearing Test Findings in Tympanic Membrane Perforation. Depending on the exact mechanism, traumatic perforations vary considerably in size, shape, and their effect on hearing (Hall & Ghorayeb, 1991). Small perforations produce surprisingly minimal hearing loss. In fact, hearing thresholds may be within normal limits (< 20 dB HL). High-pressure blast explosions, on the other hand, create large perforations with considerably greater hearing loss.

Otitis Media

Otitis media is the technical term for ear infection. The word *otitis* is derived from Latin words for "ear" (*oto*) and "inflammation" (*itis*), whereas *media* means "middle." We'll soon review the various forms of otitis media. Ear infections and other middle ear disorders are common health problems in young children. Ear infections often result in hearing loss and sometimes contribute also to a delay in the development of speech and language (Paradise et al., 2010; Roberts et al., 2004). Audiologists and speech pathologists regularly encounter children whose ear infections affect hearing and communication. Thus, we'll devote more attention to otitis media than most other middle ear diseases or disorders.

Otitis media is often referred as simply *ear infection,* but it is by no means a simple disease. Indeed, terminology used to describe ear infections is poorly understood and sometimes used incorrectly. Otitis media is really a general term for a variety of disorders that involve fluid in the middle ear space. Otitis media encompasses a spectrum of disease conditions. Over a period of weeks, or months, a child may transition from one stage of middle ear disease to another. We will now review two middle ear disorders that are most often encountered in children: *acute otitis media* and *otitis media with effusion,* abbreviated *OME.* Other middle ear disorders will be mentioned in a following section.

Acute otitis media (AOM) is caused by either a viral or, less often, a bacterial infection in the middle ear space. It often develops quite rapidly in children. Figure 11.4 illustrates the appearance of an ear with acute otitis media. Symptoms of acute otitis media may include fever, pain, irritability, crying, and a disruption in sleeping or eating patterns. Symptoms may even include vomiting and diarrhea (Post & Kerschner, 2009). Ear pain is mostly closely associated with acute otitis media. Ear examination of a child with acute otitis media shows a reddish, white, or yellow tympanic membrane that often bulges outward.

Drainage of pus into the external ear canal in patients with acute otitis media indicates perforation of the tympanic membrane. At this stage, the disease is sometimes called *purulent otitis media* because the technical term for pus is *purulence.* Repeated episodes of acute otitis media in a child are described as *recurrent acute otitis media.*

The term *otitis media with effusion* refers to fluid in the middle ear space. It is also called *serous otitis media.* The word *effusion* means an accumulation of fluid, and the term *serous* is related to *serum,* meaning a watery substance. Otitis media with effusion most often follows an episode of acute otitis media, but it may also occur without previous acute otitis media (Post & Kerschner, 2009). Otitis media with effusion does not usually exhibit the rather distinct symptoms just described for acute otitis media, such as ear

FIGURE 11.4

An ear with chronic otitis media as viewed from the external ear canal with an otoscope or a microscope. The tympanic membrane is dull and retracted. Courtesy Prof. Tony Wright/Institute of Laryngology & Otology/Science Source/Photo Researchers, Inc.

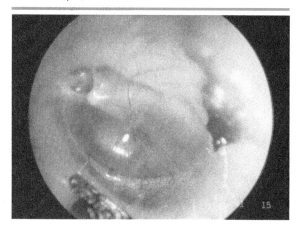

pain and fever. In fact, a child with otitis media with effusion may not complain of any symptoms. Parents or caregivers may be aware of a problem only when they notice that the child is experiencing trouble hearing.

Ear examination of a patient with otitis media with effusion usually reveals an inward retraction of a dull gray tympanic membrane, sometimes with visible air bubbles and a fluid line. Inflammation and redness are not seen in a child with otitis media with effusion unless the child is crying before or during the ear examination.

How Does Otitis Media Develop in Children? Two general explanations are offered for how otitis media develops. Both explanations involve Eustachian tube dysfunction. As you've learned, the Eustachian tube plays an important role in maintaining equal pressure between air in the middle ear space and the outside. Blockage or inadequate opening of the Eustachian tube in children results most often from an upper respiratory infection or from inflammation associated with allergies. You're also aware that the Eustachian tube in young children is more susceptible to blockage because it's smaller and oriented more horizontally than in older children and adults.

Ongoing Eustachian tube dysfunction usually leads to negative air pressure in the middle ear space. Oxygen in the middle ear space is absorbed in the mucous membranes lining the space. Eustachian tube dysfunction prevents a fresh supply of air from entering the middle ear space and air pressure begins to decrease.

Due to the effect of negative air pressure (as compared to atmospheric or ambient air pressure), fluid from the mucous membrane lining the middle ear begins to seep into the middle ear space. If the Eustachian tube dysfunction persists, the fluid in the warm enclosed middle ear space becomes an ideal environment for development of a bacterial infection. Very young children generally have an immature immune system, which increases their risk for developing an ear infection.

The other explanation for the development of otitis media posits that bacteria already in the middle ear space are the primary cause of the infection. Bacteria originating in the nose or mouth reach the middle ear space by traveling through the Eustachian tube. Again, it's likely that decreased immune reaction to middle ear bacteria in young children also contributes to the development of otitis media.

Risk Factors for Otitis Media. Some children are at greater risk for developing otitis media than others. There is no clear difference in the prevalence of otitis media between males and females. However, within the past twenty years large studies involving thousands of children have confirmed that a number of factors affect the likelihood of otitis media.

These multiple risk factors increase the chance that a child will develop otitis media. For example, a young child under the age of 2 years who is bottle fed, exposed to secondhand smoke, and spends time in a day care center with repeated exposure to other children is at considerably greater risk for otitis media than a young child who is not exposed to these factors. Otitis media is almost always found in children with certain craniofacial abnormalities such as cleft palate. The anatomical explanation is an abnormality in the insertion of the muscle that is responsible for opening the Eustachian tube.

Medical and Surgical Management. A physician examining a child for possible otitis media aims to accurately diagnose the condition and to determine whether medical management is required. Medical diagnosis of otitis media is made primarily from careful review of the child's health history, as given by a parent or caregiver. Diagnosis is confirmed with an otoscopic examination of the ear. For a diagnosis of acute otitis media, medical management may include treatment with drugs or a surgical procedure.

Even though otitis media is the most common ear disease and the most common reason children receive care from pediatricians, there is still no clear consensus on the best management (Darrow, Dash, & Derkay, 2003). Antibiotics are clearly appropriate for management of acute otitis media when bacterial infection is confirmed or highly likely. Concerns about excessively prescribing antibiotics for treatment of otitis media have, in turn, prompted the development of step-by-step guidelines by physician groups for when drugs should or should not be considered as a management option (American Academy of Pediatrics, 2004). Most types of physicians regularly prescribe medications for treatment of infections and other disorders.

Surgical management is usually considered for children with repeated episodes of otitis media despite medical treatment. Otolaryngologists are specialists who also perform surgical operations for management of otitis media. Surgical options for management of otitis media include myringotomy to create a small opening in the tympanic membrane and insertion of a tiny tube into the tympanic membrane. A tube in the tympanic membrane permits a release of pressure in the middle ear and spontaneous drainage of fluid from the middle ear space.

Various terms are used to describe the tubes, including *tympanostomy tubes, ventilation tubes,* and *pressure equalization tubes.* Figure 11.5 shows four different types of tympanostomy tubes on a penny for size comparison. The typical tube is only 1 mm in diameter.

Figure 11.6 shows a tympanostomy tube in the anterior-inferior part of a tympanic membrane. Antibiotic eardrops are administered following the procedure to minimize the chance of infection. The entire surgical procedure requires only a few minutes per ear. Insertion of ventilation tubes into the tympanic membranes of children with otitis media is one of the most common surgical procedures performed in the United States.

Otitis Media and Hearing Loss. Physicians have responsibility for medical diagnosis and management of ear disease. Audiologists are concerned about hearing loss in children with otitis media. Hearing loss in children with otitis media with effusion is typically in the range of 25 to 30 dB.

Otitis media with effusion may also occur in children with pre-existing unrelated permanent sensorineural hearing loss. The combination of a conductive hearing loss from otitis media plus the sensorineural hearing loss from a pre-existing cochlear deficit produces hearing impairment that is greater than what would be expected from either disorder alone.

Careful hearing assessment before and after medical management is important for all children with otitis media to determine the full extent of hearing loss. Hearing assessment before medical treatment will confirm or rule out the possibility of a permanent sensory deficit and will contribute to the most appropriate and timely management approach.

FIGURE 11.5

Examples of four different types of tympanostomy (ventilation) tubes used to treat otitis media and to improve hearing thresholds. The small tubes are identified with arrows and compared in size to a penny. Reproduced with permission from Otolaryngology Houston. www.ghorayeb.com

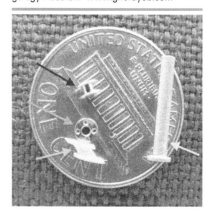

WebWatch

You can view a wide variety of surgical procedures on YouTube, including myringotomy with insertion of tympanostomy tubes. Just search the Internet with a few key words and you'll quickly locate an assortment of videos showing the surgical procedure.

FIGURE 11.6

A tympanostomy (ventilation) tube after insertion into the anterior-inferior part of a tympanic membrane. Courtesy of SPL/Science Source/Photo Researchers, Inc.

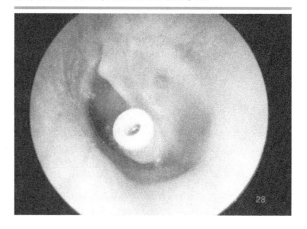

Chronic Otitis Media and Cholesteatomas

Chronic otitis media. *Chronic otitis media* is a longstanding disease process. The disease process begins with acute otitis media and a long, drawn-out course of otitis media with effusion. It is not clear whether chronic otitis media is an extension of acute otitis media or an independent pathology (Friedland, Pensak, & Kveton, 2009).

Permanent defects in the tympanic membrane are a characteristic feature of chronic otitis media. The abnormalities include perforations of the tympanic membrane and also regions that are severely retracted into the middle ear space. The infection in chronic otitis media also extends beyond the middle ear space into the tiny spaces in the mastoid portion of the temporal bone (Friedland, Pensak, & Kveton, 2009). The mastoid spaces are normally filled with air. The mastoid air spaces in chronic otitis media lack an adequate amount of air and eventually become infected.

Chronic otitis media is associated with consistent and significant hearing loss that may be moderate to severe, as great as 60 dB HL. Audiologists will almost always encounter children with chronic otitis media because of concerns about serious hearing loss. Due to the longstanding nature of the disease and its impact on communication, speech pathologists may also be involved in the assessment and management of children with chronic otitis media.

Cholesteatoma. **A cholesteatoma** is a very serious and complicated form of ear disease (Chole & Nason, 2009). A cholesteatoma may be present at birth, but most arise as a complication of chronic otitis media. A cholesteatoma is a growth of skin or a cyst in the middle ear space.

There are different theories about why and how a cholesteatoma initially forms (Arts & Neely, 2001). The growth usually arises when a portion of the tympanic membrane is pulled back or retracted into the middle ear space. Over time layers of skin are added to the initial growth. The layers of skin in a growing cholesteatoma are sometimes compared to the layers of an expanding onion. Within unchecked growth, a cholesteatoma obstructs movement of the tympanic membrane and the ossicles and leads gradually to greater degrees of hearing loss. Over time a cholesteatoma may even erode the ossicles in the middle ear, producing more hearing loss.

Health problems associated with a cholesteatoma extend far beyond hearing. In addition to permanent hearing loss due to infection of the inner ear the list of serious health complications includes dizziness, facial nerve weakness, and life-threatening infections of the skull (Arts & Neely, 2001; Chole & Nason, 2009).

 ClinicalConnection

Chronic otitis media and cholesteatoma are two of the most serious ear diseases. A variety of possible medical problems can develop if either disease goes undiagnosed and untreated. Diagnosis of chronic otitis media or a cholesteatoma cannot be made on the basis of hearing tests. An audiologist who evaluates a child or an adult with evidence of a middle ear disorder should always refer the patient directly to an otolaryngologist for complete evaluation and necessary management.

Management of Chronic Otitis Media and Cholesteatomas. Aggressive medical management of chronic otitis media and cholesteatomas is always appropriate (Friedland, Pensak, & Kveton, 2009). Surgical treatment is often required for chronic otitis media. Surgical removal of a cholesteatoma is almost always necessary. An audiologist may be the first healthcare professional to encounter the patient and detect the hearing loss associated with serious ear disease. Prompt referral to an otolaryngologist is necessary for any patient suspected of having chronic otitis media or a cholesteatoma. An otolaryngologist makes a diagnosis of chronic otitis media or cholesteatoma based on patient history, ear examination usually with a microscope, and often other medical tests like a CT scan.

Hearing Loss in Chronic Otitis Media and with Cholesteatomas. There is no single set or pattern of auditory findings for chronic otitis media or cholesteatoma. Rather, test findings

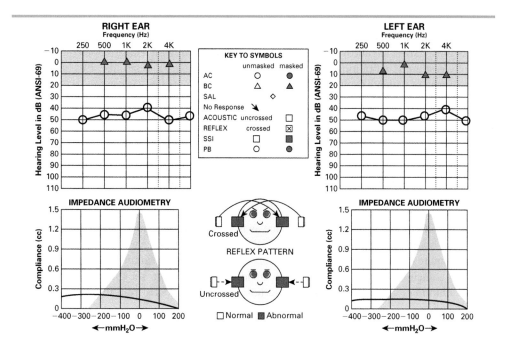

FIGURE 11.7

Audiogram and tympanograms for a child with chronic otitis media.

depend on the extent of disease and its effect on middle ear function. Figure 11.7 shows an example of hearing thresholds and tympanometry for a child with chronic otitis media. Tympanograms are abnormal (type B) for both ears and acoustic reflexes were not detected. The patient has a moderate (40 to 50 dB HL) conductive hearing loss.

There are clear and consistent differences between the pattern of hearing losses for children with otitis media with effusion and those with chronic otitis media or a cholesteatoma. Degree of conductive hearing loss is considerably greater for chronic otitis media or a cholesteatoma than for either otitis media with effusion or acute otitis media.

Fixation of the Ossicular Chain and Otosclerosis

Hearing loss may result from dysfunction involving any portion of the middle ear system, including abnormalities of the ossicular chain. The phrase *fixation of the ossicular chain* is used to describe abnormal stiffening of the connections between two or more of the ossicles in the middle ear. In most cases, fixation of the ossicular chain involves the stapes, the innermost ossicle, which resembles a stirrup. The flat footplate portion of the stapes fits into the oval window. The stapes footplate plays an important role in hearing. The stapes footplate is the final link as vibrations in the ossicular chain are transmitted to the cochlear fluids. Figures 3.3 and 3.5 in Chapter 3 showed diagrams of the ossicles and the stapes footplate.

Stiffening of the connection between the stapes footplate and oval window may interfere with vibration of cochlear fluids, in addition to reducing the amount of sound-related energy reaching the cochlea. Reduction of vibrations in cochlear fluids in turn reduces movement of the basilar membrane, resulting in a sensory hearing loss and decreased hearing on bone conduction testing. Patients with fixation of the ossicular chain who have a combination of conductive hearing impairment and also some degree of sensory hearing deficit have a mixed hearing loss.

Otosclerosis is a progressive bone disease that typically results in fixation and stiffening of the ossicular chain (Jenkins & McKenna, 2009; Roland & Meyerhoff , 2001). During the early stage of otosclerosis, the ossicles become spongy. Indeed, otosclerosis is sometimes called *otospongeosis*. Later in the disease process the spongy bone is replaced by dense bone. The origin of the word *otosclerosis* is from Greek words for "hardened ear."

As otosclerosis advances the new dense bone may occupy the entire stapes footplate and severely restrict its vibration. The bony capsule encompassing the ear may also be involved. The majority of patients show a conductive hearing loss as otosclerosis progresses. Sensory or mixed hearing loss is documented in approximately 20 to 30% of patients (Hall & Ghorayeb, 1991). The disease is known as *cochlear otosclerosis* when it produces an entirely sensory hearing loss.

Demographics of Otosclerosis. Otosclerosis is found in both ears for 80% of patients with the disease. Genetic factors play a role in the likelihood of otosclerosis (Causse & Causse, 1984). Prevalence of the disease also varies among races. It is most common in Caucasians, less common among Asians, and occurs least often in African Americans (Jenkins & McKenna, 2009). Otosclerosis affects twice as many females as males. The diagnosis is usually made sometime between the age of 30 and 50 years. Among women, the disease may progress more rapidly during a second pregnancy. Interestingly, drinking water with increased fluoride content appears to decrease the incidence of otosclerosis (Shambaugh & Scott, 1964). Fluoridation of drinking water also has a well-documented role in the prevention of tooth cavities.

Diagnosis of Otosclerosis. Otoscopic examination of an ear with otosclerosis reveals a normal-appearing tympanic membrane. In some patients with otosclerosis, however, there may be a reddish hue in the region of the promontory in front of the oval window, known as the *Schwartz sign* (Roland & Meyerhoff , 2001). Symptoms related to otosclerosis include tinnitus, a sensation of fullness in the affected ear, and a slowly progressive hearing loss (Jenkins & McKenna, 2009).

Close questioning of a patient with otosclerosis may yield a comment about a rather unusual auditory phenomenon. Patients with otosclerosis and other forms of conductive hearing loss sometimes state that they actually understand speech easier and better in the presence of background noise. In contrast, people with normal hearing sensitivity and patients with high-frequency sensorineural hearing loss invariably have better speech perception in quiet listening settings.

Paracusis willisii is the technical term for improved speech perception in background noise. Here is the explanation for this rather paradoxical symptom of otosclerosis. There is a natural tendency for normal-hearing persons to speak more loudly in noisy environments in order to better hear their own voice and also to be heard. The increased speech level is known as the *Lombard effect,* or the *Lombard voice reflex.* An increase in intensity level is just what the patient with otosclerosis needs to better understand speech. Patients with conductive hearing loss cannot hear the background noise very well. They benefit more from a favorable signal-to-noise ratio than normal-hearing persons when speakers talk loudly.

Auditory Findings in Otosclerosis. A common feature of all middle ear dysfunction is reduction of sound-related energy passing from the tympanic membrane to the inner ear. Fixation and related stiffening of the ossicular chain almost always produces a hearing loss, particularly for lower-frequency sounds. The characteristic pattern of hearing test results in patients with otosclerosis is quite useful in diagnosing the disease (Hall & Ghorayeb, 1991).

Typical auditory findings for a patient with otosclerosis were shown in a case illustrated in Figure 7.8. You'll notice in that figure a conductive hearing loss in both ears. Bone-conduction hearing in otosclerosis is generally normal, with the exception of a notch-like decrease in the bone-conduction hearing threshold at the 2000-Hz frequency. This rather unique feature of otosclerosis is called *Carhart's notch,* in honor of Raymond Carhart, who first described it (Carhart, 1950). You may recall from reading the historical information in Chapter 1 that Carhart is known as the "Father of Audiology."

A recent study of patients with otosclerosis revealed that the notch in bone-conduction thresholds is not always recorded at 2000 Hz. Notching deficits in bone-conduction hearing of patients with otosclerosis are sometimes observed in the low-, mid- or high-frequency region of the audiogram (Perez, de Almeida, Nedzelski, & Chen, 2009). Tympanograms in patients with otosclerosis are type A but abnormally shallow (Type As), reflecting a restriction in mobility of the ossicular chain. Acoustic reflexes are typically absent with the measuring probe in the affected ear, even at the early stages of otosclerosis.

Management of Otosclerosis. There are three general management options for patients with otosclerosis (Roland & Meyerhoff, 2001; Jenkins & McKenna, 2009). One is to monitor hearing status without any medical or nonmedical treatment. Although otosclerosis is a disease process, it doesn't pose a health risk aside from the hearing loss. Patients with hearing loss only in one ear or a modest bilateral hearing loss often decline treatment because they experience relatively little difficulty with communication.

Hearing aids offer another viable management option for most patients with otosclerosis. Speech perception at high-intensity levels is usually excellent in patients with conductive hearing loss, including patients with otosclerosis. Amplification of sound is typically quite effective in overcoming the reduction in hearing sensitivity produced by a conductive hearing loss (Hall & Ghorayeb, 1991).

Surgery is the third treatment option for otosclerosis (Jenkins & McKenna, 2009; Roland & Meyerhoff, 2001). The goal of surgery is to restore an effective mechanism for the transmission of vibrations from the tympanic membrane to the cochlea, with subsequent improvement in hearing sensitivity. Surgical management for otosclerosis has evolved considerably over the years, with progressively better outcomes as measured by hearing improvement. *Stapedectomy* is the technical term for the current surgical procedure used in management of otosclerosis.

An otologist first must gain access to the middle ear space by creating an opening through the tympanic membrane. Then, the distance is measured from the mid-portion of the incus to the footplate of the stapes. The middle ear muscles are cut and the joint between the incus and the stapes is separated. Using one of several techniques, the surgeon next either creates a small hole in the stapes footplate or removes most of the stapes footplate.

 WebWatch

Want to view surgical management for the hearing loss in otosclerosis? You can watch a stapedectomy surgical procedure performed on a patient with otosclerosis on YouTube and also at educational sites on the Internet. Just conduct a search with the key word "stapedectomy."

The final step in surgery is to insert a special prosthesis that provides a connection between the remaining portion of the incus and the stapes footplate and cochlea (Jenkins & McKenna, 2009; Roland & Meyerhoff, 2001).

Surgery is almost always performed on the ear with poorer hearing in patients with bilateral hearing loss due to otosclerosis (Jenkins & McKenna, 2009; Roland & Meyerhoff, 2001). Over 90% of patients undergoing stapedectomy benefit from almost complete closure of the air-bone gap. In other words, for these patients the conductive hearing loss is minimized or eliminated and hearing sensitivity is substantially improved. As with any surgical procedure, however, complications may accompany stapedectomy. Complications include the possibility of leakage of cochlear perilymph fluid from the oval window, with associated sensory hearing loss, or facial nerve injury. Among the long-term complications of surgery are the development of infection and dislocation of the prosthesis, with worsened hearing.

Disarticulation of the Ossicular Chain

Disarticulation or *discontinuity of the ossicular chain* is another cause of conductive hearing loss. The disarticulation is a break or interruption somewhere in ossicular connection leading from the tympanic membrane to the cochlea. The disarticulation or discontinuity most often occurs where the incus is connected to head of the stapes.

A common cause for disarticulation of the ossicular chain is trauma involving the temporal bone enclosing the ear. Temporal bone trauma may result from a motor vehicle accident or a blow to head with an object. In either case, the trauma breaks the normal continuity of the ossicular chain (Ghorayeb, Yeakley, Hall, & Jones, 1987). Surgical management of ossicular discontinuity is possible. The objective of surgery is to re-establish a functional connection between the ossicles so sound vibrations from the tympanic membrane can again effectively reach the inner ear.

Auditory Findings in Disarticulation of the Ossicular Chain. Disarticulation of the ossicular chain results in increased compliance or decreased stiffness, and produces a high-frequency conductive hearing loss (Hall & Ghorayeb, 1991). In contrast, most conductive hearing loss due to increased stiffness of the middle ear system is greatest for lower frequencies.

Figure 11.8 shows a pattern of auditory findings typical for a patient with unilateral right-sided disarticulation of the ossicular chain. The audiogram shows a high-frequency hearing loss by air conduction, but normal bone-conduction hearing thresholds. In the lower portion of Figure 11.8 you'll notice that the right tympanogram is a variation of type A known as type Ad. The "d" refers to deep. An Ad tympanogram reflects very high middle ear compliance, consistent with a break in the continuity of the ossicular chain. Acoustic reflexes are abnormal (not observed) in each of the four test conditions.

Trauma and Head Injury

Trauma to the head and ear may also produce a combination of different middle ear abnormalities (Hall & Ghorayeb, 1991). You have already learned that objects such as cotton tips, keys, pens, or pencils unwisely inserted into the ear canal can penetrate the tympanic membrane

FIGURE 11.8

Audiogram and tympanograms for a young adult with a history of head trauma and the diagnosis of disarticulation of the ossicular chain.

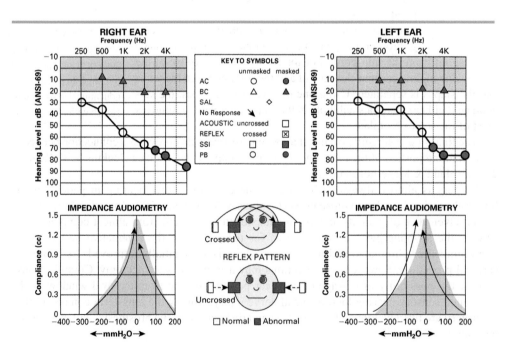

and can damage the ossicular chain. Patients with temporal bone fracture due to head trauma often have blood in the middle ear space, a problem called *hemotympanum*.

And, you just read about how head trauma can produce disarticulation of the ossicular chain in the middle ear. Hearing test results may reveal only one disorder or a combination of abnormalities. A complete patient history and physical examination by a physician, along with other medical tests such as radiological studies like a CT scan, is almost always necessary to reach an accurate diagnosis of ear disease.

Indeed, head trauma can produce abnormalities in virtually all parts of the auditory system. Trauma can damage the outer ear, the middle ear, the inner ear, the auditory nerve, and various auditory pathways within the brain. Trauma-related inner ear damage is described in the next section. Retrocochlear and central auditory abnormalities following traumatic head injury are covered in the next chapter.

Summary of Middle Ear Disorders

We've just reviewed the more common disorders involving the middle ear system. Additional abnormalities were not discussed, including rather unusual pathologies like tumors and cancer that may pose a serious health risk. It is important to recognize that one patient may have multiple disorders of the outer and/or middle ear. For example, some congenital malformations and syndromes are associated with abnormalities of the outer ear as well as the middle ear.

In summary, audiologists make four important contributions to the diagnosis of middle ear disease: (1) detection of middle ear abnormalities in patients entering the healthcare system, (2) accurate description of middle ear dysfunction, (3) testing of hearing status before and after surgery for ear disorders, and (4) management of patients with hearing loss due to middle ear disorders that cannot be adequately improved with medical or surgical intervention.

Inner Ear Disorders

Inner ear disorders produce a sensory hearing loss. The adjective **sensorineural** is traditionally used to describe hearing loss that may be due to either cochlear or eighth nerve dysfunction. For the vast majority of patients with sensorineural hearing loss the abnormality is sensory and due to abnormality in the cochlea, rather than neural and involving the auditory nerve. Retrocochlear auditory dysfunction affecting the auditory nerve is quite uncommon in both pediatric and adult patient populations. *Sensory* is a more accurate term than *sensorineural* when describing audiometric evidence of a hearing loss due to cochlear dysfunction, with no evidence of auditory nerve dysfunction.

In reading about sensorineural or, more specifically, sensory auditory dysfunction, you'll notice it differs in three main ways from the middle ear dysfunction we've just reviewed. The first and rather obvious distinction is the anatomical site of the dysfunction in the auditory system, that is, the cochlea rather than the middle ear.

Second, conductive hearing loss associated with middle ear dysfunction is almost always mild to moderate in degree and rarely exceeds 60 dB HL. Sensory hearing loss, however, may range in degree from mild to profound. Some patients with profound sensory hearing loss have no response to sound even at maximum sound intensity levels.

Finally, conductive hearing loss caused by middle ear dysfunction is less likely to be permanent. Indeed, middle ear disorder and associated hearing loss can often be minimized or eliminated with medical or surgical treatment. Cochlear dysfunction with sensory hearing loss is often permanent and generally not improved with medical management or with surgery.

Sensory hearing loss associated with many etiologies is permanent. However, fluctuations in hearing, improved hearing, or even complete reversal of hearing loss occur in some patients spontaneously or with medical treatment (Hall, Bratt, Schwaber, & Baer, 1993). As a general rule, audiologists should promptly refer patients with potentially fluctuating or progressive hearing loss to an otolaryngologist. Timely medical intervention for patients with changing sensory hearing loss sometimes leads to an improvement in hearing status (Hall, Bratt, Schwaber, & Baer, 1993).

Etiologies for sensory hearing loss are highly varied. Causes for sensory hearing loss include, for example, malformations at birth, physical damage of inner ear structures, infections, and age-related changes. And, no clear etiology can be determined for cochlear dysfunction in some patients.

The two most common causes of sensory hearing loss are exposure to excessive levels of noise and cochlear dysfunction due to advancing age. This was apparent from the summary of prevalence of hearing loss shown earlier in Table 11.1. In an elderly adult population, age-related hearing loss (presbycusis) and noise-induced hearing loss account for more than one-half of all persons with hearing impairment. Neither etiology involves active ear disease or pathology. Cochlear hearing loss may also be caused by drugs used to treat serious infection or drugs included in chemotherapy for medical management of malignant tumors.

We'll now review some of the more common etiologies for sensory hearing loss in children and adults. The review includes case reports illustrating typical hearing test results for some etiologies.

Review of the Genetics of Hearing Loss

You may have been introduced to concepts of genetics in a biology course earlier in your education. Here we'll review some genetics terminology and principles before applying them in a discussion of hereditary hearing loss. The word *genetic* is derived from the ancient Greek word *genesis,* meaning "origin." Patterns of inheritance and hereditary information are genetically encoded in *deoxyribonucleic acid (DNA)*. DNA is a double-stranded ribbon-like structure consisting of amino acids and proteins that form a connection of units called *nucleotides*. Nucleotides are molecules composed of various combinations of basic elements, such as carbon, oxygen, hydrogen, and phosphate. There are four different types of nucleotides.

Approximately 30,000 genes are located in long chains, called chromosomes, in the DNA strand. There are twenty-three pairs of chromosomes. Twenty-two are non-sex chromosomes called *autosomes*. The other is a pair of *sex chromosomes*. These two well-known chromosomes are labeled X and Y. The Y chromosome determines exclusively male characteristics. The X chromosome contains many genes. Females have two X chromosomes, whereas males have an X and a Y chromosome. So, each child has a pair of chromosomes, with one chromosome in the pair inherited from one parent and the second one from the other parent.

The pairs of genes in a chromosome are referred as *alleles*. The word *alleles* is from the Greek language and means "of one another." The alleles are described as *homozygous* if two genes, one from each parent, are identical for an inherited genetic trait. *Heterozygous* alleles include a different gene from each parent, with associated different genetic traits in a child. All living organisms, including human beings, inherit their genetic code from their parents. The genetic code consists of a sequence of genetic information coded in nucleotides in the DNA.

Historical Perspective. The modern study of genetics dates back to the mid-1800s. However, scientists, notably James Watson and Francis Crick, described the molecular structure of DNA as recently as the early 1950s. Since then, intensive research in molecular biology has produced many exciting discoveries, leading to an understanding of the genetic code.

A major research effort, the Human Genome Project, produced a description of the organization or sequencing of human genes (www.ornl.gov/sci/techresources/Human_Genome/home.shtml). Ongoing advances in molecular biology and medical genetics have led to discoveries of genetic variations associated with health and disease in humans. Many health problems, such as cancer, are linked to genetic traits and are inherited. Among the scientific advances in genetics within the past few decades is the discovery that defects in different genes are responsible for various patterns of hearing loss (Smith, Kochhar, & Friedman, 2009).

Genetic Factors in Hearing Loss. Genetic factors play a role in approximately 60% of infants with congenital hearing loss. In other words, hereditary factors help to explain hearing loss for the majority of babies when it is present from birth (Smith, Kochhar, & Friedman, 2009). Over 125 *genes for hearing loss* have been identified so far (Cohen & Phillips, 2012, Lesperance et al., 1995).

Genes for hearing loss may be dominant or recessive. A child with a genetically determined hearing loss may have one parent with the trait of hearing loss, while the other parent has normal hearing. In the heterozygous parent with the hearing loss, one allele is mutated and the other is normal. One allele dominates the other one. This is an *autosomal dominant* form of hearing loss passed on to the child from the parent with the hearing loss. The child may have a 50% chance of inheriting the hearing loss from one parent. Whether the hearing loss is present or expressed may vary. For example, even though it is passed on genetically, the hearing loss may not affect individuals of one generation. Then, the hearing loss may appear in a member of the next generation. If both parents carry a gene for an autosomal dominant form of hearing loss and actually have hearing loss, it is highly likely that their children will be born with the same form of hearing loss.

With an *autosomal recessive* form of hearing loss, both parents may carry the recessive gene even though each parent has normal hearing. A normal gene in the parents suppresses the recessive gene that would otherwise cause the hearing loss. There is a 25% chance that a child of the parents with autosomal recessive genes will show the hearing loss. The majority of children with profound hearing loss of genetic origin have parents with autosomal recessive genes for that hearing loss. Many of these children inheriting autosomal recessive genes have syndromes associated with hearing loss.

There are two other ways hearing loss can be inherited (Smith, Kochhar, & Friedman, 2009). One is called *X-linked inheritance.* A female has two X chromosomes. Even if one X chromosome is defective, the other normal gene will prevent the hearing loss from appearing. A male has only one X chromosome, since the other is a Y chromosome. Thus, if one X chromosome in a male is defective, the child is more likely to have a hearing loss.

The other form of genetically determined hearing loss is *mitochondrial inheritance.* You may recall from the discussion of outer hair cell physiology in Chapter 3 that mitochondria are energy-storing intracellular structures found in cochlear hair cells. Mitochondria contain DNA. Only affected mothers can pass mitochondrial-inherited hearing loss on to offspring, since there are no mitochondria in sperm.

Genetic factors are not only significant in congenital hearing loss in infants. Inherited genetic tendencies and DNA defects play a role in many other etiologies for hearing loss in children and also adults. Genetics may be a factor in the development of sensory hearing loss after birth and also in the likelihood of retrocochlear auditory dysfunction. The latter topic will be considered in the next chapter. The influence of genetic factors extends to diverse etiologies for cochlear auditory dysfunction, such as the likelihood of hearing loss due to exposure to high-intensity noise, age-related hearing loss, and even sensitivity to drug-induced hearing loss.

 WebWatch

There is a wealth of information on genetics and the genetics of hearing loss on the Internet. For example, websites operated by the Centers for Disease Control, or the CDC (www.cdc.gov), and the National Library of Medicine at the National Institutes of Health, or NIH (www.nlm.nih.gov) include links to the latest information and research findings. Given the speed and frequency with which new genetic findings are reported, some information in book chapters and even published articles will soon be outdated. These and some other Internet sites are sources of reliable and current information.

Prenatal, Perinatal, and Postnatal Diseases and Disorders

Prenatal. The terms *prenatal, perinatal,* and *postnatal* refer to time periods before, during, and soon after the birth of a child. *Prenatal* causes of sensory hearing loss occur before birth when the cochlea is still developing. Some forms of inherited hearing loss fit into the prenatal category, that is, a child has a gene for hearing loss from the time of conception and a hearing loss is present from birth. The term *in utero* is sometimes used to describe the early stage of the perinatal period. It is a Latin phrase meaning "in the uterus" or before the child is born.

Maternal infections, especially during the early part of pregnancy, are also classified as prenatal causes of hearing loss. Some prenatal and perinatal infectious processes identified by the Joint Committee on Infant Hearing were listed in Table 10.1 in the previous chapter. An infection in a pregnant woman may affect the unborn child by transmission through the placenta. Prenatal infections may pose a major risk for abnormal development of the cochlea and central auditory system. Several of the more common of prenatal infections may also occur later, in the perinatal and postnatal periods.

Perinatal. The term *perinatal* refers to the period of time near a child's birth. A variety of different etiologies contribute to hearing loss in this time period, ranging from inadequate oxygen or blood supply to the auditory system to exposure to medications that are potentially damaging to the cochlea. All systems in the body require a steady and adequate supply of oxygen and blood. Damage to hearing can result if the cochlea and the brain are deprived of the oxygen required for normal metabolism, even for just minutes. The term *anoxia,* literally meaning no oxygen, is used for oxygen deprivation, whereas the related term *hypoxia* refers to a decrease in the amount of oxygen.

Reduced blood flow to structures and tissues, including the cochlea and auditory regions of the brain, may also result in auditory dysfunction. *Ischemia* is the technical term for damage to tissue or organs, such as the ear or the brain, resulting from an abnormal reduction in blood flow. Medical problems causing a reduction of necessary amounts of oxygen and blood to the ear and brain are referred to as *hypoxic and ischemic events.*

Hypoxic and ischemic events affecting the central nervous system can be a complication of different diseases and of severe trauma. In the perinatal period, hypoxic and ischemic events pose a serious threat to hearing and to auditory function in general. As you might expect, the likelihood of hypoxia and ischemia is highest among infants born prematurely, with very low birth weight.

Prematurity is another perinatal factor related to hearing loss. Hearing loss is associated with problems arising from the birth of an extremely small baby, as many as twelve or thirteen weeks before the normal forty-week length of pregnancy. Prematurity with lower-than-normal birth weight is one of the most common perinatal risk factors for hearing loss.

The criterion for *low birth weight* is a weight of less than 2500 grams or 5.8 pounds at birth. Fortunately, advances in neonatal medical care and technology have contributed to higher survival rates for children who are even more premature and smaller at birth. A longstanding and common risk factor for newborn hearing screening is *very low birth weight (VLBW),* defined as weight of less than 1500 grams or 3.4 pounds at birth. As of 2006, approximately 1.5% of all babies born in the United States were VLBW, a total of over 60,000 babies each year. The term *extremely low birth weight (ELBW)* is used for even smaller infants who weigh less than 1000 grams, or 2 pounds, 3 ounces at birth. Extremely low birth weight babies are typically born at or before 27 weeks *gestational age.* Survival is now possible for infants born as young as 23 weeks gestational age, more than four months before normal-term birth!

Postnatal. Diseases and disorders that can produce sensory hearing loss in the *postnatal* period include a diverse assortment of infections that affect the inner ear and also a number of medications used to treat the infections. Some perinatal and postnatal infectious processes were also listed in Table 10.1. We'll soon review some of the more common infections that can cause hearing loss, as well as drugs used in treating infections and other medical problems that can also cause hearing loss.

Syndromes and Hearing Loss

Syndromic versus Nonsyndromic Hearing Loss. One of the simplest and most useful ways of categorizing congenital hearing loss is to describe it as either *syndromic* or *nonsyndromic* (Smith, Kochhar, & Friedman, 2009). Nonsyndromic hearing loss is most common, accounting for about 70% of all forms of inherited hearing loss. Over seventy specific gene locations have been mapped out for nonsyndromic hearing loss. Children with nonsyndromic hearing loss generally do not have a pattern of abnormalities involving other senses or systems in the body. That is, the primary problem is a deficit in hearing. In the nonsyndromic category, autosomal recessive inheritance is responsible for four out of five cases of hearing loss. Autosomal dominant forms of hearing comprise the other 20% (Dror & Avraham, 2009).

The characteristics of nonsyndromic hearing loss vary considerably from one patient to the next in both degree and configuration (Lesperance et al., 1995). The hearing loss may range from mild to profound. Hearing loss configuration also varies considerably, including high-frequency loss, low-frequency loss, or a flat hearing loss with similar thresholds across the audiometric frequencies. Nonsyndromic hearing loss may also be unilateral, affecting one ear, or bilateral. Finally, some forms of nonsyndromic hearing loss are delayed in onset and first appear later in childhood. Other forms of nonsyndromic hearing loss are progressive, with hearing thresholds gradually worsening during childhood and sometimes throughout a person's lifetime.

Syndromes Associated with Hearing Loss. Almost 600 **syndromes** may have hearing loss as a feature. Some of the more common syndromes associated with hearing loss were listed in Table 10.1, as described by the Joint Committee on Infant Hearing. The type, degree, and configuration of hearing loss in persons with these and other syndromes vary remarkably (Smith, Kochhar, & Friedman, 2009). Even though we are discussing inner ear abnormalities in this section of the chapter, it is important to note that conductive hearing loss, mixed hearing loss, and retrocochlear and central auditory nervous system abnormalities may be associated with certain syndromes. Progression of hearing loss is also a feature of some syndromes.

At least one-third of children with hearing loss have other disabilities that must be appropriately evaluated by specialists and taken into account during management (Jahrsdoerfer & Hall, 1986). The likelihood of multiple disabilities in addition to hearing loss reinforces the need for genetic consultation in families with children who have hearing impairment. Still, for over 30% of newborn infants with hearing loss there is no definitive etiology, despite intensive multidisciplinary diagnostic assessments.

Dual Sensory Impairment. At this point in our review of syndromes and hearing loss, it is appropriate to mention *dual sensory impairment (DSI).* Audiologists and speech pathologists must appreciate the unique challenges associated with the evaluation and rehabilitation of children and adults with dual sensory impairment. Dual sensory impairment is defined by abnormalities in two senses, such as the auditory and visual senses.

Usher's Syndrome, one of the syndromes listed in Table 10.6 (Chapter 10), is well known as an etiology associated with DSI. Patients with Usher's syndrome gradually, over the course of many years, experience the loss of hearing and vision. Dual sensory impairment is also found in over ten other syndromes, such as *Alport syndrome, Marshall syndrome, Stickler syndrome,* and *Pierre Robin syndrome.* The possibility of visual and auditory deficits in children is the rationale for the Joint Committee on Infant Hearing's 2007 recommendation that "every infant with a confirmed hearing loss should have an evaluation by an ophthalmologist to document visual acuity and rule out concomitant or late-onset visual disorders, such as Usher's syndrome" (pp. 907 and 908).

Young and old persons who are not diagnosed with a syndrome may also have dual sensory impairment. Visual and auditory deficits are not uncommon in a serious childhood illness called *cytomegalovirus (CMV)* infection. We'll soon talk a little more about hearing loss associated with CMV.

Ear and eye abnormalities are also two of the six features of *CHARGE association,* a rare disorder with a variety of symptoms. CHARGE is an acronym for the six features: (1) **C**oloboma (absence of eye tissue), (2) **H**eart disease, (3) **A**tresia of the choanae (an abnormal opening between the nasal cavity and the back of the throat), (4) **R**etarded growth with delayed development of the central nervous system, (5) **G**enital underdevelopment, and (6) **E**ar anomalies and hearing loss.

Dual sensory impairment does not occur only in pediatric populations. Dual sensory impairment also affects adults. For example, up to 20% of adults over the age of 70 years have dual sensory impairments (Saunders & Echt, 2007). You'll learn more in Chapter 14 about dual sensory impairment and its effect on communication.

Infections

Major infections that can cause inner ear dysfunction with hearing loss were listed previously in Table 10.1. Although these infections, identified by the Joint Committee on Infant Hearing, are clearly a risk for hearing loss in infants and young children; some may also pose a threat to hearing for older children and adults.

Bacterial Infections. **Meningitis** is a serious health problem for persons of all ages. The meninges are thin membranes that surround and protect the brain and spinal cord. Either viral or bacterial *microorganisms* can cause an infection and related inflammation of the meninges. The exact bacteria responsible for bacterial meningitis vary, depending on age of the patient. In other words, different types of bacteria typically cause meningitis in newborn infants than those that cause it in older children or in adults.

Because of the close proximity of the meninges to the central nervous system, meningitis is potentially life threatening and is always viewed as a medical emergency. Prompt and aggressive treatment with antibiotics and sometimes anti-inflammatory drugs is necessary to reduce serious complications and the possibility of neurological and cognitive deficits, and also hearing loss. Even though viral meningitis is more common, the health consequences are generally more serious for bacterial meningitis.

One in ten children who survive and recover from meningitis develop a sensorineural hearing loss (Fortnum, 1992). Here the term *sensorineural* is quite appropriate, as the hearing loss may be due to damage in the cochlea producing a sensory hearing loss or due to neural structures in the auditory nervous system. The risk for hearing loss is greater for newborn infants and young children than for older children and adults. Meningitis usually produces hearing loss in both ears, but unilateral deficits are possible (Hall, Bratt, Schwaber, & Baer, 1993).

One of the most exciting advances in medicine in recent years is the development of vaccines for prevention of infections that formerly were common causes for hearing loss in children (Yogev & Tan, 2011). There is now a vaccine for certain forms of bacterial meningitis. The meningitis vaccine, which can be given to children as young as 9 months, is 85% effective in preventing most forms of bacterial meningitis (Jodar, Feavers, Salisbury, & Granoff, 2002).

Fortunately, medical advances and public health initiatives have substantially reduced concerns about certain bacterial infectious diseases that cause hearing loss, at least in developed countries (Gulya, 2001). *Rubella* is a very good example of such a disease. Rubella, also called *congenital rubella syndrome* or *German measles,* was for many years a major cause of severe permanent hearing loss in children. An epidemic of rubella in 1964 and 1965 affected over 12 million persons and resulted in severe hearing loss for tens of thousands of children. The term *congenital rubella syndrome* is often used because of the multiple health consequences associated with the disease in addition to hearing loss, among them low birth weight, visual deficits, heart defects, and cognitive impairment.

Viral Infections. We'll now review *viral infections* and other *inflammatory disorders* (Gulya, 2001). Viral infections are another major cause for sensory hearing loss. Eight different *herpes viruses* may infect humans. Interestingly, the word *herpes* is derived from the Greek word for "creep." To be accurate, the word *herpes* is not used alone but combined with another term that describes either a specific virus or a particular region of the body that is affected. For example, *herpes simplex* is caused by one of two forms of *herpes simplex virus (HSV type I* or *HSV type II).* And, *herpes zoster* is an acute infectious disease caused by a specific virus, the *varicella-zoster virus.*

Cytomegalovirus (CMV) is one of the eight herpes viruses affecting humans. It is the most common viral cause of congenital hearing loss. Like other herpes viruses, CMV may be a lifelong latent infection. Congenital CMV is transmitted from an infected mother to the fetus. In fact, 30 to 40% of mothers infected with CMV will pass the infection on to the fetus.

Only about 10 to 15% of children born with congenital intrauterine CMV infection will have symptoms related to the disease, ranging in severity from mild to severe (Gulya, 2001). Serious symptoms include disrupted fetal growth and development, premature birth, developmental delay, and disorders affecting multiple organs and systems such as the liver, spleen, eyes, and central nervous system.

CMV is one of the most common causes of childhood hearing loss, perhaps accounting for about 15 to 20% of all cases of moderate-to-profound hearing loss in children (Gulya, 2001). Severe-to-profound hearing loss is also found in children who are otherwise asymptomatic although hearing loss is more likely in CMV-infected children with other symptoms.

Large-scale longitudinal studies at several pediatric research institutions, such as the University of Alabama-Birmingham, have revealed important aspects of the natural course of hearing loss associated with CMV (Dahle et al., 2000). For example, delayed onset of hearing loss, more than three years after birth, is quite common in children with CMV. Also, hearing loss progressively worsens in over one-half of children infected with CMV with decreases in hearing sometimes continuing well into school age.

Appreciation of the nature of hearing loss in children infected with CMV leads to five guidelines for identification, diagnosis, and management of auditory dysfunction (Hall, Bratt, Schwaber, & Baer, 1993). First, because it is so common, CMV-related hearing loss must always be suspected in all children until another diagnosis is made. Second, newborn infants who pass hearing screening at birth are still at risk for hearing loss that is delayed in onset or progressive in nature. Third, close audiological monitoring and reassessment of CMV-infected children with diagnosed or possible hearing loss must continue for years, even through school age. Fourth, hearing loss due to CMV may be unilateral or bilateral. Hearing assessment needs to include procedures and techniques that provide ear-specific information on auditory function. Follow up testing should always include both ears because children with CMV-related hearing loss in one ear are at considerable risk for later development of bilateral hearing loss.

Finally, assessment of hearing with behavioral techniques in children with CMV is complicated because of other sensory deficits, such as vision loss or dysfunction of the central nervous system. The use of objective measures of hearing, including otoacoustic emissions, acoustic immittance tests, and auditory evoked responses, is essential for timely and accurate diagnosis of hearing loss in children with CMV.

A review of viral etiologies for hearing loss would not be complete without a reference to *human immunodeficiency virus (HIV)*. HIV-infected persons are at considerable risk for various types of auditory pathology and dysfunction, including infections of the outer ear and middle ear and abnormalities involving the inner ear and central auditory nervous system (Swanepoel & Louw, 2010). We'll focus here on hearing loss due to cochlear disorders.

Cochlear disorders associated with sensorineural hearing loss are found in 20 to 50% of patients with HIV infection (Swanepoel & Louw, 2010). In some of these cases, the hearing loss also includes auditory nerve dysfunction. Importantly, sensorineural hearing loss in HIV-infected persons may be worsened if potentially ototoxic medications are used in management of life-threatening infections. HIV infection also puts the patient at higher risk for viral etiologies of sensorineural hearing loss described earlier in this chapter.

Finally, patients with HIV infection are susceptible to a variety of central nervous system diseases that, depending on location, may affect auditory functioning (Swanepoel & Louw, 2010). You'll be introduced to these and other etiologies for central auditory dysfunction in the next chapter.

Autoimmune Disease Involving the Inner Ear

The *human immune system* helps to protect the body from invasion and infection by viruses and other *pathogens*. A pathogen is any substance or microorganism that can cause disease. The body's defense mechanism for identifying and neutralizing the invading agents and preventing disease involves complex processes that go far beyond our discussion here. Substances called *antibodies* circulating in the blood and in structures like the ear serve as an early warning of potential invasion. When a viral intruder is detected in the ear, antibodies play an important role in mounting an attack to prevent or minimize disruption of inner ear function.

Autoimmune disease results from an overactive immune response. The immune system of a patient incorrectly identifies a part of the body, such as the inner ear, as a pathogen and attacks the structure (Harris, 2001; Harris, Gopen, & Keithley, 2009). There are over 100 different autoimmune diseases affecting systems and structures throughout the body, such as the skin, the joints, and the heart. Systemic autoimmune diseases involving the entire body may affect the inner ear along with other parts of the body. Examples of systemic autoimmune diseases associated with possible hearing loss include *Cogan syndrome, rheumatoid arthritis, systemic lupus erythematosus,* and inflammatory bowel disease (Harris, 2001; Harris, Gopen, & Keithley, 2009).

Autoimmune inner ear disease (abbreviated *AIED*) was first recognized as a cause for hearing loss in the 1980s (Harris, 1983). In this disease, antibodies or immune cells damage inner ear structures, particularly tissues containing the inner ear fluid endolymph. Autoimmune disease patients are most often middle-aged adults. Usually, a hearing loss develops over weeks or months in one ear, often followed months or even years later by progression of hearing loss in the other ear. Tinnitus is also a common symptom in patients with AIED. Prompt and accurate diagnosis of AIED is critical for effective treatment (Harris, 2001; Harris, Gopen, & Keithley, 2009). The bodily response to viral infections includes inflammation. Treatment includes quick administration of powerful *anti-inflammatory drugs* called *steroids*. Fortunately, AIED is quite rare, accounting for less than 1% of all forms of hearing loss (Harris, Gopen, & Keithley, 2009).

 ClinicalConnection

Any patient with a sudden sensorineural hearing loss or a hearing loss developing over a relatively short period should be referred directly to an ear specialist (an otologist). One possible explanation for the hearing loss is autoimmune inner ear disease (AIED), which may be successfully managed medically if the disorder is diagnosed promptly.

Potentially Ototoxic Medications

Physicians sometimes face a dilemma when caring for a patient with a serious health problem, such as a severe infection or a tumor that cannot be removed surgically. Aggressive medical management is required to treat or at least slow the progression of disease. However, there is a possibility that the medical management will lead to serious hearing loss. A variety of medicines are potentially **ototoxic**, that is, they may cause auditory dysfunction and produce a hearing loss (Brockenbrough, Rybak, & Matz, 2001; Campbell, 2006; Roland & Pawlowski, 2009). We'll review a small sampling of the drugs here.

You'll recall from the review of cochlear physiology in Chapter 3 that outer hair cells are capable of changes of shape called *motility*. Almost all potentially ototoxic drugs first affect function of the outer hair cells in the cochlea. The motility of the outer hair cells is dependent on a high level of metabolism. Ototoxic drugs interfere with outer hair cell metabolism and produce toxic substances in the cochlea that can cause permanent dysfunction, cell death, and corresponding hearing loss (Brockenbrough, Rybak, & Matz, 2001; Campbell, 2006; Roland & Pawlowski, 2009).

In administering drugs when treating infections and other disorders, physicians take care to adhere to proper doses or amounts of the drug. Physicians also regularly take blood samples for analysis to assure that the potentially ototoxic drug is within clinically acceptable limits. The goal is to administer enough of the drug to effectively treat the disease but not enough to pose a risk to the patient's overall health.

Unfortunately, these precautions do not eliminate the possibility of drug-induced auditory dysfunction (Brockenbrough, Rybak, & Matz, 2001; Roland & Pawlowski, 2009). Some patients are more susceptible to cochlear damage than others. A variety of factors play a role in increased susceptibility, among them kidney function, the administration of other ototoxic drugs in the past or at the same time, and genetic factors.

 ClinicalConnection

A patient history obtained by an audiologist always includes questions about medications the patient is taking. Answers to the questions are important in decisions about what hearing tests the audiologist will administer, the analysis and interpretation of tests that are performed, and how often the patient undergoes hearing testing. Information about potentially ototoxic medications might shed light on the etiology of hearing loss and related disorders like tinnitus.

Prevention of Drug-Induced Hearing Loss. Ongoing research is demonstrating that the damaging impact of ototoxic medications can be minimized or prevented entirely by prompt administration of combinations of vitamins, micronutrients, and other substances (Campbell, 2006). These substances protect the ear by reducing oxidative stress and removing or neutralizing toxic substances that damage cochlear hair cells. This breakthrough in hearing loss prevention also applies to protection from noise-induced hearing loss, as you will learn a little later in the chapter.

Aminoglycoside Antibiotics. Two antibiotics often administered to newborn infants for treatment of infection fall in the *aminoglycoside antibiotic* category of drugs. Aminogycosides are specific types of molecules that are very useful in fighting infections. *Gentamycin* is an aminoglycoside drug frequently given to newborn infants in a neonatal intensive care unit to treat an infection or as a precaution while testing is done to rule out the possibility of an infection. *Tobramycin* is another aminoglycoside antibiotic used to treat infection, including lung infections associated with the disease *cystic fibrosis.*

Aminoglycoside antibiotic drugs affect outer hair cell function and produce hearing loss at the highest frequencies (Brockenbrough, Rybak, & Matz, 2001; Roland & Pawlowski, 2009). With ongoing administration of the drug, hearing loss extends to the lower frequencies important for speech perception and communication. The damaging impact on cochlear function of multiple potentially ototoxic medications administered in combination may continue for months after the drugs are discontinued (Hall, Winkler, Herndon, & Gary, 1988).

L E A D E R S   A N D   L U M I N A R I E S

Kathleen Campbell

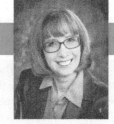

Kathy Campbell earned her bachelor's degree at South Dakota State University, her master's degree at the University of South Dakota, and her PhD at the University of Iowa. She then completed a doctoral fellowship with the Department of Veterans Affairs. Dr. Campbell is currently Professor & Director of Audiology Research in the Division of Otolaryngology, Department of Surgery at Southern Illinois University (SIU) School of Medicine, where she also has an appointment in the Department of Pharmacology. Dr. Campbell provided clinical services in audiology for over two decades, but now is fully devoted to research. She's published two textbooks and over 200 abstracts, articles, or book chapters.

Dr. Campbell has held leadership positions in the American Academy of Audiology. She received an award from American Mensa for chairing its research and awards committee and for her multiple patents. Dr. Campbell is sole inventor on five U.S.-issued patents. She regularly consults with the pharmaceutical industry and the FDA on ototoxicity issues. Dr. Campbell has discovered and patented substances that protect the ear from the damaging effects of certain drugs and from exposure to excessive noise. Her current research funding from the Department of Defense and the NIH exceeds $6 million and in previous years her external funding exceeded $9 million. Dr. Campbell exemplifies the role of clinical scholar in the profession of audiology. You'll find a 2004 interview of Dr. Campbell on Audiology Online.

Audiologists have responsibility for close long-term monitoring of hearing status in children who are receiving one or more potentially ototoxic medications.

Loop Diuretic Drugs. Loop diuretic medications are also ototoxic (Brockenbrough, Rybak, & Matz, 2001). Diuretic medicines help to remove excessive fluid in patients with a variety of disorders, including infants with pulmonary disorders. Loop diuretics alter function in a specific region of the kidney called the loop of Henle. One of the most common loop diuretic drugs is *furosemide*. It is often referred to as *Lasix*.

Most ototoxic drugs interfere directly with the function of outer hair cells in the cochlea. Furosemide disrupts metabolism of the stria vascularis and electrical activity in the inner ear (deJong, Adelman, Rubin, & Sohmer, 2012). These changes in cochlear function in turn affect outer hair cell functioning. Hearing loss due to furosemide alone may be reversible. However, permanent hearing loss is possible when furosemide is combined with certain other potentially ototoxic medications, including most aminoglycoside antibiotics.

Cancer Drugs. Some drugs used in chemotherapy for medical treatment of cancers are highly ototoxic (Brockenbrough, Rybak, & Matz, 2001; Campbell, 2006). Two common examples are the drugs *cisplatin* and *carboplatin*. Cisplatin causes sensory hearing loss due to disruption of outer hair cell metabolism, whereas carboplatin may affect inner and outer hair cells. The hearing loss associated with cisplatin is almost always observed first in the very high frequency region, above 8000 Hz (Brockenbrough, Rybak, & Matz, 2001; Roland & Pawlowski, 2009).

Patients treated with either cisplatin or carboplatin drugs should be closely monitored for ototoxic-induced auditory dysfunction. Otoacoustic emissions offer a very valuable tool for regular monitoring of auditory function in children who are treated medically with ototoxic drugs. Clinical research offers compelling evidence that otoacoustic emissions are more sensitive in early detection of cochlear dysfunction associated with cisplatin than conventional pure tone audiometry (Dhar & Hall, 2012).

Other Potentially Ototoxic Medications. The list of potentially ototoxic drugs grows longer as new medications are developed. For example, recent clinical studies suggest that long-term abuse of certain painkillers such as *OxyContin* and *hydrocodone* is linked to inner ear damage and profound sensory hearing loss. Even the common over-the-counter drug *aspirin* can cause ototoxicity (deJong, Adelman, Rubin, & Sohmer, 2012). Fortunately, auditory dysfunction following ingestion of aspirin is usually reversible. Case histories should always include questions about all prescription and over-the-counter medications a patient is taking.

Genetic Factors in Ototoxicity. Let us take a moment here to reflect back on the earlier discussion of the genetics of hearing and hereditary patterns in hearing loss. You'll recall that one form of genetically determined hearing loss is called *mitochondrial inheritance* and that mitochondria contain DNA. Recent studies confirm that a defect in mitochrondrial DNA, specifically rRNA, increases the possibility of hearing loss from aminoglycoside antibiotic medications. In other words, children or adults with this maternally inherited genetic defect are much more likely to develop a hearing loss following administration of common aminoglycoside drugs than persons without the mitochondrial fRNA genetic defect.

> **⬤ⁱ WebWatch**
>
> The Internet has made it much easier to learn more about new medications that are potentially ototoxic or interfere in any way with auditory or vestibular function. A document entitled "Adverse Drug Reactions and Audiology Practice," prepared by audiologist Dr. Robert DiSogra, is available online from the website of the American Academy of Audiology.

Ménière's Disease and Endolymphatic Hydrops

Ménière's disease is a complicated and incompletely understood medical problem. It is named after a nineteenth-century French physician, Prosper Ménière, who first reported some of the symptoms. Ironically, retrospective review of research papers from that time has shown that the patients Ménière initially described probably did not have the disease. The phrase *endolympatic hydrops* describes a buildup of fluid pressure in the cochlea. It is one of the key features of Ménière's disease.

Ménière's disease most often affects persons in the age range of 40 to 60 years, and slightly more women than men (Friedland & Minor, 2009). The disease may initially be bilateral (in about 10% of patients), but more typically one ear is affected first. For about 12% of patients with Ménière's disease, the other ear becomes involved within eight years. Ménière's disease is often misdiagnosed and sometimes over diagnosed, especially by physicians who are not otolaryngologists (Wackym, Balaban, & Schumacher, 2001).

Symptoms. Four symptoms are classically associated with the diagnosis of Meniere's disease: (1) fluctuating hearing loss, (2) episodic vertigo, (3) tinnitus, and (4) a sensation of ear fullness or pressure. We'll briefly review in a little more detail each of these four symptoms.

The *hearing loss* in patients diagnosed with Meniere's disease is sensorineural, and usually appears first in the lower-frequency region. Figure 11.9 shows hearing test findings for a typical patient with Ménière's disease. The hearing loss has a rising configuration, with thresholds gradually improving for higher test frequencies. Word recognition is reasonably good, but not 100% bilaterally. A peak of normal or at least better hearing is sometimes observed in patients with Ménière's disease, with decreased thresholds for the highest frequencies. Acoustic immittance findings like tympanometry are normal. Notably, to meet criteria for the diagnosis of Ménière's disease a patient's hearing loss must *fluctuate,* occasionally improving and worsening during the course of the disease.

FIGURE 11.9

Audiometric findings for a typical patient with Ménière's disease.

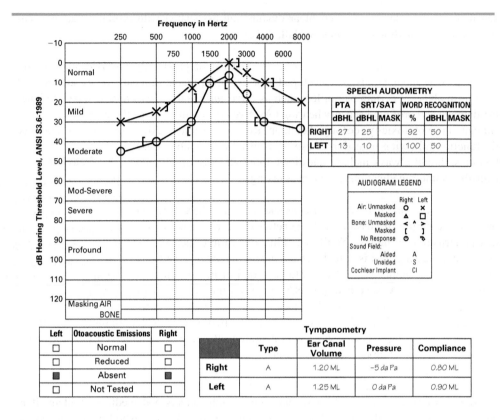

Patients use a variety of terms to describe the dizziness symptom in Ménière's disease, among them lightheadedness, disequilibrium, imbalance, and wooziness. However, true *vertigo* is the symptom that is always associated with Ménière's disease. Vertigo is the rather specific sensation of motion when the patient is still. Patients with vertigo often describe an experience in which suddenly the world is spinning around them.

Episodes of vertigo are essential for diagnosis of the disease (Friedland & Minor, 2009; Wackym, Balaban, & Schumacher, 2001). The episodes are relatively brief periods of intense spinning sensation that spontaneously resolve. The vertigo in Ménière's disease must occur spontaneously rather than following movement, such as getting out of bed. Additionally, the patient's vertigo must occur more than one time and it must last at least twenty minutes. Vertigo in Ménière's disease sometimes persists up to twenty-four hours. The vertigo may be very intense and associated with nausea and vomiting. You can easily appreciate why vertigo is the symptom that most often prompts the patient to go to a physician.

Patients with Ménière's disease typically perceive a low-frequency roaring type of *tinnitus* sound on the same side as their hearing loss, along with a sensation of ear pressure. Tinnitus loudness tends to increase along with the intensity of the other symptoms. Although patients with Ménière's disease often describe a *sensation of pressure* in the ear or aural fullness, this symptom is not required for a diagnosis. Aural fullness, when present, increases when a patient with Ménière's disease is experiencing an "attack" or episode.

Diagnostic Assessment. The diagnosis of Ménière's disease is based on these four symptoms, as well as findings on a variety of medical and audiological tests (Friedland & Minor, 2009; Wackym, Balaban & Schumacher, 2001). Vestibular testing plays an important role in the assessment of patients with possible Ménière's disease. We reviewed vestibular procedures in the preceding chapter. Certain auditory evoked responses like electrocochleography (ECochG) may also contribute to the diagnosis of Ménière's disease.

Medical Intervention. The main goal for management of Ménière's disease is to minimize or eliminate vertigo and to improve hearing status (Friedland & Minor, 2009; Wackym, Balaban, & Schumacher, 2001). Treatment strategies include medication to reduce excessive accumulation of cochlear fluids, injection of drugs to reduce vestibular function, and, less often, surgery that involves cutting the vestibular nerve on one side.

Superior Canal Dehiscence Syndrome

Superior canal dehiscence syndrome (SCDS) is a rather uncommon disorder that involves both the vestibular and the auditory systems. The term **dehiscence** refers to an abnormal thinning or even absence of the bone that covers the superior semicircular canal in the vestibular system. The opening in the bone surrounding a portion of the superior semicircular canal creates an abnormal "window" in the canal. You may recall reading about the semicircular canals in the review of vestibular system anatomy in Chapter 3. SCDS is most often unilateral, affecting only one side, but bilateral involvement is also possible (Friedland & Minor, 2009).

Symptoms in SCDS include hearing loss, vertigo, and nystagmus (Friedland & Minor, 2009). You encountered the term *nystagmus* in the previous chapter. It is used to describe rapid eye movements. The symptoms are usually brought about or intensified when the patient is exposed to loud sounds or to changes in middle ear pressure. Two abnormal phenomena in SCDS involve eye movements with auditory stimulation or pressure changes. The *Tullio phenomenon* consists of nystagmus produced by the presentation of loud sounds, whereas the *Hennebert sign* is defined as eye movements elicited by pressure changes in the external ear canal.

Loud sounds and pressure changes do not produce vestibular sensations in persons who do not have SCDS because the semicircular canals are entirely enclosed by bone. Vibrations cannot be transmitted through the thick fluid in the rigid, unyielding canals. Instead, energy from vibrations reaching the ear is transmitted through the cochlea, with release of the energy at the membranous round window in the inner ear. The? abnormal window or opening in the semicircular canal of a patient with SCDS permits vibration of fluids in the canal that, in turn, produce vestibular abnormalities like nystagmus (Friedland & Minor, 2009; Vrabec, 2001).

In addition, air-conducted sound energy that reaches the stapes footplate and would normally activate the cochlea is diverted to and dissipated by the semicircular canals. As a result, patients with SCDS show an apparent conductive hearing loss even though middle ear function is actually normal. Acoustic reflexes are typically recorded in patients with SCDS, confirming normal middle ear function. Interestingly, bone-conducted hearing may be enhanced, with thresholds for bone-conduction audiometry that are better than 0 dB. Some patients with SCDS are even bothered by their own voice, their footsteps, and the sound of their heartbeat.

Patients with SCDS may not be debilitated by the disorder. In other words, the auditory and vestibular abnormalities don't always have a serious impact on quality of life (Wackym, Balaban, & Schumacher, 2001). Patients with SCDS are generally able to avoid the high-intensity sounds and the changes in air pressure that produce disturbing symptoms. Surgery offers an effective treatment option for patients whose lives are impacted by SCDS (Vrabec, 2001). The goal of surgery is to identify the region of dehiscence and plug the opening in the superior semicircular canal.

ClinicalConnection

The anatomical abnormalities in SCDS lead to a highly unusual pattern of auditory test findings. Patients with SCDS have a very obvious air-bone gap, suggesting middle ear dysfunction, yet acoustic reflexes are entirely normal and middle ear disease is not supported by history or other test results. Therefore, the finding of normal acoustic reflexes in a patient with an obvious air-bone gap raises the suspicion of SCDS.

Idiopathic Sudden Sensorineural Hearing Loss

Idiopathic sudden sensorineural hearing loss is simply a hearing loss of unknown etiology that occurs suddenly. Hearing loss usually develops over a three-day period, but sometimes the onset is, literally, overnight. The word *idiopathic* is derived from Greek words for "personal" and "disease." It means there is no clear cause for the disorder. There are many known causes of sudden sensorineural hearing loss, such as infectious disease, meningitis, head trauma, and Ménière's disease. These and other etiologies for hearing loss are reviewed elsewhere in this chapter. *Idiopathic sudden sensorineural hearing loss (ISSHL)* is considered when other causes for the hearing loss are ruled out or eliminated by medical evaluation, history, and comprehensive diagnostic testing (Dobie & Doyle, 2009).

Causes of Idiopathic Sudden Sensorineural Hearing Loss. There are two main theories about the underlying pathology of ISSHL (Dobie & Doyle, 2009). The most likely explanation is a *viral infection* that disrupts cochlear function. As we've discussed elsewhere in this chapter, viral infections are a major cause for hearing loss in children and adults. Changes in cochlear structures following ISSHL closely resemble those documented for other viral causes for hearing loss, such as cytomegalovirus and mumps. It is possible that ISSHL reflects the abrupt reactivation of a latent or asymptomatic virus that then causes cochlear dysfunction.

The other theory for ISSHL focuses on a *vascular cause* that involves a disruption in blood flow to the cochlea (Dobie & Doyle, 2009). There are many risk factors for vascular disease involving the ear, among them high blood pressure, diabetes, cholesterol abnormalities, obesity, and even age and family history. Some of the characteristics of ISSHL, however, argue against a vascular explanation. For example, the risk factors just cited would more likely be associated with bilateral abnormalities and a higher incidence of ISSHL in men than women, yet ISSHL usually presents in only one ear, and ISSHL shows no gender preference (Dobie & Doyle, 2009).

Hearing Findings in Idiopathic Sudden Sensorineural Hearing Loss. ISSHL is defined as a decrease in pure tone hearing thresholds of more than 30 dB for at least three consecutive frequencies, such as 1000, 2000, and 3000 Hz (Dobie & Doyle, 2009). Hearing loss is typically accompanied by the perception of tinnitus and often vertigo. ISSHL is most often diagnosed in persons aged 30 to 60 years and affects males and females equally. Over 25,000 cases of ISSHL occur each year in the United States alone (Dobie & Doyle, 2009).

Hearing sensitivity recovers completely for over one-half of patients, even without aggressive medical treatment (Hall, Bratt, Schwaber, & Baer, 1993). The likelihood of hearing recovery is greater for low-frequency thresholds than for high-frequency thresholds. Nonetheless, quick and aggressive medical management is almost always recommended for patients with ISSHL. The different types of medical intervention include administration of anti-inflammatory drugs including steroids, antiviral drugs, medications to improve blood flow, and even antioxidants to enhance recovery of cochlear function.

 ClinicalConnection

The likelihood of improved hearing in sudden sensorineural hearing loss is always greater with prompt and appropriate medical management. Any patient with a sudden hearing loss must be referred immediately and directly to a physician, preferably an otologist, for evaluation and management. The chances for a good outcome are decreased considerably if intervention is delayed even for only a few days after the onset of the hearing loss.

Head Trauma

Objects penetrating the tympanic membrane can result in inner ear abnormalities, as well as middle ear damage. A different type of inner ear trauma can arise during air travel and when diving under water, including scuba diving. The common problem in both instances is the difference between the atmospheric pressure outside the ear and the pressure in the middle ear. *Barotrauma* is the technical term for pressure-related damage to the ear. Failure to equalize pressure in the middle ear with adequate passage of air through the Eustachian tube may lead to damage of the tympanic membrane, the round window membrane, or the oval window membrane. Symptoms of barotrauma include pain, dizziness, tinnitus, and hearing loss.

Head injury with trauma to the temporal bone produces varying degrees of ear damage and resulting hearing loss (Welling & Packer, 2009). Sensorineural hearing loss is almost always found in patients with fracture of the temporal bone. The degree of hearing loss is related to the extent and nature of temporal bone fractures (Hall & Ghorayeb, 1991).

Noise-Induced Hearing Loss (NIHL)

We'll conclude the chapter with a review of the two most common etiologies for hearing loss: age-related hearing loss and noise- or sound-induced hearing loss. Short-term or chronic exposure to excessive levels of sound is a common cause for hearing loss in adults (Dobie, 2001; Kujawa, 2009). Audiologists in a variety of work settings, including military audiology clinics, regularly test the hearing of adults and sometimes children who are at risk for sound-induced hearing loss.

The phrase *sound-induced* rather than noise-induced hearing loss is really more accurate because cochlear damage can be due exposure to high-intensity levels of music as well as noise. The National Institute of Deafness and Other Communicative Disorders (NIDCD) estimates that 10 million persons in the United States alone have permanent noise-induced hearing loss. Another 30 million are regularly exposed to levels of sound that are potentially damaging to the ears and hearing.

Occupational exposure to high-intensity noise accounts for about 10% of all adults with moderate hearing loss (Dobie, 2008; Nelson, Nelson, Concha-Barrientos, & Fingerhut, 2005). Billions of dollars are paid annually by the private sector, the military, and the Veterans Administration healthcare system in compensation for noise-related hearing impairment. Importantly, noise-induced hearing loss is almost always preventable. The World Health Organization (WHO) refers to noise-induced hearing loss as "the major avoidable cause of permanent hearing impairment worldwide" (WHO, 2011).

Risk for Noise-Induced Hearing Loss. Exposure to excessive levels of sound can occur during a wide variety of work and recreational activities. Military personnel in combat and noncombat settings are often at considerable risk for noise-induced hearing loss. One of the main responsibilities of audiologists serving in the U.S. Army, Navy, or Air Force is assessment of soldiers, sailors, marines, and airmen who are exposed to potentially dangerous levels of noise. Audiologists employed in Veterans Administration Medical Centers also test on a daily basis veterans with noise-induced hearing loss and related auditory disorders like tinnitus.

Industrial noise sources include heavy machinery, engines of trains, ships, automobiles, tractors, aircrafts, lawnmowers, drills, mining equipment, compressors, presses, and power tools. Recreational activities with potentially harmful sound levels include motorcycle and snowmobile riding, shooting and hunting, woodworking, and attendance at automobile races and other sports events such as football games in large stadiums.

Live and recorded music exceeding 85 dBA is potentially damaging to the ears and hearing (Dobie, 2001; Kujawa, 2009; Mueller & Hall, 1998). Hearing loss is well documented in musicians of every genre, from rock and roll to orchestral symphony music. Even playing in a school band involves risk for sound-induced hearing loss. Also, the use of personal audio players like iPods and MP3 devices at high-intensity levels may result in sound-induced auditory dysfunction (LePrell, Hensley, Campbell, Hall, & Guire, 2011). Greater exposure to high levels of sound is implicated in the rather dramatic increase of hearing loss in teenage persons in recent years (Shargorodsky, Curhan, Curhan, & Eavey, 2010).

L E A D E R S   A N D   L U M I N A R I E S

Sharon Kujawa

Sharon G. Kujawa earned her bachelor's degree from Michigan State University, her master's degree from Idaho State University, and her PhD from the University of Arizona. She then completed a post-doctoral fellowship in auditory pharmacology at Kresge Institute of Louisiana State University and another post-doctorate at in auditory neurophysiology in the Eaton-Peabody Lab at Harvard University. She currently has an appointment as an Associate Professor of Otology and Laryngology at Harvard Medical School. She also serves on the faculty of the Harvard-MIT Program in Speech and Hearing Biosciences and Technology. Dr. Kujawa is Director of the Department of Audiology at the Massachusetts Eye and Ear Infirmary in Boston. She has held a variety of leadership positions in the American Auditory Society, the Association for

Research in Otolaryngology, and the American Academy of Audiology. Dr. Kujawa is a recipient of the Academy's Distinguished Achievement Award.

Dr. Kujawa's laboratory research focuses on understanding how vulnerability to noise-induced hearing loss is shaped by genetic background, how noise exposure alters the way ears and auditory nervous systems age, and how these consequences of exposure can be manipulated pharmacologically to reveal underlying mechanisms or for treatment or prevention. She is also involved in a biomedical engineering research partnership that seeks to develop drug delivery systems suitable for chronic use in the human inner ear. Dr. Kujawa defines what is meant by the phrase "clinical scholar."

Duration of Noise Exposure and Level of Noise. Cochlear dysfunction and damage are possible whenever noise levels exceed 85 dBA (Dobie, 2001; Kujawa, 2009). There is a well-defined relation between noise levels and the maximum safe exposure time within a 24-hour period. That is, the time before there is a possibility of ear damage. A few examples of intensity levels for typical sound sources and safe exposure times will put this noise level in perspective,. Let's say you are exposed to a noise level of about 85 dBA while standing near a truck with a diesel engine running or using a lawnmower. The maximum safe exposure time to these types of noise is eight hours. Riding a motorcycle or listening to a live performance of a symphony orchestra results in exposure to sound at a level of 100 dBA with a safe exposure time of about two hours. You'll be exposed to sound of about 110 dBA while listening to a rock band. The maximum safe exposure time is only 30 minutes. And, sounds produced by firecrackers, jet engines at take-off, and gunfire exceed 140 dBA and pose immediate risk to hearing. This relationship between intensity level of noise and dose over time is referred to as the *time-weighted average (TWA)*. Very simply, the higher the intensity level of noise, the shorter the safe exposure time.

Threshold Shift Following Noise Exposure. Two types of hearing changes are associated with noise exposure, as determined by changes in pure tone hearing thresholds. *Temporary threshold shift (TTS)* is a decrease in hearing thresholds occurring during and immediately after noise exposure and persisting for a period of sixteen to forty-eight hours. Consistent exposure to high levels of sound temporarily affects metabolism in the cochlea, particularly in the outer hair cells. During this time period a person with TTS may experience tinnitus, such as ringing or other sounds in the ears. Also, speech and music may sound distorted or muffled. After a few days, hearing thresholds generally return to pre-exposure levels as normal cochlear physiology is naturally restored.

Repeated exposure to harmful levels of noise may produce *permanent threshold shift (PTS),* or irreversible hearing loss. Figure 11.10 illustrates the characteristic pattern of NIHL (noise-induced hearing loss). The audiogram shows a high-frequency sensorineural hearing loss, with maximum deficit in the region of 3000 to 4000 Hz. Notice the notching pattern for decreased air-conduction thresholds in each ear. In this case, the hearing loss is greatest at 3000 Hz in both ears. Then, hearing sensitivity improves for higher test frequencies.

A number of variables play a role in determining the effects of noise exposure on an individual person and the likelihood of permanent hearing loss. They include a history of previous noise exposure, exposure to certain chemicals like solvents, age, and genetic factors.

Cochlear Damage from Noise Exposure. Research has documented specific anatomic and physiologic changes in the cochlea with excessive noise or music exposure (Dobie, 2001; Kujawa, 2009). Some of the most obvious changes involve hair cells. Studies have confirmed mechanical damage to hair cell stereocilia, swelling of hair cells, and production of toxic substances in hair cells. The outer hair cells are most vulnerable to effects of noise exposure and show the greatest changes. Figure 11.11 shows the negative impact of noise on cochlear hair cells. Figure 11.11A is a microphotograph of stereocilia on healthy outer hair cells, whereas Figure 11.11B is an example of stereocilia on noise-damaged outer hair cells.

Other pathologic changes in the cochlea produced by exposure to excessive sound levels include swelling of the stria vascularis and collapse of supporting cells. Studies have also recently revealed that noise exposure is linked to excessive release of the primary

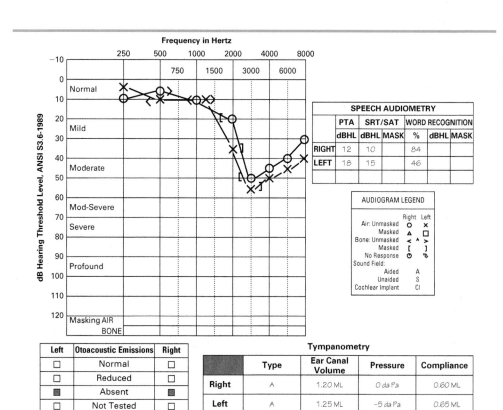

FIGURE 11.10

Audiogram for an adult with a history of chronic noise exposure and noise-induced hearing loss.

FIGURE 11.11 **A.** Photomicrograph of normal stereocilia on an outer hair cell. **B.** Photomicrograph of abnormal stereocilia on an outer hair cell damaged following excessive exposure to high-intensity noise. Images reproduced with permission from Dangerous Decibels. www.dangerousdecibels.org

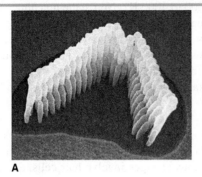
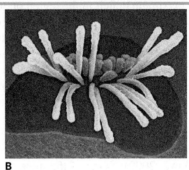

A B

neurotransmitter glutamate in the ear and to abnormal functioning of auditory nerve fibers (Kujawa, 2009; Lin, Furman, Kujawa, & Liberman, 2011).

In addition, intensive laboratory research in the past few years has revealed one of the major causes of cochlear damage by noise exposure (deJong, Adelman, Rubin, & Sohmer, 2012). High levels of noise trigger the release of destructive molecules in the cochlea (Kujawa, 2009). Molecules called *free radicals* are responsible for many of the changes in the cochlea, leading to oxidative damage and hair cell death, a condition referred to as *apoptosis*.

Traditional approaches to hearing protection and prevention of noise-induced hearing loss have focused mostly on devices like earplugs and earmuffs that attenuate or reduce the level of sound reaching the inner ear (Dobie, 2001; Kujawa, 2009).

In the past decade, research on the mechanisms of noise-induced hearing loss has led to an exciting discovery. Certain chemicals called *antioxidants* and other substances like vitamins can protect the ear against the damaging effects of free radicals (Campbell, 2006; Kujawa, 2009; LePrell, Gagnon, Bennett, & Ohlemiller, 2011; Le Prell & Spankovich, 2012). Antioxidants are found naturally in many fruits and vegetables that are rich in beta-carotene, vitamin C, and vitamin E, particularly fruits and vegetables that are colorful, especially purple, blue, red, orange, and yellow. Vitamins and micronutrients with high concentrations of antioxidants are also available for ingestion in the form of tablets or pills.

If an optimal combination of antioxidants reaches the ear within hours after excessive noise exposure, hair cells can be "rescued" from death and hearing loss can be prevented or substantially reduced (LePrell, Gagnon, Bennett, & Ohlemiller, 2011a; LePrell & Spankovich, 2012). Temporary disruption in cochlear metabolism is prevented from developing into permanent damage and hearing loss. You may have noticed that the principle underlying protection of the ear from the effects of noise exposure with antioxidants and other substances is similar to that described in our discussion of the prevention of drug-induced hearing loss (Campbell, 2006).

ClinicalConnection

The old saying "an ounce of prevention is worth a pound of cure" certainly applies to the role of audiologists in hearing conservation. Hearing conservation is the term used to describe efforts to prevent or minimize noise-induced hearing loss on a large scale in at-risk populations such as workers in industry or military personnel. The most effective approach to hearing conservation is to limit exposure to unsafe levels of sound to brief periods of time.

Presbycusis

Presbycusis is the technical term for age-related hearing loss. Another similar sounding word, *presbyastasis,* is often used in reference to age-related balance disorders. Published reports describing severe hearing loss with aging date back to the end of the nineteenth century. A gradual decrease in hearing thresholds across the age span was described in the 1920s (Bunch, 1929). Later, microscopic investigations of the temporal bones of deceased older persons confirmed specific age-related structural changes in the ear and auditory nerve (Schuknecht, 1964).

Prevalence of hearing loss in adults clearly increases with age. Less than 10% of people aged 20 to 30 years have hearing loss, whereas hearing loss affects more than one-half the population by age 75. In years to come the number of people with presbycusis will continue to increase in the United States, as the percentage of elderly people in the general population increases (Agrawal, Platz, & Niparko, 2008). According to estimates offered by the World Health Organization (WHO), by the year 2025 there will be more than 500 million persons worldwide with significant impairment from presbycusis (Sprinzl & Riechelmann, 2010).

Factors Contributing to Age-Related Hearing Loss. Presbycusis commonly describes hearing loss that reflects an accumulation of factors that can affect hearing (Mills, Megerian, & Lambert, 2009; Roland, Easton, & Meyerhoff, 2001). Factors that presumably contribute to hearing loss with aging include the following:

- Race
- Cardiovascular health and hypertension, or high blood pressure
- Dietary habits
- Exercise habits
- Smoking
- Diabetes
- Exposure to nonoccupational noise
- Ototoxic drugs
- Heredity

Research now suggests that hearing loss attributed specifically to the aging process may be determined to a large extent by genetic factors. Analysis of large amounts of data in a well-known ongoing longitudinal investigation known as *The Framingham Heart Study* suggests that hereditary factors play an important role in the likelihood of developing age-related hearing loss (Gates, Couropmitree, & Myers, 1999).

Age-Related Changes in Cochlear Structure and Function. Multiple explanations for presbycusis have been proposed. In a classic paper published in the 1960s, a well-known hearing scientist at Harvard, Harold Schuknecht, first described four different types of presbycusis, based on study of age-related changes in the auditory system (Schuknecht, 1964). They were: (1) a sensory type associated with the loss of hair cells in the high-frequency region of the cochlea, (2) a metabolic or "strial" type associated with an at least 30% loss of stria vascularis tissue, (3) a neural type caused by an at least 50% loss of neurons in the spiral ganglion region of the auditory nerve, and (4) a "conductive" presbycusis, defined by

FIGURE 11.12

Average hearing loss as shown with in an audiogram format over the decades of age from 49–59 years to 80–89 years for males **(A)** and females **(B)**. Source: Cruickshanks, K. J. et al. (1998). Prevalence of hearing loss in older adults in Beaver Dam, Wisconsin. The epidemiology of hearing loss study. *American Journal of Epidemiology, 148,* 879–886.

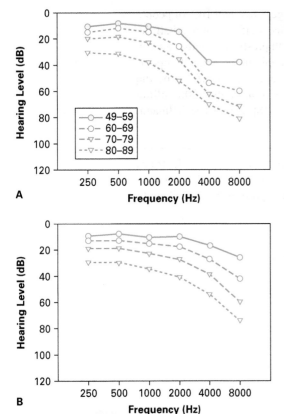

a high-frequency hearing loss with none of the changes in the cochlea or auditory nerve just described.

There is now general agreement that the gradually-sloping high-frequency hearing loss characteristic of presbycusis often involves a combination of these pathological changes. Some patients do not fit into any of the four categories described by Schuknecht (Ohlemiller, 2004). In other words, the pattern of hearing loss reflected in the audiogram often does not correlate with changes in the auditory system described by Schuknecht's four types of presbycusis (Nelson & Hinojosa, 2006).

Recent research clearly shows that hearing problems in the aging are sometimes linked to dysfunction of the central auditory nervous system (Gates & Mills, 2005; Gordon-Salant, 2005). There is also scientific evidence that age-related changes in the ear can later lead to abnormal function and even loss of neurons in the central auditory nervous system (Canlon, Illing, & Walton, 2010).

Concluding Comments about Presbycusis. Our current knowledge of age-related hearing loss supports four general statements (Mills, Megerian, & Lambert, 2009; Roland, Easton, & Meyerhoff, 2001): First, presbycusis is not limited to the elderly. Changes in hearing thresholds begin before the age of 30. Second, age-related decreases in hearing thresholds are invariably most prominent for audiometric frequencies from 4000 to 8000 Hz and higher frequencies (Cruickshanks et al., 1998). These patterns are clearly evident in the representative audiograms of different age groups in Figure 11.12. Hearing thresholds gradually decrease as test frequency increases. The hearing loss is quite symmetrical. Third, as evidence from the audiogram graphs in Figure 11.12 shows, hearing loss with aging is greater for males than females, even when the effects of noise exposure are removed (Cruickshanks et al., 1998). Finally, age-related hearing loss is to a considerable extent related to genetic or hereditary factors.

PULLING IT ALL TOGETHER

You now appreciate why audiologists, speech-language pathologists, and other healthcare professionals working with children and adults need to have an understanding of diseases and disorders affecting the ear. The information influences decisions about how to proceed with hearing assessment, the most appropriate management options and, importantly, whether the patient should be referred to a physician for medical evaluation and possible treatment.

Hearing loss is not uncommon. For example, parental concerns about ear disorders and associated hearing loss are among the top reasons why children go to pediatricians. Toward the other end of the age spectrum the majority of elderly persons have some degree of hearing impairment. You were introduced in the chapter to some principles of genetics. Also, you learned that family history and genetic factors play an important role in determining whether a child or an adult will have hearing loss. Indeed, genetics seems to be involved in a diverse assortment of disorders and diseases underlying hearing loss, and over 100 genes are directly linked to hearing loss.

After reading this chapter, you know that disorders of the outer ear range from non-pathologic problems, like cerumen in the ear canal, to serious pathology, including cancerous growths on the pinna. Some middle ear disorders like otitis media in children may occur without parental awareness, and certain growths in the middle ear space, such as a cholesteatoma, require immediate attention by an otolaryngologist.

Etiologies for inner ear dysfunction also cover a wide range. Nonpathologic etiologies include excessive noise exposure and advancing age, which account for most patients with hearing loss encountered by audiologists in an adult patient population. There are diseases requiring prompt medical attention, including autoimmune disease, Ménière's disease, and sudden sensorineural hearing loss, to cite just three. And, you now realize that certain medications used to treat infections and other serious medical problems may, unfortunately, produce ototoxic-induced hearing loss. The good news is that anti-oxidants and other substances may reduce the damaging effects of the potentially ototoxic drugs, even acoustic trauma. Throughout the chapter, you drew on information on hearing testing methods acquired earlier in the book to understand the different patterns of auditory findings associated with many and diverse outer, middle, and inner ear causes for hearing loss in children and adults.

READINGS

Bailey, B. J., Calhoun, K. H., Healy, G. D., Pillsbury, H. C., Johnson, J. T., Jackler, R. T., & Tardy, M. E. (Eds.). (2001). *Head and neck surgery—Otolarynoglogy. Volume II.* (3rd ed.). Philadelphia: Lippincott Williams & Wilkins.

Dhar, S., & Hall, J. W. III. (2011). *Otoacoustic emissions: Principles, procedures, and protocols.* San Diego: Plural Publishing

Gordon-Salant, S., Frisina, R. D., Popper, A. N., & Fay, R. R. (Eds.). (2010). *The aging auditory system.* New York: Springer.

Jerger, S., & Jerger, J. (1981). *Auditory disorders: A manual for clinical evaluation.* Boston: Little, Brown & Co.

Mueller, H. G. III, & Hall, J. W. III. (1998). *Audiologists' desk reference. Volume II. Audiological management, rehabilitation & terminology.* San Diego: Singular Publishing.

Snow, J. B. Jr., & Wackym, P. A. (Eds.). (2009). *Ballenger's otorhinolaryngology—head and neck surgery* (17th ed.). Shelton CT: BC Decker.

12

We Hear with Our Brain: Retrocochlear and Central Auditory Nervous System Disorders

LEARNING OBJECTIVES

In this chapter, you will learn:

- Some neuroscience principles and how they've contributed to the assessment of patients with disorders of the nervous system
- The meaning of the expression "retrocochlear auditory dysfunction"
- Causes of retrocochlear auditory and vestibular dysfunction in children and adults
- How retrocochlear auditory dysfunction can be identified and confirmed with diagnostic auditory tests
- About a relatively recently discovered and serious category of hearing problems called auditory neuropathy spectrum disorder (ANSD)
- About the major disorders affecting the central nervous system and how they produce auditory abnormalities
- That auditory abnormalities are found in patients with some rather common neurological diseases, such as Alzheimer's dementia
- What is meant by the phrase "auditory processing disorders" (APD)
- How auditory processing disorders are diagnosed
- That audiologists and speech pathologists work as a team in the management of patients with APD

KEY TERMS

Acoustic neuroma
Alzheimer's dementia
Auditory Neuropathy Spectrum Disorder (ANSD)
Auditory processing disorder (APD)
Brain plasticity
Cerebrovascular accident (CVA)
Dementia
Demyelinating diseases
Functional magnetic resonance imaging (fMRI)
Meningiomas
Neurodegenerative diseases
Neurofibroma (neurofibromatosis)
Neuroradiology
Paralysis and paresis
Retrocochlear
Vestibular schwannoma

CHAPTER FOCUS

At this point in the book, the phrases hearing impairment and auditory dysfunction may bring to mind an audiogram depicting pure tone thresholds that are outside of normal limits. You might also envision poor word recognition scores and even abnormal tympanograms. Such auditory findings are certainly consistent with hearing impairment due to middle ear or inner ear dysfunction. However, some patients with hearing impairment or auditory dysfunction have a normal audiogram, excellent word recognition scores, and normal tympanograms. Not all patients with hearing impairment have a conductive or sensory hearing loss.

As you'll learn in this chapter, auditory nerve dysfunction can produce dramatic abnormalities in a variety of hearing tests. Abnormalities affecting auditory pathways beyond the inner ear are often referred to as retrocochlear auditory dysfunction. Disorders involving the auditory nerve, like tumors, can pose a serious risk to health. Tumors not detected in a timely fashion are potentially life threatening. In addition, a substantial and diverse assortment of disorders affecting auditory regions in the brain can produce hearing problems. This fact supports an important principle reiterated throughout the book: *"We hear with our brain."* A hearing assessment should describe function throughout the auditory system, from the ear to the auditory regions of the temporal lobe.

You'll now be introduced to many causes of hearing loss that arise beyond the ear. The topic is extensive. Although a number of disorders are mentioned, we will focus on a handful that account for the majority of patients that audiologists and speech pathologists encounter clinically. Diagnostic assessment of retrocochlear and central auditory nervous system function with a comprehensive test battery is not a recent trend. Rather, it is a long and respected tradition in clinical audiology, dating back to the 1960s. Within the past decade, audiologists have witnessed the discovery of new etiologies for neural auditory dysfunction. There is also renewed appreciation of auditory abnormalities associated with neurological diseases that were first described over a hundred years ago.

In this chapter, we'll discuss causes of retrocochlear and central nervous system dysfunction, such as tumors affecting the auditory nerve and brain. We will also highlight relatively new discoveries, including auditory neuropathy spectrum disorder (ANSD), auditory dysfunction in neuropsychiatric disorders such as Parkinson's disease and Alzheimer dementia, and auditory processing disorders (APD) in children and adults.

We Hear with Our Brain

Historical Perspective

The typical objective in hearing assessment is detection and diagnosis of auditory problems caused by abnormalities of the ear. A focus on the ear is logical. You learned in the previous chapter about dozens of diseases affecting the outer ear, middle ear, and inner ear, diseases that account for the auditory disorders encountered most often in the clinical or educational setting.

The almost exclusive emphasis on disorders of the ear and audiogram abnormalities dates back to the very beginnings of audiology. In a classic 1954 textbook entitled *Auditory Disorders in Children: A Manual for Differential Diagnosis,* Helmer Mykelbust prompted readers to remember that "hearing is a receptive sense . . . and essential for normal language behavior" (p. 11) and, in addition, "the diagnostician of auditory problems in children has traditionally emphasized peripheral damage. It is desirable that he also include central damage" (Myklebust, 1954, p. 54). Mykelbust was a well-known psychologist at Northwestern University who was among the first to define what are now called learning disabilities. The point Mykelbust made in the 1950s is still as valid today as it was then. We should not focus only on ear-related hearing problems because, in truth, "we hear with our brain."

In the 1960s, occasional articles described patterns of test findings in persons with documented abnormalities of the auditory nervous central nervous system (Jerger, 1960; Katz, 1962). As you learned in Chapter 9, an entire specialized diagnostic test battery emerged in the 1960s and 1970s for differentiating cochlear from retrocochlear auditory dysfunction. The primary objective of diagnostic testing during that era was identification of patients with tumors affecting the eighth cranial auditory nerve (see Hall, 1991, for review).

In the 1980s, behavioral and auditory evoked response test findings were described for a variety of neurological diseases, such as multiple sclerosis, cerebrovascular accidents, and traumatic head injury (Hall, 1983, 1991, 2007a). As reviewed in Chapter 9, the Joint

Committee on Infant Hearing (JCIH) during this time period first cited neurological risk indicators for hearing impairment, including asphyxia or inadequate oxygen to the brain, meningitis, cytomegalovirus, and other diseases affecting the central nervous system in addition to the inner ear.

The Decade of the Brain

Interest in auditory function and the brain increased remarkably beginning in the 1990s, in parallel with an explosion of neuroscience research. Indeed, the period from 1990 to 2000 was officially known as "the Decade of the Brain." In the United States, then President George H.W. Bush, the Library of Congress, and the National Institute of Mental Health of the National Institutes of Health promoted a decade-long initiative to "to enhance public awareness of the benefits to be derived from brain research" through "appropriate programs, ceremonies, and activities."

Renewed emphasis on basic brain research led to an unprecedented volume of scientific publications and new discoveries. And, assuring a promising future for brain research and ongoing new clinical developments, the number of neuroscience doctoral students and persons who identify themselves as neuroscientists has steadily increased during the past twenty years. Productive researchers from other disciplines, such as molecular biology and computer science, now focus entirely on studies of the brain. As a result, techniques like functional brain imaging and measurement of brain activity during a listening task are now regularly applied in auditory neuroscience research.

An enormous number of neuroscience research questions are still not answered. The human brain is remarkably complex, with as many as 86,000 billion neurons and perhaps more. Amazingly, each neuron in the brain receives input from about 10,000 other neurons. Questions about how the brain processes sound are now regularly answered by intensive ongoing auditory neuroscience research.

Beginning around the year 1990, discoveries in one area of neuroscience quickly inspired and fueled investigations in other areas. The emphasis on neuroscience soon contributed to increased study of auditory processes in the brain. Before long newly discovered auditory neuroscience principles found clinical applications in patients with a wide variety of central auditory nervous system disorders.

Brain Plasticity

The concept of **brain plasticity** and its molecular basis was perhaps the dominant discovery during the Decade of the Brain. Changes in the brain are brought about by experience and reflected by perceptions, learning, memory, language, emotion, creativity, and the brain's response to injury or developmental deficits. The principles of neuroplasticity or brain plasticity help to answer some of the most important questions about brain development. How do synapses between neurons form? What factors influence the branching out (or arborization) of neurons and why do they reach out to other specific neurons? Why do some neurons differ from others? The concept of neuroplasticity is essential for understanding how disruptions in brain function during development, or disruptions that follow injury or disease, are not necessarily permanent.

What is the importance of these many neuroscience breakthroughs for audiologists, speech pathologists, and other professionals who work with patients who have communicative disorders? Brain plasticity provides the evidence-based rationale for almost all forms of intervention and treatment that audiologists and speech pathologists offer to persons with auditory disorders, language impairment, and related problems such as reading disorders.

In this chapter, you will learn about the diverse disorders that can affect the auditory system beyond the ear. Diseases, disorders, deficits, and developmental delays of the central nervous system are often associated with serious hearing problems and other communicative disorders like language and reading impairments. We will now discuss many disorders affecting the auditory nerve and auditory regions of the brain that can cause hearing or auditory deficits. In later chapters you'll learn about the technologies and techniques audiologists and speech pathologists use in the habilitation, rehabilitation, and management of specific populations of patients.

Retrocochlear Disorders

The adjective **retrocochlear** is often used in describing disorders involving pathways and structures between the cochlea and the brainstem. Most retrocochlear disorders are neoplasms. Neoplasm is technical term for tumor and literally means *new growth*. We will begin the review of retrocochlear disorders with mention of some of the main tests and studies physicians use to diagnose them. The same types of tests are also used to diagnose disorders affecting the central nervous system (CNS), from the lower portion of the brainstem all the way to the cerebral cortex. If it has been some time since you read in Chapter 3 about auditory system anatomy and physiology, you may wish to review information there before continuing on with this chapter.

Diagnosis of retrocochlear and CNS disorders is to a large extent based on a complete patient history. In diagnosing any disease or disorder, healthcare providers gain a great deal of information from a description of the patient's symptoms, when they were first noticed, and how they have progressed over time.

For example, a patient may describe symptoms mostly for the left side like recent difficulty using the telephone with the left ear, a ringing type of tinnitus arising from the left ear, tingling sensations and weakness on the left side of the face, and perhaps some unsteadiness. A medical specialist like an otolaryngologist or a neurosurgeon would certainly include an acoustic tumor or acoustic neuroma on the short list of possible diagnoses for a patient with such symptoms and complaints.

As you'll soon learn in more detail, an **acoustic neuroma** is a mass that originates on a vestibular nerve. The technical term for acoustic tumor is *vestibular schwannoma*. As an acoustic tumor slowly grows it often presses on the auditory nerve that leads from the cochlea to the brainstem. At this point, the patient begins to notice a disruption in hearing or related problems.

A very different diagnosis would be suspected for a patient with another set of symptoms. Take for example an elderly patient whose family members express concern about problems their loved one is experiencing, including memory loss, disorganization, and getting lost during walks in the neighborhood or when driving home from church. A physician or psychologist caring for that patient would almost certainly consider some type of dementia. Dementia is a general term for deterioration in mental and cognitive status. Findings on auditory tests in combination with information from a patient history contribute to the diagnosis of disorders involving auditory system structures and pathways beyond the ear.

Brain Imaging

Neuroradiology is an essential tool for the diagnosis of diseases and disorders involving the retrocochlear pathways and the CNS. The term **neuroradiology** encompasses various techniques for imaging or viewing the brain. Neuroradiologists are medical specialists that perform and interpret various forms of brain scanning images. Neuroradiological procedures are available in most hospitals and medical centers nowadays. The same general types of radiological procedures are used to image any part of the body, but our discussion will be limited to brain imaging.

FIGURE 12.1

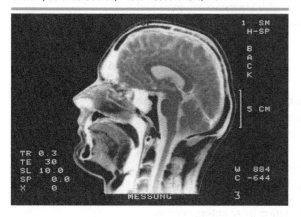

Computed tomography (CT) image of a normal brain. Courtesy of BSIP/Science Source/Photo Researchers, Inc.

Computed Tomography. Neuroradiological techniques are relatively new. Until the 1980s, imaging of the brain was not possible. Physicians were limited to examining simple X-ray scans of the skeletal system, including the skull. X-ray technology did not permit physicians to view the brain or other non-bony structures. The word *radio* in radiology actually means ray.

The development of computed tomography (CT) was a breakthrough in the diagnosis of brain abnormalities, as well as abnormalities in other parts of the body. CT technology was discovered in the 1970s. Within ten years it was widely available as a diagnostic procedure for detecting an assortment of brain abnormalities due to disease or injury.

The X-ray computed tomography or CT technique combines many X-ray scans or slices together to form two- and even three-dimensional images of the head. Part of the term *tomography* is from the Greek word *tomos* for "slice." As illustrated in Figure 12.1, CT scanning is certainly a useful tool for viewing the skull and its contents. However, the CT picture of brain tissue does not reveal detailed structure, so small masses and other abnormalities are easily missed. Also, repeat CT scanning is not without some health risk, as it exposes a patient's brain to small amounts of radiation.

Magnetic Resonance Imaging. Magnetic resonance imaging (MRI) was also discovered in the 1970s. However, MRI was not available at most hospitals until several years after the introduction of CT scanning. MRI scanning does not utilize X-ray technology. Rather, a very powerful magnet alters the movement of protons in water molecules in the brain. Water is a major component of the brain and the rest of the body. A carefully controlled and strong electromagnetic field produced by the magnet causes protons in water molecules to spin at their resonance frequency. The resonance activity of protons throughout brain tissue is detected and imaged when the magnet is turned off.

An MRI image provides a remarkably accurate view of the brain, with lifelike depiction of even small details in structure. You may recall viewing in Chapter 10 an MRI image that revealed a tumor affecting the auditory system (Figure 10.3).

The main advantage of MRI over CT scanning is a higher degree of contrast resolution. That is, with MRI it is possible to distinguish between two tissues that are quite similar and to detect small structural abnormalities within the brain. Also, MRI does not expose the patient to any radiation. Nonetheless, there are a few drawbacks of MRI scanning. MRI magnets generate very high levels of noise, reaching intensity levels of 130 dB! Patients must routinely wear earplugs when undergoing MRI scanning. Even so, some patients with extreme intolerance to loud sounds do not consent to participate in the procedure. Also, MRI scanning of patients with implanted metal devices, including some electronic hearing devices like cochlear implants, is sometimes not possible because the technique utilizes a powerful magnet. A cochlear implant consists of a metallic electrical component surgically placed under skin behind the ear, and there is metal in the electrodes that wind through the cochlea.

Functional MRI. A variation of this imaging technique known as **functional magnetic resonance imaging** or **fMRI** is a valuable research tool for studying brain activation while a patient is involved in a task such as listening to words or sentences. Using a slight modification in technique, brain scanning is performed at very rapid rates. When the normal brain is involved in a task, such as listening, increased neural activity is associated with increased demand for oxygen. As a result, bloodflow to the activated area increases and is reflected by brighter regions on the fMRI scan.

Figure 12.2 shows the visualization of increased activity in auditory regions of the brain during a listening task. There are now thousands of publications describing fMRI studies of auditory function in normal persons and patients with various CNS disorders. You'll learn about some of these exciting investigations in the following review.

Vestibular Schwannoma

Prevalence. Audiologists play a role in the early detection of tumors that cause hearing loss or related disorders, such as a vestibular disorder. Tumors affecting the retrocochlear pathways like the auditory nerve are quite rare. The prevalence of symptomatic vestibular schwannomas is low affecting only about 1 in every 100,000 people (NIH Consensus Panel, 1991). The term *symptomatic* here refers to tumors producing one or more symptoms, like hearing loss or tinnitus. To put this prevalence figure in perspective, think back about what you learned about prevalence of ear disorders in the previous chapter (Chapter 11). Hearing losses caused by exposure to excessive noise, age-related hearing loss (presbycusis), and even sudden onset sensory hearing loss and Ménière's disease are many times more prevalent than vestibular schwannoma.

FIGURE 12.2

Functional magnetic resonance imaging (fMRI) scans of normal brains averaged from eighteen persons during auditory stimulation with tones. The top row of images shows activity in auditory regions of the temporal lobe on both sides of the brain. The bottom row shows the same activity in the temporal lobe as viewed in vertical slices through the brain. Source: Figure represents original unpublished data provided by Karima Susi, Nottingham Trent University, Nottingham, UK.

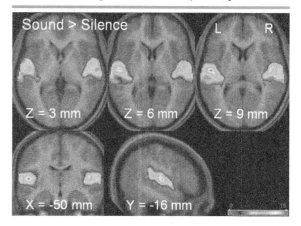

Recent studies suggest that vestibular schwannomas are not that uncommon in the general population, if one includes people who have no symptoms. As documented by MRI in persons without any symptoms or concerns about a vestibular schwannoma, the prevalence is estimated at 700 in 1,000,000, and at autopsy a remarkably high 8000 in 1,000,000, or about 8 per 1000 persons (British Association of Otorhinolaryngologists, 2002). Vestibular tumors are usually found in middle-aged persons, aged 30 to 60, and more often in females than males.

Proper Terminology. As noted already, **vestibular schwannoma** is the anatomically correct term for what's often referred to as an acoustic tumor or acoustic neuroma. Breaking the term vestibular schwannoma into portions may help you to understand its meaning. You are already familiar with the term *vestibular,* used to designate one of the systems important for balance. The term *Schwann* refers to a specialized type of cell that encompasses some nerve fibers. Schwann cells act as insulation for the nerve fibers and contribute to speedier transmission of information along the nerves. The suffix *oma* means tumor.

The commonly used term *acoustic tumor* is technically not correct because a vestibular schwannoma grows from Schwann cells surrounding vestibular nerve fibers, not from auditory nerve fibers. However, as they grow, vestibular tumors usually compress the auditory nerve and disrupt auditory function. An audiologist may be the first healthcare professional to suspect retrocochlear abnormality in a patient with auditory or vestibular problems.

Benign but a Serious Health Problem. Vestibular schwannomas are almost always benign, rather than malignant (Agrawal, Blevins, & Jackler, 2009; Brackmann & Green, 2001). The term *benign* generally means noncancerous. Audiologists and physicians, especially otolaryngologists, who are well aware of the signs and symptoms of a vestibular schwannoma, make every attempt to detect the tumor as early as possible. Why is there such concern among

FIGURE 12.3

Illustration of the structures in the internal auditory canal, including the facial nerve, the superior and inferior vestibular nerves and the auditory nerve. Also shown is a vestibular schwannoma arising from the inferior vestibular nerve.

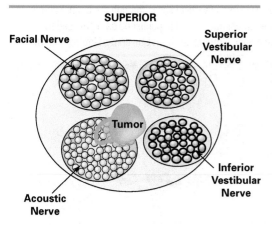

hearing healthcare professionals about early detection of a benign tumor? A review of the information on auditory anatomy in Chapter 3 will help you answer this question.

Figure 12.3 is a diagram showing a tumor growing from the outer portion of an inferior vestibular nerve that is pressing upon the auditory nerve.

As it grows and expands in the narrow inflexible internal auditory canal inside the skull, a vestibular schwannoma begins to press upon nearby structures. The vestibular nerves, the auditory nerve, the facial nerve, and the major artery leading to the cochlea all pass through the internal auditory canal. With continued growth, an undetected vestibular schwannoma often extends from the internal auditory canal in a proximal direction toward the brain into the cerebellopontine angle, abbreviated CPA. You were first introduced to this term in Chapter 3 and then again in a review of diagnostic audiology in Chapter 10.

The cerebellopontine angle is a rather small space located in the lower portion of the brainstem, bordered by the cerebellum and the pons. You may want to refer back to the diagram of central auditory nervous system anatomy in Figure 3.17 (Chapter 3) for a review of this region. Pressure of the growing tumor on the cerebellum can cause problems with gait and movement. Very large tumors may compress and affect vital cardiac and respiratory centers in the brainstem. A vestibular schwannoma can produce very serious medical problems if not detected in a timely fashion or not effectively medically managed (Agrawal, Blevins, & Jackler, 2009; Brackmann & Green, 2001). Ironically, these benign tumors can be fatal.

Auditory Symptoms. From the information just presented, you can probably anticipate some of the auditory symptoms and findings associated with vestibular schwannomas. An expanding tumor originating on a vestibular nerve usually compresses the auditory nerve. Auditory nerve fibers are organized tonotopically. Nerve fibers arising from various frequency regions in the cochlea are in different locations in the auditory nerve. This concept was reviewed in Chapter 3. Fibers carrying high-frequency information from the base region of the cochlea primarily form the outer portion of the nerve. Therefore, in most cases, compression of the auditory nerve by an expanding vestibular schwannoma initially produces a high-frequency hearing loss (Agrawal, Blevins, & Jackler, 2009; Brackmann & Green, 2001).

 ClinicalConnection

The absence of acoustic reflexes at high-intensity levels in a person with only a mild-to-moderate hearing loss is a good example of an abnormal auditory adaptation and retrocochlear dysfunction. Acoustic reflexes are clearly detected in patients with cochlear hearing loss even if hearing thresholds are as poor as 50 or 60 dB HL. In contrast, acoustic reflexes are often absent in patients with even a mild hearing loss due to neural auditory dysfunction caused by a vestibular schwannoma.

Abnormal auditory adaptation or auditory fatigue is another characteristic finding in patients with vestibular schwannomas. Auditory adaptation is the inability of the nerve fibers to continuously respond to an ongoing pure tone. Over the course of a minute or less, a patient will report that the tone fades away. Auditory adaptation is more pronounced at high stimulus intensity levels.

Tumor-related pressure on the auditory nerve also typically produces tinnitus (Agrawal, Blevins, & Jackler, 2009; Brackmann & Green, 2001). To review briefly, tinnitus is a sound like ringing or roaring that a patient hears even in the absence of an external sound and in a quiet setting. Unilateral tinnitus is a serious risk factor for possible vestibular schwannoma.

A growing tumor compressing the internal auditory artery and restricting blood flow to the cochlea often leads to a sensory hearing loss in addition to the neural abnormality. In other words, the tumor produces a *neural* hearing loss directly by affecting function of auditory nerve fibers and indirectly causes a sensory hearing loss by interfering with delivery of blood to the cochlea.

Finally, larger tumors may also produce serious nonauditory symptoms (Agrawal, Blevins, & Jackler, 2009; Brackmann & Green, 2001). An expanding tumor in the internal auditory canal may reach the facial nerve, as shown in Figure 12.3. The patient may feel a tingling sensation in the face and may also have facial muscle weakness or paralysis. The technical term for muscle weakness is **paresis**, whereas **paralysis** is the term for absence of muscle movement.

A large tumor extending from the internal auditory canal to the cerebellum and the brainstem may produce other very concerning neurological symptoms, such as an unsteady gait, headaches, and even breathing difficulties. Fortunately, prompt CT or MRI scanning of any patient with a unilateral hearing loss or unilateral tinnitus usually results in the relatively early detection of vestibular schwannomas and other tumors in the auditory system. Tumors are usually found well before a patient develops serious neurological symptoms.

Since vestibular schwannomas arise from one of the vestibular nerves, you may wonder why vertigo is not a prominent symptom. An expanding tumor pressing on the auditory nerve typically causes a hearing loss. Then why doesn't a tumor growing from a vestibular nerve produce a vestibular symptom, like vertigo? The answer to this reasonable question has to do with the very slow growth of vestibular schwannomas.

A Vestibular Schwannoma Grows Slowly. Vestibular schwannoma tumors expand very slowly, averaging less than 2 mm per year (Strasnick, Glasscock, Haynes, McMenomey, & Minor, 1994). In fact, it is not uncommon for vestibular schwanommas to show no change in size over the course of many years. As the tumor grows very slowly, the vestibular centers in the brain have ample time to adjust to the very slight changes in sensory input from vestibular nerves. The explanation for the absence of major vestibular symptoms in patients with vestibular schwannomas is based on the plasticity of the nervous system that you just learned about. The brain essentially adapts to the altered vestibular information and learns to function normally with less input from one side than the other (Agrawal, Blevins, & Jackler, 2009; Brackmann & Green, 2001).

Case Report. We will finish the discussion of vestibular schwannomas with a brief case report of an actual patient that includes a summary of auditory findings. The patient was a 27-year-old female referred to an audiology clinic. A primary care physician referred the patient to due to a complaint of left-sided tinnitus.

Figure 12.4 shows hearing test findings. Hearing thresholds were normal for the right side. There was a moderate-to-severe high-frequency sensorineural hearing loss for the left ear. Tympanograms were normal bilaterally, and acoustic reflexes were observed for both ears. Word recognition scores were poor on the left side, with rollover at high stimulus intensity levels. You'll recall from discussions in earlier chapters that rollover is decreased word recognition performance at high-intensity levels.

Following consultation with the patient's primary care physician, the audiologist immediately performed a neurodiagnostic auditory brainstem response (ABR) assessment. ABR measurement is very useful in the diagnosis of neural auditory dysfunction. ABR tests are sensitive to disruption of auditory function caused by a tumor pressing on nerve fibers. A tumor interferes with the fast passage of electrical information along auditory pathways from the cochlea through the brainstem. The disruption slows the transmission of information, resulting in longer times or latencies between the different ABR waves. Sometimes the pressure of a tumor blocks any information from passing along auditory nerve fibers, and the ABR is totally absent.

FIGURE 12.4

Hearing findings for a 27-year-old female with a vestibular schwanomma on the left side.

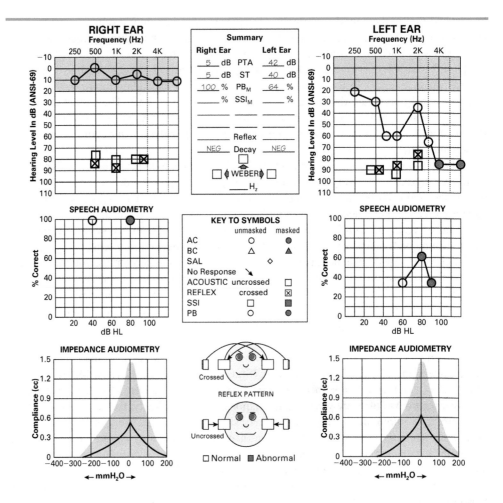

Figure 12.5 shows ABR waveforms for the patient. The ABR with right ear stimulation was entirely normal. All the major waves were clearly present at the expected times after the stimulus, that is, latency values were normal. In contrast, for left ear stimulation, there was an abnormal delay in the time interval between Wave I and Wave III. You may recall from our discussion in Chapter 11 that Wave I arises from the auditory nerve and Wave III arises from the lower portion of the brainstem. The wave I–III latency interval on the left side was prolonged at 3.66 ms, in comparison to 2.40 ms on the right.

You'll also notice in Figure 12.5 a difference in the latency values between the left and right sides for the wave I–V interval and for the wave V latency. Taken together, the ABR findings and the other hearing test results are consistent with what we would expect if there were a tumor in the left internal auditory canal pressing on the auditory nerve and disrupting the transmission of information from the cochlea to the brainstem.

An otologist working with the audiologist promptly ordered MRI imaging when informed of these hearing test findings. MRI scans for the patient revealed a tumor originating in the left internal auditory canal. Again, an MRI image confirming a tumor in the internal auditory canal, a vestibular schwannoma, was shown in Figure 10.3.

The audiologist played an essential role in detection of the patient's tumor. Suspicion about left-sided neural auditory dysfunction arose from the patient's complaint of tinnitus in her left ear plus the asymmetrical results of the hearing assessment. Of special concern were

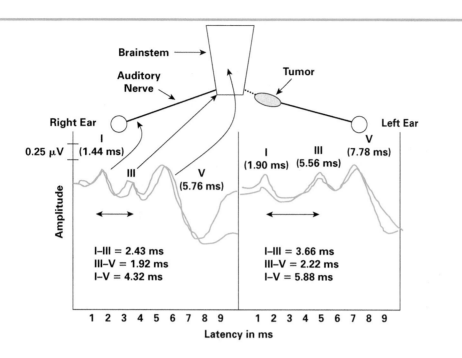

F I G U R E   1 2 . 5

Auditory brainstem response (ABR) findings for a 27-year-old female diagnosed with a vestibular schwanomma on the left side.

the left ear hearing loss and the poor word recognition scores and rollover. The concern intensified with analysis of the ABR findings, specifically of a delay in the latency between Wave I and later waves. MRI confirmed the diagnosis of a vestibular schwannoma.

The tumor was successfully removed surgically in an operation performed by an otologist and a neurosurgeon. The audiologist was on hand in the operating room to make repeated ABR measurements during the surgery to minimize the likelihood of complications as the tumor was removed. You'll learn more in Chapter 16 about the role of audiologists in management of special patient populations, including patients with tumors affecting the auditory system.

Neurofibromas

Neurofibromatosis is a genetically transmitted autosomal dominant disease. The term means "fibrous tumors on a nerve." There are two types of neurofibromatosis, type I and type II. Over 95% of patients with tumors affecting the auditory nerves have neurofibromatosis type II, abbreviated NF2. Hearing impairment is found in more than nine out of ten patients with NF2, and in one-half of these patients it is the first complaint.

Diagnosis and Management. The diagnosis and management of patients with NF2 who have bilateral neural auditory dysfunction present some challenges to audiologists. We will review briefly the diagnostic challenges here. Patients with a vestibular schwannoma typically have unilateral or asymmetrical symptoms and auditory abnormalities that contribute to early detection and diagnosis. However, most etiologies affecting the auditory system produce bilateral hearing loss and abnormalities. The bilateral abnormalities in NF2 can initially be mistaken for those found in sensory and non-tumor etiologies for hearing loss such as Meniere's disease. Comprehensive diagnostic hearing assessment, including the auditory brainstem response, is usually necessary to differentiate between sensory and neural auditory dysfunction.

Case Report. Another brief case report will help to clarify the distinctions in auditory findings for patients with the diagnosis of NF2 and those diagnosed with a vestibular schwannoma. Figure 12.6 shows hearing test results for an 19-year-old university student who was complaining of difficulty using the telephone with his left ear and problems with clumsiness. His audiogram showed a low-frequency hearing loss bilaterally, with greater hearing loss on the left side. Tympanograms were normal bilaterally, but acoustic reflexes were not observed when the stimulus was presented to the left ear. Also, word recognition performance was unusually poor (0%) for the left ear.

Distortion product otoacoustic emissions (DPOAEs) were present despite the patient's hearing loss. DPOAE amplitude values for both ears were within normal limits for test frequencies from 500 to 8000 Hz. A neural problem must be suspected whenever a patient has normal otoacoustic emissions and the audiogram shows a hearing loss.

Figure 12.7 shows ABR waveforms for the patient. ABR recording failed to produce a reliable response at high click stimulus intensity levels for the right or the left ear even with manipulation of test parameters. Bilateral absence of an ABR despite reasonably good hearing sensitivity was a clear abnormality and raised the suspicion of NF2.

Based on these multiple retrocochlear auditory findings, a consultation was immediately arranged with an otologist, who promptly ordered an MRI.

FIGURE 12.6

Hearing findings for a 19-year-old male with bilateral neurofibromas.

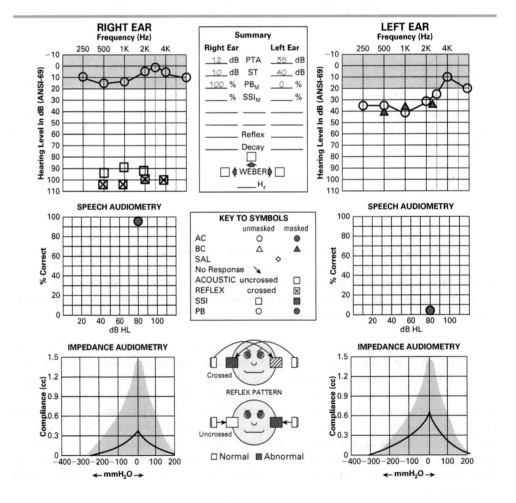

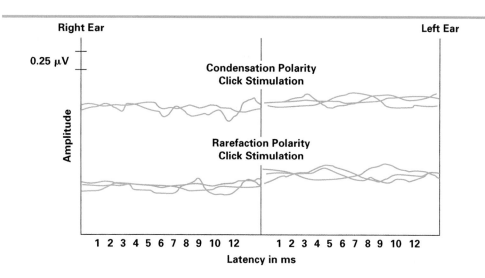

FIGURE 12.7

Auditory brainstem response (ABR) waveforms for a 19-year-old male with bilateral neurofibromas. The patient's audiogram is shown in Figure 12.6.

The MRI scan was available to the audiologist and otologist within three hours after the patient first entered the audiology clinic. Figure 12.8 clearly shows a tumor affecting the auditory nerve on each side. The left-sided neurofibroma was considerably bigger than the one on the right. The large tumors were also compressing the patient's brainstem. MRI images of the spine showed other neurofibromas.

The patient underwent two types of intervention for the tumors. The larger tumor on the left side was removed surgically. Hearing was lost during surgery but facial nerve function was preserved. A special type of radiation was used to shrink the tumor on the right side, with preservation of hearing and facial nerve function.

The bilateral and progressive nature of hearing loss in NF2 makes effective audiological management rather challenging. You'll learn in the final chapter (Chapter 16) about different options available to audiologists for management of patients with NF2.

Meningiomas

Meningiomas may be found in various locations in the skull. The meninges are membranes covering and protecting the brain and spinal cord. **Meningiomas** are tumors arising from the meninges. We will focus this brief discussion on meningiomas that arise in the cerebellopontine angle (CPA) region, where they may affect the auditory system.

Meningiomas are more common in females than males and usually appear later in life. A meningioma involving the auditory nerve is sometimes difficult to distinguish from a vestibular schwannoma. Meningiomas do not always produce a hearing loss because they originate and grow only in the space bordered by the cerebellum and pons, rather than in the relatively constricted internal auditory canal. As a meningioma grows, it usually produces findings similar to those for vestibular schwannomas, such as acoustic reflex decay or word-recognition rollover.

FIGURE 12.8

Brain magnetic resonance imaging (MRI) scan for a 19-year-old male with bilateral neurofibroma.

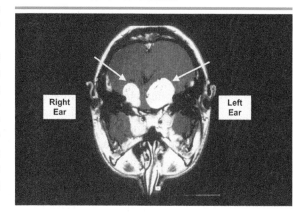

Two Other Retrocochlear Disorders

Vascular Loop. You've now been introduced to the three types of tumors that audiologists encounter clinically: vestibular schwannomas, neurofibromas, and meningiomas. However, there are other types of retrocochlear auditory abnormalities that are not neoplasms or tumors. One example is a disorder referred to as cochleovestibular nerve compression syndrome and also vascular loop syndrome. The vascular loop consists of the U-shaped portion of a blood vessel abnormally protruding from the cerebellopontine angle region into the internal auditory canal and pressing on the auditory nerve (Schwaber & Hall, 1992). The blood vessel is the anterior inferior cerebellar artery, which is important for circulation of blood to the brainstem. Auditory symptoms and findings in vascular loop syndrome closely resemble those for tumors affecting the auditory nerve. MRI scans can differentiate these two retrocochlear disorders.

Vestibular Neuritis. Vestibular neuritis is one of the most common causes of severe dizziness that prompts a person to seek medical care and often a visit to a hospital emergency department (Friedland & Minor, 2009). This serious problem is not due to a tumor, but rather to inflammation of a vestibular nerve. Symptoms include the sudden onset of intense vertigo, lasting days, spontaneous nystagmus, and an imbalance disturbance related to posture. The exact mechanism of vestibular neuritis is not well understood, but possible explanations include viral inflammation of the vestibular nerve and reduced blood flow to the vestibular portion of the ear.

Vestibular neuritis produces severe vestibular abnormalities, but hearing is typically not affected. Management of vestibular neuritis is generally not a direct treatment of the disease process. Instead, the patient is given medicines to reduce nausea, fluid replacement if there is a problem with vomiting, and drugs to suppress the symptom of vertigo (Friedland & Minor, 2009). Once a patient with vestibular neuritis has passed through the acute phase of the disease, vestibular rehabilitation by a physical therapist or audiologist is sometimes needed to help the patient regain balance.

Auditory Neuropathy Spectrum Disorder (ANSD)

Discovery

Auditory neuropathy spectrum disorder (ANSD) is in reality a collection of disorders involving the region of the auditory system from the cochlea to the auditory nerve. The typical combination of test findings suggesting the possibility of ANSD is the presence of normal otoacoustic emissions with absence of the auditory brainstem response. This odd combination will soon be explained.

ANSD was not formally discovered or recognized until the 1990s. At that time the disorder was simply referred to as auditory neuropathy. Clinical experience and research over the past fifteen to twenty years confirmed that dysfunction in patients diagnosed with auditory neuropathy was not limited to the auditory nerve. The site of dysfunction may also be the inner hair cells in the cochlea or the synaptic region between inner hair cells and auditory nerve fibers. The inclusive term *auditory neuropathy spectrum disorder,* or ANSD, is a more accurate way to describe the collection of disorders.

What factors led to the identification of a new auditory disorder more than fifty years after the beginnings of audiology? Before the discovery and regular clinical application of otoacoustic emissions, hearing assessment of children and adults was performed only with procedures that depended on integrity of the auditory nerve. In analyzing abnormal findings for conventional behavioral test procedures and even the auditory brainstem response, audiologists generally assumed that the auditory nerve was intact.

Auditory nerve disorders were viewed as very rare in the adult population and almost unheard of in infants and older children. Analysis of test findings then was quite simplistic. A severe cochlear abnormality was presumed if a patient had no behavioral response to even high-intensity pure tone or speech signals or if no ABR was elicited with high-intensity sounds. Auditory nerve dysfunction was simply not suspected.

In the years before 1990, patients who did not respond to sound in behavioral hearing testing or who did not produce a response on an objective test like ABR were diagnosed with severe or profound sensorineural hearing loss. The patients were then managed as if that was the cause of the hearing problem. For example, a child with no response on behavioral tests or during ABR measurement was typically fit with powerful hearing aids. Depending on the age when hearing loss was identified and the patient's language status, some children with apparent severe-to-profound sensorineural hearing loss were enrolled in schools for the deaf.

For some children with presumably profound hearing loss, management with powerful hearing aids was often ineffective for no apparent reason. In some cases, children simply refused to wear the hearing aids. In retrospect, we now realize that a proportion of children with apparent severe sensory hearing impairment actually had pure neural auditory abnormality with normal cochlear function.

You may recall learning in Chapter 8 about the discovery and clinical implementation of the OAE technique. Clinical instrumentation for measurement of otoacoustic emissions was available to most audiologists beginning in the mid-1990s. OAE measurement then gained popularity as a clinical procedure particularly for auditory assessment of infants and young children. During that time period, audiologists around the world were surprised to observe a seemingly paradoxical pattern of findings. Perfectly normal OAEs could be recorded in patients with no behavioral response to sound and no ABR at maximum intensity levels!

By 1996 there was an explosion of presentations at scientific conferences and a growing number of published articles describing this new and confusing pattern of auditory findings. Also in this year, a well-respected neurologist and auditory researcher named Arnold Starr published with several other well-known audiologists a paper that described normal outer hair cell function yet no ABR for a series of patients with neurological diseases affecting the auditory nerve and other cranial nerves (Starr, Picton, Sininger, Hood, & Berlin, 1996). Starr and colleagues coined the term *auditory neuropathy* in reporting on the unusual collection of findings.

 WebWatch

You'll find a wealth of information on ANSD with an Internet search using the key words *auditory neuropathy spectrum disorder*. Here are just two of the many websites related to the topic: www.nidcd.nih.gov/health/hearing/neuropathy.htm and The Children's Hospital. At the second website you can search for ANSD-Guidelines to access and download a comprehensive evidence-based clinical guideline for identification, diagnosis, and management of ANSD.

ANSD was poorly understood and not well defined for a number of years after the initial recognition of the disorder. Indeed, the term *auditory neuropathy* was used incorrectly for a diverse collection of disorders associated with abnormal ABR findings. In 2008, an international panel of experts prepared a detailed and evidence-based clinical guideline on the topic and recommended that *"auditory neuropathy spectrum disorder" (ANSD)* replace the term *auditory neuropathy*.

The definition in the monograph entitled *Identification and Management of Infants and Young Children with Auditory Neuropathy Spectrum Disorder* is clear and concise yet complete.

[ANSD] is a relatively recent clinical diagnosis used to describe individuals with auditory disorders due to dysfunction of the synapse of the inner hair cells and auditory nerve, and/or the auditory nerve itself. Unlike patients with sensory hearing loss who show clinical evidence of impaired outer hair cell function, patients with "auditory neuropathy" show clinical evidence of normally functioning outer hair cells. Individuals with "auditory neuropathy" typically demonstrate impaired speech understanding, and show normal to severely impaired speech detection and pure tone thresholds.

It has been shown that "auditory neuropathy" affects an individual's ability to process rapidly changing acoustic signals, known as auditory temporal processing. (p. 3)

Identification of ANSD

Suspicion or identification of possible ANSD usually occurs when OAEs are recorded in a patient who has no detectable ABR. Figures 12.9 and 12.10 depict this combination of findings. Waveforms in the figure are for an infant who did not pass hearing screening with an automated ABR technique in the intensive care nursery (ICN) or neonatal intensive care unit (NICU). Follow up diagnostic assessment at 3 months after birth again revealed normal OAEs and no ABR. On close examination of the ABR tracings in Figure 12.9 you'll notice a series of peaks and valleys early in the waveform.

How can we be sure that these clear waves are not components in an ABR? Again looking closely at the figure, you'll read a notation next to different waveforms about the polarity of the click stimulus used to elicit the waveforms. ABR waveforms were recorded separately for rarefaction polarity click stimulation and for condensation polarity clinical stimulation. As you learned in Chapter 2, condensation polarity stimuli reflect higher density of air molecules produced with outward movement of the diaphragm of an earphone, whereas rarefaction polarity stimuli reflect lower density of air molecules produced with inward movement of the earphone diaphragm. The positive and negative polarity sounds in the ear canal reach the tympanic membrane. Corresponding vibrations are transmitted from the tympanic membrane through the middle ear ossicles to the stapes footplate and the cochlear fluids.

Returning to Figure 12.9, you'll notice with close inspection of the waveforms for condensation and rarefaction stimulation that the peaks in the waveforms of one polarity (either condensation or rarefaction) are exactly lined up with the valleys in the waveforms of the opposite stimulus polarity. We would expect ABR waveforms to be nearly the same for the two opposite stimulus polarities, but in the figure the waveforms are totally reversed. You may recognize these inverting waveforms for rarefaction and condensation stimulus as cochlear microphonic (CM). The CM is an electrical response produced by outer hair cells. It was described in a review of cochlear function in Chapter 3 and in Chapter 9 in the section on electrocochleography (ECochG).

The cochlear microphonic response is produced by the outer hair cells. The response is not part of the ABR. OAEs are also a reflection of outer hair cell activity. Normal OAE findings

FIGURE 12.9

Auditory evoked responses in a 3-month-old child with auditory neuropathy spectrum disorder (ANSD). Within days after birth, the child had failed newborn hearing with an automated auditory brainstem response technique.

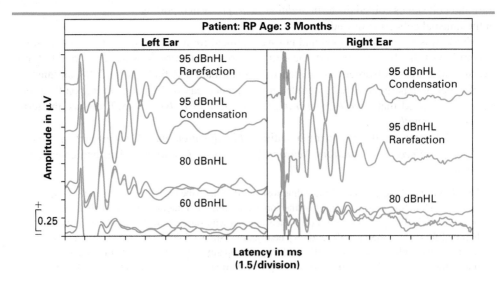

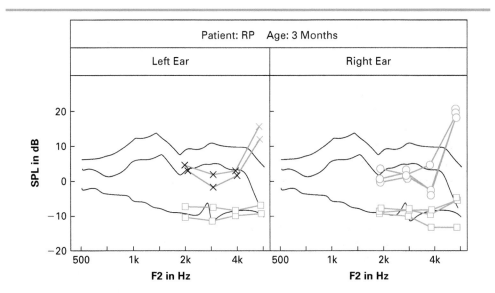

FIGURE 12.10

Otoacoustic emissions (OAEs) recorded from a 3-month-old child with auditory neuropathy spectrum disorder (ANSD). Auditory evoked response findings for the child are shown in Figure 12.9.

for the patient are shown in Figure 12.10. Both otoacoustic emissions and CM are pre-neural auditory responses. They arise from outer hair cells and do not depend on activation of the auditory nerve. In contrast, ABR and most other auditory measures are dependent on auditory nerve function. Once this concept is grasped, the combination of normal OAEs and absence of a behavioral response or an ABR to sound seems quite logical.

The OAEs shown in Figure 12.10 and the cochlear microphonic activity shown in Figure 12.9 clearly document outer hair cell function, which is one of the defining requirements of ANSD. These findings in combination with the absence of reliable ABR in this infant raise the suspicion of ANSD.

Diagnosis of ANSD. ANSD is identified most often in infants who are graduates of an intensive care nursery and who are at risk for neurological dysfunction. However, ANSD is also sometimes encountered in well babies and in older children and even adolescents. The disorder is most often bilateral, but unilateral ANSD is a possibility. ANSD is diagnosed in up to 15% of all of children with confirmed hearing loss who spent time in an intensive care nursery after birth (Ramesh, Panwar, Nilkanthan, Nair, & Mehra, 2012). The prevalence of ANSD is considerably higher than suspected in the past. ANSD is rather unusual in otherwise healthy children born in the well-baby nursery. In such cases, family history of hearing loss and perhaps genetic consultation often suggest the possibility of a genetic etiology for ANSD. As you will soon learn, the risk for ANSD increases in children with neurological diseases affecting the central nervous system.

Identification of ANSD is necessarily followed by additional testing to confirm the diagnosis. Auditory assessment for a diagnosis of ANSD is quite challenging. It requires an extensive test battery consisting of numerous behavioral and objective auditory procedures, including most of the procedures reviewed in Chapters 8 and 9. The 2008 clinical guidelines for ANSD include detailed recommendations for test procedures to be administered during the diagnostic process and describe the role of nonaudiology diagnostic procedures such as magnetic resonance imaging.

Auditory findings and characteristics in patients with ANSD are summarized in Table 12.1. A key feature of ANSD is very poor word recognition performance. Research and clinical experience during the past few decades clearly confirm that ANSD is not a single

TABLE 12.1

Features of auditory
neuropathy spectrum
disorder (ANSD)
including findings on
hearing tests and other
characteristics

- Otoacoustic emissions are present and often normal.
- Auditory brainstem response cannot be recorded, including the absence of wave I.
- Cochlear microphonic activity is recorded.
- Acoustic reflexes are generally not present or recordable.
- Hearing thresholds vary from one patient to the next, ranging from normal to the absence of a behavioral response to high intensity sounds.
- The most common audiogram configuration is a low-frequency hearing loss.
- The patient has very poor word recognition scores, even in quiet settings.
- Background noise severely disrupts speech perception.
- Bilateral abnormalities are typical but there are cases of one-sided ANSD.

or homogeneous type of auditory abnormality. In other words, encompassed under the label ANSD are three or four distinct types of auditory dysfunction. Consequently, the findings on the many procedures in the test battery vary considerably from one patient to the next.

The main goal of the diagnostic process for ANSD is to determine as precisely as possible the location of dysfunction in the auditory system. Specifically, it is important for the diagnosis and management of ANSD to differentiate between three sites of dysfunction: (1) inner hair cells, (2) synapse between the inner hair cells and auditory nerve fibers, or (3) auditory nerve fibers.

Etiologies Associated with ANSD

A wide range of nonauditory disorders and diseases are linked to ANSD. Many are very serious and some can be fatal unless promptly diagnosed and properly managed medically. An audiologist involved in newborn hearing screening and diagnostic follow up testing is often the first healthcare professional to suspect a possible neurological disorder. Babies in the intensive care unit who do not pass an ABR hearing screening are regularly screened with OAEs as recommended by the Joint Committee on Infant Hearing (2007). As a result, it is not uncommon for suspicion or identification of ANSD to occur within days after a child leaves the nursery.

LEADERS AND LUMINARIES

Linda Hood

Dr. Linda J. Hood is a Professor in the Department of Hearing and Speech Sciences at Vanderbilt University and an Honorary Professor at the University of Queensland, Australia. She earned her bachelor's degree in Speech and Hearing from Bowling Green State University (Ohio), her master's degree in Audiology from Kent State University, and her PhD from University of Maryland. Dr. Hood also completed an NIH Post-Doctoral Fellowship at Kresge Hearing Research Laboratory, LSU Health Sciences Center, New Orleans, where she was a faculty researcher for over twenty years. During that time Dr. Hood was involved in work that led to the description of auditory neuropathy/dys-synchrony (AN/AD). Since then many of her research and teaching activities continue to focus on issues related to the evaluation and management of AN/AD, now known as auditory neuropathy spectrum disorder (ANSD). Additional research areas include auditory physiologic responses, efferent auditory function, hereditary hearing loss, and aging of the auditory system. Dr. Hood has participated in review and working groups of the NIH and has leadership roles in several professional organizations.

Diagnosis of ANSD may occur within months after birth. Part of the full diagnostic process includes referral of the infant to medical specialists, including neurologists, otolaryngologists, eye specialists, and genetics experts (Children's Hospital of Colorado, 2008). Recognition of ANSD allows the possibility of early identification of neurological and other diseases in infants. Audiologists contribute importantly to this process. A person who has been diagnosed with diseases affecting the central nervous system should be referred for diagnostic testing, to include the numerous procedures already mentioned. Audiologists play a primary role in the management of ANSD. In Chapter 16, you'll learn about management options for ANSD and how audiologists and speech pathologists collaborate to manage patients with this challenging spectrum of communication problems.

Central Auditory Nervous System (CANS) Disorders

Summary of CANS Disorders

The central auditory nervous system begins in the pons region of the brainstem. The precise demarcation between the peripheral auditory system and the central auditory system is where auditory nerve fibers form a synapse with neurons in the cochlear nucleus of the lower brainstem.

A diverse collection of disorders in the central nervous system may affect auditory pathways and hearing function. Seven major categories of etiologies involving auditory pathways and centers in the central nervous system include: (1) *tumors* involving nerves and other brain cells, (2) *vascular abnormalities* involving blood vessels and affecting blood flow to the brain, (3) *degenerative disease*s producing a progressive worsening of neurological function, (4) *demyelinating diseases* involving myelin that surrounds nerve fibers, (5) *dementias* and other neuropsychiatric diseases that affect cognitive functioning, (6) *trauma* with resulting brain injury, and (7) *developmental disorders* in children.

In each of these categories, disorders are often further classified or organized according to some other feature like the location of the tumor, the type of brain tissue involved, or patient age or gender. In this section, we'll review some of the disorders in each of the categories. Along the way, you'll be introduced to general features of central nervous system diseases and disorders that will help you better understand this rather complicated topic. The reason for including this discussion in a book about audiology is quite straightforward. You've already learned that we hear with our brain. Disorders affecting the brain are sometimes associated with difficulties in hearing and with communication disorders.

Role of Audiologists and Speech Pathologists

Audiologists and speech pathologists in many work settings encounter patients with central auditory nervous system disorders. In some cases, another healthcare professional refers a patient who is already diagnosed with a central nervous system disorder. Referrals of patients to audiologists and speech pathologists often come from physicians or psychologists. Referrals are made to determine whether the brain disorder affects hearing, auditory function, speech, or language function.

Let's say a medical specialist such as a pediatric neurologist has diagnosed a brainstem tumor in a young child. The neurologist then refers the patient to an audiologist and a speech pathologist. The audiologist performs a series of diagnostic procedures to evaluate auditory function. If comprehensive testing confirms a hearing impairment or some type of auditory dysfunction, the audiologist develops a plan for management. Similarly, a speech pathologist evaluates speech/language function and recommends treatment as appropriate.

Or, to cite another example, a physical rehabilitation physician, a psychologist, or a speech pathologist may refer a veteran with combat-related traumatic brain injury to an audiologist for hearing assessment. In some cases, the patient has already been diagnosed with language impairment and cognitive dysfunction. The reason for the referral is to determine whether the auditory system is also involved. The audiologist takes into account information supplied with the referral, such as the patient's medical diagnosis, the results of brain imaging, and speech/language test findings. The audiologist then decides on the best techniques and strategies for evaluating the patient's hearing.

Patients with complaints of hearing problems often seek help directly from an audiologist or speech pathologist without referral from a physician and with no previous medical diagnosis. An audiologist or speech pathologist first obtains a complete history from the patient and then performs a diagnostic assessment. Based on the history or certain test findings on the assessment, the audiologist or speech pathologist may have concerns about possible central nervous system dysfunction that prompt additional diagnostic testing.

If an audiologist or a speech pathologist is the first healthcare professional to evaluate a patient with communication problems, the next step is almost always referral to an appropriate medical specialist like an otolaryngologist, a neurologist, or a psychiatrist. The physician is responsible for medical diagnosis of brain diseases or disorders. The patient may later return to the audiologist or speech pathologist for additional diagnostic testing or for management. Over the years, clinical experience and research reported in published papers have clearly proven that auditory abnormalities are sometimes associated with each of the central nervous system disorders reviewed in this chapter (Musiek & Baran, 2007).

ClinicalConnection

Audiologists and speech pathologists must remain vigilant about the possibility of central nervous system disorders. Concerns are addressed with appropriate diagnostic assessment using procedures that are sensitive to central auditory nervous system dysfunction, including the diagnostic speech tests and auditory evoked responses reviewed in Chapter 9. Audiologists and speech pathologists in this way contribute to early detection and accurate diagnosis of central nervous system diseases and disorders. Early detection and diagnosis are always important steps leading to proper management and optimal patient outcome.

Tumors

We'll begin with a brief discussion of brain tumors sometimes associated with auditory dysfunction. Brain tumors are clearly a serious medical condition. However, addressing tumors first does not imply that other central nervous system disorders are less serious or concerning. All of the different central nervous system disorders covered in this review pose a major risk to health and to quality of life.

Types of Tumors. Brain tumors can be classified or organized in different ways (Kleihues, Burger, & Scheithauer, 1993; Tarazi & Schetz, 2011). One approach is based on the type of brain cell or tissue that gives rise to the tumor. For example, tumors found on the meninges are called meningiomas, whereas those arising from astrocyte cells are astrocytomas. Another strategy is to categorize tumors according to their typical location in the brain, such as the brainstem, the cerebellum, or the cerebral cortex.

Interestingly, the likelihood of a specific tumor depends to a large extent on a patient's age. A sizable proportion of brain tumors (from 80 to 90%) occur in adult patients over the age of 16 years. Only about 2% of brain tumors occur in young children, between birth and 3 years. Gliomas arising from the glial cells in the brain account for about 75% of tumors in children, but they are rare in adults. In contrast, meningiomas almost exclusively affect adult patients and are rarely found in children (Tarazi & Schetz, 2011).

Hearing Assessment Strategies. Information about the likelihood of brain tumors in different patient groups is helpful in determining the best approach to hearing evaluation.

Information about brain tumors helps an audiologist select which procedures to include in the test battery and how to interpret abnormal auditory findings. A case scenario might help to clarify this point.

Let's say a child with a brain tumor is referred for hearing assessment. A team of medical specialists at a children's hospital make a specific diagnosis of brainstem tumor before the referral. An audiologist would most likely begin the hearing assessment with tests that assess auditory brainstem functioning. Children with brainstem tumors are often treated with chemotherapy, including a drug that can cause hearing loss. Children receiving chemotherapy may be very fatigued, sleepy, and unable to remain alert during behavioral hearing testing. Accurate evaluation of auditory function and detection of brainstem auditory dysfunction would be enhanced with objective hearing tests like acoustic immittance measures, OAEs, and the auditory brainstem response.

The same test strategy is valuable for a child not yet diagnosed with a brain tumor. Abnormalities on objective tests of brainstem function raise concern about the possibility of brainstem abnormality. An audiologist obtaining such findings would generally communicate with the child's physician, who would in turn refer the child for a neurological evaluation with studies like an MRI. Knowledge of the nature of brain tumors is important whether medical diagnosis is made before or after the hearing assessment. The knowledge contributes to an audiologist's decisions about the most effective test strategy and protocol for hearing assessment.

Vascular Abnormalities

Cerebrovascular Accident. Audiologists and especially speech pathologists often encounter patients with vascular abnormalities involving the central nervous system. Each year hundreds of thousands of persons suffer a **cerebrovascular accident (CVA)** or stroke in the United States alone, and over one-third of the victims die (NINDS, 2013). Arteries serving the brain may become blocked or occluded, preventing adequate flow of blood. Cerebrovascular diseases involving disruption of blood flow to the brain and damage to brain tissue are the third leading cause of death in the United States. They often cause language impairment and they may also be associated with auditory disorders.

Arteriovenous Malformation. Arteriovenous malformations (AVMs) are another type of cerebrovascular disease. Most commonly, the disease consists of a tangle of blood vessels involving both arteries and veins (Tarazi & Schetz, 2011). Rupture of an abnormally enlarged blood vessel may seriously damage brain tissue. A bulging blood vessel is known as an aneurysm. The likelihood of specific types of cerebrovascular disease and disease location in the brain varies considerably with age. For example, 90% of aneurysms rupture between ages 30 and 70 years. In contrast, rupture of an aneurysm under the age of 15 is unusual. Risk factors for these cerebrovascular accidents include high blood pressure, an age of greater than 65, health habits like smoking, heart disease, diabetes, and birth control pills.

Patterns of Vascular Abnormalities. The patterns of auditory dysfunction and language impairment with cerebrovascular diseases depend on which arterial system is affected. Disruption in blood flow to the cerebral cortex via the middle cerebral artery system affects auditory function at the level of the temporal lobe.

On the other hand, cerebrovascular disease involving blood flow to the lower regions of the brain via the vertebrobasilar system causes auditory dysfunction in the brainstem and even in the ear. The term *vertebrobasilar* refers to blood vessels serving the spinal region and vertebral structures, plus the base or basilar region of the brain. The internal auditory artery supplying blood to the cochlea is a branch of the vertebrobasilar arterial system. Some forms of cerebrovascular disease actually result in total deafness due to a disruption of blood flow to the cochlea.

Auditory dysfunction is only one health problem in cerebrovascular disease. Cerebrovascular disease produces different forms of language impairment and a variety of serious neurological signs and symptoms, such as headache, gait problems, abnormalities of the cranial nerves, eye movement abnormalities, and limb weakness (Tarazi & Schetz, 2011).

Demyelinating Diseases

Auditory problems are sometimes found in patients with demyelinating diseases. **Demyelinating diseases** affect the myelin sheath of neurons, but not the axons of neurons (Tarazi & Schetz, 2011). There are two forms of these neurological diseases. The disease process in one form disrupts function of the insulating myelin sheath around a nerve.

Multiple sclerosis (MS) is one well-known demyelinating disease. It is the most common type of demyelinating disease and a major cause of neurological impairment in young to middle-aged adults. Onset is between ages 20 and 40 for about 50 to 70% of patients. MS in children is extremely rare. MS is more common in females, with a male-to-female ratio of about 1:1.7. The disease has a slow and progressive course that is characteristically irregular, with a patient experiencing fluctuating periods of exacerbation or worsening and then remission of specific symptoms (Tarazi & Schetz, 2011). Large and irregular lesions on myelin sheaths anywhere in the CNS are a dominant feature of MS. For reasons not completely understood, MS is most prevalent in colder climates. Auditory dysfunction is not a consistent feature of MS but some patients have hearing loss and other auditory disorders.

Demyelinating diseases in the *dysmyelinating* category are characterized by defective myelin metabolism (Tarazi & Schetz, 2011). In other words, myelin is present but it does not function normally. The most common dysmyelinating diseases are categorized as *leukodystrophies*. Leukodystrophies are one of the etiologies associated with auditory neuropathy spectrum disorder (ANSD).

Degenerative Diseases

A wide variety of neurological diseases progressively worsen over time (Tarazi & Schetz, 2011). They are known as **neurodegenerative diseases**. Here you'll be introduced to a small sample of these serious health conditions that audiologists and speech pathologists may encounter in clinical practice. Two degenerative diseases sometimes diagnosed in patients with ANSD or central auditory dysfunction include Friedreich's ataxia and hereditary motor sensory neuropathy. The audiologist's role in early detection of ANSD was thoroughly discussed earlier. In the same way, an audiologist is sometimes instrumental in initiating medical management of children with various degenerative neurological diseases. Prompt and appropriate medical referrals ultimately contribute to improved patient outcome.

Dementias. The general term **dementia** refers to a progressive and irreversible decline in mental state that interferes with daily activities and tasks. Audiologists and speech pathologists working with older adults can expect to regularly provide services to patients with dementia. There are many reasons and neurological explanations for deterioration of mental functioning. There are also a variety of specific types of dementia.

We will focus on the most common type of dementia known, as **Alzheimer's dementia**. Alzheimer's disease is definitely caused by brain pathology, but the exact cause and nature of the brain pathology and dysfunction are not yet known (Tarazi & Schetz, 2011). Alzheimer's dementia is associated with loss of neurons, disruption in the communication between neurons, neurofibrillary tangles located inside nerve fibers, and growths or plaques on neurons.

These brain abnormalities are found in different regions of the central nervous system, including auditory regions of the cerebral cortex.

Although memory loss is a feature of Alzheimer's dementia, criteria for diagnosis includes more than memory loss. The presence of memory loss in an aging adult does necessarily mean the person has Alzheimer's dementia. It is also important to point out that Alzheimer's dementia is not a normal feature of aging (Tarazi & Schetz, 2011). You might be surprised to learn that Alzheimer's dementia is a terminal disease, meaning it ends with death. In fact, it is the sixth leading cause of death in adults.

The many symptoms of Alzheimer's disease include problems recalling recent events, declining cognitive functioning, and long-term memory loss that progresses over time. Other symptoms of Alzheimer's dementia are confusion, irritability, mood swings, aggression, a tendency to wander, language impairment with reduced vocabulary, apathy, and withdrawal from social engagement.

Research in the past fifteen years clearly documents abnormalities in auditory dysfunction with Alzheimer's dementia (Gates et al., 2008; Strouse, Hall, & Berger, 1995). Specifically, patients with Alzheimer's dementia show abnormal performance on diagnostic speech audiometry procedures in comparison to normal subjects of the same age and gender and with similar audiograms. Patients with Alzheimer's dementia have lower scores on tests of speech perception in noise, on dichotic listening tasks, and on tests of auditory sequencing. There is also longstanding evidence that Alzheimer's and other forms of dementia are associated with language impairment (Miller, 1989).

Some of the symptoms of Alzheimer's dementia are psychosocial problems often associated with hearing impairment. Unrecognized auditory dysfunction in persons with Alzheimer's dementia probably intensifies these symptoms. A recent large-scale study with hundreds of subjects confirmed that hearing deficits are among the earliest difficulties experienced by persons who are or will be diagnosed with Alzheimer's dementia. The findings of the study led the well-known researcher George Gates to conclude: "We recommend that central auditory testing be considered in the evaluation of older persons with hearing impairments as part of a comprehensive, individualized program to assist their needs in both the aural rehabilitative and the cognitive domains" (Gates et al., 2008, p. 771).

An appreciation and understanding of these many symptoms is important in the evaluation of hearing in elderly patients with Alzheimer's dementia or other forms of dementia and cognitive deficits in general. An audiologist or speech pathologist needs to take special care in evaluating patients with dementia. It is important to assure that patients with cognitive impairment understand test instructions and the task involved in the test. Audiologists sometimes need to re-instruct patients with decreased memory or to shorten test sessions for patients with limited ability to sustain attention. Communication between the tester and the patient requires more effort and time. Patients with advanced dementia may even be unwilling to participate in the test process or may demonstrate aggressive behavior toward the tester. In short, audiologists and speech pathologists must modify many aspects of the testing process to accommodate an individual patient's status and obtain valid results. Reliance on objective tests is often the best strategy for auditory assessment of patients with advanced dementia.

Patterns of Central Auditory Dysfunction

An appreciation of four principles will help you understand the different patterns of auditory abnormalities found in disorders of the central nervous system. First, simple hearing tests often do not detect auditory dysfunction caused by disorders of the central nervous system. Hearing thresholds and speech reception thresholds are often normal in patients with disorders involving the higher levels of the nervous system. Word recognition scores in a quiet condition are sometimes 100% for each ear. Diagnostic procedures that put greater demands on auditory function are required to detect abnormalities in the central pathways.

Second, central nervous system disorders are often reflected by bilateral deficits on auditory tests, with some degree of abnormality observed for each ear. In contrast, diseases affecting the ear or auditory nerve often produce unilateral abnormalities.

Third, the relation of the side of auditory abnormalities to the side of a central nervous system tumor varies, depending on whether the tumor is involving the auditory pathways in the brainstem or the temporal lobe in cerebral cortex. Disorders located entirely on the right side of the central nervous system may be associated with hearing test abnormalities in the right ear, the left ear, or both ears. A tumor in the brainstem is more likely to produce bilateral deficits on auditory tests, although abnormalities are often greater for one ear or the other. In contrast, patients with tumors involving auditory regions of the temporal lobe usually have auditory abnormalities for the ear contralateral to the side of the tumor, that is, on the other side from the tumor. A patient with a left temporal lobe tumor is likely to show abnormal auditory test results when signals are presented to the right ear.

Finally, diagnostic assessment of auditory function in patients with disorders involving the central nervous system is quite challenging for a variety of reasons. We've already talked about the insensitivity of simple hearing tests to central auditory dysfunction. Special diagnostic auditory tests must be administered in this patient population. Also, patients with diseases and disorders involving the central nervous system may have nonauditory deficits that can interfere with hearing testing or affect the test results. The disorders summarized in this chapter may be associated with patient symptoms such as fatigue, irritability, emotional distress, inattention, and cognition impairments like poor memory, attention, and slower processing speed.

Auditory Processing Disorder (APD)

Audiologists and speech pathologists are involved in the detection, diagnosis, and management of children and adults with auditory processing disorders. Diagnosis of auditory processing disorders is the responsibility of the audiologist, whereas audiologists and speech pathologists share the responsibility for management. Disruption in the transmission and processing of auditory information can occur anywhere in the auditory system, from the inner ear to the highest levels of the auditory cortex.

You were introduced in the previous chapter to a variety of outer and middle ear disorders that reduce the level of sound that reaches the inner ear. We also discussed many diseases that affect cochlear function and disrupt the normal hearing process. We will focus in this final section on a category of hearing problems commonly described as auditory processing disorders or APD.

An **auditory processing disorder (APD)** is defined as "a deficit in the processing of auditory information that is specific to the auditory modality" (Jerger & Musiek, 2000) and a reduction in the effectiveness and efficiency in auditory processing (ASHA, 2005). Auditory processing disorders in children interfere with school performance and academic success. Adults with auditory processing disorders may encounter serious problems communicating in work settings and during social activities.

Table 12.2 shows characteristics and behaviors often reported for children with auditory processing disorders. Patients with auditory processing disorders have problems in discriminating between different but similar sounds, difficulty recognizing the correct sequence of sounds, problems separating or integrating auditory signals presented simultaneously to each ear, and abnormalities in the perception of speech in the presence of background sound. Another characteristic of auditory processing disorders is slower-than-normal processing of auditory information.

- Says "huh" or "what" a lot
- Trouble listening in noise
- Responds inappropriately in the classroom
- Reluctant to participate in class discussions
- Difficulty following multi-step directions
- Seems to have a hearing loss but audiograms are normal
- Teacher concern about hearing and listening abilities
- Poor reading and spelling skills

TABLE 12.2
Behaviors and characteristics of patients with auditory processing disorders

APD and Scope of Practice

Audiologists and speech pathologists are the professionals with primary responsibility for caring for patients with auditory processing disorders. "Evaluation and management of children and adults with auditory-related processing disorders" is within the scope of practice for audiologists (American Academy of Audiology, 2004; ASHA, 2007). The scope of practice for speech pathologists includes "providing intervention and support services for children and adults diagnosed with auditory processing disorders" (ASHA, 2007).

Distinction between APD and Hearing Loss

Auditory processing disorders differ in three important ways from the other types of auditory dysfunction we've discussed up to this point. First, hearing sensitivity on an audiogram is often within normal limits in patients diagnosed with APD. Second, patients with APD typically have excellent word recognition performance in quiet listening conditions. Word recognition scores are often 100% for each ear. Third, the majority of patients with APD do not have specific central nervous system pathology such as a tumor, a vascular abnormality, or a brain injury. Nonetheless, APD can have a major impact on hearing and communication. The consequences of unrecognized or untreated APD in children include difficulty in communicating, reading disorders, poor academic performance, and psychosocial problems.

Etiologies for APD

APD in young children may be associated with a specific etiology, such as a perinatal incident of hypoxia, a head injury, or some other risk for neurological dysfunction (Chermak & Musiek, 2011). However, APD in children most often reflects a disruption in the normal development of central auditory nervous system function, with no documented pathology or risk for neurological disorder. We will take a moment to explore developmental factors contributing to auditory processing disorders.

Developmental Explanations

Neuroscience research has in recent years shed light on developmental processes that are critical for normal auditory development, particularly the critical role of auditory stimulation and experience. We reviewed some neuroscience principles at the beginning of this chapter. The concept of auditory system plasticity is crucial for the understanding of auditory processing and auditory processing disorders in children. Specifically, the concept of brain plasticity helps to explain why auditory nervous system development is disrupted in some children. Brain plasticity also offers an opportunity for improvement with appropriate treatment of disrupted auditory processing.

Most children diagnosed with APD also have coexisting disorders, that is, other problems related to central nervous system functioning. Examples of disorders coexisting with auditory

LEADERS AND LUMINARIES

Teri James Bellis

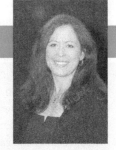

Teri James Bellis earned her bachelor's degree at the University of Northern Colorado, her master's degree at the University of California, and her PhD at Northwestern University. Dr. Bellis is Professor and Chair of Communication Sciences and Disorders at the University of South Dakota, and director of the USD Speech-Language-Hearing Clinics. An international expert on the topic of central auditory processing disorders, she chaired the American Speech-Language-Hearing Association Working Group on CAPD and also served on the American Academy of Audiology Task Force, which developed clinical guidelines for diagnosis of an intervention for the disorder. Dr. Bellis is the author of many peer-reviewed journal articles as well as the textbook *Assessment and Management of Central Auditory Processing Disorders in the Educational Setting* and a popular consumer book entitled *When the Brain Can't Hear: Unraveling the Mystery of Auditory Processing Disorder.*

processing disorders include difficulties or deficits in attention, language, learning, and reading (AAA, 2010). Research also clearly shows that struggles in school associated with auditory processing disorders in children can lead to multiple psychosocial problems, like anxiety, aggression, withdrawal, and even depression (Johnston, John, Kreisman, Hall, & Crandell, 2009; Kreisman, John, Kreisman, Hall, & Crandell, 2012).

APD in Adults

In an adult population, APD is more often due to a specific central nervous system disorder like traumatic brain injury (TBI). Audiologists and speech pathologists are increasingly focused on detection, assessment, and management of APD and other communicative disorders in military personnel and veterans with TBI resulting from combat exposure to explosive blasts (AAA, 2010; Hall & Bellis, 2008; Hall et al., 1983). As noted earlier in this chapter, central auditory dysfunction and APD are also common findings in patients with degenerative neurological conditions like Alzheimer's dementia. In addition, age-related changes in the central nervous system can lead to auditory processing deficits in older adults (Hall, 1983; Jerger, Oliver, & Pirozzolo, 1989).

ⓘ WebWatch

Full versions of evidence-based and peer-reviewed technical reports and clinical guidelines on auditory processing disorders can be downloaded from the Internet. "Diagnosis, Treatment, and Management of Children and Adults with (Central) Auditory Processing Disorders" is the most recent document describing clinical guidelines on (central) auditory processing disorders. A task force commissioned by the American Academy of Audiology (AAA) completed the guidelines in 2010. The task force summarized research findings in support of recommendations. Guidelines are available from the American Academy of Audiology (AAA) and the American Speech-Language-Hearing Association (ASHA) websites.

Assessment of APD

Since the "Decade of the Brain" in the 1990s, research interest in and clinical focus on APD has steadily increased. Assessment and management of APD is now clearly within the scope of practice of audiology and speech pathology as defined by professional organizations. Documents stating the scope of practice for audiology can be reviewed or downloaded from the websites of the American Academy of Audiology or the American Speech Language Hearing Association. In addition, several panels of experts have developed evidence-based and peer-reviewed technical documents and monographs on all aspects of APD (AAA, 2010; ASHA, 2005).

Team Approach. Assessment and management of APD requires a multidisciplinary approach, involving audiologists, speech pathologists, psychologists, school representatives, physicians, and sometimes professionals such as occupational therapists. A test battery approach is essential for assessment of APD in children and adults. However, the procedures included in a test battery for evaluation of a specific patient depend on a number of factors, like the patient's age, audiogram pattern, cognitive abilities, and ability to maintain attention during the testing (AAA, 2010).

Test Battery. Some general principles guide the selection of procedures included in a test battery for the assessment of APD. The tests should be appropriate for the patient's age. The test battery should include verbal tests consisting of words and sentences but also nonverbal tests utilizing simple signals like tones or broadband noise. The test battery must consist of behavioral tests like speech audiometry and also objective auditory tests. Examples of objective tests for the evaluation of auditory processing include otoacoustic emissions, acoustic immittance measures, and auditory evoked responses (AAA, 2010; Dhar & Hall, 2012; Hall, 2007b). You learned about each of these procedures in Chapters 8 and 9. Finally, the test battery must include procedures that assess most major auditory processes identified by research and specified in published clinical guidelines (AAA, 2010; ASHA, 2005).

We've focused here on the nature and diagnosis of auditory processing disorders. In Chapter 16 you'll learn about the intervention strategies for auditory processing disorders. We will specifically review the roles of audiologists and speech pathologists in developing and implementing appropriate and effective management strategies.

PULLING IT ALL TOGETHER

The chapter began with a brief review of important discoveries in brain research that accelerated in the 1990s and continue even today. Newly discovered neuroscience principles like brain plasticity have had a direct impact on assessment and management of patients with central auditory nervous system dysfunction, including auditory processing disorders. Audiologists and speech pathologists now have a greater appreciation for the connection between cognition, hearing, and communication in persons of all ages. Awareness of brain plasticity has led to renewed efforts to provide diagnostic and rehabilitative communication services to all persons at risk for central nervous system dysfunction, from premature newborn infants to veterans with traumatic brain injury and aging adults.

You learned in this chapter that a diverse collection of disorders affecting the auditory nerve or the central nervous system may disrupt normal auditory function and result in hearing impairment. In some cases, the abnormalities are tumors verified with neuroradiologic techniques like CT or MRI scanning. Two examples are vestibular schwannomas and neurofibromas. Other neurological diseases can interfere with auditory function, including demyelinating and degenerative diseases and different types of dementia.

You were also introduced in this chapter to two forms of auditory disorder that involve multiple sites in the auditory system, specifically auditory neuropathy spectrum disorder (ANSD) and auditory processing disorders (APD). There are multiple important distinctions between ANSD and APD. However, both types of auditory disorder require a team approach for accurate diagnosis and effective management.

Throughout the chapter you've had the opportunity to review patterns of auditory findings associated with disorders affecting the auditory nerve or the central nervous system.

You now appreciate the importance of comprehensive diagnostic assessment of auditory function with a battery of tests in certain patient populations. Each of the tests is specifically selected to provide the information needed for accurate diagnosis, proper referral to other healthcare professionals, and appropriate management. One point is clear: hearing assessment of patients with suspected central auditory disorders and auditory processing disorders must extend far beyond the audiogram.

READINGS

American Academy of Audiology. (2010). Clinical practice guidelines: Diagnosis, treatment and management of children and adults with central auditory processing disorder. Accessed August 24, 2010 from audiology.org.

American Speech-Language-Hearing Association. (2005). (Central) auditory processing disorders [Technical Report]. Retrieved from asha.org

Bailey, B. J., Calhoun, K. H., Healy, G. B., Pillsbury, H. C., Johnson, J. T., Jackler, R. T., & Tardy, M. E. (Eds.), *Head and neck surgery—otolarynoglogy. Volume II.* (3rd ed.). Philadelphia: Lippincott Williams & Wilkins.

Bantwal, A. R., & Hall, J. W. III. (2011). Pediatric speech perception in noise. *Current Pediatric Reviews, 7,* 214–226.

Bellis, T. J. (2003). *Assessment and management of central auditory processing disorders in the educational setting: From science to practice* (2nd ed.) New York: Thomson and Delmar Learning.

British Association of Otorhinolaryngologists – Head & Neck Surgeons Clinical Practice Advisory Group. (2002, Spring). Clinical effectiveness guidelines acoustic neuroma (vestibular schwannoma) BAO-HNS Document 5. London: The Royal College of Surgeons of England.

Chermak, G. D., & Musiek, F. E. (Eds.). (2007). *Handbook of (central) auditory processing disorders: Comprehensive intervention (Volume 2).* San Diego, CA: Plural Publishing.

Chermak, C. D., & Musiek, F. E. (2011). Neurological substrate of central auditory processing deficits in children. *Current Pediatric Reviews, 7.*

Hall, J. W. III, & Mueller, H. G. III. (1997). *Audiologists' desk reference. Volume I. Diagnostic audiology: Principles, procedures & practices.* San Diego: Singular Publishing.

Jerger, S., & Jerger, J. (1981). *Auditory disorders: A manual for clinical evaluation.* Boston: Little, Brown & Co.

Musiek, F. E., & Baran, J. A. (2007). *The auditory system: Anatomy, physiology, and clinical correlates.* Boston: Allyn & Bacon.

Musiek, F. E., & Chermak, G. D. (Eds.). (2007). *Handbook of (central) auditory processing disorders: Auditory neuroscience and diagnosis (Volume 1).* San Diego, CA: Plural Publishing.

Myklebust, H. R. (1954). *Auditory disorders in children: A manual for the differential diagnosis.* New York: Grune and Stratton.

Snow, J. B. Jr., & Wackym, P. A. (Eds.). (2009). *Ballenger's otorhinolaryngology—head and neck surgery* (17th ed). Shelton CT: BC Decker.

Tarazi, F. I., & Schetz, J. A. (Eds.). (2011). *Neurological and psychiatric disorders.* New York: Humana Press.

13 Audiological Management: Technology

LEARNING OBJECTIVES

In this chapter, you will learn:

- New terminology about hearing aids
- About major developments in hearing aid technology
- The components of modern hearing aids
- The types of hearing aids today
- The difference between analog and digital hearing aids
- How hearing aids are selected
- How hearing aid operation is verified
- The multiple benefits of amplification and hearing aid use
- About new hearing devices that are surgically implanted
- New terminology about cochlear implants
- The components of cochlear implants
- Which patients are candidates for cochlear implants
- New terminology about assistive listening devices
- What an FM system is and how it improves communication

KEY TERMS

Assistive listening devices (ALDs)
Baha (bone-anchored hearing aid) devices
Behind-the-ear (BTE)
Candidacy
Cochlear implants
Completely-in-the-canal (CIC)
Compression
Digitally programmable
Ear mold
Ear mold impression
Electroacoustical measurement
Feedback
Gain
Hearing aid selection
Hearing assistance technology (HAT)
In-the-canal (ITC)
In-the-ear (ITE)
Linear amplification
Prescriptive hearing aid fitting
Receiver
Receiver-in-the-canal (RIC)
Validation
Verification

CHAPTER FOCUS

An impressive array of technology is now available for improvement of communication in persons with hearing impairment. Hearing aids are the most common management option. Although modern hearing aids come in various shapes and sizes, most incorporate digital technology and features that permit precise amplification of sound for children and adults with varying degrees and configurations of hearing loss.

In this chapter, you will first read about the development of hearing aids over the years. You'll then learn about the basic components found in all modern hearing aids, and about a half-dozen types of hearing aids that differ in size, location, and other features. Some of the newer features permit computer control of amplification so that soft sounds are amplified more than loud sounds. Patients have the option of selecting specific hearing aid programs for use in different kinds of listening environments. Problems that sometimes arise during hearing aid use are noted, as well as some solutions to the problems. You'll also be introduced to techniques audiologists use to determine whether a patient might benefit from amplification and whether the hearing aid once fit is actually providing the desired benefit.

CHAPTER FOCUS *Concluded*

Hearing aids are not the only technology available for improving communication function in children and adults. Some patients are not candidates for hearing aids due to the severity of their hearing loss. Cochlear implants are an option for children or adults with profound hearing loss who cannot be helped with hearing aids. You will read about the different components of cochlear implants and which patients are candidates for implantation. Other surgically implantable devices are also mentioned in this chapter. Fortunately, there are now technological options for improving communication for almost every person with hearing impairment, regardless of the type or severity of the impairment.

Hearing is always more difficult in the presence of background noise and when the speaker is at a considerable distance from the listener. One solution to these problems is hearing assistance technology. The final section of the chapter includes a review of personal assistive devices that improve listening performance for a single person and also classroom or group amplification systems that improve listening for many people. You will also be introduced to some of the many different forms of hearing assistance technology available to persons with hearing impairment in addition to hearing aids, implantable devices, and assistive devices.

Amplification 101

We'll spend much of this chapter talking about hearing aids and other devices and instruments designed to assist with hearing. Hearing aids are now incredibly sophisticated and heavily dependent on digital and computer-based technology. There is no doubt that hearing aids offer the most effective management tool for the vast majority of persons with hearing loss. We should keep in mind, however, that hearing performance is also quickly and inexpensively enhanced with some simple techniques and strategies. In fact, you've probably employed some of these techniques and strategies in certain difficult listening environments.

The common practice of cupping your hands behind your ears is a very simple and cost-free method for aiding hearing. Your hands are low-tech hearing instruments that capture sound and increase or amplify sound at some frequencies. The sound intensity of a speaker's voice is also increased quite noticeably as you move closer to a speaker. In fact, the intensity level of speech in a free field setting like an open area is increased by about 6 dB every time you reduce the distance to the speaker by one-half, such as from a distance of 6 feet to 3 feet.

Another very effective approach for improving speech perception in a noisy setting is to simply relocate with the speaker to a quieter place. Speech perception is invariably improved when the signal speech to noise difference is increased. It is easier to understand what a person is saying when the background noise level is lower.

Finally, we've all enjoyed improvement in hearing with electronic amplification when we turn up the volume of a radio, personal audio player, television, or CD player. These examples illustrate that the goal of amplification is improvement of hearing ability. Electrical devices like hearing aids are one tool for accomplishing this goal.

Historical Perspective

Ear Horns and Trumpets. The history of aids for hearing is usually traced far back to the use of animal horns as simple amplifiers. The animal horn approach for amplification led to the design of early ear trumpets that were partly or entirely made out of metal. A person with a hearing impairment placed the open narrow end close to the ear canal while the speaker's mouth was placed near the wide portion of the horn. Animal horns and ear trumpets were "low-tech" devices that effectively magnified the natural ear-related funnel and resonance to further enhance and amplify perception of sound, especially speech.

Horns and trumpets are mechanical or acoustical devices for hearing enhancement. The development of electrical engineering and the creation of electrical devices like the light bulb in the late nineteenth century opened up new possibilities for amplification of sound. Introduction of electrical amplification devices was a major breakthrough leading to the design and manufacture of hearing aids.

Early Electronic Hearing Aids. Electronic hearing aid developments can be grouped into four eras. In the first era, from 1900 to about 1940, sound was amplified by rudimentary carbon hearing aids. Carbon can be used to amplify electrical energy. Carbon hearing aids were big and very basic by later standards, but they were a major improvement over earlier acoustical and mechanical devices.

The next generation of electrical hearing aids relied on *vacuum tube* technology for amplification of sound. A vacuum tube is an airtight glass enclosure with air removed, containing electrodes or terminals. Power applied to one terminal permits control and amplification of electrical current or voltage between the other two terminals. Vacuum tubes became increasingly more common in electrical devices from the early 1920s to the 1950s, just as the profession of audiology was forming. Home radios in large wooden cabinets and even audiometers operated with vacuum tube technology. Vacuum tubes permitted much higher-quality amplification than earlier electronic hearing aid devices, but the technology did little to reduce their size. In fact, early vacuum tube hearing aids were so big they were placed on a table and not worn on the body.

Transistor Hearing Aids. The transistor was one of the most important inventions of the twentieth century. Development of the transistor in the 1950s ushered in a third era in hearing aid technology. Transistor technology is referred to as solid-state or semiconductor electronics. The transistor was a logical outgrowth of vacuum tube technology as it also had three terminals. Electrical circuits with transistor technology eliminated the need for bulky, power-consuming glass vacuum tubes.

During an exciting era of investigation and discovery, researchers at Bell Telephone Laboratories in Murray Hill, New Jersey, conducted many of the studies on transistor technology with the specific goal of creating audio amplifiers for speech (Berger, 1984; Gertner, 2012). Three scientists at Bell Labs involved in the invention of transistors and solid-state electronics, John Bardeen, William Shockley, and Walter Brattain, received the Nobel Prize for physics in 1956.

Not surprisingly, during the 1950s, transistors rapidly became an essential component in hearing aids as well as radios and a wide variety of other electrical devices. The small size of transistors immediately contributed to a new generation of smaller hearing aids.

Figure 13.1 shows examples of rather large body-worn transistor hearing aids and smaller ear-level transistor hearing aids. Some of these were powerful hearing aids, permitting amplification of sound for persons with severe hearing loss.

Body-worn hearing aids had one main disadvantage in addition to their large size. The microphone on the hearing aid was located in an unnatural location, in front of the chest and far from the ear. The microphone is the part of a hearing aid that detects sound. A cord led from the hearing aid box to receivers in ear pieces where amplified sound was then delivered to each ear. Sometimes the cord was split into two separate components, one leading to each ear, called a "Y-cord" because of its shape.

FIGURE 13.1

Transistor-based hearing aids worn on the body (top of display) and at ear-level (bottom right portion of the photograph). Courtesy of Wayne Staab.

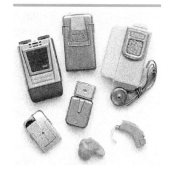

WebWatch

There are several collections of vintage hearing aids in museums within the United States. You can view an impressive and very interesting array of old hearing aid styles at a website for a Washington University Hearing Aid Museum.

Transistor hearing aids were the first to be worn on the ear and even in the ear canal, rather than on the body (Staab & Lybarger, 1994).

Modern Hearing Aid Technology

Hearing aid technology is constantly changing and evolving. New features, options, and advances in hearing aid design are introduced on an annual basis, often at major audiology professional conferences. There are currently three general categories of hearing aid technology: (1) analog, (2) digitally programmable, and (3) digital. Early hearing aids utilized analog technology. A combination of analog and digital technology was introduced in the 1980s (Schweitzer, 1997; Staab & Lybarger, 1994). These are usually referred to as digitally programmable hearing aids. Digital hearing aids are the most recent and the most common category of hearing aid technology (Kochkin, 2009, 2010).

Analog Hearing Aids. All hearing aids were built with *analog* technology for many years (Staab & Lybarger, 1994). Even today analog hearing aids are almost always simpler and less expensive for the consumer. The word *analog* is derived from the Greek word for "proportional." The acoustic signal is detected by a microphone, converted into an electrical signal, and amplified by a certain or proportional amount. Then the amplified electrical signal is converted back to sound at the receiver and delivered to the person's ear. With external controls an audiologist can make some minor modifications in analog hearing aids. For example, filters can be changed to increase or decrease amplification in certain frequency regions, depending on the person's hearing loss.

Most analog hearing aids utilize **linear amplification**. It is helpful to use the terms *input* and *output* in describing amplification. Input is the sound entering the microphone of the hearing aid and output is the amplified sound leaving the hearing aid receiver. With linear amplification, the output sound is proportional or directly related to the input sound. The extent of linear amplification doesn't change according to the intensity level of input sound. As the level of sound in the environment increases or decreases, the amount of sound heard by the patient also increases and decreases. Put another way, soft sounds and loud sounds are amplified by the same amount.

The linear or constant amplification of all sounds creates problems for some patients in certain listening conditions. The analog hearing aid user often notices that low background sounds in noisy settings are louder and more annoying. At the other extreme, sudden high-intensity sounds in the environment amplified with linear technology are often uncomfortably loud.

Analog linear amplification is illustrated in Figure 13.2. An audiologist considers three main hearing aid functions with analog technology. The first is the overall gain or amplification from the input to the microphone to the output of the receiver. The second is the slope or rate of amplification. In other words, the amount of output or amplification produced by the hearing aid for every decibel of sound coming into the hearing aid. Third, an audiologist determines and documents in dB the maximum output of the hearing aid. That is, what is the maximum sound intensity produced by the hearing aid at the highest possible amplification setting?

Since analog hearing aids are older and simpler, it is tempting to consider them inferior to sophisticated and complex digital counterparts. However, the quality of sound amplified by analog hearing aids is sometimes equal to or even better than digitally amplified sound. Users of analog hearing aids may describe the sound as more natural and less distorted. This positive perception of analog audio technology is certainly not limited to amplification and hearing aids. As the music industry transitioned from analog to digital technology, similar positive

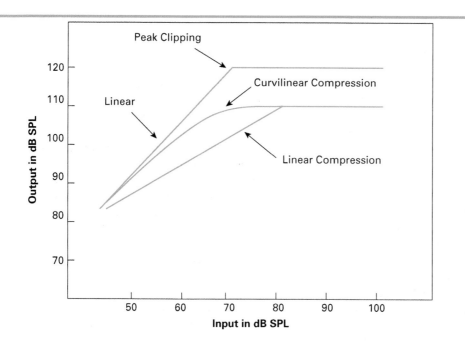

FIGURE 13.2

Diagram of linear
amplification, nonlinear
amplification, and
compression in
amplification.

comparisons were made between the older analog recordings and those made and mixed in the digitally format.

Analog/Digital Hearing Aids. Advances in electronic circuitry and hearing aid design in the mid-1980s led to the introduction of hearing aids that combined analog and digital technology (Berger, 1988; Levitt, 1987; Staab & Lybarger, 1994). Analog/digital devices are often referred to as **digitally programmable** hearing aids. They rely on traditional analog amplification circuits to process sound. However, multiple different analog processing strategies can be built into a single hearing aid and stored in separate digital memories. Using an external remote control device, the hearing aid wearer can quickly select among the stored programs for the sound processing system that is best suited to the listening environment, such as a quiet or a noisy setting. Digitally programmable hearing aids remain a reasonable flexible, moderately priced, and effective hearing aid option for many people.

Digital Hearing Aids. The current era of modern hearing aid design incorporates *digital technology* and the capacity for *digital signal processing,* abbreviated *DSP* (Levitt, 1987; Lunner, Hellgren, Arlinger, & Elberling, 1998; Murray & Hanson, 1992; Schweitzer, 1997). Digital hearing aids first came on the market in the late 1980s and early 1990s. Today's hearing aids are really tiny computers consisting of specially programmed computer chips. Digital hearing aids can be custom tuned, fit, and adapted to different types and degrees of hearing losses and a wide variety of listening situations (Chung, 2004a, b). Our discussion about hearing aids and how they work will now focus on this latest technology.

Advances in digital signal processing technology have greatly expanded the possibility for a wide array of additional hearing aid features and hearing aid flexibility (Schaub, 2008; Schweitzer, 1997; Murray & Hanson, 1992). Digital hearing aids can be precisely fitted to persons with hearing loss of virtually every type, degree, and configuration to improve communication performance in a variety of listening settings and environments. Incoming sound is immediately converted to a digital signal, before amplification takes place.

The list of current features and potential future options for digital hearing aids is almost endless (Chung, 2004a,b). The amount of amplification in a digital hearing aid is manipulated depending on the level of sound entering the hearing aid (Kates, 2005; Levitt, 1987; Lunner et al., 1998). For example, amplification is greater for very soft sounds to assure that they are audible, whereas loud sounds are amplified less or not at all. Greater amplification for lower-intensity input sound than for higher-intensity sound is called **compression**. The amount of amplification is decreased or compressed as sound levels increase. Figure 13.2 shows the concept of compression in amplification.

Other amplification strategies are also available with digital hearing aids. For example, the amount of amplification can be precisely controlled for different frequency regions, bands, or channels. A digital hearing aid can be adjusted with a computer in order to provide appropriate amounts of amplification across the audiogram frequency range (Schaub, 2008). Varying the amount of amplification for different frequencies is, for example, quite helpful for a person with normal hearing in the low-frequency region and a hearing loss that progressively worsens for the higher-frequency sounds.

Digital technology with a wide array of hearing aid options permits flexible fitting of persons with diverse hearing needs. Some digital options include signal-processing algorithms to reduce the negative impact of steady background noise, to control problems with feedback, and even to digitally enhance speech signals versus non-speech noise (Bentler & Chiou, 2006; Chung, 2004a, b; Kates, 2005). Digital hearing aids also permit the incorporation of sophisticated microphone technology, including multiple microphones to detect sound and microphones that detect the direction of sound (Amiani, 2001; Ricketts, 2000; Ricketts & Mueller, 1999).

FIGURE 13.3

Major components of an in-the-ear (ITE) hearing aid (top) and behind-the-ear (BTE) hearing aid (bottom) including the microphone, amplifier, receiver, and battery. The abbreviation "O-T-M" refers to the switch for turning the hearing aid off (O), or to the telephone (T) or microphone (M) settings.

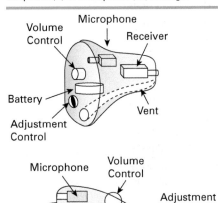

Basic Hearing Aid Components

A variety of features and options are available in modern hearing aids. First we'll review the four components common to all hearing aids. Then you'll be introduced to types and features of hearing aids. Figure 13.3 depicts each of the four hearing aid components. The figure includes simplified drawings of an in-the-ear hearing aid that fits within the external auditory canal (top of figure) and a **behind-the-ear (BTE)** hearing aid that is so named because the body of the hearing aid is located behind the pinna (bottom of figure).

Microphone. One essential hearing aid component is a *microphone*. At least one microphone is necessary to detect sounds and to convert them to electrical signals. Some modern hearing aid designs may actually have multiple microphones. The location of the microphone or array of microphones varies depending on the type of hearing aid. Figure 13.3 shows a microphone for both types of hearing aids.

Amplifier. The *amplifier* is really the heart of the hearing aid. It is an important part of the electrical circuit enclosed within a hearing aid case. Electrical energy produced by sound passing through the microphone is increased or amplified by a specific amount. The amplification process can be quite complex yet also remarkably flexible in modern hearing aids. For example, the amount of amplification can be separately controlled for different frequency bands or for other characteristics of sound.

A common strategy is to progressively increase the amount of amplification for higher frequencies with relatively less or even no amplification for lower frequencies (Staab & Lybarger, 1994). This approach is appropriate for patients whose hearing loss is mostly for higher-frequency sounds. Also, the amount of amplification can be increased or decreased depending on the intensity level of sound entering the hearing aid. Most persons with a hearing loss have difficulty hearing soft sounds. All modern hearing aids include the option for amplifying soft sounds considerably more than louder sounds (Ricketts, De Chicchis, & Bess, 2001; Staab & Lybarger, 1994).

Receiver. The third general component of the hearing aid is the **receiver**. The receiver *receives* amplified electrical energy from the amplifier and changes it back to sound. The location of the receiver varies from one hearing aid design to the next. Depending on the style of the hearing aid, the receiver may be included in the hearing aid casing or in the ear canal. For many years the receiver was almost always embedded in the hearing aid. Amplified sound was then routed into the ear canal via tubing coupled to an ear mold. Figure 13.3 shows a conventional behind-the-ear hearing aid with a plastic ear-hook that is connected to tubing leading to an ear mold. With newer hearing aid designs, the receiver may be located in the ear canal even though the rest of the hearing aid fits behind the patient's ear.

Battery. A *battery* is the fourth essential component common to all hearing aids. Typical placement of a battery for an in-the-ear hearing aid and in a behind-the-ear hearing aid was also shown in Figure 13.3. Batteries provide power that hearing aids require to amplify and process sound. Today's hearing aids are powered with zinc air batteries that are available from a number of manufacturers.

Hearing aid batteries of different sizes are shown in Figure 13.4. The slightly wider flat positive terminal of a hearing aid battery is called the *cathode* and the narrower rounded negative terminal is the *anode*. The cathode in a zinc battery is activated by air that releases electrical energy in the form of electrons. The energy travels to the anode that is connected to electrical circuitry in the hearing aid.

New batteries are usually packaged in the factory with stickers covering the cathode that forms the wider side of the battery. The sticker on the cathode keeps the battery "fresh." A battery is activated when a hearing aid user or the parent of a child who uses hearing aids removes the sticker. Battery life ranges from seven to fourteen days, depending on hearing aid type and features and assuming the hearing aid is used for about sixteen hours each day. Before activation, hearing aid batteries stored in a cool and dry location stay fresh for up to three years.

Batteries are usually available for sale in audiology clinics. They can also be purchased from vendors online or in pharmacies, grocery stores, and other retail outlets. Each size is color-coded. The smallest hearing aid battery is size 5 and coded red. The largest is size 675 and coded blue.

Rechargeable hearing aid batteries are now available from a number of different manufacturers. Figure 13.5 shows a relatively recently developed low-cost and eco-friendly hearing aid. The innovative hearing aid is very durable and incorporates batteries that are rechargeable with solar power. It is manufactured for millions of

FIGURE 13.4

A sample of hearing aid batteries of different sizes.

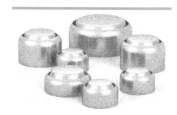

FIGURE 13.5

An example of a device designed for recharging batteries with solar energy. A small solar panel is shown to the left. A hearing aid and several hearing aid batteries are shown to the right. Courtesy of Solar Ear.

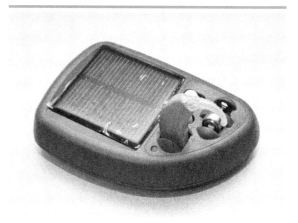

hearing-impaired persons in developing countries where conventional batteries are not readily available or affordable (McPherson, 2011). Indeed, the hearing aid shown in Figure 13.5 is called the "Solar Ear."

Battery Information. One step in fitting a hearing aid is to provide information about batteries. Battery education is particularly important for first-time users. The information is given directly to adult patients and to parents or caregivers of pediatric patients. Most patients and parents require instructions on insertion and removal of batteries.

Information on battery safety is also essential. Batteries consist of toxic materials that are very harmful and potentially fatal if swallowed by children or by pets. Unfortunately, ingestion of hearing aid batteries remains a concern in any home where someone wears hearing aids. Swallowing a battery is a medical emergency requiring immediate attention. Used hearing aid batteries should be disposed of properly, like any other type of battery. Instructions for appropriate disposal are often printed on the battery packaging. One acceptable disposal option is to include the batteries with other objects that are taken to a local household hazardous waste site.

Ear Molds

Hearing aids are often coupled or connected to the ear with an **ear mold** that is custom-fit to the patient's external ear canal. A permanent ear mold is manufactured at a commercial laboratory from an **ear mold impression** that an audiologist makes in the clinic or office. The ear mold impression is made before the hearing aid fitting.

Figure 13.6 shows supplies used to make ear mold impressions. The ear mold impression is made with a substance that has a consistency similar to toothpaste. A soft *oto-block* made of cotton or sponge-like material is first inserted into the ear canal. A penlight is used to illuminate the external ear canal and to push the oto-block inward down the external ear canal. The oto-block prevents the ear mold impression material from going too far into the external ear canal.

An audiologist then prepares the impression material. The impression material generally consists of two substances that slowly harden after they are mixed together. Containers of the impression materials and a packet of the two impression materials are shown in Figure 13.6.

An audiologist stuffs the soft impression material into a syringe like the one at the bottom of Figure 13.6. Then, using the syringe, the audiologist injects the soft impression material into the ear canal. The entire ear canal from the oto-block out to the concha is filled with ear mold impression material. The impression material hardens in several minutes to take on a rubbery consistency. An audiologist gently removes the hardened ear mold impression.

Ear molds are made from several different types of material. Silicone is relatively soft, and some materials like Lucite or acrylic are harder. Nontoxic and hypoallergenic ear mold materials are available for patients who have skin allergies. Depending on the characteristics of a person's hearing loss, an ear mold may or may not totally fill the concha of the outer ear.

FIGURE 13.6

Supplies and equipment for making ear mold impressions including from top to bottom two containers of impression material, a packet of impression materials, several sizes of foam oto-block (identified with arrows), a penlight for illuminating the external ear canal and inserting oto-block, and a syringe for injecting the material into the external ear canal.

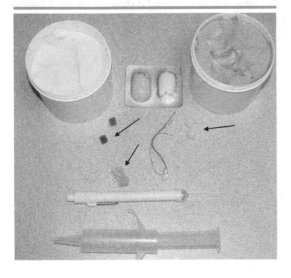

Types of Hearing Aids

We'll now review briefly each of the five main types of modern hearing aids: (1) conventional behind-the-ear (BTE), (2) open-fit behind-the-ear (BTE), (3) in-the-ear (ITE), (4) in-the-canal (ITC), and (5) completely-in-the-canal (CIC). These hearing aid types differ considerably in their appearance. However, each consists of a hard plastic case that encloses and protects electronic components within.

Behind-the-Ear (BTE). The *BTE* design dates back to the 1950s when transistors were first incorporated in hearing aids. Figure 13.1 showed an early BTE hearing aid in the lower right corner. A typical modern BTE hearing aid is shown in Figure 13.7. Many people probably envision a BTE style like the one in the figure when they think of hearing aids. The concave shaped hearing aid case enclosing electronic circuitry rests on and behind the ear. The plastic case of BTE hearing aids is available in different colors. Adult patients often prefer hearing aids that blend in with their skin and hair color, whereas children may be attracted to very bright, creative, and colorful hearing aid appearances.

A plastic tube leads downward from the front of the case to the external ear canal so amplified sound can be delivered to the ear. The tube of some hearing aid styles is connected or coupled to the ear with an ear mold that is custom-made to fit the patient's ear.

The BTE style is best suited for young children who require hearing aids. There are at least four reasons why the BTE hearing aid style is best for children. First, BTE hearing aids offer the most powerful option for amplification, so they are appropriate even for children with a severe degree of hearing loss. Second, BTE hearing aids offer maximum flexibility, so adjustments can be made as more information about a child's hearing becomes available.

Third, a child can wear the same hearing aids for relatively long periods of time, even with physical growth. New ear molds are easily and inexpensively made to accommodate age-related changes in the size of a child's ear. The new ear molds are simply coupled with new tubing to the child's existing hearing aids. Ear mold materials are chosen to maximize comfort and function of the hearing aid.

Finally, children sometimes lose hearing aids and ear molds. When a hearing aid is lost, the child is fit with an appropriately selected temporary "loaner" BTE hearing aid. A loaner hearing aid is connected to newly made ear molds until the replacement hearing aid is available.

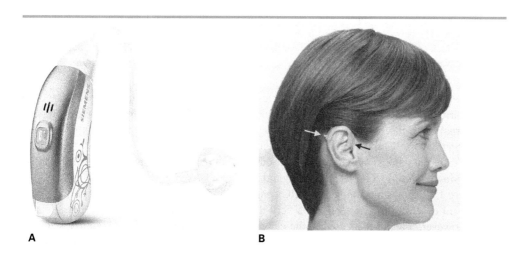

A   **B**

FIGURE 13.7

A modern open-fit behind-the-ear (BTE) hearing aid **(A)**. The same hearing aid is shown as worn by a patient **(B)**. The arrow toward the back points to the hearing aid whereas the arrow toward the front points to the tiny tube leading to the external ear canal. Photos courtesy of Siemens Hearing Instruments.

Open-Fit BTE. The open-fit style is the most recent version of BTE hearing aids. This popular hearing aid style was shown in Figure 13.7A. Look closely at the end of the tubing of the hearing aid in Figure 13.7A, and you will notice that there is no ear mold. A soft dome- or cone-shaped piece directs sound into the ear canal without occluding or plugging up the ear canal. There is no need for manufacturing a custom permanent ear mold from an ear mold impression. As a result, it is possible for a patient to undergo a hearing aid consultation and walk out of an audiology clinic with an open-fit hearing aid on the same day.

Over a period of about two decades, the popularity of conventional BTE hearing aids consistently diminished because patients were attracted to smaller devices that were enclosed in the ear canal. This trend began to reverse dramatically in the year 2005 with the introduction of the modest-sized open-fit BTE hearing aids, often simply called open-fit hearing aids.

Why are open-fit BTE hearing aids so popular? Discrete appearance, small size, and lightweight are certainly factors that contribute to the popularity of open-fit BTE hearing aids. An open-fit BTE hearing aid is considerably smaller and less noticeable than its conventional BTE counterpart, and the very thin clear plastic tubing connecting the hearing aid to the ear canal is almost invisible. Looking again at Figure 13.7, it's hard to see the hearing aid or the tubing that leads to the external ear canal.

Patients also appreciate the comfort of an open-fit hearing aid. In addition, patients benefit from access to sound directly entering the ear canal, with natural amplification provided by the pinna and external ear canal. Low-frequency sounds in the environment are not blocked out by an ear mold or a hearing aid filling the ear canal. Instead, low-frequency sounds reach the ear freely and naturally as they do for persons who are not wearing a hearing aid. Also, patients who tend to build up excessive cerumen need not be concerned about blockage of openings in hearing aids or ear molds.

Open-fit hearing aids are for all of these reasons an appropriate and appealing option for the sizable number of persons with mild-to-moderate high-frequency hearing loss. The popularity of open-fit hearing aids is likely to increase as the need for amplification extends to millions of aging and technologically savvy baby boomers (Cruickshanks et al., 1998; Wiley, Chappell, Carmichael, Nondahl, & Cruickshanks, 2008).

A consumer-oriented newspaper article with the catchy title *Lilliputian Aid All the Rage among the Slightly Hard-of-Hearing Set,* published in 2006, soon after open-fit hearing aids arrived on the market, captures the excitement about this new option for amplification:

> It's tiny, it's sleek, and consumers are raving about its great sound. The latest iPod model? No, it's a new type of hearing aid. Made with the latest in digital technology and nearly invisible when worn, the device is intended for people with high-frequency hearing loss. It has been on the market for less than a year, but one leading company says sales of the new hearing aid have been four times higher than expected. The new devices can best help people with only mild to moderate high-frequency hearing loss, which accounts for about 20% of hearing impairment cases. ..." (Russel Berman, Staff Reporter of the New York Sun, February 7, 2006)

Receiver-in-the-Canal (RIC). With the original BTE hearing aid and the newer open-fit BTE hearing aids, sound produced by the hearing aid is delivered down a plastic tube to the external ear canal. A new variation of the open-fit BTE features a receiver that is not in the hearing aid itself but, instead, located remotely in the ear canal. This hearing aid style goes by different names, including post-auricular canal hearing aid and speaker-in-the-ear or **receiver-in-the-canal** (**RIC**) BTE hearing aid.

Figure 13.8 shows a example of a RIC hearing aid. The electrical signal amplified by the hearing aid is sent to the receiver via a very thin wire. In contrast to other BTE hearing aid styles, however, a receiver located in the ear canal produces the amplified sound. As seen in Figure 13.8A, the receiver is sometimes held securely in place with a small retention device

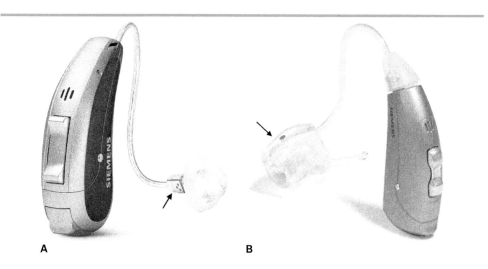

A   B

FIGURE 13.8

Two receiver-in-the-canal (RIC) hearing aids including an open-fit design **(A)** and a design featuring an ear mold **(B)**. Arrows point to the hearing aid receivers. Photos courtesy of Siemens Hearing instruments.

that does not block the entrance to the external ear canal. Or, the receiver may be enclosed within an ear mold that fits in the external auditory canal as shown in Figure 13.8B.

For some patients, the RIC hearing aid style offers at least three advantages over the open-fit BTE. First, availability of RIC hearing aids extends the range of hearing loss that can be managed with open-fit hearing aids. RIC hearing aids are not only appropriate for persons with a mild high-frequency hearing loss, but also for those with severe hearing loss in the high frequencies and even low-frequency hearing loss. Second, the intensity and quality of amplified sound tends to be higher when delivered directly to the ear canal rather than through narrow plastic tubing to the ear.

Finally, the receiver producing amplified sound is located some distance away from the microphone that detects sound, minimizing the possibility of a squealing sound, called **feedback**. *Feedback* is the term used to describe sound from the receiver in the hearing aid being fed back into the microphone and then re-amplified.

In-the-Ear (ITE). **In-the-ear** (ITE) hearing aid designs were introduced in the 1980s. Figure 13.9 shows an example of an ITE hearing aid. ITE hearing aids are enclosed in a hard plastic case or shell that is custom made for each of the patient's ears. An ear mold impression must first be made for the patient, using the technique described earlier. The ear mold impression material is injected so that it entirely fills the external ear and the outer portion of the ear canal. Then, the ear mold impressions are sent off to a hearing aid manufacturer where the electronic components are built into a permanent case. One to two weeks later the new hearing aids return to the clinic from the manufacturer and the patient is scheduled for a hearing aid fitting.

The outer portion of an ITE hearing aid has a very small opening that leads to the microphone. Nearby is a volume control knob just barely visible in Figure 13.9. Location of the microphone at the entrance of the ear canal is an advantage of ITE-type hearing aids. The ear canal is a natural place for sound to enter the ear. Properly fit ITE hearing aids are comfortable and they are appropriate for

FIGURE 13.9

An in-the-ear (ITE) hearing aid on a patient. The arrow points to the hearing aid within the ear. Photo courtesy of Siemens Hearing Instruments.

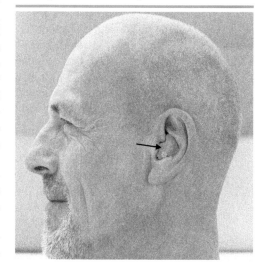

patients with hearing loss ranging from mild to severe in degree. And, ITE hearing aid controls are not difficult to operate due to their adequate size. Unfortunately, ITE and other custom hearing aids that require service must be shipped to a manufacturer, leaving the patient without amplification for sometimes a week or more.

In-the-Canal (ITC). An **in-the-canal (ITC)** hearing aid is located entirely in the ear canal. The ITC style is a smaller version of the ITE hearing aid. All electrical components are squeezed in a more compact space. The ITC hearing aid design is an option for persons with a mild-to-moderate hearing loss. It is also custom manufactured for a patient from an ear mold impression made deep in the external ear canal.

Because the microphone on the outer face of an ITC hearing aid is necessarily located in the external ear canal, the patient benefits from the natural sound-enhancing features of the pinna and external ear. Insertion and routine care and operation of ITC hearing aids requires more manual dexterity and coordination than is needed for operating controls on BTE or ITE types of hearing aids. Operation of the controls and battery replacement may be difficult for some patients, particularly elderly persons who have reduced manual dexterity.

Completely-in-the-Canal (CIC). The **completely-in-the-canal (CIC)** hearing aid is the smallest and most deeply located in the external ear canal. The CIC style is cosmetically appealing for patients who prefer to wear a hearing aid that is "out of sight." It is custom manufactured from a very deeply made ear mold impression. CIC hearing aids can only be removed with a small fishing-line string on the outer edge that is barely visible.

CIC hearing aids are certainly not appropriate for all patients. The tiny hearing aids require considerable manipulation for a comfortable and consistent fit in the ear canal. Repair problems related to cerumen are more likely with CIC hearing aids. On the positive side, there are no external controls to adjust on the CIC hearing aids. People with CIC hearing aids often determine the source of environmental sounds quite well and rather easily use the telephone while wearing hearing aids. Also, some problems affecting users of other hearing aid types do not arise with CIC fittings, such as the occlusion effect and annoying wind noise.

 ClinicalConnection

Hearing aids are the most common management option for patients with sensorineural hearing loss. Diagnostic hearing testing is important in determining whether a patient is a candidate for amplification. Then, results from hearing testing are critical for hearing aid selection and fitting, including measures such as hearing threshold levels, word discrimination scores, and loudness discomfort levels.

Contralateral Routing of Signals (CROS) Hearing Aids. Before we begin a review of hearing aid features is a good time to mention a special type of hearing aid developed years ago. The *contralateral routing of signals CROS* hearing aid design is intended for people with no usable hearing in one ear and normal hearing or only a mild hearing loss in the other ear. With a CROS hearing aid, sound at the impaired ear is picked up with a microphone and then routed to a hearing aid located on the better hearing ear. The hearing aid is coupled to the better hearing ear without blocking the external ear canal using an open ear mold or simply some tubing.

With earlier versions of CROS hearing aids, the signal from the microphone on the poorer hearing ear reached the BTE hearing aid on the opposite side via a wire that went around the back of the head. Nowadays, the signal is routed from one ear to the other using wireless technology. CROS hearing aids offer benefits for certain patients in certain listening conditions. You will soon be introduced to a new generation of surgically implanted bone-conduction hearing devices that are also an option for persons with severe or profound hearing loss in only one ear.

Hearing Aid Problems and Solutions

Hearing aids are complex electronic devices that are worn in various environments and locations. Digital hearing aids are tiny but sophisticated computers that must function consistently for sixteen or more hours each day. Consequently, problems sometimes arise with hearing aid operation. Audiologists typically have the responsibility for determining what is wrong with a hearing aid.

Table 13.1 summarizes common hearing aid problems and likely solutions. In some cases, an audiologist can identify and then solve a specific hearing aid problem. However, hearing aids with electrical or digital malfunctions must often be sent off to the manufacturer for repair. We'll now review some of the most frequently encountered reasons for hearing aid malfunction.

Cerumen and Moisture. Hearing aid problems for many patients are caused by cerumen in the ear canal or are related to excessive moisture. It is not uncommon for cerumen to block the tiny openings or ports in hearing aids or in ear molds where sound from the receiver travels into the ear canal toward the tympanic membrane. A variety of products are now available to eliminate or minimize hearing aid problems related to cerumen.

Moisture in the air enclosed in the ear canal can affect function of electronic components of hearing aids. Problems related to moisture are most often encountered with hearing aids that totally occlude the external ear canal, such as ITE, ITC, and CIC hearing aids. Other sources of moisture affecting the operation of any hearing aid include sweat from the patient and water in the environment. Hearing aid users have access to devices designed to remove moisture from hearing aids. In fact, some modern hearing aids are designed to be waterproof. Hearing aid users can also take advantage of devices that disinfect hearing aids.

TABLE 13.1 Guidelines for troubleshooting some common problems with hearing aids.

Problem	Example of a solution
Feedback	Modify the ear mold or the tubing from the hearing aid to the ear mold
	Modify the hearing aid frequency response
Tinny sound	Educate and counsel the patient about expectations for amplification
	Modify the ear mold
	Reduce high frequencies in the hearing aid's frequency response
Occlusion effect	Create an opening (a vent) in the hearing aid or ear mold
	Lengthen the ear mold
Weak output	Inspect the tubing and ear mold for cerumen and remove as necessary
	Replace the battery
Intermittent sound	Clean the battery contacts
	Replace the battery
	Return the hearing aid to the manufacturer for repair
Hearing aid is "dead"	Verify status of the battery
	Clean cerumen and debris from tubing and the receiver
	Return the hearing aid to the manufacturer for repair

Adapted from Mueller, H. G., III & Hall, J. W., III. *Audiologist's Desk Reference* (Vol. II, pp. 263–265). San Diego: Singular Publishing Group, 1998.

Acoustical Problems. Patients with hearing aids that block or occlude the ear canal often complain that their voice doesn't sound natural. Complaints of poor sound quality also arise when the ear canal is blocked with an ear mold coupled to a BTE hearing aid. The problem has to do with the occlusion effect. The occlusion effect was described in the review of bone-conduction hearing in Chapter 5.

Sound of the speaker's voice reaches the enclosed external ear canal via bone conduction. The speaker's voice is unnaturally enhanced because the ear canal is occluded. Low-frequency sounds cannot escape the enclosed external ear canal. The increased loudness of low-frequency sounds is usually bothersome for a patient. Problems arising from the occlusion effect are often minimized with modifications in the ear mold or the hearing aid. Acoustic problems related to the occlusion effect are not a concern with open-fit BTE hearing aids because the ear canal is not blocked.

Mechanical Problems. Mechanical and other problems are inevitable with complex modern hearing aids. Malfunctions related to hearing aid circuitry or digital software require shipment of the hearing aid to the factory for diagnosis and repair. However, an audiologist or a hearing aid technician can often solve more common mechanical hearing aid problems right in the office or hearing aid laboratory. Patients with hearing aid problems schedule an appointment with an audiologist to evaluate the cause of the malfunction and to determine the best approach for solving the problem.

A surprisingly high number of patients who report mechanical problems with hearing aids do not realize that the explanation is related to the batteries. Batteries should always be checked when a hearing aid is not functioning. At least four battery-related problems can be solved inexpensively, simply, and quickly: (1) there is no battery in the hearing aid, (2) the battery is dead and needs to be replaced, (3) a battery with the proper size is placed incorrectly in the hearing aid, usually upside down, and (4) the battery is the wrong size for the hearing aid.

Battery problems are encountered with hearing aid users across the age spectrum, from infants to the elderly. However, they are perhaps more common in older patients with cognitive deficits who depend on others for help with daily activities: for example, a patient who does not remember to check battery status with an inexperienced caregiver who is unable to offer assistance. Battery problems are common among older adult hearing aid users in skilled nursing facilities and other long-term care settings.

Troubleshooting. A hands-on and on-the-spot approach for solving hearing aid problems is referred to as *troubleshooting*. Indeed, the term *troubleshooting* is used to describe the process of identifying and solving any technical problem in audiology. Graduate students usually find the experience interesting, challenging, educational, and sometimes actually fun. First-hand interaction with patients to solve hearing aid problems helps to reinforce information about amplification acquired from textbooks and lectures in the classroom.

Students in Doctor of Audiology programs are often required to provide troubleshooting services during the walk-in hours at a university or hospital clinic. *Walk-in clinics* are common in clinical practices where hearing aids are dispensed. A block of time each week, perhaps a Friday afternoon, is set aside for the walk-in clinic. Any patient with a hearing aid from the facility can simply come in for a service visit, without an appointment. Based on the patient's description of the problem and an inspection and in-office diagnostic testing, an audiologist, student, or technician attempts to identify the cause or causes of the problem. Some of the hearing aid problems encountered in a walk-in clinic simply involve batteries.

Damage and Loss. Hearing aids are sometimes destroyed or seriously damaged. For example, they may be crushed under foot, inadvertently cycled through the washer and dryer, dropped in a toilet bowl, or eaten by a loving pet who is attracted by their owner's scent. Children and even adults sometimes lose hearing aids.

The likelihood of hearing aid damage or loss is reduced when an audiologist routinely provides the patient and family members with verbal and written information about routine care and maintenance. Patient education also increases the longevity of hearing aid operation and satisfaction with hearing aid use (Kochkin, 2010, 2011). One or two hearing aids are a substantial financial outlay for an adult patient who makes the purchase out of pocket. The cost to the patient for two digital hearing aids is at least $3000 and usually considerably more. Hearing aid warranties and insurance are available to protect this investment.

Wireless Connectivity for Hearing Aids

We've now reviewed hearing aid technology, types of hearing aids, and hearing aid problems and solutions. Discussion of modern hearing aid technology would not be complete without mentioning options for and benefits of wireless connectivity. Modern-day communication involves a variety of devices such as telephones, televisions, and personal audio music players. Audio signals are also transmitted via Bluetooth wireless technology. Until recently hearing aid users could not take advantage of the latest wireless technology. Some types of hearing aids included a feature called a T-coil for communication between the hearing aid and conventional landline telephones, but it could not be used with cell phones. Connectivity with hearing aids often relied on cables and cords or devices designed for persons with hearing loss rather than for the general population.

Users of modern hearing aids can enjoy the benefits of Bluetooth wireless technology with the help of special accessory devices. The devices facilitate communication between a hearing aid and a wireless device like a cell phone or a telephone. Advances in connectivity offer many benefits for hearing aid users, including communication between two hearing aids for persons with bilateral hearing loss, higher-quality sound that improves speech understanding, fewer technical difficulties when using telephones and televisions, increased mobility when using telephones, and greater convenience when watching television with others (Schum, 2010). You'll learn more about enhanced connectivity for persons with hearing loss later in the chapter, in a discussion of communication devices that can be used with or without hearing aids.

Hearing Aid Candidacy

We will now briefly review the hearing aid fitting process. Figure 13.10 shows each of the four steps involved in hearing aid fitting. The entire process of hearing aid fitting combines *technology* for audiological habilitation or rehabilitation with the *techniques* used in audiological habilitation or rehabilitation. Technology is the topic of this chapter. Techniques for habilitation and rehabilitation, including the critical role of family counseling, are covered in the next chapter.

Who is a candidate for a hearing aid? The simple answer to this question is: A person with a hearing loss. **Candidacy** of a patient for a hearing aid is almost always based on the presence of a hearing loss and its

FIGURE 13.10

Sequence of steps in hearing aid assessment and fitting and selected factors in each step.

Patient Candidacy

- Degree and type of hearing loss
- Impact of hearing loss on quality of life
- Acceptance of hearing loss
- Motivation for hearing aid use

Hearing Aid Selection

- Hearing aid style and size
- One or two hearing aids
- Hearing loss degree and configuration
- Tolerance for loud sounds
- Listening demands
- Patient preferences (adult)

Verification

- In-ear measurements of amplification
- Measurement of hearing aid output
- Frequency response of hearing aid
- Sound is audible to patient
- Sound is comfortable (not too loud)
- Patient's perception of sound

Validation

- Hearing aid orientation and counseling
- Patient satisfaction with hearing aids
- Improved communication abilities
- Improved quality of life
- Reduction of handicap

negative impact on communication. Adult patients have responsibility for deciding to proceed with a hearing aid consultation and fitting. The adult patient's decision is often made after discussions with family members.

A hearing aid or two hearing aids are selected once the patient makes a decision to proceed with amplification and family members are in agreement with the decision, or at least informed about the decision. A variety of factors go into the **hearing aid selection** process. An audiologist generally recommends specific hearing aid features that are likely to result in optimal performance for the patient. However, a patient may prefer a specific style of hearing aid based on its size and discreet appearance.

The process of selecting a hearing aid differs considerably with age, that is, whether the patient is a young child, an older child, or an adult. Indeed, determination of hearing aid candidacy is quite different in the pediatric population. Candidacy in children is determined based mainly on the results of comprehensive diagnostic assessment confirming a hearing loss that interferes with speech and language acquisition and communication. Parents and other family members of a child with a hearing loss make the decision to move forward with hearing aids based on information, support, and advice from an audiologist.

Candidacy in Adults. A variety of factors determine which patients are candidates for a hearing aid. We'll begin by considering adult patients with hearing loss. The first step in the hearing aid fitting process is always a complete hearing assessment. The patient is informed following documentation of a hearing loss with diagnostic hearing assessment. An audiologist simply and clearly describes the hearing loss to the patient and to significant others accompanying the patient to the clinic.

The explanation of hearing test findings is followed by a summary of the likely benefits of amplification. Even when an audiologist recommends hearing aids for an adult patient, the final decision to proceed with amplification rests with patient, often with advice or encouragement from family members.

A patient's perception of the impact of hearing loss on communication plays a pivotal role in his or her decision to proceed with or to reject amplification (Pacala & Yueh, 2012). Imagine a person with a hearing loss clearly documented on an audiogram. The patient also yielded poor scores on word recognition, confirming difficulty with speech perception. Family members strongly encouraged their loved one to begin using hearing aids. According to family reports and inventories completed in the clinic, the patient struggles on a daily basis to communicate in various listening settings, at work, at home, and in social activities. You might think that such a patient would immediately and unequivocally wish to proceed with the hearing aid fitting process.

Unfortunately, the majority of adults with hearing impairment initially decide against hearing aids (Kochkin, 2007, 2012; Mueller & Hall, 1998). Only approximately one in five persons with hearing loss who would benefit from amplification actually wears hearing aids. Clinical experience suggests that the average adult with hearing impairment who finally decides to purchase one or two hearing aids takes seven years to make the decision! For the adult population, the process of selecting hearing aids can begin only after the patient has accepted amplification as appropriate, necessary, and worth the effort and cost (Meyer & Hickson, 2012; Pacala & Yueh, 2012).

Candidacy in Children. It is appropriate to emphasize here that candidacy for amplification is approached very differently for children than for adults. The process begins with confirmation of hearing loss in the child following a comprehensive diagnostic assessment. An audiologist or a physician explains the results of the hearing assessment to parents and often other family members. In one or more counseling sessions, the audiologist or physician answers family questions and addresses family concerns regarding hearing and management. Then the audiologist strongly recommends amplification and, with support from the family, the fitting process is initiated as soon possible.

The benefits of early intervention for hearing loss in infants and young children are well documented (Yoshinaga-Itano, Sedley, Coulter, & Mehl, 1998). The most obvious benefit of amplification in infants and young children with hearing impairment is enhanced speech and language development. The decision to proceed with hearing aids, with input and approval from the child's family, is usually reached quickly and confidently. In addition, selection of hearing aid style and features for young children is based exclusively on data and factors such as the child's age and hearing loss characteristics, rather than the patient's preferences. Older children, especially adolescents, often participate in decisions regarding certain hearing aid options, such as color or even style.

Hearing Aid Selection

Some of the many factors important in selection of hearing aids for a specific patient were illustrated in Figure 13.10. You've already been introduced to a variety of different hearing aid designs and styles. How is a specific hearing aid selected for a specific patient? A few of the factors that enter into selection were noted earlier in the discussion of types of hearing aids.

Degree of Hearing Loss. Degree of hearing loss greatly influences hearing aid selection. A hearing aid must have enough power to adequately amplify sound for the patient's hearing loss. Indeed, one of the basic selection goals is to choose a hearing aid with an appropriate amount of amplification. A hearing aid must be capable of increasing the intensity of conversational speech so that it can be heard comfortably. That is, amplified conversational speech should be not too soft or too loud.

One or Two Hearing Aids? Another rather basic question must be answered. Should one or two hearing aids be selected? Past debate and even controversy regarding the benefits of *monaural versus binaural hearing aid fittings* has given way to universal agreement that two hearing aids are generally best (Kochkin & Kuk, 1997; Mueller & Hall, 1998). Table 13.2 summarizes reasons that support the use of two hearing aids, rather than one, in the management of bilateral hearing loss.

- Improved speech perception in quiet and sometimes in noisy listening environments
- More accurate determination of the direction of sound
- Sounds from greater distances can be detected
- Reduction in deterioration in auditory function associated with auditory deprivation
- Communication requires less effort and is less stressful
- Hearing seems more natural and balanced
- Loud noises are usually not as uncomfortable
- Feedback problems are minimized because less amplification volume is required
- Perception of tinnitus is reduced
- Patients with bilateral hearing loss prefer binaural hearing aid fitting
- Satisfaction with amplification is enhanced with the use of two hearing aids

TABLE 13.2

Reasons why two hearing aids are better than one for persons with bilateral hearing loss.

Binaural amplification results in a more natural hearing experience. In comparison to monaural hearing aid fitting, two hearing aids increase the loudness of sound. Two hearing aids also help the patient to determine the source of sound and enhance hearing in background noise. In 2010, almost three-fourths (74%) of hearing aid fittings were binaural (Kochkin, 2010). A hearing aid was fit to each ear of the patient in the same clinic visit.

Other Factors. As summarized earlier in Figure 13.10, assorted other factors also influence hearing aid selection for a given patient. For example, the size of the hearing aid enters into the decision process. This factor is particularly relevant for hearing aid fittings in older patients. A patient must have adequate manual ability to insert the hearing aid and ear mold, to replace batteries, and to operate the hearing aid controls.

Hearing Aid Verification

Verification of hearing aid performance is an important step in the process of hearing aid fitting. The goal of verification is to make sure that the hearing aid is properly amplifying sound. Verification confirms that amplified sound is appropriate for the patient and the patient's hearing loss. Selection of a specific hearing aid with specific features is followed by precise adjustments or "tweaking" in hearing aid operation.

Each decision in the hearing aid selection and verification process is made with the goal of optimizing amplification for the patient. The time and effort required for verification and validation of hearing aid performance is well spent. Research confirms that the verification process enhances patient satisfaction with amplification and reduces the number of visits the patient makes to the clinic for adjustments (Kochkin, 2011; Mueller & Hall, 1998).

Successful hearing aid selection and fitting requires experience and close attention to technical details. The verification process provides evidence that a hearing aid is providing the intended benefit to the patient. The process sometimes reveals that hearing aid settings are less than optimal for the patient. That is, there is room for improvement in the hearing aid fitting. An audiologist then adjusts certain hearing aid settings and again verifies hearing aid performance. The process of making adjustments in hearing aid settings and then rechecking or verifying the patient's response is repeated until the hearing aid is providing the intended benefit to the patient. The two-way double-ended arrow in Figure 13.10 shows this adaptive, or trial-and-error, approach to hearing aid fitting.

Electroacoustical Hearing Aid Measurement. A variety of procedures and strategies are used in the hearing aid verification process. One important procedure is **electroacoustical measurement** of the characteristics of amplified sound in the patient's ear canal. Electroacoustical measurement involves precise documentation of the features of amplified sound produced by hearing aids. There are accepted guidelines for electroacoustical evaluation of hearing aids (ANSI, 2003). The measurements are made with specialized equipment connected to a hearing aid.

Figure 13.11 shows typical equipment used for electroacoustical measurements. Hearing aid performance is measured in a special sound-treated box.

Probe-Microphone Measures. *Probe-microphone recordings* are one example of electroacoustical measurements (Mueller, Hawkins, & Northern, 1992). Figure 13.11 also shows a device for making the measurements. The audiologist inserts a very narrow and flexible rubber probe tube deeply into the external ear canal so that the end of the tube is located within a few millimeters from the tympanic membrane. The other end of the tube is connected to a microphone that detects sound in the external ear canal and to instrumentation for measuring and quantifying the intensity of sound across a wide range of frequencies. The wires leading

FIGURE 13.11 Equipment for electroacoustical hearing aid analysis. Measurements are made with a hearing aid in the sound-treated box in the left portion of the photograph identified with an arrow. Sound used in measurement is produced with a speaker in front of the patient, also indicated with an arrow. The cables attached to the patient lead from small probe tubes located deep within each external ear canal to the electroacoustical measurement device just to the patient's right side. Courtesy of Frye Electronics, Inc., Tigard, OR.

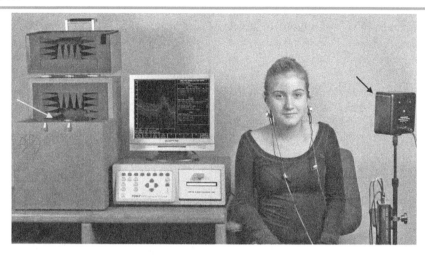

from the subject in the figure carry information from the probe tube in her ear canal to the equipment just to her right side.

Probe-microphone measurements of sound in the external ear canal can be made with the hearing aid in place on the ear and also in an open ear canal with no hearing aid on the patient. You'll recall from our discussion of anatomy and physiology of the ear in Chapter 3 that sound intensity is increased at some frequencies as it travels through the ear canal to the tympanic membrane. It is quite helpful when fitting a hearing aid to know how the patient's ear canal acoustics influence sound produced by the hearing aid.

LEADERS AND LUMINARIES

Ruth Bentler

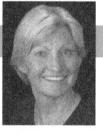

Ruth Bentler earned her bachelor's, master's, and PhD degrees in Speech and Hearing Sciences from the University of Iowa. She has held an academic position at the University for the past forty years and an appointment as Professor since 2002. Dr. Bentler's career combines research, teaching, and professional service. She serves as Chair of the Department of Communication Sciences and Disorders at the University of Iowa and teaches graduate students there in courses related to hearing aids and adult auditory rehabilitation. As Director of the Hearing Aid Laboratory for Basic and Applied Research in the Department of Communication Sciences and Disorders, Dr. Bentler's research has focused on a variety of hearing aid related topics, such as directional microphones, digital noise reduction, and, currently, frequency-lowering algorithms. Her research has led to over 100 articles and chapters on hearing aid technology and fitting practices. Dr. Bentler is a Fellow of the American Speech-Language-Hearing Association and the American Academy of Audiology. You can read an informative interview of Dr. Bentler at the American Speech-Language-Hearing Association website.

With the probe-microphone technique, hearing aid output is precisely measured at various settings to verify that the desired amount of amplification is achieved. Three basic recorded hearing aid measures, or parameters, made with the probe-microphone technique are (1) frequency response, (2) gain, and (3) maximum output.

 ClinicalConnection

Use of probe-microphone measurements is standard of care for hearing aid fitting in children and adults (Valente et al., 2006). The proportion of audiologists utilizing probe-microphone measurement in hearing aid fitting has increased over the years, but it not yet a regular component of clinical practice.

Hearing Aid Frequency Response. A frequency response curve shows the amount of amplified sound in the patient's ear canal produced by a hearing aid at different frequencies. The intensity level of the sound that goes into the hearing aid is referred to as the input and it is specified in dB SPL. An audiologist specifies the intensity level of the input sound, such as 50 dB SPL or 60 dB SPL. Different types of input sound are used to measure hearing aid performance. A hearing aid response documenting amplification of sound is displayed on a test equipment screen like the one shown in Figure 13.11. The level of sound produced by the hearing aid is amplified across the frequency region with hearing aid output exceeding the sound input for all frequencies.

Hearing Aid Gain. The term **gain** refers to the amount of amplification produced by a hearing aid. Gain is the increase in sound intensity that occurs between the input, when sound arrives at the microphone of the hearing aid, and the output, when amplified sound from the receiver enters the external ear canal. Hearing aid gain varies across the frequency range of the speech sound.

A number of different gain measurements can be made in hearing aid verification, including measures at different input intensity levels, such as 50 and 70 dB SPL. During electro-acoustical measurements of a hearing aid in the clinic, gain is also measured with the volume control at the highest level to determine the maximum amount of amplification produced by a specific hearing aid. Measurement of the maximum amount of amplification for a hearing aid is done at a specific high-intensity input level.

Prescriptive Hearing Aid Fitting. This is an appropriate point for the introduction of the technical phrase **prescriptive hearing aid fitting**. An audiologist develops a "prescription" for amplification with the hearing aid that is most likely to yield the greatest benefit for a specific patient. The term *target output* is used to describe the desired amount of amplified sound to be produced by the hearing aid for a given patient. The prescription is based on the patient's degree and configuration of hearing loss and includes components of hearing aid selection that we've already reviewed, such as the amount of gain and the maximum level of amplified sound. An audiologist establishes targets for these hearing aid parameters, or goals that should be met.

Actual measurements of hearing aid performance made with probe-microphone techniques can then be compared to prescriptive targets in hearing aid fitting. Differences between actual measurements and prescriptive targets are minimized by further adjustments in hearing aid settings. Systematic use of prescriptive strategies for hearing aid fittings is now standard of care and essential when determining amplification needs of children with hearing loss (AAA, 2003; JCIH, 2007).

A variety of different prescriptive methods are available for hearing aid fitting in children and adults (Bagatto & Scollie, 2011; Humes, 1996; Mueller & Hall, 1998). The prescriptive approach to matching actual hearing aid performance to the desired goals or targets contributes to more accurate and effective hearing aid fitting for any patient. Verification and validation of hearing aid performance in the adult population relies to a large extent on the patient's description of sound and perceived benefit from amplification.

The outcome of paper-and-pencil or sometimes computer-based inventories and self-assessment scales are also very helpful in verification of hearing aid performance with adult patients. These techniques for verification and validation are clearly not feasible for infants and young children. Prescriptive hearing aid fitting is essential for infants and young children (Bagatto & Scollie, 2011).

Precise application of a well-researched prescriptive hearing aid fitting technique is a critical step for verification of desired hearing aid performance with children. Indeed, one of the most popular computer programs for hearing aid fitting in children is called *Desired Sensation Level* or *DSL* (Bagatto & Scollie, 2011; Cornelisse, Seewald & Jamieson, 1995; Seewald, 1992;). Data on the child's hearing threshold levels and values from probe-microphone measurements are entered into the DSL program. The program then predicts target settings for amplification across the speech frequency region that will allow the child to hear low-, mid-, and high-frequency sounds. DSL also estimates the amount of amplified sound that is comfortable for the child so that uncomfortably high levels of sound can be avoided.

 WebWatch

There is a website dedicated to Desired Sensation Level (DSL) that is filled with information about the prescriptive hearing aid fitting technique. This website includes access to published and unpublished references about DSL.

Other Approaches for Hearing Aid Verification. Hearing aid fitting can be verified in other ways in addition to electroacoustical measurements (Humes, 1996; Mueller & Hall, 1998). Strategies for selecting hearing aids and verifying hearing aid fittings can be traced back to the 1940s, before audiology was a profession (Carhart, 1946).

A longstanding simple measure of amplification is called *functional gain*. The patient's hearing thresholds for pure tones or for spondee words are estimated first without hearing aids and then with amplification. During the verification process, hearing aid settings and controls may be manipulated to produce an improvement in these measurements.

Other verification approaches require the patient to make judgments about the quality or intelligibility of speech heard with the hearing aid(s). For example, does speech sound clear and natural? How well and how easily can the patient perceive different kinds of speech signals like words or sentences in quiet and noisy conditions? Verification may also involve documentation of a patient's speech perception scores with and without hearing aids.

 WebWatch

There are dozens of videos on YouTube illustrating hearing aid fitting techniques with children and with adults.

Hearing Aid Validation

The final step in the hearing aid fitting process is **validation**. It is important to understand the distinction between hearing verification and validation. The goal of verification is to make sure that the hearing aid is properly amplifying sound. The goal of validation is to assure that the patient is getting as much benefit as possible from amplification in daily communication. The ultimate goal in hearing aid fitting is not simply close correspondence between the targets for hearing aid performance and the amplified sound in a patient's external ear canal. Three more important purposes of hearing aid fitting and intervention in general are reduction of the disability created by hearing loss, enhanced communication, and improvement in quality of life.

Self-Assessment Scales and Inventories. Whether or not the goals of hearing aid fitting are achieved is typically evaluated by carefully questioning the patient and by administering self-assessment scales or inventories for determining benefit from and satisfaction with amplification (Bentler & Kramer, 2000; Mueller & Hall, 1998; Valente, 2002). An inventory is a carefully selected list of questions that are usually answered with "yes," "no," and "sometimes," or "maybe." There are a variety of widely accepted inventories used to validate hearing aid fitting. Research has shown that these inventories are valid measures of hearing handicap and hearing aid benefit (Mueller & Hall, 1998, pp. 512–531).

A small sample of the dozens of inventories now available for use in hearing aid validation include the Abbreviated Profile of Hearing Aid Benefit, or APHAB (Cox & Alexander, 1995), the Satisfaction with Amplification in Daily Life, or SADL (Cox & Alexander, 1999), the Hearing Handicap Inventory for the Elderly, or HHIE (Weinstein, Spritzer, & Ventry, 1986), and the Client Oriented Scale of Improvement, or COSI (Dillon, James, & Ginis, 1997).

Client Oriented Scale of Improvement (COSI). To illustrate how inventories are applied in the validation of a patient's performance with hearing aids, we will briefly review the COSI. The COSI is an instrument developed at the National Acoustic Laboratories in Australia (Dillon et al., 1997; National Acoustic Laboratory website). The COSI form is shown in Figure 13.12. At the first clinic visit for hearing aid selection an audiologist asks the patient to

FIGURE 13.12 The Client Oriented Scale of Improvement (COSI) for assessing outcome with hearing aid use. Reproduced from NAL.gov.au, courtesy of the National Acoustic Laboratory (NAL), Sydney, Australia.

National Acoustic Laboratories
A division of Australian Hearing

NAL

CLIENT ORIENTED SCALE OF IMPROVEMENT

Name : ______________ **Category.** **New** ____
Audiologist : ______________ **Return** ____
Date : **1. Needs Established** ______
2. Outcome Assessed ______

Degree of Change

Final Ability (with hearing aid)

Person can hear

10% 25% 50% 75% 95%

SPECIFIC NEEDS

Indicate Order of Significance

Specific Needs	Worse	No Difference	Slightly Better	Better	Much Better	CATEGORY	Hardly Ever	Occasionally	Half the Time	Most of Time	Almost Always
☐											
☐											
☐											
☐											
☐											

Categories
1. Conversation with 1 or 2 in quiet
2. Conversation with 1 or 2 in noise
3. Conversation with group in quiet
4. Conversation with group in noise
5. Television/Radio @ normal volume
6. Familiar speaker on phone
7. Unfamiliar speaker on phone
8. Hearing phone ring from another room
9. Hear front door bell or knock
10. Hear traffic
11. Increased social contact
12. Feel embarrassed or stupid
13. Feeling left out
14. Feeling upset or angry
15. Church or meeting
16. Other

identify five very specific listening situations that are troublesome, in which the patient wants to hear better. For example, the patient might state, "I want to hear better when I'm speaking with my wife at our favorite restaurant."

Five listening conditions are listed in the left portion of the COSI form (Figure 13.12) and ranked in order of importance. A selection from the sixteen categories at the bottom of the COSI form in the figure is entered into each box under Specific Needs. A professional man or woman might select the category "conversation with group in noise" (number 4) if he or she was particularly concerned about hearing during generally noisy business meetings.

Later, after the hearing aid fitting and verification process is complete, the patient is asked to judge the amount of change in hearing for each of the five listening situations. Last, the patient is encouraged to rate his or her "final ability" to hear with amplification in each of the listening conditions using the descriptors to the right of the COSI form, from "hardly ever" to "almost always." The patient is guided by the percentages corresponding to each category shown in the right portion of Figure 13.12.

Advantages of Inventories. Before the formal hearing aid fitting process begins, self-assessment inventories provide valuable information about a patient's communication handicap and whether the patient is really a candidate for amplification. Scores on inventories completed before hearing aid fitting can later be compared with scores following a period of hearing aid use. Self-assessment scales and inventories have a number of advantages in audiology in general, and specifically in hearing aid fitting. They do not require much time. They are easy for the patient to understand and complete and for the audiologist to score. Importantly, inventories offer a means of quantifying subjective judgments of benefit and satisfaction with amplification.

Validation with Infants and Young Children. A very different approach for validation must be used with infants and young children who cannot describe the quality of sound or their satisfaction with the hearing aid fitting. The stakes for hearing aid fitting in infants and

L E A D E R S   A N D   L U M I N A R I E S

Harvey Dillon

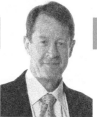

Harvey Dillon earned his undergraduate degree in electrical engineering and his PhD in psychoacoustics at the University of New South Wales in Sydney, Australia, in 1979. He is currently Director of the National Acoustic Laboratories (NAL) and Adjunct Professor at Macquarie University, both in Sydney. Dr. Dillon has conducted research involving many aspects of hearing aids. At various times he has also been responsible for the design of hearing aids and for the coordination of clinical audiology services.

Most recently, Dr. Dillon's research has concerned signal-processing schemes for hearing aids, prescription of hearing aids, evaluating the effectiveness of rehabilitation, electrophysiological assessment, auditory processing disorders, and methods for preventing hearing loss. He has authored over 180 publications, including the comprehensive and internationally popular textbook on hearing aids, now in its second edition, entitled simply *Hearing Aids.* You'll find an interesting 2001 interview of Dr. Dillon at the AudiologyOnline website.

young children are very high. Hearing aid performance in a child is verified with electroacoustical procedures like probe microphone or real ear measurements. Real ear measurements are made with a tiny microphone in the child's ear canal using equipment illustrated earlier in Figure 13.11. Validation of the benefit of amplification for infants and young children goes far beyond electroacoustical measurements of hearing aid performance.

Successful hearing aid fitting of an infant is most importantly reflected by acquisition of speech and language skills. Accuracy of hearing aid fitting has a long-term and major impact on the development of effective communication. Validation of the hearing aid fitting is based largely on the child's responsiveness to sound and careful documentation of speech and language development. Description of responsiveness to sound is based on observations of the child in the clinic and also reports of parents and other family members who are with the child on a daily basis.

Examples of speech and language measures are documentation of the speech sounds a child produces and the number of words in the child's vocabulary. Audiologists and speech pathologists collaborate in this effort. Hearing aid performance must be measured regularly and speech and language acquisition monitored closely to assure that the child is receiving optimal benefit from amplification.

Hearing Aid Laboratory in a Clinic. Most clinical facilities that dispense hearing aids have one or more rooms equipped with computers for electroacoustical measurements. The computers also have special software programs supplied by manufacturers for customized hearing aid fitting. Another room is generally used as a hearing aid laboratory.

A typical hearing aid laboratory includes a wide variety of supplies, instruments, and tools used in the hearing aid fitting process. There are wall hooks for stethoscopes for listening checks and storage bins for tubing, batteries, special tools, and ear mold impression materials and supplies.

Figure 13.13A shows a hearing aid stethoscope. The hearing aid is coupled to the soft rubber connector at the end of the stethoscope. An audiologist or technician uses a specially designed stethoscope to listen to hearing aid output.

Most hearing aid labs also contain tools and machines for modification of hearing aids and ear molds, including drills and polishers. Figure 13.13B shows a machine for hearing aid and ear mold modifications.

Patient and Family Education. Patient education about hearing aids and related topics is not simply a step in hearing aid fitting but, rather, an integral feature throughout

FIGURE 13.13   Photograph of two types of hearing aid laboratory equipment. A special stethoscope **(A)** is used for performing listening checks of hearing aid output. The hearing aid is connected to the end of the tubing indicated with an arrow. The machine shown in **(B)** is used to make hearing aid modifications.

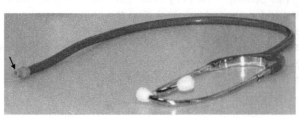

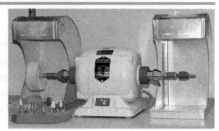

A   B

the process. Patient and family education, orientation, and counseling are very important, beginning with the audiologist's first encounter with a patient. Topics covered may include:

- An explanation of hearing in general and specifically of the patient's hearing loss
- Helping the patient to accept his or her hearing loss
- How a hearing aid will help the patient in different communication settings
- Battery information and warnings
- Practical information about the use and care of hearing aids and batteries
- Fostering realistic patient expectations about benefit from amplification
- Reviewing options for other hearing devices and aural rehabilitation

Counseling and education of parents and family members of children with hearing impairment is an essential part of the management and rehabilitation process. We'll review in more detail in the next two chapters these and other topics important to management of persons with hearing impairment.

 ClinicalConnection

The importance of patient and family education and counseling in the hearing aid fitting of children and adults cannot be overestimated. Indeed, patient outcome is determined as much by education and counseling as by hearing aid technology. This important topic is reviewed further in Chapter 14.

How Important Is Verification and Validation?

Completion of the verification and validation process results in fewer patient visits back to the audiologist after hearing aid fitting. This observation is based on a recent analysis of findings for a group of 533 patients wearing hearing aids (Kochkin, 2011). In 2010 almost 2.7 million hearing aids were sold in the United States. Consistent use of verification and validation procedures for the entire hearing aid market in the United States is associated with over 500,000 fewer return visits to audiologists for adjustments or refitting of hearing aids that are not providing the expected benefit.

Fewer follow-up visits are certainly good for patients. Reducing the number of follow-up visits also saves audiologists many hours of valuable time that can be devoted to other patients. Unfortunately, the same study (Kochkin, 2011) revealed that audiologists completed both verification and validation ("V & V") in only 36% of their patients. Verification alone was completed for 9% of the group, whereas validation alone was done for 34%.

 ClinicalConnection

A wide assortment of inventories and other tools are available for validation of hearing aid fitting. Most inventories are designed for use with pediatric or adult patient populations. Some are most appropriate for select groups of patients, such as elderly adults. Regular use of inventories in hearing aid fitting is an important component of best practices in the rehabilitation of persons with hearing impairment.

Surgical Options for Amplification of Sound

Surgically implanted amplification devices are now an alternative to conventional hearing aids. Various electrical hearing devices are designed for implantation into the ear or near the ear during a surgical operation. Candidacy for surgically implantable hearing aids is based on the findings of hearing tests. Audiologists play an important role in the diagnostic assessment of patients before a decision is made to consider an implanted amplification device for management of hearing loss. In some cases, either a conventional hearing aid or an implantable hearing device is an appropriate and effective option for improving communication. For other patients, however, an implantable hearing device is clearly the best and perhaps the only treatment option.

We'll take a moment now to make a distinction between conventional hearing aids and surgically implantable hearing devices, including cochlear implants. As you have already learned, a conventional hearing aid is an external device that amplifies sound for patients with hearing loss. A patient typically wears hearing aids during waking hours, when communication is important. Hearing aids pick up and amplify all environmental sound, including speech. The amplified sound is delivered via air conduction to the patient's ear canal. Energy from sound is then transmitted through the middle ear to the inner ear. The hearing process for a patient with conventional amplification is similar to the process for someone with normal hearing. A conventional hearing aid user removes it at the end of the day and doesn't wear the hearing aid while sleeping. Hearing aids are also removed before certain physical activities that involve water such as bathing and swimming.

Surgically implanted hearing aid devices include an external component to pick up sound in the environment, an amplification system, and a component that is surgically inserted in or near the ear. Patients do not remove the entire implanted hearing device at the end of each day. Following implantation the devices remain in place permanently. They may be activated or inactivated depending on listening needs.

Cochlear implants are a type of implantable hearing device. Briefly, a cochlear implant converts sound in the environment into electrical signals. Electrical signals activate the auditory nerve directly by means of special electrical wires surgically inserted into the damaged and nonfunctioning inner ear. This is the main distinction between conventional or implantable hearing aids versus cochlear implants. Conventional and implantable hearing devices deliver amplified sound to the inner ear, whereas cochlear implants electrically stimulate the auditory nerve directly, bypassing the inner ear in the hearing process. Cochlear implants are reviewed in more detail in the next section of the chapter.

You will now be introduced to the two general types of implantable hearing devices—bone-anchored hearing aids and middle ear implant devices.

Implantable Bone-Conduction Devices

Implanted bone-anchored hearing devices delivery energy to the inner ear via bone conduction. These devices were originally abbreviated *BAHA* for *b*one-*a*nchored *h*earing *a*id, but more recently they have been referred to simply as **Baha devices**. Bone-anchored hearing devices are available from several manufacturers.

Design. Baha devices consist of a small speech-processing component worn externally on the head. The speech-processing component includes a microphone for picking up sound. It can be programmed with special computer software for a patient's specific listening needs.

The speech processor is connected to a small titanium component or abutment anchored in the mastoid bone behind the ear. Soon after implantation, the metal abutment portion of the device fuses with the bones of the head. Sounds including speech are converted to vibrations that are transmitted via bone conduction from the abutment to the inner ear.

Candidacy. Bone-anchored hearing devices may be appropriate for at least three different types of patients with hearing loss (Doshi, Sheehan, & McDermott, 2012; Dun, Faber, de Wolf, Cremers, & Hol, 2011; Hodgetts, 2011; Snik, Verhaegen, Muder, & Cremers, 2005). One group includes patients with chronic ear infections or with a constant problem with excessive cerumen in the external ear canal. Conventional hearing aids are not appropriate for patients with infection and possible drainage of pus into the external ear canal or patients with excessive cerumen in the external ear canal.

Bone-conduction hearing devices are certainly an option for patients with conductive hearing loss, particularly children with conductive hearing loss associated with certain ear malformations (Hodgetts, 2011; Ricci et al., 2011). Congenital malformations of the ear were discussed earlier, in Chapter 11. Bone conduction energy from a Baha device bypasses the abnormal middle ear system to directly activate the inner ear. A newer non-implanted version of the device called the Baha Softband is now available for infants and young children who cannot undergo surgical implantation due to certain medical conditions (Dun et al., 2011; Hodgetts, 2011; Verhagen et al., 2008).

Single-Sided Deafness. Considerable research evidence confirms that patients with total hearing loss on one side benefit from implantation of a bone-anchored hearing aid (Lin et al., 2006; Pai et al., 2012; Rasmussen, Olsen, & Nielsen, 2012; Stewart, Clark, & Niparko, 2011; Wazen et al., 2003). A complete unilateral hearing loss is often referred to as *single-sided deafness,* abbreviated *SSD.* Sound arriving on the side of the hearing loss is rerouted via bone conduction to the normal hearing inner ear on the opposite side. Some published studies offer data suggesting that Baha devices improve a patient's ability to localize the source of sounds and also improve speech perception (Pai et al., 2012). Other studies, however, raise questions about these auditory benefits of the Baha devices and about criteria for candidacy (Grantham et al., 2012). According to recent papers, some patients with bilateral deafness might also benefit from bone-anchored hearing aids (Colquitt et al., 2011; Doshi, Sheehan, & McDermott, 2012).

 ClinicalConnection

Information from diagnostic hearing assessment is vital in determining whether a surgically implanted device is an appropriate treatment option for a patient with hearing loss. The decision is based to a large extent on the pattern of findings for air- and bone-conduction hearing testing and speech audiometry. Audiologists play a critical role in evaluation of possible candidates for surgically implanted devices, including bone-anchored hearing aids and middle ear implants.

Middle Ear Implants

Implantable middle ear devices are another option for hearing-impaired patients who cannot benefit from conventional hearing aids or who prefer a more permanent alternative to conventional forms of amplification (Briggs et al., 2008; Haynes, Young, & Wanna, 2010). Technology for surgically implantable middle ear devices was developed in the 1990s and the first patient was implanted in 1996. The Food and Drug Administration (FDA) approved a middle ear amplification device for patient use in 2002.

Design. Most middle ear implants consist of an external component worn behind the ear and an internal component mounted on one of the ossicles in the middle ear space. The programmable external processing component detects sound and converts the sound to digital signal. In this way the devices function much like a hearing aid or the sound processor of a bone-anchored hearing aid.

Other middle ear devices are entirely implanted. All components are located in the ear. There is no external sound processor. With this type of surgically implanted device, environmental sound enters the external ear canal and vibrates the tympanic membrane as it does in normal-hearing persons. The tympanic membrane functions as a microphone for the middle ear implant system. The device then uses one of several strategies for amplifying vibrations of the ossicles. Middle ear implants use batteries for power. Unlike hearing aid batteries that must be replaced every one or two weeks, batteries powering middle ear implants are designed to last up to five years.

Candidacy. Persons with varying degrees of hearing loss are candidates for middle ear implant devices. The hearing loss can range from mild to severe, with word recognition scores of 50% or better (Gerard, Thill, Chantrain, Gersdorff, & Deggouj, 2012; Wolframm, Giarbini & Streitberger, 2012). Persons considering middle ear implants must be at least 18 years old. Candidates include patients with hearing loss who for various reasons cannot or do not choose to wear conventional hearing aids. Recent clinical research suggests middle ear implants

ⓘ WebWatch

With an Internet search, you can quickly access information about middle ear implants from manufacturer websites, including photographs and even videos of surgical implantation of the devices.

are also appropriate for certain patients with conductive or mixed hearing loss (Verhaegen, Mulder, Cremers, & Snik, 2012; Verhaert, Fuchsmann, Tringali, Lina-Granade, & Truy, 2011).

Middle ear implant devices have advantages in comparison to conventional hearing aids for the amplification of sound. And, as already noted, among surgically implanted devices there are clear differences between bone-anchored hearing aids and middle ear implants. It is important to evaluate the benefits of any hearing device based on research evidence from independent investigations that is published in scientific literature.

A New Nonsurgical Alternative for Management of Hearing Loss

Research and development of innovative technology for helping persons with hearing impairment is advancing steadily and rapidly. One new and novel approach transmits sound via the teeth.

Figure 13.14 shows the relatively new Sound-Bite Hearing System. It consists of two components. One is a behind-the-ear component, with a microphone located deep in the ear canal. Figure 13.14A illustrates the behind-the-ear component and Figure 13.14B shows how it is worn discreetly at ear level. The other component of the Sound-Bite Hearing System is a removable in-the-mouth (ITM) device that is custom fit to the patient's teeth (Doshi, Sheehan, & McDermott, 2012; Popelka, 2010). Figure 13.14C depicts the device that fits in the mouth. Sound detected by the external component is converted into vibrations that are delivered via the teeth to the bones of the head and then transmitted directly to each cochlea.

The Sound-Bite Hearing System is a nonsurgical and noninvasive prosthetic bone conduction device for persons with conductive hearing loss and total unilateral hearing loss, or single-sided deafness. It is also appropriate for persons with conductive hearing loss. One obvious advantage of the approach taken with the Sound-Bite Hearing System is elimination of the need for surgery. A dental impression is required for fitting a Sound-Bite device.

According to published reports, the in-the-mouth component is comfortable and does not interfere with talking, drinking, or biting down when eating (Popelka, 2010). Research suggests that the frequency response of the Sound-Bite Hearing System extends to 12,000 Hz (Popelka et al., 2010). Studies in persons with unilateral hearing loss offer evidence that the device enhances the ability to localize the direction of sound and also improves speech perception in quiet and in background noise (Murray, Miller, Hujoel, & Popelka, 2011).

FIGURE 13.14   The Sound-Bite Hearing System including the behind-the-ear microphone **(A)**, the microphone device as worn on a patient **(B)**, and the bone conduction prosthetic device that transmits sound via the teeth **(C)**. Photos courtesy of Sonitus Medical.

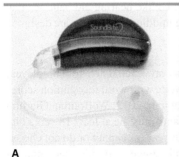   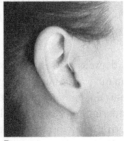   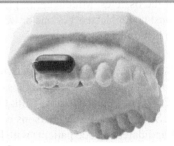

A   **B**   **C**

Cochlear Implants

Cochlear implants are certainly one of the most exciting technological advances in the management of hearing loss. Thousands of published articles describe research studies on cochlear implants in children and adults, with over 100 papers appearing each year (Wackym & Runge-Samuelson, 2009; Waltzman & Roland, 2009). Surgical techniques for implantation and procedures for programming or mapping cochlear implants by audiologists are described in detail in dozens of book chapters and books. The terms *programming* and *mapping* are used to describe the process of adjusting the cochlear implant operation to best meet the needs for a specific patient.

Before cochlear implants were first introduced in the early 1980s, effective verbal communication was rarely an option for persons with profound sensory hearing loss and deafness due to serious cochlear damage or dysfunction. Even powerful hearing aids provide little or no benefit for persons who cannot hear sound even at maximum intensity levels.

Prior to the advent of cochlear implants, intervention for children identified with profound hearing loss often combined *oral* and *manual techniques*. The oral component of habilitation included hearing aids in an attempt to provide the patient with some sensation of sound, supplemented with intensive lip or speech reading instruction. The manual communication technique included instruction in a form of sign language. A sizable proportion of children with profound hearing impairment or deafness received instruction only in manual communication, essentially deriving no benefit from sound. Aural rehabilitation techniques and strategies, including methods for education of children with hearing impairment, are reviewed in the next chapter. Cochlear implants revolutionized the management of patients with severe and profound hearing loss.

Historical Perspective

The first cochlear implants were developed in the 1970s at the House Ear Institute in Los Angeles. The devices were very simple and even primitive by today's standards. Patients wore a large box-shaped device that looked like a body-style hearing aid. It included a microphone for detecting sound and converting it to electrical signals. Electrical signals were routed via a cable to a smaller button-shaped external component usually worn behind and slightly above one ear. The external component was located over a similar-sized internal component that had been surgically inserted under the skin. The external and internal components were held together by means of a magnet.

The surgeon implanting the internal component under skin behind the ear also inserted a thin wire into the damaged cochlea during the same operation. The thin wire curled around each turn in the cochlea and functioned as an electrode. Electrical signals related to sounds in the environment were sent from the little button-shaped external component to the implanted component that, in turn, produced electrical pulses related to sound stimulation. Electrical pulses delivered with the single wire electrode in the cochlea activated nearby auditory nerve fibers and produced the sensation of sound.

Stimulation of auditory nerve fibers normally follows activation of thousands of inner hair cells in the cochlea. You'll recall from our review of auditory anatomy in Chapter 3 that hair cells in different regions of the cochlea from the base to the apex are responsive to different frequencies. This tonotopic organization of frequencies is maintained by different auditory nerve fibers and throughout the central auditory nervous system. In essence, with the earliest cochlear implant the complex and frequency-specific tonotopic auditory information conveyed by thousands of hair cells in the cochlea was replaced by one electrode stimulating many auditory nerve fibers at one time.

Remarkably, patients benefited from the early single-electrode cochlear implants. The sound sensations reflecting speech produced by the cochlear implants was nothing like normal hearing. However, most patients were able to communicate reasonably well following aural rehabilitation and considerable experience, supplemented with the use of visual cues such as lip reading.

Intensive engineering and clinical research since the 1980s, continuing today, has resulted in steadily advancing cochlear implant technology. Cochlear implants are now highly sophisticated electrical devices that are custom programmed for each patient to optimize processing of auditory and electrical information. Almost all patients, including children and adults, develop effective communication with appropriate rehabilitation. In this section, you will be introduced to modern cochlear implant technology and design. Management of cochlear implant patients, including how cochlear implants are programmed to provide maximum communication benefit to adults and children with profound hearing loss, is reviewed in the final chapter (Chapter 16).

Evaluation and Criteria for Candidacy

Cochlear implants are appropriate for persons with severe-to-profound sensory hearing loss who do not receive adequate benefit from hearing aids (Miyamoto & Kirk, 2001; Wackym & Runge-Samuelson, 2009). Specific criteria for cochlear implant candidacy are listed in Table 13.3. Although the term *sensorineural hearing loss* is often used in the clinical setting, such hearing loss is rarely due to neural dysfunction. As you learned in Chapter 11, cochlear damage and dysfunction is the most common cause of permanent hearing loss. The main role of the cochlea is to convert energy from sound into activity in auditory nerve fibers. We reviewed the process in Chapter 3. In very simple terms, a cochlear implant performs the same general function, thus replacing the role of the cochlea in hearing.

Criteria for cochlear implant candidacy continue to evolve with increased knowledge about the benefits of cochlear implants and technological advances (Miyamoto & Kirk, 2001; Wackym & Runge-Samuelson, 2009). For example, in years past children under the age of 12 months were not approved for cochlear implantation, according to Food and Drug Administration (FDA) regulations. Because of research confirming the benefits of

TABLE 13.3
Criteria for cochlear implant candidacy in children and adults.

Children
• No health contraindications to surgery
• Age greater than 12 months (there are medical exceptions for younger implantation)
• Bilateral severe-to-profound sensory hearing loss
• Minimal benefit from hearing aids after a period of at least three months, including failure to develop speech and language
• Education that includes aural rehabilitation
• Family support, commitment, and appropriate expectations
• Radiographic confirmation of cochlear and auditory nerve anatomy

Adults
• No health contraindications to surgery
• Bilateral severe-to-profound sensory hearing loss
• Post-lingual hearing impairment in the ear to be implanted
• Minimal benefit from appropriate amplification
• Appropriate expectations about the outcome of cochlear implantation
• Radiographic confirmation of cochlear and auditory nerve anatomy

early intervention for hearing impairment in infants, some children are implanted earlier. In such cases, approval is given for cochlear implantation of the child under the age of 12 months.

Components of Cochlear Implants

There are three major manufacturers of cochlear implants. Cochlear implant design varies somewhat from one manufacturer to the next and even within the product line for each manufacturer. New technologies and clinical devices are introduced quite often because cochlear implant manufacturers devote substantial resources to research and development.

Figure 13.15 shows the major components common to all cochlear implants. The components are (1) an external sound processor and transmitting cable, (2) an external transmitting device often referred to as a radiofrequency coil, (3) an internal receiving device, (4) an internal stimulator, and (5) an electrode array.

Each of the components for cochlear implants marketed by different manufacturers varies in size and shape. The components also differ somewhat in terms of how auditory and electrical information is transmitted and processed. Nonetheless, there are similarities in the overall function of each the components. Our discussion of cochlear implants will be supplemented with photographs and simple diagrams supplied by manufacturers.

As you read about each of the components of a cochlear implant, take a moment to examine and review the photographs and diagrams. You will readily appreciate similarities and differences in the design of cochlear implants on the market today. The differences in appearance

> **ClinicalConnection**
>
> Audiologists and speech pathologists are involved in each step of the management of cochlear implants. Results from diagnostic hearing testing largely determine whether a patient is a candidate for cochlear implantation. Following cochlear implant surgery audiologists and speech pathologists have responsibility for providing habilitation in implanted children and rehabilitation in implanted adults.

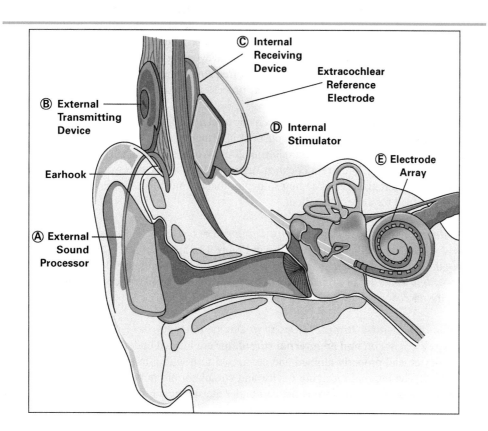

FIGURE 13.15

Components of all cochlear implants, including **(A)** external sound processor, **(B)** external transmitting device, **(C)** internal receiving device, **(D)** internal stimulator, and **(E)** electrode array. Courtesy of Cochlear Americas.

FIGURE 13.16

An example of an external sound processor for a cochlear implant. Courtesy of Cochlear Americas.

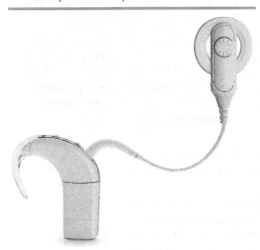

for each cochlear implant brand are paralleled by internal distinctions in electronics and details of signal processing.

Component 1: External Sound Processor. The *external sound processor* and the hook for attaching it to the ear look like a behind-the-ear hearing aid. Figure 13.16 shows an external sound processors for a cochlear implant available from one manufacturer. The microphone located in the external sound processor detects sounds in the environment and converts them into digital electrical signals that are then amplified. The information undergoes digital processing that precisely codes each of the three main properties of the incoming sound: (1) intensity, (2) frequency, and (3) duration. Batteries are used to power external sound processing units.

Digital processing of the properties of sound is quite different for cochlear implants than for hearing aids. Digital hearing aids convert environmental sound like speech into electrical signals. The electrical signals are processed and amplified. Then the electrical signal is converted back into sound. The amplified sound leaving the digital hearing aid receiver and entering the external ear canal consists of the same three properties—intensity, frequency, and temporal features—as the sound entering the hearing aid microphone.

The external processor component of a cochlear implant must convert sound from the environment into electrical pulses that activate auditory nerve fibers. It is not possible to precisely represent each and every aspect of a complex sound like speech in electrical pulses. However, there is a reasonably close correspondence between the intensity level of environmental sound and the amplitude or magnitude of the electrical pulses produced by the cochlear implant (Miyamoto & Kirk, 2001; Wackym & Runge-Samuelson, 2009). Much of the temporal or timing information in sound is conveyed via the electrical pulses that stimulate the auditory nerve fibers. The thousands of frequencies in the acoustical signal representing external sound that reaches the external processor are divided into frequency bands or segments called channels.

Much of the extensive research on cochlear implants has focused on the development of more effective strategies for coding acoustical information into electrical pulses (Miyamoto & Kirk, 2001; Wackym & Runge-Samuelson, 2009; Wolfe & Schafer, 2011). Multiple coding strategies are available in current cochlear implants. With assistance from manufacturer representatives, audiologists select coding strategies that are most likely to improve communication performance for a specific patient.

Component 2: External Transmitting Device. Let's return for a moment to the components of a cochlear implant shown earlier in Figure 13.15. The coded electrical signal representing the intensity, frequency, and timing information in environmental sounds is sent along a *transmitting cable* to an *external electromagnetic transmitting device* that rests upon skin behind the ear.

Components 3 and 4: Internal Receiving Device and Internal Stimulator. An *internal receiving device* or *coil* **and an internal stimulator** are located underneath the external transmitting device and properly aligned and connected to it with a magnet. Figure 13.17 shows an example. The internal receiving device and stimulator are quite thin, usually less than 6 mm in thickness. A surgeon inserts the unit under the skin in a little depression created in the temporal bone during the cochlear implantation operation. These components of the cochlear implant are in an airtight biocompatible silicone case that is designed to seal out bodily fluids and minimize rejection by the body.

In the past, patients with cochlear implants could not undergo magnetic resonance imaging because of the magnet used to connect the external and internal coils. The very powerful magnet in a magnetic resonance scanner poses a serious health risk to patients with magnets imbedded in their head. However, the latest generation of cochlear implants features removable magnets so that implanted patients can safely undergo brain scanning as indicated for diagnostic purposes.

Component 5: Electrode Array. The electrical pulse signals representing acoustical information in the environment, particularly speech, pass from the internal receiving device and stimulator to an *array of electrodes* surgically implanted in the cochlea, from the base toward the apex. The location of the array of electrodes was shown earlier in Figure 13.15.

Modern cochlear implants have between sixteen and twenty-four electrodes. Figure 13.17 showed a close-up view of the internal receiving device and the electrodes for a cochlear implant manufacturer. When properly inserted, the intracochlear electrodes remain quite close to auditory nerve fibers. The electrical pulses encoded with sound information are presented at remarkably fast rates, over 30,000 pulses per second (Miyamoto & Kirk, 2001; Wackym & Runge-Samuelson, 2009). The presentation rate varies considerably among different manufacturers.

Electrical pulses for each of the frequency channels created by the external sound processor are delivered to different electrodes located along the electrode lead. Information for higher-frequency channels reaches electrodes located nearer the base of the cochlea and stimulates nearby auditory nerves, whereas lower-frequency channels reach more apical auditory nerve fibers via electrodes located deeper in the cochlea and more toward the apex. In this way, modern cochlear implants provide some of the tonotopical organization and auditory nerve stimulation that is a characteristic feature of the cochlea.

Interface Device. Another component of cochlear implant systems is an *interface device* that permits communication between the cochlear implant and the computer used to program the cochlear implant. The interface device is installed whenever the patient is in the audiology clinic for programming, including at the time of initial activation of the system following cochlear implantation surgery.

Recent Developments in Cochlear Implant Technology

As already noted, cochlear implant technology is rapidly advancing. Modern cochlear implant components are smaller than earlier versions. Now constructed with substances such as silicon, titanium, and platinum, cochlear implants are remarkably durable and reliable. Cochlear implant malfunctions and breakdowns are rare. Such problems occur in a very small proportion of patients, generally less than 0.05% (Miyamoto & Kirk, 2001; Wackym & Runge-Samuelson, 2009).

Cochlear implant electrodes are now designed to facilitate surgical insertion, to minimize damage to structures in the cochlea, and to assure that the electrode contacts are located close to auditory nerve fibers. Like modern digital hearing aids, some cochlear implant sound processors have multiple microphones to improve speech perception performance in noisy settings (Wolfe & Schafer, 2011).

FIGURE 13.17

Example of a cochlear implant internal receiving device and electrode array. Image courtesy of Advanced Bionics LLC.

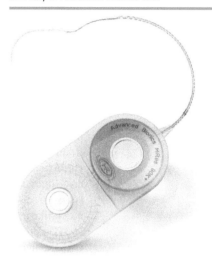

 WebWatch

You can readily access via the Internet color photographs of cochlear implants and also videos of cochlear implantation surgery. You will find considerable information on the websites of the three major manufacturers of cochlear implants, Advanced Bionics, Cochlear Americas, and Med-El.

One other recent technology development is the so-called *hybrid cochlear implant system,* sometimes referred to as *combined electrical and acoustical stimulation* or *EAS* (Gantz et al., 2010; Wackym & Runge-Samuelson 2009; Woodson, Reiss, Turner, Gfeller, & Gantz, 2010). Patients with relatively better hearing at lower frequencies and a steeply sloping severe high-frequency hearing loss have traditionally posed a serious management challenge. These patients were not good hearing aid candidates because of the severity of the high-frequency hearing loss. Even powerful hearing aids were incapable of amplifying high-frequency sounds enough to provide the patient with improved communication. Cochlear implantation was also not an option because of usable hearing at lower frequencies. Insertion of a conventional cochlear implant would damage the apical or low frequency region of the cochlea, producing a profound hearing loss across the audiometric range.

The hybrid hearing aid-cochlear implant approach utilizes a shorter cochlear implant electrode. The shorter electrode extends only partially into the cochlea and activates only higher-frequency auditory nerve fibers (Wackym & Runge-Samuelson 2009; Woodson et al., 2010). High-frequency hearing is thus improved with cochlear implantation. The sound processor also functions as a hearing aid in the same ear. An acoustical portion of the cochlear implant sound processor amplifies low-frequency sounds and delivers them into the external ear canal much like a typical hearing aid.

Research has shown promising findings in speech perception and communication outcome with the hybrid hearing aid-cochlear implant approach. Also, just as two hearing aids are now regularly recommended for patients with bilateral hearing loss, there is increased appreciation of the benefits of binaural cochlear implants (Gantz et al., 2010; Gordon & Papsin, 2009; Wackym & Runge-Samuelson 2009). As an alternative, the patient may benefit from what is referred to as *bimodal hearing,* with a hearing aid worn on one ear and a cochlear implant on the opposite side (Cullington & Feng, 2011).

Hearing Assistance Technology (HAT)

You've learned about diverse technologies that can be utilized to improve communication and quality of life for persons with varying degrees of hearing impairment. Hearing aids, implanted amplification devices, and cochlear implants are invaluable tools for managing many children and adults with hearing impairment. Now we will review other technologies that play an important role in connecting persons with hearing impairment to audio devices and the world of sound around them.

Hearing assistance technology (HAT) is important for improving communication of persons with hearing loss. Other phrases used to describe the technology include **assistive listening devices (ALDs)** and *assistive listening systems (ALS).* Hearing assistance technology is useful in a variety of settings and venues, including the home, school classrooms, places of worship, workplaces, and concert halls.

Hearing assistance technology often consists of a single system for communication between a speaker and a listener. The listener takes responsibility for supplying part of the system to the speaker and initiating its use. Increasingly, however, public places are fitted with an *induction loop* for transmission of signals to anyone who uses either hearing aids or an assistive listening device.

An induction loop consists of a coil of wire located around a public area, such as an auditorium, theater, or a church sanctuary. Loops may be installed under the carpet or along the tops of the walls of a room. The loops are connected to an amplifier and a microphone. Sounds entering the microphone are broadcast throughout the looped area. Hearing aid wearers can access sound information transmitted via the loop by means of the same tele-coil option used for telephone conversations.

Who Benefits from HAT?

There are two general groups of patients who require technology options beyond conventional hearing aids or surgically implanted devices. One group includes persons with difficulty hearing and communicating effectively who are not candidates for other hearing devices or who are not motivated to pursue them. For example, some school-age children with entirely normal hearing thresholds experience serious difficulty hearing what their teachers are saying in noisy classroom settings. Or, some elderly patients with a modest amount of age-related hearing loss are simply not ready to consider amplification. Still, they struggle to understand friends and family members during telephone conversations or when watching television.

The other group consists of patients who require the use of assistive technology in addition to hearing aids, implanted amplification devices, and cochlear implants. Patients in this group have hearing impairment and receive considerable benefit from one of the three treatment options. However, communicative performance is inadequate in certain listening environments or circumstances. One example is a hearing-impaired child who can easily understand speakers in quiet settings with amplification or a cochlear implant but experiences serious difficulty in all noisy listening environments like classrooms. Another example is an adult with profound hearing loss who uses a cochlear implant very effectively during the day but who has concerns about hearing a doorbell, a telephone, or a fire alarm at night when the cochlear implant sound processor is not in place.

We'll review in the final section of the chapter a wide array of technologies that are available for augmenting hearing and enhancing communication, including those with normal hearing sensitivity and those with varying degrees of hearing impairment.

 ClinicalConnection

Assistive listening or hearing assistance technology is underutilized in pediatric and adult patient populations. Audiologists and speech pathologists play an important role in educating patients and families about the availability of ALDs and HAT. In public school settings, audiologists and speech pathologists have the primary responsibility for fitting and maintenance of FM technology in children.

Classroom Amplification

All children in an educational setting require an adequate acoustical environment for optimal learning. The teacher's voice must exceed background noise for children to clearly and effortlessly hear during classroom instruction, discussions, and conversations. The difference between the teacher's voice and the level of background noise is often described in terms of a signal-to-noise ratio or difference. *Classroom amplification* improves the acoustical environment and listening performance for all school children. Younger children require more favorable or larger signal-to-noise ratios than older children to perform adequately in the classroom setting. Therefore, kindergarten and other elementary school children benefit most from a quieter acoustical learning environment (Crandell, Smaldino, & Flexer, 1992).

Unfortunately, the typical classroom is not an ideal acoustical or learning environment. Noise sources include student activity, heating and air conditioning systems, and environmental noise like traffic sounds from outside the classroom. The signal-to-noise difference tends to be smaller and more adverse in older schools. Noise levels are usually higher in classrooms containing younger students, like kindergarten and first-grade classes, and in classrooms with a greater number of children. Steps to reduce classroom background noise arising from various sources are inadequate in many school buildings. In noisy classrooms, even children with normal auditory function experience daily difficulty in clearly and effortlessly hearing classroom instruction and discussions unless they are seated relatively close to the teacher. Children with hearing loss or auditory processing disorders struggle even more to listen in a typical classroom.

Classroom amplification with FM technology is one effective and reasonably economical solution to the problem of noisy acoustic learning environments. Figure 13.18 shows a classroom amplification system in operation. The teacher wears a microphone located about six inches from the mouth. The microphone may be connected with a wire to a small transmitter

FIGURE 13.18

A classroom amplification system including microphone for the teacher, a belt-worn transmitter, and a light-weight movable loudspeaker (identified with an arrow) just to the left of the teacher. Courtesy of Phonak.

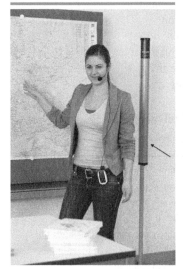

device also worn by the teacher or the microphone and transmitter may be integrated in a single component, as illustrated in Figure 13.18.

The teacher's voice is converted to a *frequency modulated (FM)* or infrared signal that is then transmitted to one or more loudspeakers usually placed closer to the students in the classroom. The intensity of the teacher's voice is based on the distance between the students and the loudspeakers, rather than between the teacher and the students. Also, the teacher's voice can be amplified by the system for greater enhancement of the signal-to-noise ratio.

Classroom FM systems can be purchased from a handful of manufacturers, each offering different design options for microphones and speakers. All classroom amplification systems enhance the acoustical environment by increasing the signal-to-noise ratio for all of the students. Research has consistently shown benefits in academic performance with the use of FM technology, at a very modest cost per student (Crandell, Smaldino, & Flexer, 1992; Holstad, 2011; Hornickel, Zecker, Bradlow, & Kraus, 2012; Johnson, Benson, & Seaton, 1997). Additional advantages of classroom amplification include improved classroom behavior and less teacher vocal fatigue.

Personal FM Technology

A personal FM device includes the same general components as a classroom amplification system. A microphone is located about 6 inches from the speaker's mouth. The person speaking may be a teacher, a religious leader, a parent, or a friend. The microphone and transmitter are sometimes combined in a single device. Or, the microphone may be connected via a wire to a small box-like transmitter device that is worn on a belt or placed in a pocket.

With a personal FM device, sound is not delivered via a large loudspeaker located several feet from the listener. With a personal FM device, sound reaches the listener via a headset or receiver worn at ear level or even through a receiver located in the ear canal. The headset or earpiece picks up the FM signal from the microphone/transmitter. Children and adults readily accept the modern style and small size of the earpiece.

Recent studies have clearly confirmed the added benefits of delivering FM-transmitted sound as close as possible to the ear. Personal FM systems are associated with improvements in signal-to-noise ratio of more than 10 dB (AAA, 2010; Johnston, John, Kreisman, Hall, & Crandell, 2009; Lewis & Eiten, 2011). One study showed that daily use of an ear-level personal FM system by school-age children with auditory processing disorders (APD) resulted in better scores for speech perception in noise, improved academic performance, and resolution of psychosocial problems (Johnston, Kreisman, Hall, & Crandell, 2009). Perhaps most importantly, regular use of the personal FM system over the course of a school year resulted in higher scores for speech perception in noise, even when testing was conducted without the FM system. Evidence suggests that consistent auditory experience with a favorable signal-to-noise ratio contributes to more efficient auditory processing in school-age children.

FM Technology with Hearing Aids and Cochlear Implants

The principles of FM technology just described for classroom amplification and personal devices are also applicable to hearing aid users and persons with cochlear implants (Holstad, 2011; Wolfe & Schafer, 2010). The overall objective remains enhancement of communication by increasing the signal-to-noise ratio in adverse listening settings. Consistent with most forms of FM technology, the speaker wears a microphone or a microphone is located relatively close to multiple speakers. Also, as described for classroom and personal devices, speech detected by the microphone is transmitted as an FM signal. However, the FM signal is received by the patient's hearing aid or cochlear implant, rather than a loudspeaker or separate ear-level device.

L E A D E R S   A N D   L U M I N A R I E S

Carol Flexer

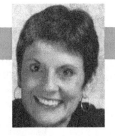

Carol Flexer earned her bachelor's degree in speech and psychology at Metropolitan State College in Denver, her master's degree from the University of Denver, and her PhD in Clinical Audiology, aural rehabilitation, and psychology from Kent State University. She held a position at the University of Akron for twenty-five years as a Distinguished Professor of Audiology in the School of Speech-Language Pathology and Audiology. Dr. Flexer lectures extensively nationally and internationally about pediatric audiology issues. She has authored more than 155 publications and co-edited and authored twelve books. Dr. Flexer is past president of the Educational Audiology Association, past president of the American Academy of Audiology, and past president of the Alexander Graham Bell Association for the Deaf and Hard of Hearing Academy for Listening and Spoken Language. She is a Certified Auditory-Verbal Therapist and a licensed audiologist. Dr. Flexer has received three prestigious awards for her research on and advocacy for children with hearing loss. You can learn more about the many accomplishments of Dr. Flexer at her website (carolflexer.com). There you'll also find links to her series of YouTube videos and other video clips.

Some hearing aids and cochlear implants can be adapted to FM technology. The FM signal representing the speaker's voice is received by a small attachment called a "boot" that is plugged into the lower portion of the hearing aid or cochlear implant speech-processing component. Patients with hearing aids or cochlear implants thus benefit from amplification and perception of all sound. In addition, patients may enjoy the added benefit of enhanced signal-to-noise ratio for selected speakers, like a teacher or speech pathologist in a noisy listening environment.

Other Assistive Listening Options

In addition to the forms of FM technology just reviewed, there over a hundred types of other hearing assistance technologies designed to enhance hearing and improve communication for persons with and without hearing loss. These include alerting devices for people with profound hearing loss. Examples of alerting devices include smoke alarms, alarm clocks, baby monitors, and doorbells with visual or vibratory (rather than conventional auditory) signals for easy detection by the hearing impaired person.

We'll conclude the chapter with a brief review of other assistive listening or hearing assistance options for enhancing hearing and improving communication in persons with and without hearing loss. The technology shares features with the FM systems just described. Most devices electronically bring, in some way, the speaker's voice or the sound of interest closer to the listener. A telephone with an amplification option is one of the most common forms of hearing assistance technology. Numerous vendors offer amplified telephones with volume controls, including some with recording machines that also amplify sound.

Figure 13.19 shows another simple form of hearing assistance technology called a pocket talker. The portable device includes a microphone placed near the speaker or any sound source, like a television. The microphone is

FIGURE 13.19

A hearing assistance technology like a Pocket Talker can be used in any communication setting, including hospitals and skilled nursing home facilities. The speaker's voice is picked up with a microphone in a transmitter device (see dark arrow on table), amplified, and then transmitted via a wire to a headset or some other type of earphone worn by the listener (see lighter arrow). Photo courtesy of Williams Sound.

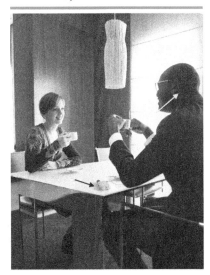

FIGURE 13.20

A popular form of hearing assistance technologies is a wireless TV listening device. **(A)** shows a close-up of a set of TV Ears, whereas **(B)** shows a person using TV Ears. Photos courtesy of TV Ears Inc.

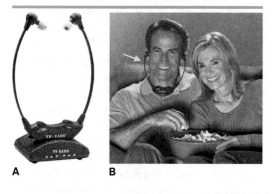

A   B

connected to an amplifier with a cable ending in a socket where a headset or earpieces can be plugged in. A pocket talker is a handy option for improving communication in a setting away from home, such as a hospital or skilled nursing facility where a hearing impaired patient needs to regularly communicate with physicians, nurses, and other healthcare personnel. Pocket talkers are an inexpensive and simple form of hearing assistance technology for persons with normal hearing or with hearing loss.

Figure 13.20 shows another popular example of hearing assistance technology, a wireless TV listening device. The device includes a component that plugs directly into the television audio output socket. An infrared signal is then transmitted through the air to a stethoscope-like headset shown in Figure 13.20A. A Bluetooth TV listening aid is also now available. A hearing-impaired person using the TV listening device shown in Figure 13.20B can hear a television, a radio, or any sound source at an appropriate intensity level without disturbing normal hearing listeners who are in the same area.

There are also specialized assistive listening devices or hearing assistance technologies designed for healthcare professionals. Perhaps the best example is a stethoscope, which amplifies body sounds. Custom earpieces for persons who regularly use stethoscopes further enhance the intensity and quality of sound, while also increasing wearer comfort.

PULLING IT ALL TOGETHER

Over the years as hearing aids have diminished in size, they have expanded in terms of appearance and the options available for providing amplification to persons with varying degrees and types of hearing impairment. You can now identify different hearing aid styles and the acronyms used to identify them. You've learned about behind-the-ear (BTE) hearing aids, open-fit hearing aids, including the receiver-in-the-canal (RITE) type, in-the-ear (ITE) hearing aids, in-the-canal (ITC) hearing aids, and completely-in-the-canal (CIC) hearing aids. You also understand some basic concepts of hearing aid function, such as the difference between linear and nonlinear amplification and the role of digital signal processing (DSP).

After reading the chapter, you know that problems can interfere with hearing aid operation and that the most common problems involve batteries. You also learned about criteria audiologists use to determine whether a patient is a hearing aid candidate. You have an appreciation for the importance of verifying hearing aid performance and then validating the benefit the patient obtains from hearing aid use.

You were introduced in the chapter to the design of different types of implantable hearing devices, including cochlear implants, bone-conducted hearing aids, middle ear implantable hearing aids, and even a device that uses the teeth for auditory stimulation.

Working in collaboration with otolaryngologists, audiologists and speech pathologists play an important role in the selection of patients with severe hearing loss who are good candidates for cochlear implantation or for other surgically implantable devices. You are now aware that audiologists and speech pathologists have responsibility for habilitation and rehabilitation of children and adults with implants, leading to effective communication.

The chapter concluded with a review of assistive listening technology and hearing assistance technology that contributes importantly to improved communication and quality of life. Assistive listening technology and hearing assistance technology is helpful even for patients who are not candidates for or are not interested in management with hearing aids or implantable devices. You now understand that one or more form of technology can help almost all children and adults who have hearing loss and communication problems.

READINGS

American National Standards Institute. (2003). *American National Standard for specification of hearing aid characteristics.* ANSI S3.22-2003. New York: Author.

Carmen, R. (Ed.). (2009). *The consumer handbook on hearing loss and hearing aids: A bridge to healing.* Sedona, AZ: Auricle Ink Publishers.

Crandell, C. C., Smaldino, J. J., & Flexer, C. (1992). *Sound-field FM applications: Theory and practical applications.* San Diego: Singular Publishing.

DiGiovanni, J. J. (2010). *Hearing aid handbook.* New York: Cengage Learning.

Dillon, H. (2001). *Hearing aids.* New York: Thieme Medical Publishers.

Gordon, K. A. (2011). Cochlear implants for children: Promoting auditory development with electrical pulses. In R. Seewald & A. M. Tharpe (Eds.), *Comprehensive handbook of pediatric audiology* (pp. 565–584). San Diego: Plural Publishing.

Hall, J. W. III, & Johnston, K. N. (2009). Diagnostic audiology, hearing instruments and aural habilitation. In J. B. Snow Jr. & P. A. Wackym (Eds.). *Ballenger's otorhinolaryngology-head and neck surgery* (17th ed., pp. 115–130). Shelton CT: BC Decker.

Madell, J. R., & Flexer, C. (2011). *Pediatric audiology casebook.* New York: Thieme Medical Publishers.

Mueller, H. G. III, & Hall, J. W. III (1998). *Audiologist's desk reference. Volume II. Amplification, management, and rehabilitation.* San Diego: Singular Publishing.

Mueller, H. G., Hawkins, D. B., & Northern, J. L. (1992). *Probe microphone measurements: Hearing aid selection and assessment.* San Diego: Singular Publishing.

Niparko, J. K. (Ed.). (2009). *Cochlear implants: Principles and practices.* New York: Lippincott Williams & Wilkins.

Schaub, A. (2008). *Digital hearing aids.* New York: Thieme Medical Publishers.

Seewald, R., & Tharpe, A. M. (Eds.). (2011). *Comprehensive handbook of pediatric audiology.* San Diego: Plural Publishing.

Taylor, B., & Mueller, H. G. III. (2011). *Fitting and dispensing hearing aids.* San Diego: Plural Publishing.

Valente, M. (Ed.). (1996). *Hearing aids: Standards, options, and limitations.* New York: Thieme Medical Publishers.

Valente, M. (Ed.). (2002). *Strategies for selecting hearing aids and verifying hearing aid fittings.* New York: Thieme Medical Publishers.

Wackym, P. A., & Runge-Samuelson, C. (2009). Cochlear and auditory brainstem implantation. In J. B. Snow Jr. & P. A. Wackym (Eds.), *Ballenger's otorhinolaryngology—head and neck surgery* (17th ed., pp. 363–388). Shelton CT: BC Decker.

Waltzman, S. B., & Roland, J. T. Jr. (2009). *Cochlear implants.* New York: Thieme Medical Publishers.

Wolfe, J., & Schafer, E. C. (2010). *Programming cochlear implants.* San Diego: Plural Publishing.

14 Audiological Habilitation and Rehabilitation

LEARNING OBJECTIVES

In reading this chapter, you will learn:

- What audiological rehabilitation (AR) is and why it is important
- The difference between rehabilitation and habilitation
- How audiologists and speech pathologists help persons with hearing loss
- How hearing impairment can affect quality of life
- That a person's hearing impairment also impacts family members
- Different ways hearing loss in a child can affect each family member
- About counseling in audiology
- About the roles of audiologists and speech pathologists in counseling
- When patients should be referred to professional counselors
- What is meant by "psychosocial" problems
- About auditory training
- About the critical importance of counseling in hearing aid fitting
- The meaning of the phrases "Deaf community" and "Deaf Culture"
- Why a patient's cultural background must be considered in assessing and managing hearing loss

KEY TERMS

American Sign Language (ASL)
Auditory-oral approach
Auditory training
Auditory-verbal
Content counseling
Cued speech
Deaf community
Deaf Culture
Earobics
Fast ForWord
Hearing Handicap Inventory for the Elderly–Screening Version (HHIE-S)
Information counseling
Listening and Communication Enhancement (LACE)
Manual approaches
Natural auditory-oral approach
Oral approach
Signing Exact English (SEE or SEE2)
Total communication

CHAPTER FOCUS

The focus of this chapter is in many respects the focus of clinical audiology. As we review each of the major steps of audiological rehabilitation, you'll learn about the ways audiologists and speech pathologists work together to help people with hearing loss and their families communicate more effectively. Audiological rehabilitation must involve the families of persons with communicative disorders. Humans don't communicate in isolation. Hearing loss in a young child differentially impacts each family member. Mother, father, siblings, and grandparents respond differently to the news that their loved one has a hearing loss. Family-centered counseling to facilitate personal adjustment to hearing loss is a critical aspect of effective audiological rehabilitation. You'll also appreciate after reading this chapter the special challenges associated with management of patients at each end of the age spectrum, specifically young children and elderly adults.

Over hundreds of years educational methods for developing communication in children with profound hearing loss and deafness have been introduced, refined, and debated. To appropriately and effectively

CHAPTER FOCUS *Concluded*

manage children with profound hearing loss, audiologists and speech pathologists need to have a firm grasp of current options available for education and habilitation. Sensitivity to cultural, ethnic, and other aspects of patient diversity is also essential in today's complex society. These and other humanistic issues are included in the following review of audiological rehabilitation.

Overview of Audiological Rehabilitation and Habilitation

Audiology, like other healthcare professions, is now remarkably "high tech." You learned in preceding chapters that sophisticated technology is increasingly applied in the assessment and management of hearing loss, and related disorders like vestibular and balance disturbances. Advances in instrumentation have certainly contributed to more accurate and timely diagnosis of hearing loss, especially in infants and young children. And, with ongoing improvements in hearing aids, cochlear implants, and other treatment devices more children and adults with varying degrees and types of auditory dysfunction have the opportunity to benefit greatly from audiological rehabilitation.

Audiologists, speech-language pathologists, and all healthcare professionals must continuously strive to maintain a balanced perspective about sophisticated technology. There is no doubt that the latest technology and techniques contribute to more accurate diagnosis and management of hearing loss. Nonetheless, it is also very important to provide patients with information about how to use residual hearing and with counseling to facilitate adjustment to hearing loss. Nontechnical approaches to rehabilitation improve communication abilities and help patients to live well with their hearing loss.

Family-centered counseling for hearing impairment substantially improves long-term patient outcome, including improved communication and quality of life. Counseling is not something that is done only when an audiologist has some extra time in a busy clinic schedule or when a patient or family member is clearly worried, angry, or discouraged. Counseling should be viewed as the central and essential component of audiological rehabilitation. Put simply, *counseling is intervention*.

The importance of collaboration between audiologists and speech pathologists in rehabilitation of persons with hearing impairment and related disorders cannot be overstated. Rehabilitation knowledge and skill is essential for successful improvement of hearing and communication in children and adults. An emphasis on rehabilitation in audiology and speech pathology is also critical for the autonomy and future of the professions.

Audiologists and speech-language pathologists have the educational background and the clinical skills required for managing persons with communicative disorders. They are well prepared to assume responsibility for the challenging process of rehabilitating children and adults with hearing impairment and related disorders.

The information reviewed in this chapter is, therefore, at the heart of the profession of audiology, and much of it is also within the scope of practice for speech pathologists. You'll recall from Chapter 1 that aural rehabilitation and auditory training of hearing-impaired military personnel and veterans were the main responsibilities of persons who were instrumental in the creation of the profession of audiology. The current resurgence of interest in fundamental rehabilitation services is in some ways taking the profession of audiology back to its roots.

Initial Patient Encounter

We will now take a step-by-step look at the big picture of the audiological rehabilitation process. Rehabilitation usually begins with the audiologist's initial encounter with a patient, the first of the steps in the rehabilitation process shown in Figure 14.1.

Venues for the Initial Patient Encounter. Often an audiologist first meets a pediatric or adult patient in the waiting room of an outpatient clinic or a private practice office. The encounter may also take place in a wide variety of other settings. Audiologists in hospital settings may make their initial contact with a patient in a well baby or neonatal intensive care

FIGURE 14.1   Major steps in the audiological rehabilitation process. Technology used in rehabilitation and habilitation, and technology information and orientation was reviewed in Chapter 13.

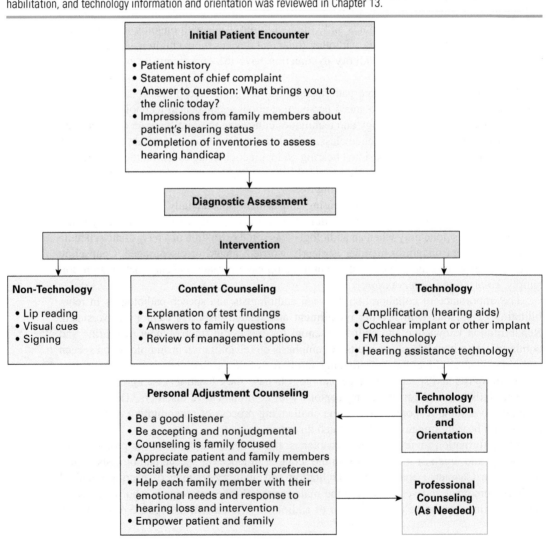

nursery, a hospital room, or even in an operating room with the patient already anesthetized and unconscious.

Other possible venues for the first patient encounter include hearing screening sites like a preschool or Head Start facility, a public school, an industrial setting, a mobile healthcare van, or an assistive living facility for the elderly. Military audiologists have even participated in triage of combat-injured service personnel in hospitals located in war zones. With modern modes of communication, patients may begin to benefit from audiological rehabilitation before the first face-to-face encounter with an audiologist. For example, an audiologist can begin to help an anxious patient with a brief but informative telephone call or a reassuring email communication.

Why the First Patient Encounter Is Important. The first patient encounter contributes importantly to the creation of an effective working relationship between an audiologist or speech pathologist and the patient and the patient's family. In many respects, the initial interaction with the patient and family members forms the foundation for the diagnostic and rehabilitation services to follow. You learned in Chapter 4 about creating, developing, and maintaining a humanistic and patient- or family-centered relationship in providing audiology services. The practice of audiology and speech pathology requires knowledge extending far beyond technical skills required for assessment and management of hearing loss.

The Patient's Chief Complaint. The chief complaint is a patient's main concern, that is, the reason the patient is seeking healthcare. An audiologist or speech pathologist can rather quickly learn about the patient's chief complaint with a review of the patient's health history or medical chart, by actively listening as the patient describes the complaint, and with careful questioning. Valuable information can almost be elicited from adult patients with the simple question: "What brings you to our clinic today?" Questions should also be posed to family members who accompany the patient to the clinic, especially when the patient is a young child or when family members accompany an adult with reduced cognitive abilities.

Social and Emotional Impact of Hearing Loss. A paper-and-pencil scale or inventory administered at the time of the first encounter is useful in estimating the impact of a patient's hearing loss. One or more validated communication scales or inventories contribute valuable information about a patient's hearing problem and its impact on daily activities.

A commonly used self-report communication scale is called the **Hearing Handicap Inventory for the Elderly–Screening Version**, abbreviated **HHIE-S** (Ventry & Weinstein, 1982). In several minutes a patient can complete the ten items. The HHIE-S consists of five items that focus on the social impact of hearing loss and another five on the patient's emotional response to hearing loss.

The HHIE-S provides useful qualitative information on how the patient's hearing loss affects quality of life. When also administered after intervention, such as a hearing aid fitting, the HHIE-S provides a quick quantitative measure of improved outcome. However, the HHIE-S is certainly not a substitute for formal hearing screening or assessment.

Information Counseling

Information counseling or **content counseling** is an essential component of the rehabilitation process. Content or information counseling is explaining the results of the hearing assessment and what should be done next. When the hearing assessment process is complete, an audiologist usually describes test findings to the patient and/or the patient's family.

An audiologist typically counsels a patient and family members soon after completion of a hearing assessment. Figure 14.1 shows the typical sequence of steps in information or content counseling. This form of counseling is very common in audiology (Clark & English, 2004; Kricos, 2000a, b).

If the patient has a hearing problem, the audiologist also offers an explanation of appropriate options for management or perhaps the importance of referral to another professional, like a physician, a speech-language pathologist, or another audiologist. An audiologist most often refers a patient to another healthcare professional for additional diagnostic assessment or for medical or nonmedical management. During time allotted for content counseling, the patient and family members have an opportunity to ask questions about the test results and the management plans.

Content counseling might sound quite simple and straightforward. Effective counseling, however, requires considerable skill, experience, and sensitivity to the emotional state and needs of the patient and family members.

Challenges in Content or Informational Counseling. Research shows that information recalled by a patient and the patient's family after the initial content counseling session is often incomplete and inaccurate (Clark & English, 2004; Margolis, 2004; Martin, Krueger, & Bernstein, 1999). By some estimates, up to 80% of the information is almost immediately forgotten. And, about one-half of the information that is retained is inaccurate. According to the well-known counseling expert David Luterman (Luterman, 2008), patients and family members are more likely to recall irrelevant details of the counseling session, like the clothing worn by the audiologist, than information about hearing loss and the most appropriate management options. Ironically, effectiveness of information counseling may actually decrease when a patient or family is given more detailed information.

Most patients and family members are unfamiliar with the topics and terminology included in a content counseling session. Patients and family members are not familiar with anatomy of the auditory system, with hearing tests regularly used by audiologists, and with the vocabulary an audiologist uses in describing test results. Consequently, the patient and family often understand and remember little of the detailed explanation of test results.

L E A D E R S   A N D   L U M I N A R I E S

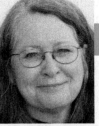

Kristine English

Dr. English earned her bachelor's, master's, and PhD degrees from San Diego State University. She is a professor at the University of Akron/NOAC (Northwest Ohio Audiology Consortium). Dr. English is very active in the profession of audiology. She has served on many committees and boards for the American Academy of Audiology the Educational Audiology Association.

Dr. English has been teaching and writing about audiological counseling since 1996. She coauthored with John Greer Clark *Counseling in Audiologic Practice,* the most popular textbook on counseling for audiologists. Dr. English's first teaching assignment on the topic opened up fascinating and important questions. What is the help-seeking process and how does it apply to persons with hearing loss? What is the role of the audiologist as patients seek or resist help? Patients look for reasons to trust us before they move forward, so how does counseling help us earn that trust? What is empathy? Can everyone learn to be an effective counselor? The answer to the last question is *yes.* It is the inspiration for Dr. English's commitment to audiologic counseling.

In fact, as the detailed explanation of test results continues, patients and family members may "tune out" while focusing on one or two points the audiologist makes early in the counseling session. As cleverly and appropriately stated by Robert Margolis (Margolis, 2004), information provided during audiological counseling may "go in one ear and out the other." Counseling is more effective when information is presented slowly, simply and without technical terms or jargon, and in an organized format (Margolis, 2004; Martin, Krueger, & Bernstein, 1999).

Improving Content or Information Counseling. A variety of factors influence the amount of counseling information that is recalled by a patient and family members (Clark & English, 2004; Kricos, 2000a, b). Counseling is more effective for persons who are familiar with hearing and hearing loss terminology, maybe from a previous visit to an audiologist or following informal research via the internet. In general, elderly persons retain less information than younger persons. Patients who are anxious, worried, or in denial about their hearing problem are less likely to retain information from a counseling session (Clark & English, 2004).

Information retained from counseling is inevitably increased when the face-to-face verbal explanation of test findings and management options is supplemented with a written summary. The written summary may be in the form of a handout with general information on hearing and hearing loss or a written report of the patient's test findings and recommendations for management.

The impact of counseling style on the information retained by a patient may be best appreciated with two brief examples. The first scenario is actually an example of "what not to do" in an content counseling session. The second scenario with the same patient illustrates a more effective counseling approach. Let's assume the patient is a 75-year-old woman who has just completed a hearing assessment. The patient was seeking help from an audiologist for the first time. Let's assume the patient has a high-frequency hearing loss in each ear like the one depicted in an audiogram you saw in Chapter 7 (Figure 7.7).

Counseling Scenario 1: What Not to Do. In this first scenario, the patient's counseling session was filled with a surplus of detail and technical terminology. Imagine a session in which information is presented rapidly and in a matter-of-fact manner by a newly graduated and rather inexperienced audiologist sitting across a big desk from the patient. During most of the session the young audiologist looks down at many sheets of paper containing test results and appears ill at ease counseling an elderly patient. The patient is given little opportunity to ask questions or to request clarification of confusing information. The exhaustive review of test findings and management options is lengthy, going on for more than 10 minutes. Only excerpts of the counseling discussions are provided here.

> Mrs. Johnson, now I'd like to explain the hearing test findings to you. We began in the sound booth with pure tone audiometry where I tested you with both air-conduction and bone-conduction stimulation. Today's tests shows that you have a mild-to-moderate hearing loss bilaterally in the frequency region from 250 Hz to 1000 Hz, with a moderate sloping to severe hearing loss bilaterally for test frequencies from 2000 to 8000 Hz. There is no air-bone gap, so the hearing loss is sensorineural in nature. Your pure tone average is 40 dB HL in the right ear and 45 dB HL in the left ear. Let's see, your speech discrimination—I mean word recognition— scores were pretty good in each ear, in the range of 84% to 92% at an intensity level of 65 dB and going up to 96% at an intensity level of 80 dB. We also performed tympanometry to determine how your middle ear was functioning. You had a type A tympanogram in each ear. That probably rules out any ear disease.
>
> Okay. Now I'd like to talk with you about hearing aids.

Counseling Scenario 2: Effective Counseling. Compare for the same elderly patient the foregoing detailed and rapid-fire counseling session with the following relaxed and simple explanation of test results and management options. Picture a smiling and confident audiologist sitting upright in a chair near the patient, speaking slowly with occasional pauses, and frequently making eye contact with the patient and her husband.

> How are you holding up, Mrs. Johnson? You may be a little tired because the hearing assessment was quite thorough and you had to concentrate for such a long time as you listened to all the sounds. We have some good information about your hearing. I'm going to explain the results to you now, and then we'll talk about different strategies that will help you hear better. You'll probably have some questions. You and Mr. Johnson should feel free to ask a question anytime. [Pause]
>
> If you miss something or if anything I say isn't clear, please ask me to explain it again. Don't be concerned if you forget some of this information. I'll be mailing you a written report that summarizes your test results and what we've talked about here today.
>
> You do have a hearing loss in each ear. Test results confirm that you have more difficulty hearing high-pitched sounds than low-pitched sounds. It appears from today's test results that your hearing loss may be caused by a problem in the inner ear. [The audiologist then points out the inner ear on a simple figure of the auditory system.]
>
> We often see this pattern of hearing loss in people who are about your age. A hearing loss often develops over the years as a person ages. I'll stop at this point and ask if you or your husband have any questions. [The patient or her husband at this point might ask whether the hearing loss is permanent or whether it might improve with medicine or surgery.]
>
> I suspect that you struggle to understand what some people are saying, particularly when you can't see their face or if there is background noise like in a restaurant or at a social event at church. [The audiologist pauses to allow the patient or her husband to speak.]
>
> You may also have some trouble understanding speech when you're talking on the telephone. Fortunately, our test results confirm that you did very well repeating words in the quiet of the sound booth. [The audiologist pauses again to give Ms. Johnson time to comment about her hearing difficulties.]
>
> Now let's talk about what can be done to help you to hear more effectively and to communicate more easily. First of all, we have group meetings once each month at our clinic. At these meetings people with hearing loss like yours learn communication strategies, like lip reading, and share experiences about their hearing loss. [Pause] Also, based on my clinical experience, I'm quite sure you would benefit from the use of hearing aids. Here are samples of modern hearing aids that could be adjusted specifically for your hearing loss. I'll stop again because you probably have some questions about hearing aids and the other options we have to help you hear better. [The audiologist sits back and waits for questions from the patient or her husband.]

The audiologist reviews the patient's responses on the Hearing Handicap Inventory for the Elderly that was administered before the hearing assessment. The audiologist then has a comfortable conversation with the patient and her husband about hearing aids, including how they work and how much they will cost.

Content or Information Counseling Is Essential. Counseling and education about the hearing loss before and after appropriate hearing aid fitting or cochlear implant programming is an essential component of the typical rehabilitation process (Kricos & McCarthy, 2007). Counseling often includes information about rehabilitation techniques and computer programs for developing communication skills, in addition to the discussion about hearing devices. **Auditory training** or listening training is often helpful to assure that persons with hearing loss take full advantage of amplification and their residual or remaining hearing (Sweetow & Sabes, 2006). The phrase *auditory retraining* may be more appropriate in a discussion about audiological rehabilitation of adults who are born with normal hearing and later develop a hearing loss (Kricos & McCarthy, 2007).

Technology Information and Orientation

Many patients benefit from intervention using some form of technology, such as hearing aids, a cochlear implant, an FM system, or hearing assistance technology. Patients almost always require more information about these various devices and forms of technology. Figure 14.1

indicated that technology information is typically provided when intervention with hearing aids, cochlear implants, and/or FM technology is first implemented.

You learned in the previous chapter that a patient's candidacy for hearing aids, cochlear implants, and other devices is determined with information gathered during the initial encounter in combination with findings on the diagnostic assessment. For adult patients, factors such as interest, motivation, perceived need, and financial concerns may also enter into the decision to proceed with formal intervention.

Let's assume that results from the initial encounter and hearing assessment indicated the need for intervention and that the patient elected to pursue the appropriate management option, in this case hearing aids, recommended by the audiologist. An appointment is usually scheduled to review in some detail the operation and care of hearing aids, including insertion and safe disposal of hearing aid batteries. One goal of counseling is to foster realistic patient expectations for benefit from amplification or cochlear implants. An audiologist also reviews with the patient and family members' options for assistive listening devices. In some cases, the audiologist discusses likely benefits of an auditory training or aural rehabilitation program. Time and effort devoted to providing patients with technology information and orientation contributes importantly to patient satisfaction and improved outcome. Adequate information and orientation also reduces the chance that a patient will encounter difficulties with hearing aids or other technology.

Psychosocial Problems Associated with Hearing Loss

Untreated hearing loss has serious consequences that are often described as *psychosocial problems*. Psychosocial problems are negative emotional responses to hearing loss that greatly impact quality of life. Psychosocial problems also interfere with effective communication and hinder rehabilitation efforts.

Some common emotional responses or reactions of persons with hearing loss and their families, listed in alphabetical order, include:

- Anxiety
- Anger
- Bitterness
- Confusion
- Denial
- Depression
- Fear
- Frustration
- Guilt
- Hopelessness
- Isolation
- Low self-esteem
- Self-consciousness
- Shock

Not all patients have all of these psychosocial problems. However, most children and adults with hearing loss do experience one or more psychosocial difficulties (Clark & English, 2004; Kricos, 2000a, b). The psychosocial problems interfere with a patient's adjustment to hearing loss and benefit from rehabilitation efforts.

Childhood Hearing Loss Impacts the Entire Family. Understandably, a child with hearing loss experiences psychosocial problems such as a sense of loss, disappointment, and frustration. The psychosocial problems associated with hearing loss change at different periods in the child's life. For example, psychosocial issues are typically different for preschool children than for children just beginning school, and different for adolescents than for younger children. Family-centered counseling is an important step toward empowering family members and maintaining or rebuilding positive family relationships and a healthy family system (Kricos, 2000a; Luterman, 2008).

Hearing loss that is newly identified in an infant or a young child affects the entire family, including the mother, father, siblings, and grandparents. The family goes through a process of grieving that may include a combination of traditional stages, such as denial, anger, bargaining, depression, and, hopefully, acceptance (Clark & English, 2004; Kricos, 2000a; Van Hecke, 1994).

Clinical Connection

Clinical experience supported by research evidence confirms the impact of hearing impairment and related auditory disorders on emotional health and psychosocial status. Counseling is an essential tool in the management of children and adults who have hearing loss.

Parents experience added stress during the period following the confirmation of hearing loss in their child. The stress is associated with a need to make important decisions and the demands on family time and financial resources. Restrictions on daily activities and new educational requirements for the child also contribute to family stress. Confirmation of hearing loss in a child has a clear impact on family dynamics and often especially strains the relationship between the patient's mother and father. Additionally, the self-image of fathers in particular may suffer from the knowledge that their child is not perfect (Kricos, 2000a; Luterman, 2008).

Normal-hearing siblings of a child with hearing loss may resent the increased attention directed to their brother or sister, or the reduction in privacy as professionals help with the care of their family member (Kricos, 2000a, b; Luterman, 2008). Brothers and sisters often experience feelings of shame and annoyance. On the other hand, sibling emotions may also include love, empathy, and pride.

Grandparents are not immune to the affects of hearing loss. Indeed, grandparents grieve about their grandchild's hearing loss and also have concerns about the impact of the grandchild's hearing loss on their own children as well as other grandchildren (Kricos, 2000a; Luterman, 2008). On the positive side, grandparents may provide valuable emotional, practical, and sometimes financial support to the family of a child with hearing impairment. Grandparents may help to maintain family resilience and optimal family communication and bonds.

Adult Hearing Loss Also Affects the Family. Hearing loss in an adult patient also affects the spouse, children, and other family members. Hearing loss in an adult almost always interferes with patterns of communication between the patient and his or her spouse, with an associated diminishment of quality of life. Annoyance and frustration are two common emotional responses to hearing loss in a spouse. It is important that both marital partners attend counseling sessions whenever possible.

Fortunately, the psychosocial consequences of hearing loss can be minimized, and in some cases eliminated, with appropriate rehabilitation steps (Clark & English, 2004; Johnston et al., 2009; Kricos, 2000a). We will now review personal adjustment counseling and how it helps persons with hearing loss and their families.

Personal Adjustment Counseling

Personal adjustment counseling is very helpful for patients with hearing loss and their family members (Clark & English, 2004). Audiologists optimally implement personal adjustment counseling soon after the diagnosis or confirmation of hearing loss. The typical timing of personal adjustment counseling in the rehabilitation process was shown earlier in Figure 14.1.

LEADERS AND LUMINARIES

David Luterman

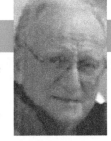

David M. Luterman is a clinician and educator who has dedicated his career to an understanding of the psychological effects and emotions associated with communication disorders. Through many workshops and publications Dr. Luterman has urged and educated speech and hearing professionals and students to incorporate effective counseling strategies in their clinical interactions. His seminal counseling text, now in its fifth edition, is used in many audiology and graduate programs. As a result of the book, Dr. Luterman has greatly influenced the effectiveness of audiologists and speech pathologists in their clinical interactions with clients and their family members. Dr. Luterman is a 2011 recipient of the Frank R. Kleffner Lifetime Clinical Career award for outstanding lifetime achievement in human communication sciences and disorders from the American Speech and Hearing Association.

Personal adjustment counseling includes efforts to resolve confusions about the patient's diagnosis and to help patients and family members to acknowledge and express their feelings about hearing loss. Personal adjustment counseling assists patients and family members as they work through disappointment and emotional pain. Counseling also clarifies rehabilitation plans and solves practical problems related to the hearing loss. Finally, personal adjustment counseling minimizes worries and concerns about the prognosis for communication and outcome of management (Clark & English, 2004, pp. 6-8; Kricos, 2000a). The overall goal of personal adjustment counseling is to resolve psychosocial responses to hearing loss in patients and their family members.

Professional Counseling

Who Performs Professional Counseling? Audiologists and speech pathologists are not formally educated or trained as counselors. Audiologists and speech pathologists can still be effective in helping most patients and family members adjust to the psychosocial impact of hearing loss. In some cases, however, professional counseling is required. A professional counselor may be a formally trained counselor, a psychologist, or a psychiatrist. In most states, professional counselors have certain credentials, such as a graduate academic degree and fulfillment of appropriate course requirements. An audiologist or speech pathologist needs to know when professional counseling is required for a patient, that is, when the patient and perhaps family members should be referred to a professional counselor (Clark & English, 2004).

When Is Professional Counseling Necessary? Professional counseling is indicated if a patient has a need or requirement for help that is outside the bounds or limits of an audiologist's or speech pathologist's education, training, experience, or scope of practice. Professional counseling is also indicated when there is a risk of harm to the patient if the need is not adequately addressed. In addition, professional counseling should always be considered for patients who are depressed as a result of their hearing loss or related auditory disorder, like tinnitus. A referral for professional counseling is required for patients with prolonged and persistent depression, resulting in a major personality change and affecting daily activities, such as work or school.

Speech Reading

Speech reading is a component of intervention in the non-technology category. Speech reading is sometimes referred to as lip reading. The goal is to determine what a person is saying from visual cues associated with movement of the structures that produce speech, including the lips, the tongue, and the mouth. Speech (lip) reading was featured in the summary of rehabilitation shown in Figure 14.1.

Speech reading is a natural strategy to enhance communication of persons with hearing loss and also normal hearers. For example, we all find ourselves looking more intently at the speaker's face and lips when involved in a conversation in a noisy setting. Persons with hearing loss gain essential information from speech reading and also from other nonverbal cues like facial expressions and body language. Speech reading minimizes the negative impact of hearing loss on communication.

Several books on speech or lip reading with guidelines for instruction and exercises are available for patients and professionals (Kaplan, Garretson, & Baily, 1985; Nitchie, 2007).

Advantages and Limitations. Speech reading definitely augments information obtained through hearing, but speech reading alone is not adequate for communication. Not all speech sounds are differentiated or even detected visually. Sounds produced by the lips, such as /m/, /p/, and /b/, are easily seen and often differentiated with visual cues alone. Other sounds produced toward the back of the vocal tract, like /h/, /g/, and /k/, can't be seen.

WebWatch

With an Internet search you'll find websites dedicated to lip-reading information, instruction, and exercises, as well as a variety of interesting and educational speech-reading videos on YouTube.

Speech-reading skills and the benefits of speech reading in communication are developed with instruction and exercises, supplemented with plenty of real-world experience. Speech-reading instruction with adult patients is most effective when integrated into an overall program of audiological rehabilitation that also includes counseling, the use of residual hearing with proper amplification, and formal auditory training.

Speech Reading and Children. This is an appropriate time to mention speech reading in children. Most instructional materials on speech reading are directed to adults with acquired hearing loss. Still, young children with hearing loss should be encouraged to utilize visual cues, and given general instruction to develop their speech-reading skills.

Recent research confirms that even infants utilize facial cues when exposed to speech (Lewkowicz & Hansen-Tift, 2012). Infants between the ages of 6 and 12 months closely watch the speaker's lips and eyes. Results from the study also suggest that speech reading during infancy plays an important role in the development of speech and language (Lewkowicz & Hansen-Tift, 2012).

Audiological Habilitation and Rehabilitation of Children with Hearing Loss

Family-Centered Management

Historical Perspective. In the years before the introduction of widespread newborn hearing screening in the 1990s, parents were almost always the first to suspect hearing problems in their child, well before anyone else. Parental concerns were initially based on their child's reduced or inconsistent response to sound and limited vocalization during the first year of life. Speech and language delay was a later and serious concern. Parents then turned to the child's pediatrician or family doctor for confirmation of their suspicion of a hearing loss.

Unfortunately, in the era before universal newborn hearing screening, months and often years passed before an audiologist formally diagnosed hearing loss. Given their ongoing concern about hearing, parents were sometimes relieved upon hearing the diagnosis of hearing loss. Intervention for infant hearing loss was provider centered, that is, coordinated and directed by the audiologist with the help of the child's physician. Audiologists made decisions regarding the child's care, rather than the child's family.

Family-Centered Intervention. With the advent of universal newborn hearing screening, audiological rehabilitation evolved to a patient-centered and then to the current evidence-based *family-centered approach* (Clark, 2007; Clark & English, 2004; Kricos, 2000a). A word about terminology would be helpful here. The term *habilitation* rather than re*habilitation* best describes comprehensive intervention for infants. Rehabilitation refers to restoration of communication function, whereas the term *habilitation* is more appropriate for infants who have not yet developed communication.

Family-centered intervention was lent considerable support by passage in 1986 of Public Law 99-457 (Education of the Handicapped Act Amendments) and in 1991 by passage of Public Law 102-119 (Individuals with Disabilities Education Act Amendments). These federal laws also addressed educational needs of preschool children.

Diagnosis of hearing loss is now generally made within months after a child's birth, well before parents suspect a problem. Parents and other family members may be surprised, and even shocked, to learn that the child has a hearing loss. As you have just learned, the unexpected news about hearing loss often leads to other emotional or psychosocial responses in parents and family members. It is important for audiologists to carefully and compassionately counsel family members as much as necessary to help them respond effectively and positively to the child's hearing loss (Clark & English, 2004; Kricos, 2000a; Walsh, 1996).

Table 14.1 summarizes other important principles of family-centered rehabilitation. Audiologists and speech pathologists are accepting, nonjudgmental, and respectful of the family's preference and ability to participate in the rehabilitation process (Clark & English,

---

- Parents are provided with honest, unbiased, and complete information so they can make informed decisions
- Families are included in each component of intervention, including decision making, planning, assessment, and service delivery
- The audiologist and the parents assume responsibility for intervention
- Intervention takes into consideration the needs of the entire family, as well as the child
- The audiologist anticipates and proactively meets the family's counseling and intervention needs
- Goals and services in the intervention process follow the family's priorities
- The audiologist respects the family's level of participation in their child's intervention program
- Strengthening function of the family system is a primary goal
- Communication and networking among parents of children with hearing impairment is encouraged, facilitated, and supported
- The family's strengths are identified and utilized during intervention
- The audiologist respects each family's unique characteristics and strategies for coping with hearing loss

TABLE 14.1
Main features of family-centered intervention for hearing impairment in children.

Adapted with permission from Patricia Kricos, PhD, University of Florida.

2004). Services are provided to the entire family, not only the child. Family needs and priorities are consistently considered in setting rehabilitation goals and in delivery of services for the child. And, importantly, families are empowered with information and closely involved in the decision-making process (Girgia & Sanson-Fisher, 1995). Rehabilitation activities take place not just in a clinical or educational setting, but also at home. With the assistance, support, and resources provided or facilitated by audiologists and speech pathologists, parents develop teaching skills and effective techniques for interacting with their child.

Special Challenges in Habilitation of Children

Habilitation of infants and young children with hearing loss is among the most challenging and also most rewarding activities in audiology (Clark & English, 2004; Kricos, 2000a; Luterman, 2008). To reiterate an important point, the goal of rehabilitation is restoration of function in a person who is handicapped. The overall objective of audiological rehabilitation is to help a person who has lost hearing function to again use hearing effectively in communication and, thereby, improve the person's quality of life (Harris, Van Zandt, & Rees, 1997; Kricos, 2000a).

Audiological habilitation or rehabilitation involves education, auditory therapy or training, and sometimes speech reading. These important components of habilitation or rehabilitation are typically coupled with the application of technology, such as hearing aids, FM devices, and/or cochlear implants. The phrase *aural rehabilitation* was used in past years for what is now known as audiological rehabituation. Thus, the phrase *audiological habilitation* is commonly used to describe intervention with infants and young children who have never heard normally (Clark & English, 2004). The goal of the process is to optimally develop hearing function and communication in the child, rather than to restore the use of hearing.

Five Specific Challenges. Audiological habilitation of infants and young children is particularly challenging for at least five reasons. First, information on hearing cannot be acquired via conventional behavioral test techniques like pure tone or speech audiometry due to the child's young age. Estimation of auditory thresholds must instead be made with objective measures of hearing, such as the auditory brainstem response (ABR).

Second, intervention is optimally started before the child is 6 months old, assuming hearing loss is identified soon after birth. The initial hearing aid fitting must be based on auditory thresholds estimated from ABR rather than pure tone audiometry.

Third, accuracy of the initial hearing aid fitting is verified with careful measurements of sound in the external ear canal, since an infant's initial responses to sound provide limited feedback on hearing aid performance. Fourth, hearing aid performance must be closely and regularly monitored and adjusted as the size and acoustic of the child's ear canal change with growth. As the external ear canal size increases with maturation, ear molds for hearing aids must also be replaced regularly.

Finally, hearing aid satisfaction cannot be determined with inventories or reflected by patient comments, as it is in older children and adults with hearing loss. Instead, outcome of audiological habilitation in infants is documented by periodically and precisely assessing speech and language acquisition.

Consequences of Habilitation in Children. The consequences of audiological habilitation in infants and young children cannot be overemphasized (Clark & English, 2004; Kricos, 2000a). The stakes are extremely high. Children with all degrees of hearing loss can develop speech and language with a timely and properly implemented diagnostic and habilitation process. That is, hearing loss is accurately estimated in an infant, appropriate hearing aids are accurately fit using a prescriptive method within the first six months after birth, and hearing aid performance is closely monitored and adjusted as necessary during the first few years of life. You learned in Chapter 13 about the hearing aid fitting process. Accurate hearing aid fitting gives the infant an opportunity to benefit from constant, consistent, and comfortable audibility of speech sounds. Consistent auditory stimulation contributes importantly to development of the auditory regions of the central nervous system. Intense audiological habilitation efforts during infancy produce for the hearing-impaired child a lifelong positive impact on communication, academic success, and quality of life.

Children with Unilateral Hearing Loss

Up to this point, we've discussed the management of children with bilateral hearing loss. Sensorineural hearing loss in one ear is actually three times more prevalent than bilateral sensorineural hearing loss (Bess & Tharpe, 1983; Tharpe, 2007). You learned in Chapter 11 about some well-appreciated etiologies for unilateral hearing loss, including trauma, inner ear structural abnormalities like a large vestibular aqueduct, mumps, and hereditary forms of hearing loss. However, unilateral hearing loss for the majority of children has no clear or proven etiology.

We will now address some practical questions about children who have a hearing loss in one ear and hear normally in the other ear. Do children with a hearing loss in one ear require audiological management or can they rely on their better-hearing ear to communicate effectively? What kinds of problems do children with unilateral hearing loss encounter? What are the indications for intervention in children with unilateral hearing loss? Finally, what kind of intervention is most helpful for children with unilateral hearing loss?

Impact of Unilateral Hearing Loss. Persons with unilateral hearing loss invariably experience difficulties localizing the source of sound in space and hearing in the presence of background noise. These problems may interfere with daily activities, classroom performance, and psychosocial status. It is important to identify difficulties with speech perception in background noise during hearing testing and to manage them accordingly.

Some children with complete unilateral hearing loss have poorer language abilities than normal-hearing children (Bess & Tharpe 1986; Lieu, 2004; Lieu, Tye-Murray, Karzon, & Piccirillo,2004). Research shows that as many as one-third of children with unilateral hearing loss fail at least one grade, compared with less than 4% of normal-hearing children (Bess & Tharpe 1986).

Interestingly, children with unilateral hearing loss in the right ear are more at risk for auditory, language, and educational difficulties (Bess & Tharpe 1986; Lieu, 2004). This observation is not unexpected, given the more prominent central auditory pathways in the central nervous system leading from the right ear to the typically language-dominant left cerebral hemisphere.

Management of Unilateral Hearing Loss. Audiological management of unilateral hearing loss begins with close monitoring of auditory and speech-language status. Children born with a hearing loss in one ear are considerably more likely to show a delayed or progressive hearing loss in the other initially normal ear. Monitoring should also include regular measures of auditory and speech-language development (Bess & Tharpe 1986; Tharpe, 2007). Information counseling is important for parents of infants and young children with newly identified unilateral hearing loss. Educational efforts for parents of children with unilateral hearing loss should include strategies for enhancing auditory function. A key strategy is to assure that the child is in the optimal location for hearing during family meals, in the classroom at school, and while participating in sports.

WebWatch

The Ida Institute, located north of Copenhagen in Denmark, is an independent nonprofit educational institution. The stated mission of the Ida Institute is "To foster better understanding of the human dynamics associated with hearing loss." Also, "the challenge of the Ida Institute is to provide greater insight and a more holistic understanding of the complex journey of hearing loss to better assist hearing care professionals and hearing impaired persons." More information is available at the Ida Institute's website.

Decisions about additional intervention for children with unilateral hearing loss are influenced by several additional factors, such as the child's age, degree of hearing loss, hearing in the better ear, performance with amplification, family preferences, and the overall impact of intervention on the child's quality of life (Tharpe, 2007).

Speech and language delay is a possible consequence of unilateral hearing loss in young children (Lieu, 2004; Lieu et al., 2004) Documentation of evidence of auditory deficits or speech-language delay warrants one or more intervention options, including a personal FM system, a hearing aid for the poorer-hearing ear, a hearing aid-FM combination, or sound-field classroom amplification for school-age children.

Audiologists sometimes take a "wait-and-see" approach to management of children with unilateral hearing loss. That is, management other than monitoring is deferred as long as auditory responses, speech-language status, and school performance is age-appropriate. Delayed audiological management is supported with research findings suggesting that children with unilateral hearing loss do not consistently benefit from amplification (McKay, Gravel, & Tharpe, 2008). In fact, some children demonstrate poorer performance with amplification in noisy listening conditions.

 ClinicalConnection

It's tempting to assume that children with normal hearing in one ear will have no problems with communication. Clinical experience and research findings, however, confirm that some children with unilateral hearing loss do have language delays and experience difficulties in school. Audiologists must always carefully assess the impact of unilateral hearing loss on communication and academic performance, while educating other professionals like teachers and physicians about the topic.

Counseling and Education of Adult Hearing Aid Patients

Most Adults with Hearing Loss Aren't Interested in Hearing Aids

The majority of adults with hearing loss do not for a variety of reasons pursue amplification. We reviewed this point in the preceding chapter. Of the many persons with hearing impairment, only one in five actually wears hearing aids. And, the average person who now wears a hearing aid took approximately seven years to decide that help in the form of amplification would be beneficial and would warrant the effort and expense.

Following identification and diagnosis of hearing loss, audiologists often devote considerable time and effort educating adult patients about their hearing problem and how they might benefit from hearing aids (Clark & English, 2004; Kricos & Holmes, 1996). Some patients appear ready to consider hearing aids following appropriate education and counseling. These patients ask for more information about hearing aids and ask which hearing aid would be best for them.

However, most patients are not yet ready to make a decision when initially provided with information about their hearing loss and rehabilitation options. A patient may opt to take more time to "think about it." Or, a patient may state with certainty that his or her hearing loss has little impact on communication and day-to-day activities and that he or she simply will not consider hearing aids (Kricos, 2000b).

Counseling Time Is Well Spent

Is the time an audiologist spends with such patients wasted and of no value? Not at all! With proper education and counseling, a hearing-impaired patient can learn to hear and listen more effectively in different situations and conditions even without the benefits of amplification (Boothroyd, 2007). Even though they are not ready for amplification, patients may elect to use hearing assistive technology like amplification for the telephone or a device to improve hearing while watching the television. Hearing-impaired patients who are bothered by tinnitus

L E A D E R S   A N D   L U M I N A R I E S

Patricia Kricos

Patricia Kricos, PhD, is Professor Emeritus at the University of Florida. She received her bachelor's degree from the University of Texas at El Paso and her master's and PhD degrees from The Ohio State University (1973). She has taught in the audiology program at the University of Florida since 1981. Her major clinical and research interest is audiological rehabilitation in adults. Dr. Kricos has published a number of articles and chapters on audiological rehabilitation for older adults. She is currently writing a book entitled *Audiologic* *Rehabilitation for Adults: Concepts, Applications, and Management.* Dr. Kricos is a past president of the American Academy of Audiology. She serves on the Advisory Council of the Better Hearing Institute and the Ida Institute (Denmark), and as Professional Advisor for the Hearing Loss Association of Florida. She is currently serving as a member of the Board of Trustees of the Hearing Loss Association of America.

can acquire strategies for minimizing the impact of the tinnitus on their quality of life. And, importantly, patients begin to understand the importance of hearing protection for prevention of further hearing loss.

The information given to a patient who is not yet ready to use hearing aids can be the catalyst that eventually leads to a decision to pursue amplification. In reality, the time spent by an audiologist counseling and educating an adult patient about hearing and hearing loss almost always results in improved quality of life for the patient. And improved communication and quality of life is what audiological rehabilitation is all about (Boothroyd, 2007).

After Hearing Aid Fitting

Counseling and education reaps additional rewards once a patient does decide to acquire hearing aids (Boothroyd, 2007; Kricos & Holmes, 1996). Research clearly confirms that thoughtful counseling and education about hearing aids results in enhanced patient satisfaction and substantially reduces the likelihood of unsuccessful hearing aid use. Education about hearing aids is often referred to as "hearing aid orientation." It is a big factor in reducing hearing aid returns (Bratt, Rosenfeld, & Williams, 2007).

Persons with hearing loss now have an option to purchase hearing aids directly via the Internet without the professional assistance and service provided by an audiologist. Unfortunately, this apparently cost-effective approach eliminates the most important determinant of hearing aid success and satisfaction—counseling and education by a qualified professional. Audiologist participation in the hearing aid dispensing process adds value by maximizing the patient's benefit from amplification (Boothroyd, 2007). The audiologist also plays a critical role in the detection and diagnosis of diseases and other conditions that require treatment prior to safe hearing aid use.

Special Challenges in Rehabilitation of Elderly Adults

A number of factors make audiological rehabilitation of elderly adults with hearing loss more challenging that rehabilitation of younger adult patient (Kricos, 2000b). Table 14.2 summarizes auditory and non-auditory factors. As you review the information in Table 14.2, consider different ways an audiologist might assess hearing and manage hearing loss in an older patient rather than a college-age person or someone in their thirties or forties.

TABLE 14.2

Age-related factors to consider in audiological rehabilitation of elderly patients with hearing loss.

Auditory Factors

- Decreased audibility of sound
- Deficit in word recognition ability
- Poorer comprehension of connected speech
- Other auditory processing deficits, such as:
    - Reduced ability to discriminate frequency information
    - Reduced ability to rapidly process auditory information
    - Deficit in speech perception in background noise

Visual Factors

- Dual sensory loss (loss of vision and hearing)
- Deficit in perception of auditory-visual speech information
- Reduction in speech (lip) reading ability

Cognitive Factors

- Changes in cognitive abilities including:
    - Speed in processing information
    - Memory
    - Attention
- Reallocation of cognitive resources to help with compromised auditory processing abilities

Adapted with permission from Patricia Kricos, PhD, University of Florida.

Factors Influencing Rehabilitation of Elderly Adults. There are at least three categories of factors to take into account in the audiological assessment and management of elderly patients. First, speech perception deficits are more common and more complicated in elderly patients. Findings for pure tone audiometry and for word recognition testing in quiet for an elderly patient may not adequately evaluate hearing function or document the full extent of auditory processing difficulties. Additional diagnostic testing may be required, including measures of auditory processing and speech perception in background noise. The audiogram shows only one age-related change in hearing—the loss of normal audibility.

Second, visual acuity and processing must be considered in older patients undergoing hearing assessment (Kricos, 2007; Saunders & Echt, 2007). Age-related vision impairment is quite common. Most persons with hearing impairment tend to rely more on visual cues for communication. For example, scores on tests of speech perception are typically much higher when a person with hearing impairment can see the face and especially the mouth of the speaker. An elderly person with dual sensory loss, combining age-related hearing and vision deficits, does not benefit as much from the advantage of visual cues in speech perception (Saunders & Echt, 2007).

Finally, age-related cognitive decline adversely impacts auditory functioning in multiple ways (Kricos, 2009; Pichora-Fuller & Singh, 2006). For example, the older patient may experience difficulty maintaining adequate attention while communicating. Memory deficits may prevent the patient from recalling important auditory information, even during a conversation. Short-term or working memory deficits may further disrupt auditory processing. In addition, an older person with a hearing loss must allocate or devote more cognitive resources like attention and memory to

 ClinicalConnection

Management of elderly adults who have hearing loss is quite challenging for many reasons. The impact of hearing loss on communication and quality of life is often enhanced by age-related problems with vision and cognitive functioning. Audiologists take a different approach to the evaluation and management of elderly hearing-impaired patients than to children or younger adults with hearing loss.

communication than a normal hearer. The result is often inadequate cognitive resources for understanding and comprehending speech.

Devastating Impact of Multiple Deficits. A worst-case scenario communication disorder emerges when there are age-related deficits in multiple areas. A patient's inadequate ability to communicate effectively results from a devastating combination of factors, including reduced ability to hear normal levels of speech, inability to rapidly process what is said, extreme difficulty with speech perception in everyday background noise, inability to augment or enhance hearing with visual information, and reduced ability to maintain attention and remember auditory information.

Unfortunately, this combination of deficits is not uncommon among elderly patients. Auditory, visual, and cognitive deficits must be recognized and addressed. An audiologist recognizing and adequately managing or co-managing these deficits can often restore effective communication in an elderly patient. With this comprehensive rehabilitation approach an audiologist will also significantly improve the patient's psychosocial status and quality of life.

Group Counseling

There is considerable value in organizing and coordinating audiological counseling, education, and rehabilitation for groups of people, rather than individuals (Clark & English, 2004). The group may consist of the patient and family members or, more traditionally, a collection of patients with hearing loss. Patients in the group setting can share knowledge, experiences, and feelings related to hearing loss and its management. Organizing a series of group meetings of persons with hearing loss who were recently fit with hearing aids can have educational and therapeutic value that would be hard to match with individual one-on-one counseling.

The group counseling approach is particularly effective with older patients who, because of their hearing loss, may experience psychosocial problems like frustration, isolation, loneliness, discouragement, and even depression. Often an audiologist or another designated person moderates or leads the group session to assure that the overall counseling goals are met and each patient has an opportunity to participate.

Group Counseling Is Uncommon. Research and clinical experience supports the value of group sessions in audiological rehabilitation. Group counseling sessions are strongly supported by counseling experts (e.g., Clark and English, 2004). You may be surprised to learn that this component of rehabilitation is rarely implemented in clinical practice.

A variety of explanations are commonly cited for the reluctance of audiologists to include group counseling in their management plans. One clear disincentive to group counseling is time. To quote Benjamin Franklin, "Remember that time is money." Many patients can't afford to take time out of their busy lives or time away from work to periodically attend group-counseling meetings. When group sessions are offered as part of a rehabilitation process, those mostly likely to attend are elderly patients who are retired.

Most audiologists are also reluctant to or simply unable to devote busy clinic time to moderating or leading a group counseling session. In typical audiology practice settings today there is considerable ongoing demand for a high level of productivity. Each hour of the health professional's workday must be filled with either direct reimbursable patient contact or patient-related administrative activities, such as clinical report preparation.

You may be confused by these apparently contradictory statements. Given the emphasis on clinical productivity, wouldn't it be good use of an audiologist's time to moderate a group counseling session with multiple patients rather than providing diagnostic or rehabilitation services to each patient individually? Group counseling sessions are certainly an efficient way to help many patients within a relatively short time period.

Unfortunately, third-party payers such as private or government-supported healthcare insurance carriers do not reimburse adequately for time spent with patients during group rehabilitation sessions. The major reason that group counseling is rarely included in audiological rehabilitation programs is directly related to lack of reimbursement or payment by health insurance carriers for professional time spent in group counseling and education sessions, and the lack of health insurance coverage of the service for the participating patient. In other words, audiologists cannot afford to devote clinic time to the group sessions, and patients are unwilling to pay privately for the service.

Strategies for Implementing Group Counseling.   Creative solutions can probably be found for these time and financial problems associated with group counseling sessions. One solution is to assign properly prepared support staff, such as an audiology assistant or technician, the responsibility of leading the counseling sessions. An audiologist develops the schedule or agenda for the group sessions and oversees their operation. However, the audiologist may remain highly productive in other clinical activities while support staff personnel led the group session.

Research has repeatedly shown that patient counseling and education during and following hearing aid fitting is associated with greater acceptance of hearing aids, increased patient satisfaction, fewer patient-initiated clinic follow-up visits, and lower hearing aid return or rejection rates (Boothroyd, 2007; Bratt, Rosenfield & Williams, 2007; Kricos & Holmes, 1996).

Advances in social networking and computer-based conferencing techniques form the basis for other innovative approaches to group counseling sessions. For example, an audiology clinic might offer weekly or monthly virtual "meetings" or chats to selected patients. Virtual sessions offer patients most if not all of the benefits of face-to-face meetings; they are more convenient for patients and eliminate driving and parking expenses. A clinic could also create a social networking sites or pages for patients who might benefit from group counseling, such as those recently fitted with amplification.

Computer-Based Auditory Training

Audiology Goes Back to Its Roots.   Audiology as a profession is rooted in rehabilitation. You will recall from the Chapter 1 that Raymond Carhart and other active-duty healthcare professionals in the U.S. Army and Navy in military hospitals, immediately after World War II, were assigned the task of helping military personnel with hearing loss. In most cases, the hearing loss was due to noise exposure and was not treatable medically or surgically. In the next decade, audiological rehabilitation continued in the Veteran's Administration medical system. Hearing aids during this era were quite primitive by today's standards, providing limited flexibility for fitting and little benefit to communication. The primary focus of rehabilitation efforts for military personnel and veterans was to optimize through education and auditory training their use of residual hearing function.

Auditory Training Today.   Now there is renewed and really unprecedented clinical interest in applying the latest audiological rehabilitation technology and techniques to help patients with hearing loss maximize their hearing abilities. To a large extent, the current emphasis on auditory training in rehabilitation is a byproduct or outgrowth of neuroscience research. You were introduced in Chapter 12 to the concept of brain plasticity, also referred to as neuroplasticity. Throughout life the brain is capable of change due to environmental stimulation. Neuroplasticity is the scientific foundation of auditory training.

Auditory training is essentially a well organized, focused, and intensive form of environmental stimulation designed to maximize neural changes necessary to improve hearing function (Kricos & McCarthy, 2007; Sweetow & Sabes, 2006; Tye-Murray, 2004). Neuroplasticity is the fundamental scientific principle underlying rehabilitation of all types, including auditory training during rehabilitation of persons with hearing impairment (Sweetow & Palmer, 2005).

Audiologists and Speech Pathologists Work as a Team. Because of their respective areas of clinical knowledge and skills, audiologists and speech-language pathologists often work together as a team for audiological rehabilitation of children and adults with hearing loss. Audiologists tend to utilize "bottom-up" auditory training techniques that focus on the acoustic content and features of sound and development of various speech perception skills.

Speech-language pathologists, on the other hand, are usually involved in "top-down" forms of auditory training that maximize the role of language processing in the perception and comprehension of speech. Maximum benefits in communication enhancement are achieved with a balanced combination of bottom-up and top-down auditory training techniques and strategies.

Computer-Based Auditory Training for Children

Several software programs are available for auditory perceptual training of children with hearing loss, deficits in auditory processing, and related disorders such as reading disorders. Audiologists and speech pathologists apply the computer-based auditory training programs in the management of children with various communication disorders, including hearing loss, auditory processing disorders, language impairment, and reading disorders. Although based on scientific research with the main purpose of developing auditory skills, the computer programs are designed to be like computer games and, therefore, engaging and interesting to young children.

Earobics and Fast ForWord. Two rather popular computer-based auditory training programs for children are **Earobics** and **Fast ForWord** (Merzenich et al., 1996; Pokorni, Worthington, & Jamison, 2004; Russo et al., 2005, 2010). Auditory training programs designed for children are appropriate to remediate auditory perceptual deficits in children with auditory processing disorders and also to augment the benefits of technology, such as hearing aids and cochlear implants, in children with hearing loss.

Earobics uses a multisensory approach to developing auditory and reading readiness skills. It offers auditory and visual stimulation. Intensive auditory stimulation is combined with attractive and age-appropriate graphics. Auditory skill categories included in the Earobics program are:

- Rhyming
- Phoneme identification
- Phonological manipulation
- Blending
- Segmentation
- Discrimination
- Auditory performance in competing noise
- Auditory sequential memory

Children enrolled in the interactive Earobics program work at their own pace through each sub-program, beginning at a simple level and progressing to more challenging levels of difficulty. One of the Earobics versions is designed for pre-kindergarten, kindergarten, and first-grade students. The other version is appropriate for second- and third-grade students and older struggling readers.

ClinicalConnection

The development of computer technology has opened up new avenues for effective and also cost-effective auditory training of persons with hearing loss and auditory processing disorders. Audiologists and speech pathologists now often include computer-based programs for auditory training as part of the habilitation or rehabilitation of children and adults with hearing loss.

WebWatch

The Internet is the source of a wealth of information about Earobics, Fast ForWord, and other computer-based auditory training programs. The websites include video demonstrations of these interesting auditory training programs. Websites for manufacturers describe their products and provide links to supporting research. Other websites summarize evidence in support of and against the program.

FIGURE 14.2

Example of a screen from the LACE (Listening and Communication Enhancement) computer-based auditory training program for children and adolescents. Courtesy of Neurotone.

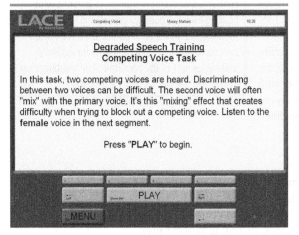

Fast ForWord includes a variety of computer-based programs for the development of attention, auditory processing rate, memory, auditory sequencing, and reading skills (Merzenich et al., 1996). Children participate in intensive daily exercises that require the identification of computer-generated speech sounds. Completion of a Fast ForWord program usually takes four to sixteen weeks. A unique feature of the training program is sounds that are slowed down with longer-than-normal temporal characteristics. As a child progresses through Fast ForWord, temporal processing becomes more challenging as the speech-time difference is decreased.

Computer-Based Auditory Training for Adults

There are now a variety of software programs for development of auditory perceptual skills in adult patients with hearing loss, including those fit with hearing aids. One program that incorporates bottom-up and top-down training techniques and strategies is the Speech Perception Assessment and Training System (SPAT). Another recently developed program with the unique abbreviation CASPERSent and the even more unusual name "Computer-Assisted Speech PERception testing and training at the SENTence level" combines auditory and visual training exercises. Other recently developed auditory training programs include Seeing and Hearing Speech by Sensimetrics, ReadMyQuips by Sense Synergy, Inc., and I Hear What You Mean, developed at Washington University School of Medicine.

Listening and Communication Enhancement (LACE). A program called **Listening and Communication Enhancement (LACE)** is among the most popular commercially available computer-based options for auditory training in adults with hearing impairment (Sweetow & Palmer, 2005; Sweetow & Sabes, 2006). Figure 14.2 shows a typical screen from one of the LACE programs. Robert Sweetow, a well-known audiologist, developed LACE. Along with other programs, LACE has contributed considerably to the renewed interest in auditory training as an important component of audiological rehabilitation.

 WebWatch

You can participate in a free demonstration of LACE and view a video of the program used with a patient on the Neurotone website. LACE is also featured in a number of YouTube videos.

LACE addresses auditory and non-auditory skills. Practical advantages of LACE include the option for adapting the level of difficulty of a listening task to the patient's level of performance and the everyday nature of the auditory training materials. We are likely to witness in the years to come an increase in the availability of evidence-based and commercially available software programs for development of auditory skills, for inclusion in rehabilitation of adults with hearing loss.

Importance of a Multicultural Approach

Cultural Differences in Patients

Audiologists and speech pathologists practicing in the United States and many other Western countries now provide diagnostic and rehabilitation services to culturally diverse patient populations. According to the 2010 census, the U.S. population continues to become more diverse in many dimensions. Racial and ethnic diversity is increasing as an estimated one million immigrants enter the United States each year, including a high proportion of persons of Hispanic or Asian background.

Complex and changing interactions among race, ethnicity, and age are also occurring in the United States. For example, younger persons tend to be more racially and ethnically diverse, whereas the older population is predominantly white. Also, an increasing number of audiologists who are U.S. citizens either work in culturally different countries or travel abroad regularly to contribute to outreach clinical projects in a variety of countries lacking adequate audiology services.

Diversity in patient populations includes the influences of language, religion, country of origin, socioeconomic level, sexual preference, age, and educational background. Values, attitudes, beliefs, and customs may vary among any of these diverse domains.

Sensitivity to and tolerance of the beliefs, traditions, and values of specific cultures is expected and essential in all interactions with patients and family members (Clark & English, 2004, pp. 165–172). Appreciation of cultural differences in patients and their families is consistent with a humanistic approach to clinical services. Interacting with patients and family members in a culturally sensitive manner enhances quality of care. In certain circumstances, sensitivity to and understanding of cultural factors by an audiologist or a speech pathologist will determine whether a patient agrees to participate in the diagnostic and rehabilitation process (Roseberry-McKibbin, 1997).

Graduate education of audiologists and speech pathologists includes formal instruction on cultural diversity and issues. Audiologists and speech pathologists are well advised to devote time to preparation for multicultural challenges in the provision of clinical services (Clark & English, 2004, pp. 165–172).

The Deaf Culture

The phrase **Deaf Culture** is not found among the many dictionary definitions or examples of the word *culture*. There exists, however, a longstanding and proud community of persons who are Deaf and who proudly share a well-defined identity and, importantly, the same language. Individuals who belong to this community are typically described as Deaf, with a capital "D," rather than a lower case "d." The more inclusive phrase **Deaf community** will be used in the following discussion.

The Deaf community is in most respects unlike other cultures. The Deaf community is not recognizable by similarities in history, geographical origin, cuisine, or clothing. Although there are diverse religious beliefs in the Deaf community, many individuals do choose to attend a Deaf church, that is, the branch of an established denomination where the service is conducted or interpreted in sign language.

Bonds in the Deaf Community

Members of the Deaf community have many strong common bonds. Among the most important bonds is their childhood education, often in a residential school for the deaf. Important aspects and values in the Deaf community, in addition to language, may be passed down from parents to children. Since most children who are Deaf are born of hearing parents, distinct characteristics of persons in the Deaf community are sometimes passed from one Deaf child to another in a residential educational setting.

Persons who are Deaf interact primarily with each other during daily activities, such as social events, religious services, performing arts, travel, and sports, and even in Deaf Clubs. In addition, a number of social customs are unique to those in the Deaf community. For example, touching another person is quite acceptable before or during conversation, whereas this practice is not permitted in certain other cultures. Deaf persons typically stare intently at the person they are communicating with while signing. Individuals who are Deaf and the

Deaf community in general have traditionally and sometimes aggressively resisted efforts by "oralists" or "audists" and hearing persons to become assimilated into the much larger hearing society. In part, the rather firm independence expressed by the Deaf community reflects awareness that many in the hearing community perceive them as persons who are handicapped by a hearing disability.

Residential and College Education

Residential schools for the Deaf throughout the United States and elsewhere are available for education of persons from preschool years through high school. A handful of universities also have a longstanding tradition of higher education for individuals who are Deaf. Universities well known among the Deaf community and the general population include Gallaudet University in Washington, DC, the National Technical Institute for the Deaf at Rochester Institute of Technology, and the California State University at Northridge.

Intervention with Individuals with Deafness

Discussion and debate about the best communication mode and training approach for persons with profound hearing loss and deafness has persisted for many hundreds of years. In reality, no single communication modality is optimal for all children with hearing impairment or acceptable to all parents of children with hearing impairment. Family-centered decisions about intervention for profound hearing loss must be made on a case-by-case basis, taking into account a variety of issues. Some of the factors influencing decisions about the intervention strategy include characteristics of the child, available community resources, commitment of the family to the child, and the chosen communication modality.

We will now review briefly major traditional communication options and methods employed in rehabilitation of persons with deafness. There are, of course, variations in and combinations of these methodologies (Brinkley, 2011; Marschark, Lang, & Albertini, 2006).

Oral Approach

An **oral approach** is one option for intervention with children who have profound hearing impairment and deafness. The term *oral* means the production of speech and language for communication with the mouth and vocal system. The homonym *aural* is used to describe reception of information through the auditory modality. An oral approach is based on the assumption that children with hearing impairment can develop effective communication, including receptive and expressive language skills, regardless of the degree of hearing loss.

Three forms or variations of oral English instruction in practice today are the auditory-verbal approach, the auditory-oral approach, and the natural auditory-oral approach. The **auditory-verbal** philosophy places an emphasis on the child's residual hearing through the use of amplification with the goal of developing listening skills through natural communication. With this approach, the child is placed in mainstream education beginning in preschool years.

The **auditory-oral approach** emphasizes the development of amplified residual hearing and spoken language utilizing speech-reading cues as a supplement to the auditory signal. With this approach, the child is usually enrolled in an oral education program until he or she can be appropriately mainstreamed.

Natural Auditory-Oral Approach

The **natural auditory-oral approach** is a family-centered variation of the auditory-oral strategy that maximizes normal daily parent-child interaction to promote development of effective communication, rather than reliance on professionals to "teach" speech and language skills (Clark, M., 2007). The natural auditory-oral approach is based on the assumption that a child's language develops through meaningful interaction with significant adults, such as family members. In other words, hearing-impaired children develop language most effectively when they are in a meaningful environment that provides language-learning opportunities.

Another premise of the natural auditory-oral approach is that "children who hear more will talk more themselves" (Clark, M., 2007). That is, the amount of parental talking during daily routines and life experiences significantly increases language development. Hearing-impaired children of mothers who talk more during daily activities develop a larger vocabulary than the children of mothers who do less talking. Examples of daily activities are eating at mealtime, bathroom activities, dressing, and play.

With the natural auditory-oral approach, hearing professionals, including audiologists, speech-language pathologists, and educators of hearing-impaired persons play an important role by encouraging and teaching parents effective strategies for playing, talking, and interacting verbally with their children. Most often the mother is the primary caregiver involved in the natural auditory-oral approach.

The book entitled *Practical Guide to Quality Interaction with Children Who Have Hearing Loss* is a straightforward and current review of oral education for hearing-impaired children. Morag Clark, the author of the book, is a woman who has successfully implemented such programs in developed and developing countries around the world.

Changes in Oral Deaf Education

Oral educational approaches have steadily become more common in the past few decades. Historically, the distinction between "hard of hearing" and "deafness" was based on the degree to which a person could use hearing for communication. Children who were hard of hearing with hearing thresholds better (lower) than 90 dB often developed effective oral communication with appropriate hearing aids and other habilitation. On the other hand, children with deafness, defined then as hearing thresholds of 90 dB or greater, were far less likely to develop effective oral communication and were dependent almost entirely on the visual modality and manual or sign language for communication.

Widespread implementation of universal infant screening programs and the resulting early identification of profound hearing loss have greatly influenced the course of oral education. An increasing proportion of deaf children undergo cochlear implantation before 18 months of age and many children undergo cochlear implantation at 12 months of age. Consequently, the majority of children with deafness using cochlear implants are entering mainstream educational environments in the first grade.

Manual Approaches

Manual approaches for education of children with profound hearing loss and deafness are distinctly different from oral educational strategies. The word *manual* is derived from the Latin word for "hand." As the name implies, manual education emphasizes the development of and reliance on sign language for communication, with little or no use of residual hearing abilities.

American Sign Language (ASL). In the United States, **American Sign Language (ASL)** is the common language of the Deaf community. It is a vast lexicon of hand shapes and motions or signs, with its own syntax and grammar. Figure 14.3 depicts signs representing the manual alphabet of ASL. Additionally, ASL places a heavy emphasis on the facial expressions and body language of the signer.

ASL is actually a unique language, as there is no simple or direct translation to oral English language. Proponents of ASL maintain that it is an easier and more natural mode of communication for children with profound hearing loss or deafness. Acquisition of communication skills with ASL certainly facilitates membership in and acceptance by the Deaf community.

FIGURE 14.3

Manual alphabet used with American Sign Language (ASL).

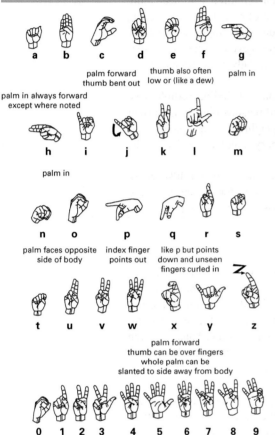

There are two potential limitations of ASL. One is the counterpart to the role played by ASL in acceptance of a hearing-impaired child into the Deaf community. In contrast to the child educated successfully with an oral approach, the child dependent on ASL will not be able to communicate effectively with most normal hearers and persons who are hearing impaired yet not deaf. Also, since syntax does not contribute to development of the English language, reliance on ASL for communication detracts from acquisition of spoken language and reading skills.

Signing Exact English. In an attempt to minimize the difficulties arising from English language learning through manual communication, some educators have developed other English-based sign systems. The most popular form of the English-based sign systems is **Signing Exact English (SEE or SEE2)**. SEE2 utilizes much of the same vocabulary as ASL, but adds grammatical features and follows English syntax. The SEE2 system is most appropriate for preschool and younger elementary-school-age children. It provides them with access to English instruction during the important language learning years. Opponents of the SEE educational approach argue that the avoidance of ASL is essentially a denial of Deaf culture. That is, SEE communication methods impose standards of the hearing world on the deaf child.

Total Communication. A blend of the oral and manual approaches is referred to as a combination approach. The most popular combination approach is **total communication**. Total communication involves the use of one or more modes of communication at any given time in the child's educational program, whether it is manual, oral, auditory only, or written. The stated objective of this approach is to utilize whatever communication modality is most appropriate for the child at that stage of development or for a given situation, allowing the child access to all means of communication.

Few educational programs actually implement a true combination educational approach due to practical challenges, such as the communication skills of the instructor and the challenge of combining more than one method at the same time. Also, consistently combining communication modalities may over stimulate or confuse some children, interfering with rather than enhancing the development of effective communication.

Cued Speech. Cued speech is a less-often-implemented combination approach. **Cued speech** is a visual communication system that employs eight hand shapes placed at four different locations near the mouth. Some sounds are not visible or distinguishable by watching lips. The hand shapes are designed to supplement spoken language and speech reading cues. The cued speech approach enhances the child's ability to see and hear English language as it is spoken.

One major limitation of the cued speech approach is the scarcity of educational programs and "transliterators," the individuals that cue what an instructor is saying. Also, unless they learn ASL, persons who master the cued speech technique are unable to communicate with persons in the Deaf community. You might wish to take a few minutes to view one or two of the many YouTube videos demonstrating the cued speech technique.

Bilingual-Bicultural Education. There is increased interest in the development of *bilingual-bicultural education* for children who are deaf. This approach is designed to educate the child in the values, customs, practices, and language of the hearing world and the Deaf culture. The term bilingual usually refers to an ability to communicate in either of two oral languages, such as English or Spanish. Here the term is used to describe acquisition of a manual and an oral form of communication.

In bilingual-bicultural educational programs, a child is generally taught ASL as his or her first language, providing a base for later oral language learning. Early access to language is designed to promote increased literacy and academic skills. The child also benefits from ongoing education with an auditory-oral educational approach. Since bilingual-bicultural educational programs are relatively new, formal data are not yet available on long-term acquisition of effective communication in children with hearing impairment.

You have now been introduced to a variety of educational methods now available to parents of children with profound hearing impairment or deafness. Parents and other family members select the educational approach for the child during a period of emotional turmoil. Family members experience intense psychosocial responses to hearing loss along with the child. As you learned during the review of family-centered counseling for children with hearing impairment, parents naturally view the identification of a hearing impairment in their child as a loss and may grieve accordingly. A clear understanding of hearing loss, its implications, and available remedial interventions facilitates the family's effective response to the news that their child has a serious hearing impairment.

Family-centered counseling may be particularly challenging for an audiologist or speech pathologist when the parents of a child with profound hearing loss are themselves deaf. Few audiologists are "fluent" in ASL. Audiologists and speech pathologists must readily employ the services of a skilled and experienced sign language interpreter when communicating with family members who are deaf, just as an interpreter would be relied upon for communication with a non-English speaking family. The use of a qualified sign language interpreter is not only good clinical policy. It is required under Americans with Disabilities Act (ADA) legislation.

PULLING IT ALL TOGETHER

Management of persons with hearing loss involves far more than technology like hearing aids and cochlear implants. You now know that audiologists and speech pathologists employ a variety of techniques to help patients make the most of their hearing and live with hearing loss. In reading this chapter, you gained an appreciation for the importance of family-centered counseling in management of children and adults to facilitate adjustment to hearing loss and to address psychosocial consequences of hearing loss. You are aware that some patients require the services of professional counselors, psychologists, or psychiatrists. You realize that instruction in speech reading helps patients use nonverbal information while communicating.

We reviewed in the chapter the multiple challenges involved with habilitation of infants and children with hearing loss, and the importance of prompt and appropriate management by audiologists and speech pathologists. You also learned about the possible consequences of unilateral hearing loss for auditory function, language development, and academic performance. The role of computer-based auditory training in children with hearing impairment was also noted.

The benefits of counseling and education for adult hearing aid patients and even those patients who are not yet ready for amplification were also addressed in this chapter. You read about the special challenges associated with management of elderly patients, including multiple auditory deficits, cognitive factors, and dual sensory loss. You learned that computer-based auditory training programs are also available for the development of hearing and listening abilities in adult patients.

Toward the end of the chapter, you gained an appreciation for cultural differences among patients and how audiologists and speech pathologists can respectfully provide clinical services to culturally and ethnically diverse patients and their families. Finally, you were introduced to Deaf Culture and to varied approaches available for education and development of communication in persons with deafness.

READINGS

Alpiner, J., & McCarthy, P. (Eds.). (2000). *Rehabilitative audiology: Children and adults* (3rd ed). Philadelphia: Lippincott, Williams & Wilkins.

Bellis, T. J. (2003). *Assessment and management of central auditory processing disorders in the educational setting: From science to prac*tice. San Diego: Singular Publishing.

Brinkley, D. (2011). *Supporting deaf children and young people: Strategies for intervention, inclusion and improvement.* New York: Continuum Press.

Butler, J. P., & Hauber, M. J. (Eds.). (2000). *Rehabilitative audiology.* Baltimore MD: Lippincott, Williams & Wilkins.

Clark, J. G., & English, K. M. (2004). *Counseling in audiologic practice: Helping patients and families adjust to hearing loss.* Boston: Pearson.

Clark, M. (2007). *A practical guide to quality interaction with children who have hearing los*s. San Diego: Plural Publishing.

Hall, J. W. III, & Johnston, K. N. (2009). Diagnostic audiology, hearing instruments and aural habilitation. In J. B. Snow Jr & P. A. Wackym (Eds.), *Ballenger's otorhinolaryngology—head and neck surgery* (17th ed., pp. 115–130). Shelton CT: BC Decker.

Holland, A. L. (2007). *Counseling in communication disorders: A wellness perspective.* San Diego: Plural Publishing.

Hull, R. H. (2009). *Introduction to aural rehabilitation.* San Diego: Plural Publishing.

Kaplan, H., Garretson, C., & Baily, S. (1985). *Speech reading: A way to improve understanding.* Washington DC: Gallaudet University Press.

Marschark, M., Lang, H. G., & Albertini, J. A. (2006). *Educating deaf students: From research to practice.* London: Oxford University Press.

Luterman, D. (2008). *Counseling persons with communication disorders and their families* (5th ed.). Austin TX: ProEd.

Madell, J. R., & Flexer, C. (2011). *Pediatric audiology casebook.* New York: Thieme Medical Publishers.

Mueller, H. G. III, & Hall, J. W. III. (1998). *Audiologist's desk reference. Volume II: Amplification, management, and rehabilitation.* San Diego: Singular Publishing.

Nitchie, E. B. (2007). *Lip-reading principles and practice.* Melbourne, Australia: Book Jungle.

Schow, R. L., & Nerbonne, M. A. (2006). *Introduction to audiologic rehabilitation* (5th ed). Boston: Allyn & Bacon.

Seewald, R., & Tharpe, A. M. (Eds.) (2011). *Comprehensive handbook of pediatric audiology.* San Diego: Plural Publishing.

Tye-Murray, N. (2008). *Foundations of aural rehabilitation: Children, adults, and their family members* (3rd ed). Clifton Park, NY: Delmar Cengage Publishing.

15 Exaggerated and False Hearing Loss, Tinnitus, and Hyperacusis

LEARNING OBJECTIVES

In this chapter, you will learn:

- The meaning of the term *pseudohypacusis*
- Why it is important to accurately diagnosis false or exaggerated hearing loss
- About hearing test findings that are clues for possible false or exaggerated hearing loss
- About risk factors for false or exaggerated hearing loss
- Strategies for management of patients with false or exaggerated hearing loss
- That tinnitus is a symptom and not a disease
- About characteristics of patients with bothersome tinnitus
- Why tinnitus bothers some patients more than others
- Steps in hearing assessment of patients with bothersome tinnitus
- Strategies for management of bothersome tinnitus
- That the term *hyperacusis* means intolerance to loud sounds
- About possible explanations for hyperacusis
- That hyperacusis is a characteristic or symptom of certain diseases
- How audiologists assess children and adults with hyperacusis
- Strategies for management of patients with hyperacusis

KEY TERMS

Erroneous hearing loss
Exaggerated hearing loss
False hearing loss
Functional hearing loss
Hyperacusis
Malingerer (malingering)
Misophonia
Nonorganic hearing loss
Phonophobia
Pseudohypacusis
Psychogenic hearing loss
Stenger test
Tinnitus

CHAPTER FOCUS

This chapter is devoted to a review of four interesting patient populations. You will learn here that some patients who complain of hearing loss actually have normal auditory function or less hearing loss than an audiogram suggests. We will begin with a discussion of false or exaggerated hearing loss. Audiologists occasionally encounter children or adults who appear to have a hearing loss, yet the test results don't quite make sense. Comprehensive diagnostic assessment of patients with false hearing loss inevitably reveals normal auditory function. You will discover in this chapter that there are different explanations for false hearing loss. Audiologists can play an important role in helping these patients who do not really have a hearing loss.

Patients with exaggerated hearing loss are also quite interesting. We will discuss in this chapter the reasons why someone would exaggerate hearing loss and how audiologists accurately describe auditory function in such patients.

CHAPTER FOCUS *Concluded*

Every audiologist sees patients who complain about hearing annoying sounds like ringing or cricket sounds. Tinnitus is a major health problem. In reading this chapter you will appreciate the valuable role that audiologists play in helping people with bothersome tinnitus. You'll learn about the causes of tinnitus and why tinnitus is so distressing for some patients. We'll also discuss techniques and strategies for accurate diagnosis and effective management of patients with bothersome tinnitus.

Toward the end of the chapter we will focus on patients who cannot tolerate the loudness of everyday sounds. Hyperacusis is a very serious problem for some children and adults. Building on your new knowledge of tinnitus, you will discover an audiologist can greatly improve the quality of life for patients with hyperacusis.

False or Exaggerated Hearing Loss

Not all patients with apparent hearing loss have dysfunction somewhere in the auditory system. Audiologists sometimes encounter patients who complain of a hearing loss, but careful and comprehensive assessment fails to document an anatomical or physiological explanation for the hearing loss. The phrase **false hearing loss** is used to describe this clinical finding.

In some cases, behavioral test results may initially suggest a hearing loss that is greater than the patient's actual hearing loss. That is, a patient willingly or unconsciously exaggerates or enhances the extent of the hearing loss. This condition is referred to as **exaggerated hearing loss**. Audiologists often refer to false or exaggerated hearing loss as **pseudohypacusis**. You've already encountered the root *cusis,* meaning hearing. Broken down, the rather unusual word *pseudohypacusis* means false decrease in hearing.

Published reports of auditory findings in patients with false and exaggerated hearing loss date back to the early years of formal hearing assessment (Dixon & Newby, 1959; Doerfler & Stewart, 1946; Martin, 1946). In the 1950s and 1960s identification and diagnosis of the problem remained challenging because hearing was assessed only with test procedures that required a behavioral response from the patient. A number of studies during this era described the rather unique patterns of behavioral test findings we now associate with false and exaggerated hearing loss (Berk & Feldman, 1958; Carhart, 1961; Goldstein, 1966; Harris, 1958; Lehrer, Hirschenfang, Miller, & Radpour, 1964; Rintelmann & Harford, 1963).

Even today false or exaggerated hearing loss is not always identified immediately when patients are evaluated in a clinical setting. Failure to promptly diagnose a false hearing loss leads to an incorrect assumption of sensorineural auditory dysfunction. Failure to recognize exaggerated hearing loss leads to an inaccurate definition of the degree of hearing loss. In either case, the result often results in mismanagement of the patient and inappropriate allocation of healthcare resources (Peck, 2011). We will begin this chapter with a review of false and exaggerated hearing loss, with an emphasis on techniques for prompt and accurate diagnosis of auditory function as well as appropriate strategies for effective management.

Terminology

There is no consensus or agreement on the preferred term for apparent hearing loss that is not due to actual dysfunction in the auditory system (Peck, 2011). Terminology is somewhat confusing, often inaccurate, and frequently debated by hearing healthcare professionals. Terms are interpreted and used inconsistently by different audiologists. The problem with terminology probably stems from the diverse nature of the disorder. In other words, no single term appropriately or accurately describes the condition for all patients with false or exaggerated hearing loss.

Numerous terms have accumulated over the years since formal hearing testing began early in the twentieth century (Peck, 2011). You will begin to appreciate from the following brief review why hearing healthcare professionals cannot agree on a single most appropriate term.

Pseudohypacusis. Audiologists most often use the term *pseudohypacusis* in referring to the diverse collection of patients with false or exaggerated hearing loss. The term has some drawbacks. The meaning of *pseudohypa*cusis is not always clear even to healthcare professionals. Also, the term implies that the hearing loss shown on an audiogram is false when it may be an exaggeration of an existing hearing loss.

Nonorganic Hearing Loss. The phrase **nonorganic hearing loss** is popular among audiologists in referring to patients with false or exaggerated hearing loss. It is quite accurate for patients with an apparent hearing loss that is not confirmed by comprehensive diagnostic assessment. The phrase *nonorganic hearing loss* implies that there is no anatomical or physiological abnormality in the auditory system. This descriptor is not appropriate, however, for patients who actually do have a sensory hearing loss, while hearing test results suggest a greater degree of hearing problem. These patients do have an organic or physiological explanation for some of their hearing loss. A common example of this type of patient is someone with a history of noise exposure whose hearing testing initially shows severe hearing loss, while further assessment confirms a lesser degree of hearing loss.

Functional Hearing Loss. **Functional hearing loss** is another common phrase that is sometimes used interchangeably with nonorganic hearing loss. The phrase implies abnormal hearing test results with no apparent physiological or anatomical basis. This phrase shares several limitations with the phrase nonorganic hearing loss. Why use "hearing loss" if auditory function is entirely normal? Also, functional hearing loss implies normal auditory function, yet the patient may actually have a true or organic hearing loss that is less than the degree indicated by behavioral hearing tests.

Malingering. Patients who are feigning or faking a hearing loss are often referred to as **malingerers** by audiologists and other hearing healthcare professionals. A malingering patient is assumed to be intentionally and deliberately producing false hearing test results, often for personal monetary gain. The gain may be financial compensation for hearing loss allegedly caused by an accident, related to work in a noisy setting, or acquired during military service. In some cases, the motivation for falsification of hearing loss is to avoid some activity the patient considers undesirable. The term *malingerer* has a very negative connotation. It essentially implies that the patient is untrustworthy and a liar (Peck, 2011). With rare exceptions, it is best to avoid use of the terms *malingering* and *malingerer* in referring to patients with apparent false or exaggerated hearing loss.

Psychogenic Hearing Loss. The phrase **psychogenic hearing loss** is no longer commonly used. It implies a documentable psychological cause for the hearing loss. Related terms are *conversion disorder involving hearing loss* or *hysterical deafness,* both of which implicate a serious psychological impairment that is manifested as a hearing loss. Each of these terms describes a person who is not consciously or willingly feigning a hearing loss or exaggerating a true hearing loss. Rather, the patient is sincerely convinced that he or she has a hearing impairment. One could argue that only professionals with formal education and training in psychology or psychiatry are qualified to make the diagnosis of psychogenic hearing loss, a conversion disorder, or hysterical deafness (Peck, 2011).

Erroneous Hearing Loss. **Erroneous hearing loss** is another phrase introduced to describe "an apparent hearing loss without any organic disorder or with insufficient pathological evidence to explain the extent of the hearing loss" (Martin & Clark, 2012, p. 354). This phrase avoids the limitations associated with the older terms we've just reviewed.

Risk Factors

You have already been introduced to risk factors for hearing loss due to etiologies involving the external, middle, or inner ear. A good example is the rather lengthy list of 2007 Joint Committee on Infant Hearing indicators for infant hearing loss. You also learned that information obtained from a thorough patient history sometimes suggests the possibility of a specific etiology or type of hearing loss. A thorough patient history is also useful in identifying patients who are at risk for false or exaggerated hearing loss. A short list of risk factors includes:

- A history of accidental injury, with representation by an attorney
- A history of noise exposure, with an attempt to secure financial compensation for hearing loss
- Sudden onset of hearing loss with no clear diagnosis
- Ongoing psychiatric care, with complaint of hearing loss
- A history of physical, sexual, or emotional abuse, especially in children
- Unexplained unilateral or bilateral hearing loss, particularly in adolescent girls

As the list suggests, there is no singular profile for patients with false or exaggerated hearing loss (Drake, Makielski, McDonald-Bell, & Atcheson, 1995; Holenweg & Kompis, 2010; Psarommatis et al., 2009; Riedner & Efros, 1995).

Assessment of Patients with False or Exaggerated Hearing Loss

Test Battery Approach. The test battery approach for diagnosis of hearing loss generally works very well for early identification and accurate diagnosis of false or exaggerated hearing loss. Figure 15.1 shows an evidence-based approach for the diagnosis and management of false or exaggerated hearing loss. We will now follow the flow chart, beginning with review of information from the patient history. The chief complaint is invariably a hearing loss. Sometimes the referral source provides a hint about possible false or exaggerated hearing loss. Examples would include a lawyer representing a patient or an audiologist who reports inconsistent test findings on a previous hearing assessment.

Answers to the first questions in an adult patient history often provide a clue as to the possibility of a false or exaggerated hearing loss. For example, an audiologist asking the question "When did you first notice your hearing loss, Mr. Johnson?" receives the response "I noticed the hearing loss immediately after a loud bang in the warehouse where I work" or "The hearing loss began when my car was rear-ended as I was driving home from work last Tuesday."

Clues for children with false or exaggerated hearing loss are rarely so obvious. The history may include risk factors as listed above. An audiologist is more likely to obtain a detailed history from parents after a comprehensive hearing assessment shows evidence of false or exaggerated hearing loss. Risk factors indicating the possibility of false or exaggerated hearing loss guide the selection of procedures for the test battery. The inclusion of objective hearing tests in the initial assessment of a patient with possible false or exaggerated hearing loss is important to assure prompt and accurate diagnosis.

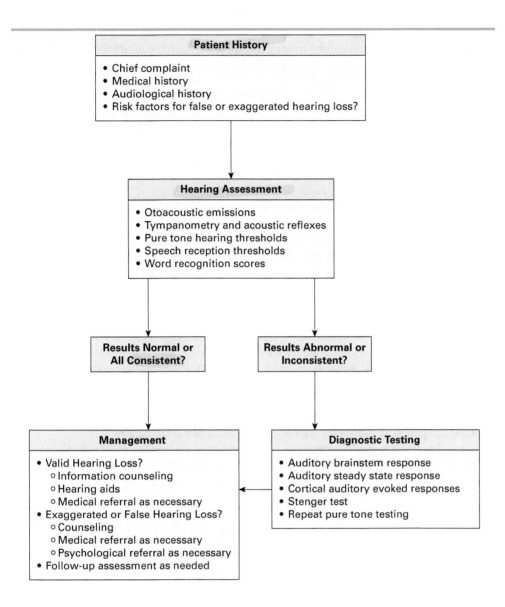

FIGURE 15.1

Flowchart for assessment and management of false or exaggerated hearing loss (pseudohypacusis).

We will now consider information in the box labeled "Hearing Assessment" in Figure 15.1. You will notice that objective tests like otoacoustic emissions and acoustic immittance measures are listed before pure tone audiometry. A finding of normal otoacoustic emissions is not consistent with most forms of hearing loss, especially those resulting from exposure to excessive noise.

Otoacoustic emissions play a vital role in the early detection and diagnosis of false or exaggerated hearing loss (Balatsouras, 2003; Dhar & Hall, 2012; Holenweg & Kompis, 2010; Musiek, Bornstein, & Rintelmann, 1995). Audiologists immediately consider the possibility of a false or exaggerated hearing loss in patients with normal otoacoustic emissions who then yield abnormal hearing thresholds during pure tone testing.

Other objective procedures like acoustic reflexes and auditory evoked responses are also important for efficient and accurate estimation of hearing status in patients with false or exaggerated hearing loss (Gelfand & Silman, 1993; Hall, 2007; Hall & Swanepoel, 2010).

Acoustic reflex threshold measurement with broadband noise stimulation is particularly helpful in distinguishing between normal hearing and some degree of hearing loss, as reviewed in Chapter 8. Acoustic reflex thresholds for broadband noise stimulation are usually higher than 80 dB HL for persons with hearing loss.

Test Indicators of False or Exaggerated Hearing Loss. Comprehensive audiological assessment typically reveals multiple clues or "red flags" that raise the suspicion of false or exaggerated hearing loss. Some of the more common suspicious findings are listed in Table 15.1. Certain combinations of test findings are not logically explained by dysfunction in any region of the auditory system. The pattern of results is simply not compatible with a true hearing loss. A false or exaggerated hearing loss must be considered.

No result for a single test analyzed in isolation leads to the diagnosis of false or exaggerated hearing loss. Indeed, abnormal findings for any one of the hearing tests are generally consistent with the presence of a true hearing loss that reflects an abnormality in the auditory system. A consistent pattern of abnormal findings for each of the tests confirms a true or valid hearing loss and usually leads to a description of the type and degree of hearing loss. The diagnosis of a valid hearing loss leads to management options like those we reviewed in Chapters 13 and 14.

Illustrative Case. Let's consider audiological indicators of false or exaggerated hearing loss for a 55-year-old adult seeking compensation for a hearing loss. He works at a commercial vehicle repair shop. The patient claims his onset of hearing loss occurred when he was exposed to an accidental explosion of a large truck tire. Figure 15.2 shows the patient's initial audiogram. Pure tone hearing test results suggest a moderate 50 to 60 dB hearing loss bilaterally, with thresholds quite similar for all test frequencies. Several findings, however, raise the suspicion that pure tone thresholds are not an accurate reflection of hearing status.

You will notice a large discrepancy between the pure tone average of 58 dB HL in each ear and the speech reception thresholds of 25 dB HL in the right ear and 30 dB HL in the left

TABLE 15.1 Indicators for false or exaggerated hearing loss based on patterns of hearing test findings.	
	• The patient's ability to carry on an informal conversation seems better than expected based on the audiogram
	• Inconsistent and unreliable pure tone hearing threshold levels
	• Absence of cross-hearing (crossover of test signals to nontest ear) in cases of total unilateral nonorganic hearing loss
	• The pure tone average (PTA) exceeds the speech reception threshold SRT by more than 10 dB, e.g., PTA is 50 dB HL and SRT is only 30 dB HL
	• Good performance on word recognition tests at an intensity level near pure tone hearing thresholds or repetition of any words at an intensity level that is better than pure tone thresholds
	• Otoacoustic emissions findings are normal or better than expected for the patient's degree of hearing loss
	• Acoustic reflexes are recorded at normal levels (85 dB or better) even with a broadband noise signal
	• Positive finding on the Stenger test
	• Positive finding on the Lombard test
	• Auditory thresholds estimated with the auditory brainstem response (ABR) or other auditory evoked responses are normal or considerably better than those for pure tone audiometry

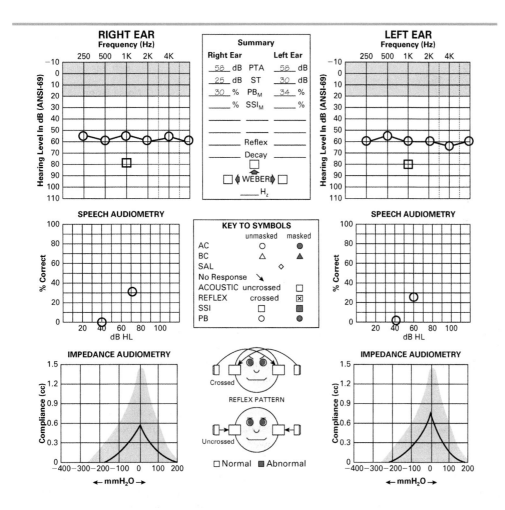

FIGURE 15.2

Audiogram for a 55-year-old male who was seeking monetary compensation for a self-reported hearing loss. Distortion product otoacoustic emissions findings for the patient are shown in Figure 15.3. Discrepancies among test findings raise the suspicion of false or exaggerated hearing loss (pseudohypacusis) as described in the text.

ear. It is not possible for a patient to accurately repeat spondee words presented an intensity level more than 25 dB better (lower) than the best pure tone hearing thresholds in the speech frequency region. In fact, a patient with a true hearing loss of 50 to 60 dB wouldn't even hear speech at an intensity level of 25 to 30 dB HL. Also, word recognition scores are remarkably good (30 to 34% correct) when testing is conducted at an intensity level within about 10 dB of the patient's alleged pure tone thresholds.

Concern about the validity of the audiogram is confirmed by findings on two objective auditory tests. As shown in Figure 15.2, acoustic reflex thresholds for a 1000-Hz tonal stimulus are recorded at an intensity level of 80 dB HL, as they would be in a person with normal hearing sensitivity. Figure 15.3 shows distortion product otoacoustic emissions findings for the patient. Amplitudes for otoacoustic emissions for both ears were well within normal limits for test frequencies up to 4000 Hz. Normal otoacoustic emissions are not consistent with noise-induced hearing loss due to cochlear and specifically outer hair cell dysfunction.

An audiologist must rule out operator errors, technical problems, and other explanations for an invalid hearing loss before considering the possibility of false or exaggerated hearing loss. Explanations for invalid hearing test results were reviewed earlier in Chapter 4. Examples of technical problems with equipment include defective earphones or earphone cables or earphones that are not properly plugged into an audiometer or sound booth panel.

FIGURE 15.3

Distortion product otoacoustic emissions (DPOAEs) for a 55-year-old male who was seeking monetary compensation for a self-reported hearing loss. Normal DPOAE findings are consistent with hearing sensitivity within normal limits. The patient's audiogram is shown in Figure 15.2.

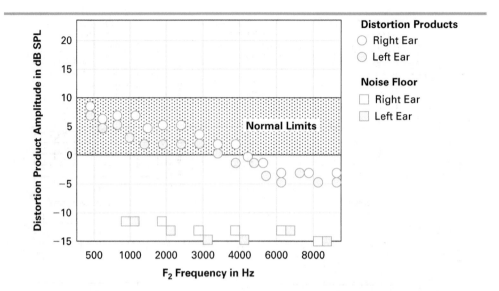

Listener variables that affect hearing test results include low motivation, attention deficits, fatigue, depressed cognitive functioning, anxiety, and medications affecting mental functioning. False or exaggerated hearing loss is considered only after these other explanations for invalid hearing test results have been eliminated.

Diagnosis of False or Exaggerated Hearing Loss. Diagnosis of false or exaggerated hearing loss is made with a comprehensive test battery consisting of behavioral and objective test procedures. This step is shown in the lower right portion of Figure 15.1. Discrepancies in the initial hearing test findings often confirm the likelihood of a false hearing loss or an exaggerated hearing loss. The purpose of diagnostic testing is to prove that a person with false hearing loss in fact has normal hearing sensitivity and normal auditory function. Diagnostic testing confirms actual hearing thresholds for a person with an exaggerated hearing loss.

Diagnostic testing often consists of objective measures of hearing thresholds. We reviewed objective hearing tests in Chapters 8 and 9. The same tests used to estimate hearing thresholds in infants and young children are well suited for objective assessment of auditory function in persons of any age who may have false or exaggerated hearing loss. In past years, several behavioral hearing tests were developed specifically for the evaluation of false or exaggerated hearing loss (Peck, 2011). These behavioral tests have been replaced with more accurate objective test procedures.

Audiologists still employ one behavioral test for false or exaggerated hearing loss. The **Stenger test** is used for evaluation of patients with unilateral hearing loss or when there is considerably greater hearing loss (e.g., > 25 dB) in one ear than the other. The test is named for the Stenger principle: When two tones of the same frequency are presented to both ears, a person hears only the tone that is perceived to be louder.

A two-channel audiometer is needed to perform the Stenger test. The results of pure tone hearing testing are generally available when the Stenger test is performed. If not, hearing thresholds for the test tone must first be measured for each ear. The patient is instructed to respond whenever he or she hears the tone by pressing a button or raising a hand. The Stenger test begins with the presentation of the tone to the "better-hearing ear" at an intensity level 10 dB above the threshold for the tone. Following the patient's response to the tone, the same tone is presented to the other ear at an intensity level 10 dB below the patient's hearing threshold on the audiogram. The patient will not respond to the tone if the intensity level is really below hearing threshold, but the patient may also not respond because he or she is feigning the hearing loss.

Next, the two steps are combined. That is, a tone is presented 10 dB above threshold for the better hearing ear at the same time it is presented to the "poorer" hearing ear at an intensity level 10 dB below threshold. The patient with a true hearing loss in the poorer ear will respond to the tone because it is clearly heard in the better-hearing ear. A patient with a false or exaggerated hearing loss in the "poorer" hearing ear does not respond. The patient hears the tone heard more loudly in the ear with the false or exaggerated hearing loss. However, the patient doesn't acknowledge hearing the sound in the ear with the false or exaggerated hearing loss. The patient's lack of response with stimulation of both ears is referred to as a "positive Stenger test."

The Stenger test process can continue with presentation of tones at various frequencies and at progressively lower intensity levels, even at 0 dB, in the "poorer" ear. In the interest of minimizing test time and increasing test accuracy, a positive Stenger test at a single frequency can be followed with estimation of hearing thresholds using an objective test procedure like the auditory brainstem response or the auditory steady state response. These techniques were reviewed in Chapter 9.

Management of False or Exaggerated Hearing Loss

Diagnosis Leads to Management. Management of false or exaggerated hearing loss is represented in the lower left portion of Figure 15.1. Intervention strategies for individual patients vary considerably, depending on the underlying explanation for hearing loss. Management may also differ for patients with a false hearing loss who really have normal hearing sensitivity from that for patients with an exaggerated version of an actual hearing loss. Management often goes beyond the scope of audiology practice. Patients with false or exaggerated hearing loss often require professional counseling, including the services of a psychologist or psychiatrist.

Management is no less important for false or exaggerated hearing loss than for other etiologies of hearing loss. This point is made well by James Peck in a recent book on the topic (Peck, 2011): Audiologists should actively manage patients with false or exaggerated hearing loss. It is important to consider psychosocial problems as an explanation for the "hearing loss." As Peck notes, in patients with false or exaggerated hearing loss an audiologist must assess or initiate assessment of "psychosocial problems in order to best manage the situation" (Peck, 2011, p. 192).

Recent clinical research confirms the serious consequences of mismanagement of children who are misdiagnosed as hearing impaired (Holenweg & Kompis, 2010; Peck, 2011). In combination, these studies confirm that the failure to document normal hearing sensitivity in children with false hearing loss may lead to expensive and unnecessary diagnostic procedures, such as blood tests and brain scans, and potentially dangerous inappropriate intervention with hearing aids, medical treatment with anti-inflammatory drugs like steroids, and even exploratory surgical procedures.

These published studies and clinical experience also confirm that the availability of accurate diagnostic test findings can in some patients facilitate resolution of the false or exaggerated hearing loss. Following an audiologist's or physician's clear and complete explanation of normal findings for objective hearing tests to the patient and family members, follow-up behavioral hearing testing often yields consistent and valid normal findings, including a normal audiogram.

Tinnitus

Tinnitus is sound heard by a person that is not produced by an external sound. In fact, the perception of tinnitus is usually most prominent in a quiet environment. Tinnitus is sometimes defined as a "phantom auditory perception." The word *phantom* means the perception of tinnitus is not a typical response to a sound in the environment. However, the perception of tinnitus is real and the result of activation of different regions in the brain.

The word *tinnitus* is derived from the Latin word for "ringing." However, a variety of types of sounds are commonly heard as tinnitus. Table 15.2 lists some of the more common tinnitus sounds that patients describe. The type of sound a patient hears isn't related to the diagnosis of tinnitus, the severity of the tinnitus, or its impact on quality of life. For example, one patient who hears a ringing-type sound will not express any concern. He may acknowledge that most his friends also hear ringing sounds some of the time. The ringing sound doesn't interfere with the patient's daily activities or sleep and has no impact on his quality of life. Another patient with ringing-type tinnitus may feel that the sound is unbearable. The tinnitus interferes with all daily activities as well as sleep. In short, the ringing sound is strongly affecting the patient's quality of life.

Research dating back fifty years strongly suggests that tinnitus is a normal experience. In 1953, an otologist named Heller and an audiologist named Bergman carried out a classic study with eighty subjects who had normal hearing and no evidence of ear disease (Heller & Bergman, 1953). Subjects were placed for a short time in a very quiet sound-treated environment and asked to describe what they heard. According to the researchers, "Audible tinnitus was experienced by 94% of the 80 apparently normally hearing adults when placed in a testing situation having an ambient noise level no greater than 18 decibels." Heller and Bergman (1953) concluded from their study that "The kinds of head noises described by patients with impaired hearing as a symptom associated with their deafness and those sounds described by normally hearing healthy adults, elicited while in a sound-proof room, appear to be similar . . . . Tinnitus, which is subaudible, may be a physiological phenomenon in an intact auditory apparatus" (Heller & Bergman, 1953, p. 82).

TABLE 15.2
Types of tinnitus noted in 120 patients undergoing diagnostic assessment at a tinnitus and hyperacusis center. Some patients reported more than one type of tinnitus.

Description of Tinnitus	Number of Patients
Ringing	47
Cricket sound	21
High-pitched tonal sound	17
Hissing	13
Humming	13
Roaring	6
Static noise	5
Buzzing	4
Pulsing	4
Clicking	2
Frying sound	2
Other	7

L E A D E R S   A N D   L U M I N A R I E S

Rich Tyler

Richard Tyler earned his bachelor's and master's degrees at the University of Western Ontario and his PhD in psychoacoustics at the University of Iowa. He worked initially at the Institute of Hearing Research in the United Kingdom. Dr. Tyler is now a professor in the Department of Otolaryngology at the University of Iowa. He has an international reputation for his research and publications on the topics of tinnitus and cochlear implants. Dr. Tyler sees tinnitus and hyperacusis patients weekly and also hosts an annual Tinnitus Treatment Workshop. He edited the first textbook on tinnitus, entitled *The Tinnitus Handbook: A Clinician's Guide,* the book *Tinnitus Treatment: Clinical Protocols,* and a self-help guide entitled *The Consumer Handbook on Tinnitus.* Based on Dr. Tyler's testimony, the Workers Compensation Code in the state of Iowa was changed, permitting compensation of workers with tinnitus and/or hyperacusis independent of hearing loss. Dr. Tyler has served on committees reviewing tinnitus, including those of the World Health Organization and the Institute of Medicine, as well as a Veteran's Administration committee attempting to increase awareness of the disabilities caused by tinnitus and hyperacusis.

In other words, in a very quiet environment even persons with entirely normal hearing and auditory function may hear sounds that resemble tinnitus. Unfortunately, some patients perceive tinnitus as a loud sound that is bothersome and may affect quality of life.

A Symptom, Not a Disease

Tinnitus is not a disease itself but, rather, the symptom of a disease or disorder (Baguley, 2002; Hall & Haynes, 2000; Jastreboff, Gray, & Gold, 1996; Hall, 2004). We are all familiar with symptoms of disease. For example, pain and fever are common symptoms of many different types of illness. Tinnitus can be a symptom of systemic health problems (such as high blood pressure) that are not directly related to hearing loss. Tinnitus is most often a symptom of diseases or disorders that involve the inner ear. You learned in Chapter 11 about diseases and disorders affecting inner ear function as well as some drugs that can cause hair cell damage in the inner ear. Tinnitus may also occur when a patient takes certain medications, including ototoxic drugs that may affect cochlear functioning. The two most common etiologies for tinnitus in patients seen in an audiology clinic are noise-induced hearing loss and age-related hearing loss. Fortunately, neither etiology is a disease.

Explanations for Tinnitus

Formal investigation of tinnitus dates back over eighty years (Wegel, 1931). Before the 1990s, however, little was known about the causes or mechanisms of tinnitus. The general connection between hearing loss and tinnitus was well appreciated, but it didn't explain a perplexing clinical observation. Some persons with severe hearing loss are not bothered at all by tinnitus. However, other persons experience very bothersome tinnitus even though they have very mild hearing loss or even normal hearing sensitivity. Furthermore, there was in the past no clear explanation for extreme intolerance to sound reported by some persons with normal hearing sensitivity.

Intensive laboratory research with animal models and clinical research with patients who experience tinnitus has led to improved understanding of the mechanisms of tinnitus, that is, the anatomical and physiological processes that underlie the perception of bothersome sound (Baguley, 2002; Baguley & Andersson, 2007; Eggermont & Roberts, 2004; Jastreboff, Gray, & Gold, 1996; Hall & Haynes, 2002; Lockwood, Salvi, & Burkard, 2003).

Current Explanation for Tinnitus. The origin for tinnitus is almost always in the cochlea. Dysfunction of cochlear hair cells disrupts the stimulation of the auditory nerve and central auditory pathways and centers (Baguley, 2002; Eggermont & Roberts, 2004; Kaltenbach, 2007, 2011; Norena & Farley, 2012). The technical term for this process is *peripheral deafferentiation*. You learned in Chapter 3 that the afferent pathways in the auditory system carry information from the ear and auditory nerve to the brain. The reduction of input to the nervous system produces a release of excessive amounts of excitatory neurotransmitters in the central nervous system. The result is increased sensitivity of the brain to sound, even the "phantom" tinnitus sounds.

Over the course of weeks and months after the onset of cochlear damage, certain auditory regions in the brainstem begin to reorganize so that neurons are active even when there is no external sound stimulation. As a result, the patient hears sounds in the absence of any external stimulus, especially in quiet settings.

The foregoing explanation accounts for the persistent tinnitus sounds of many persons. Additional information is needed to explain why a proportion of patients are extremely bothered by tinnitus. In the 1980s, an auditory neuroscientist named Pawel Jastreboff developed a model for tinnitus that included an explanation for the emotional and fearful response some patients have to tinnitus (Jastreboff, Gray, & Gold, 1996; Jastreboff & Jastreboff, 2000). Tinnitus in some patients triggers activity in the *limbic regions* of the brain that are involved in the emotional response to sound and the *autonomic regions* of the brain associated with the "flight or fight" response to danger sounds. You were introduced in Chapter 3 to these interesting and important parts of the brain.

Since its original description, the *neurophysiological model* of tinnitus proposed by Jastreboff has been supported by research findings, including brain fMRI studies of tinnitus patients (Lockwood et al., 1998).

The anatomic and physiological explanations for tinnitus just summarized are admittedly complex. However, an understanding of the causes of tinnitus is necessary for effective management of this commonly encountered condition.

Tinnitus Is a Common and Serious Health Problem

According to the American Tinnitus Association (ATA), approximately 10 million adult Americans seek medical attention for tinnitus each year. Tinnitus is debilitating for an estimated 2 million Americans. Troublesome tinnitus is far more common in adults than in children (Baguley et al., 2012).

Debilitating tinnitus has a major affect on quality of life and interferes with daily activities, such as work, social functions, and even sleep. At the extreme, some patients with tinnitus are so distressed that they feel life is no longer worth living. A small proportion of patients with troublesome tinnitus have suicidal ideations. Sadly, there are documented cases of suicide among this group of patients.

Table 15.3 summarizes typical tinnitus patient complaints and highlights the impact of tinnitus on quality of life. You will recognize some of the characteristics from our review in Chapter 14 of psychosocial disturbances associated with hearing loss and auditory processing disorders. Debilitating tinnitus often leads to a sense of hopelessness. Professional intervention is essential for patients with debilitating tinnitus. Audiologists provide the intervention, with support in some cases from other health professionals like psychologists and physicians.

It is relevant to point out here that tinnitus is a very common problem among military personnel and veterans, especially those with combat experiences and exposure to blast injuries (Henry,

- Extreme and constant fatigue
- Restlessness
- Irritability
- Anger
- Fear
- Guilt about "causing the problem"
- Difficulty concentrating
- Nervousness
- Excessive crying
- Absence of pleasures or joys
- Persistently sad mood
- Depression
- Sleeping problems, including sleep deprivation
- Hopelessness—"life is not worth living"

TABLE 15.3
Characteristics of persons with bothersome tinnitus.

Zaugg, Myers, & Kendall, 2010). Tinnitus is among the top reasons for disability and compensation for military veterans and closely related to post-traumatic stress disorder or PTSD (Fagelson, 2007).

Diagnosis of Tinnitus

Figure 15.4 summarizes the major steps in assessment and management of tinnitus. The process begins with a complete patient history, with an emphasis on factors contributing to tinnitus and quantifying the impact of tinnitus on the patient's life. One of the first goals is to determine whether the patient has a disease that includes tinnitus as a symptom. Some physicians refer patients with tinnitus to audiologists after medical examination of the patient has ruled out the presence of a disease. Other patients come directly to an audiologist because of their concerns about tinnitus or hearing loss.

If a patient with tinnitus has not yet undergone an examination by a physician, audiologists usually make a medical referral to rule out disease as the cause. Audiologists work closely with otolaryngologists and other medical specialists in the assessment and management of tinnitus. Fortunately, over 80% of patients with tinnitus show no evidence of disease or pathology on a medical examination (Hall & Haynes, 2000; Hall & Mueller, 1997). As already noted, tinnitus in the majority of patients is not due to disease or pathology but, rather, secondary to auditory dysfunction related to noise exposure and/or aging.

Drugs and Tinnitus. The history must include a review of prescription and over-the-counter medications the patient is taking. Over 100 different drugs have tinnitus as a possible side effect (DiSogra, 2008). In Chapter 12 you learned that some potentially ototoxic drugs cause hearing loss. The same drugs may also be associated with the onset of tinnitus. The association between tinnitus and most other non-ototoxic drugs is not strong and occurs in less than 3% of those who take the drug. Drugs rarely associated with tinnitus tend to alter the perception of existing tinnitus rather than cause it.

One exception is a common over-the-counter drug. Aspirin is among the drugs that can produce the perception of tinnitus. It is important to stress here that audiologists do not make

 WebWatch

Tinnitus? There's an app for that! You will find dozens of tinnitus-related applications online. Some can be used to describe a wide variety of tinnitus sounds while others with names like "sleep sound," "soothing sounds," and "quiet noise" are designed for self-guided tinnitus therapy.

FIGURE 15.4

Flowchart for assessment and management of tinnitus.

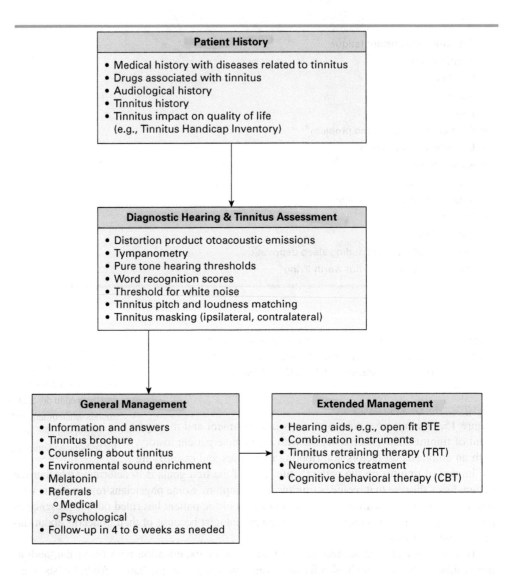

Patient History

- Medical history with diseases related to tinnitus
- Drugs associated with tinnitus
- Audiological history
- Tinnitus history
- Tinnitus impact on quality of life
  (e.g., Tinnitus Handicap Inventory)

Diagnostic Hearing & Tinnitus Assessment

- Distortion product otoacoustic emissions
- Tympanometry
- Pure tone hearing thresholds
- Word recognition scores
- Threshold for white noise
- Tinnitus pitch and loudness matching
- Tinnitus masking (ipsilateral, contralateral)

General Management

- Information and answers
- Tinnitus brochure
- Counseling about tinnitus
- Environmental sound enrichment
- Melatonin
- Referrals
  ○ Medical
  ○ Psychological
- Follow-up in 4 to 6 weeks as needed

Extended Management

- Hearing aids, e.g., open fit BTE
- Combination instruments
- Tinnitus retraining therapy (TRT)
- Neuromonics treatment
- Cognitive behavioral therapy (CBT)

recommendations about medications to any patients. That is not within the scope of audiology practice. Audiologists typically alert the patient's family physician about the possible link between tinnitus and medications.

Impact of Tinnitus on Quality of Life. One main objective in the patient history is to document the impact of tinnitus on quality of life. History forms designed for use with patients who complain of tinnitus include various questions about daily activities. Examples include: "How would you rate the impact of the tinnitus on your life, using a scale of 0 to 10 with 0 being 'no effect' and 10 for 'my life is totally ruined'?" Or, "During a typical day what percentage of your waking hours are you aware of the tinnitus?"

A number of inventories or questionnaires are available for quantifying the impact of tinnitus on quality of life (Henry, Zaugg, Myers, & Kendall, 2010; Newman, Jacobson, & Spitzer, 1996; Tyler, 2005). The Tinnitus Handicap Inventory (THI) is one of more widely used questionnaires (Newman, Jacobson, & Spitzer, 1996). It consists of twenty-five questions that the patient answers with either "yes," "maybe," or "no." The questions fall into one of three categories. Twelve questions address the impact of tinnitus on day-to-day function. For example, "Because of your tinnitus do you have trouble falling to sleep at night?" Eight questions probe the emotional reaction the patient has to tinnitus. For example, "Does your tinnitus make you angry?" Five questions in the catastrophic category provide information about the patient's hopelessness and despair. For example, "Do you feel that you cannot escape your tinnitus?"

Tinnitus Handicap Inventory scores range from 0, indicating that tinnitus has no impact on quality of life, to 100, confirming that tinnitus is having a major impact on quality of life. Patients seeking services in an audiology clinic with expertise in tinnitus often have Tinnitus Handicap Inventory scores in the range of 40 to about 80 (Hall & Haynes, 2000).

Diagnostic Hearing Test Battery. The diagnostic test battery for assessment of patients with bothersome tinnitus is similar to the test battery used for comprehensive hearing testing of other patients. Figure 15.4 also summarizes important components of the test battery. Tympanometry is important in determining whether the patient has middle ear dysfunction that requires medical attention. Middle ear disorders often increase the perception of an existing tinnitus. Acoustic reflexes are not usually measured in the hearing assessment because testing involves the presentation of high-intensity sounds. Sensitivity or intolerance to loud sounds is quite common in patients with bothersome tinnitus.

The test battery includes pure tone audiometry and assessment of word recognition performance. Distortion product otoacoustic emissions are an important part of the test battery. For most patients the perception of tinnitus originates from dysfunction in the cochlea. Distortion product otoacoustic emission findings help to confirm the cochlear origin of tinnitus.

Tinnitus Evaluation. Evaluation of patients with bothersome tinnitus includes several measurements not included in a typical diagnostic test battery (Hall & Haynes, 2000; Hall & Mueller, 1997; Henry, Zaugg, Myers, & Kendall, 2010). The additional tests are listed in Figure 15.4. Audiologists determine the patient's threshold for broadband noise. The test battery also includes an estimation of the pitch and the loudness of a patient's tinnitus.

Finally, testing includes an estimation of the amount of broadband noise that is required to cover up or mask the patient's tinnitus under different conditions. For example, the patient is asked to report when tinnitus is no longer heard in one ear as the audiologist presents gradually increasing levels of broadband noise to the same ear. Then the process is repeated with the audiologist presenting broadband noise to the opposite ear.

Management of Tinnitus

The plan for management of tinnitus is based on the patient's history and results of a comprehensive diagnostic assessment of auditory function. Figure 15.4 includes a summary of steps for general management of most patients with bothersome tinnitus, and also options for more extended management as necessary.

General Management. Management usually begins immediately after diagnostic testing with an in-depth counseling session involving the patient and often one or more family members (Hall & Haynes, 2000; Henry, Dennis, & Schechter, 2005; Hall, 2004). The audiologist dispenses accurate and up-to-date information on tinnitus to the patient and family members. Audiologists often provide the patient and family with written information about tinnitus that includes accurate but simple explanations of the causes of tinnitus and the availability of effective treatment options. Figure 15.5 shows several informational brochures available from the American Tinnitus Association (ATA). The adage "Knowledge

 ClinicalConnection

You have read in the preceding chapter (14) about family-centered treatment for communication disorders, with the goal of empowering the patient and family to optimize rehabilitation. Clinical experience confirms that effective management of tinnitus and hyperacusis depends to a large extent on education of the patient and family members about the disorders.

FIGURE 15.5

Brochures for patient education about tinnitus available from the American Tinnitus Association (available online). Courtesy of American Tinnitus Association.

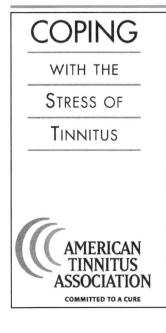

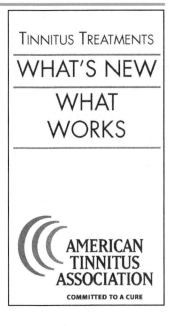

is power" is particularly relevant for patients with tinnitus and their families. You learned in Chapter 14 about the role of informational counseling in management of hearing loss. Counseling is a critical component in any strategy for management of patients with bothersome tinnitus.

Questions from the patient or family members are answered directly and honestly. Patients often have serious misconceptions about tinnitus that contribute to excessive anxiety and fear. It is normal for any person with a mysterious symptom to experience anxiety and fear until a proper diagnostic assessment offers an explanation for the symptom. Successful management of bothersome tinnitus depends to a large extent on minimizing or eliminating a patient's anxiety and fear about tinnitus.

Several other components in the general management of tinnitus were listed in Figure 15.4. Research shows that patients with bothersome tinnitus benefit from consistent exposure to soft and pleasant environmental sound (Henry, Dennis, & Schechter, 2005; Henry, Trune, Robb, & Jastreboff, 2007; Jastreboff, Gray & Gold, 1996; Jastreboff & Jastreboff, 2000). Environmental sound enrichment reduces the patient's perception of tinnitus. Relaxing background sound produced by environmental sound devices mixes in with the tinnitus sounds. Inexpensive sound devices are available at many different stores and from a variety of vendors online.

A variety of manufacturers also market ear-level sound devices designed for patients with bothersome tinnitus. Figure 15.6 shows an example of a small and discrete open-fit behind-the-ear device that produces sound that can be shaped and adjusted to meet the needs of a specific patient. The device resembles the open-fit hearing aids you learned about in Chapter 13.

 WebWatch

Information about tinnitus is readily available on the Internet. The websites for the American Academy of Audiology and the American Tinnitus Association are particularly useful. The American Academy of Audiology website includes a position statement on tinnitus and access to the Academy store that features a pamphlet written specifically for patients with bothersome tinnitus.

With constant exposure to uninteresting and unimportant sound, a person naturally begins to become less aware of the sound. We've all had the experience of gradually disregarding repetitive and unimportant background sounds like air conditioner noise, ticking clocks, and initially annoying environmental noise from traffic, trains, and airplanes. The technical term for this phenomenon is *habituation*. Over the course of weeks and months of consistent exposure to background sound, patients often report that they are less aware of tinnitus and the tinnitus is less bothersome.

Extended Management. Most patients with bothersome tinnitus respond very positively to the general management strategies just described. Figure 15.4 listed some other commonly recommended treatment options. Patients with tinnitus and hearing loss often receive considerable benefit from the use of hearing aids. Following appropriate counseling patients often find that hearing aids amplify sounds that are important for communication while at the same time minimizing perception of tinnitus sound (Del Bo & Ambrosetti, 2007; Surr, Montgomery, & Mueller, 1985; Trotter & Donaldson, 2008).

Several hearing aid manufacturers also now offer devices that combine amplification for hearing loss with the option of sound therapy for tinnitus. The combination devices allow an audiologist to manipulate aspects of the sound therapy so it is most effective in minimizing the perception of tinnitus while maximizing hearing and communication. Combination BTE hearing aid/tinnitus devices are available from multiple manufacturers.

A review of all available options for management of bothersome tinnitus is far beyond the scope of our discussion. Several tinnitus management techniques were listed toward the bottom of Figure 15.4. Books devoted to tinnitus and tinnitus management are listed at the end of this chapter. Review articles are also a concise source of information about tinnitus causes, assessment, and management (Henry, Dennis, & Schechter, 2005; Lockwood, Salvi, & Burkard, 2003). Research on effective techniques and strategies for management of tinnitus is ongoing. The American Tinnitus Association (available online) is a good source of information on current tinnitus research.

We will conclude this section on tinnitus with a case scenario. The following series of typical questions from a hypothetical patient and evidence-based answers from an experienced audiologist may help you appreciate the nature and value of a counseling session in the management of persons with bothersome tinnitus.

FIGURE 15.6

Ear-level sound device for use in management of persons with tinnitus and/or hyperacusis. Arrows point to small behind-the-ear sound device and tube leading to open fit dome in the external ear canal. Photo courtesy of Amplisound.

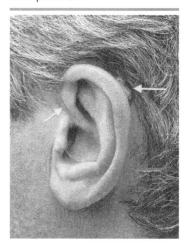

Case Scenario: Tinnitus

Patient: I'm very worried about my tinnitus.

Audiologist: Please tell me more about your concern.

Patient: Dr. Jones said there's nothing wrong with me, that I have normal hearing. Maybe he thinks I'm crazy!

Audiologist: Our very thorough diagnostic testing showed you do have a hearing loss, but only a slight problem hearing high-pitched sounds. The hearing loss is related to the exposure to loud sounds you described earlier. Our tests and the brain scan Dr. Jones ordered showed that the slight hearing loss is not caused by disease or pathology. In the first test room, we did a very sensitive test of how your ear works, an otoacoustic emissions procedure. Dr. Jones didn't perform this procedure. The test confirmed that there is a little damage to some of the delicate little hair cells in your inner ear shown in this figure [the audiologist shows the patient a graph of the ear]. It's a very common problem in men about your age and in people exposed often to loud noises. The slight damage to your inner ear is playing a role in causing your tinnitus.

Patient: Then I guess I'm not crazy.

Audiologist: I know you really hear the tinnitus sounds in your brain. Research with brain imaging techniques shows that when a person hears tinnitus, the hearing parts of the brain are activated, just like they are now while you are hearing my voice.

Patient: Dr. Jones said the tinnitus means I'm going to lose my hearing. I'm very worried about losing my hearing. If I lose my hearing, I won't be able to work. If I can't work, I won't be able to support my family. I have three young children. That will be a disaster for me. Am I going to lose my hearing?

Audiologist: No! You will not lose your hearing because of the tinnitus. I have no reason to suspect that your hearing will change, as long as you use ear protection devices whenever you're around loud sounds. That's what Dr. Jones meant when he advised you to "avoid being around noises." But you should try to avoid real quiet places, like the sound-treated room in this clinic room (chuckle). Always surround yourself with soft pleasant sounds. Whenever you are in a quiet place, like your living room or bedroom, you should use a machine that plays relaxing environmental sounds.

Patient: O.K. I guess there's nothing you can do for my tinnitus . . . I'll just have to live with it.

Audiologist: No, we can help you. Everyone with tinnitus can be helped. You should be very hopeful. There is no magic pill you can take for tinnitus. But today we will explain why the tinnitus is making you so anxious and concerned. Then we'll give you specific recommendations for how to reduce the perception of your tinnitus sound most of the time, maybe entirely. We have plenty of experience with the management of tinnitus just like yours. We'll also provide suggestions for how you can get better sleep at night. There are now a variety of techniques for management of tinnitus. I think our initial recommendations will be very helpful for you.

Patient: What kinds of techniques are you talking about?

Audiologist: We'll talk more about them in the next few minutes, but the first four things I will recommend are these. (1) Always surround yourself by soft and pleasant sound, like music or environmental sounds. You should buy a desktop sound device like this [the audiologist demonstrates operation of an actual sound device]. It costs about $25 or less. (2) Take a melatonin tablet before bedtime each night to reduce the tinnitus sounds and to help you sleep better. You can buy melatonin, a natural substance, over the counter in any drug store. Check with Dr. Jones to be sure he has no concerns about your taking melatonin. Recent studies show it's effective in reducing tinnitus and enhancing sleep. (3) Connect the desktop environmental sound device to a sound pillow [the audiologist connects the sound device to a sound pillow] to further reduce the tinnitus sounds and help you sleep. (4) Remember our discussion about how tinnitus affects many people and is not the symptom of a disease or pathology or anything that you need to be concerned about.

Patient: What if I try these techniques and my tinnitus is still really bothering me?

Audiologist: I'm quite sure you will find these simple techniques very helpful. However, if your tinnitus is still a problem for you in about a month, we'll talk about other strategies and treatment programs for the tinnitus.

Patient: Can you give me a few examples of these additional techniques?

Audiologist: Sure. First, you would benefit from consistent daily use of a tiny hearing aid type of tinnitus device (shown earlier in Figure 15.6) to help you hear high-pitched sounds more easily. The device would also reduce your awareness of your high-pitched tinnitus.

Second, if the tinnitus continues to be a problem for you, I will suggest that you consult with a psychologist who specializes in a technique called cognitive behavioral therapy (CBT). Studies of CBT have proven that it helps persons develop more positive attitudes about tinnitus. Finally, we'll talk more about two other longer-term treatment options. One is called Tinnitus Retraining Therapy and the other is Neuromonics Tinnitus Treatment. Either technique would gradually retrain your brain to no longer hear the tinnitus sounds. I'm not sure you will require one of these techniques, but they are available if you do.

Patient: I don't think I can remember everything you just told me.

Audiologist: Don't worry, I'm going to give you some written information to read about these tinnitus treatment options [the audiologist hands the patient a tinnitus educational pamphlet from the American Academy of Audiology]. I'll also summarize all of our discussions in a report that you will receive in the mail in a few days.

Patient's: Thank you for spending this time with my spouse and me today. No one has
Spouse explained tinnitus to us before. I think you really understand the effect of the tinnitus on my spouse's life—and mine.

Audiologist: I'm happy to help. Here's one of my business cards. Don't hesitate to contact me by email or call this telephone number if you have any questions or concerns after you leave the clinic today.

Counseling is remarkably effective in the management of tinnitus. Research comparing the impact of tinnitus on quality of life before and then six months after a single counseling session, with the implementation of several simple recommendations for management (included in the preceding patient-audiologist exchange), confirms that the majority of patients no longer consider tinnitus a serious problem. In other words, the tinnitus no longer has an important impact on their quality of life, even for patients who initially were debilitated by their tinnitus.

Hyperacusis

Hyperacusis is an abnormal intolerance to everyday sounds. The term first appeared in a publication as early as the 1930s (Perlman, 1938). For patients with hyperacusis, common sounds such as a telephone ringing or sounds produced by a hair dryer, vacuum cleaner, or a slamming door are often very annoying and almost unbearable. David Baguley and Gerhard Andersson succinctly and clearly define hyperacusis as "the experience of inordinate loudness of sound that most people tolerate well, associated with a component of distress" (Baguley & Andersson, 2007, p. 7). The term *hyperacusis* is somewhat confusing as it implies super or better-than-normal hearing. Most patients with hyperacusis have normal hearing sensitivity as determined with pure tone hearing testing, but hearing thresholds are rarely better than normal.

Hyperacusis Is a Symptom
Hyperacusis like tinnitus is a symptom of a variety of diseases and disorders. Table 15.4 lists some of them. Hyperacusis is a common characteristic of selected disorders like William's syndrome and persons with autism spectrum disorder (Baguley & Andersson, 2007; Hall, 1998). However, hyperacusis is not always a symptom in patients diagnosed with the health problems listed in Table 15.4. And, most patients who seek services from audiologists because of intolerance to loud sounds do not have any of the diseases or disorders. As with tinnitus, the onset of hyperacusis is sometimes associated with certain medications (DiSogra, 2008).

TABLE 15.4
Conditions associated
with hyperacusis.

- Central nervous system disorders including
  - Depression
  - Migraine
  - Chronic fatigue syndrome
  - Post-traumatic stress disorder (PTSD)
  - Ramsay-Hunt syndrome
  - Multiple sclerosis
- Lyme disease
- Facial paralysis
- William's syndrome
- Autism spectrum disorder
- Autoimmune disorders
- Selected medications

Related Terms

Three terms are used to describe other problems some patients experience with loud sounds. *Loudness recruitment* is an abnormally rapid growth of loudness that usually begins at a person's threshold for sound. It is directly related to cochlear dysfunction, specifically involving the outer hair cells. In contrast, patients with hyperacusis typically have normal cochlear function.

The second term is **phonophobia**, which refers to fear of sound or certain sounds. Patients with hyperacusis have difficulty tolerating loud sounds in general whereas patients with phonophobia experience a rather intense fear of certain sounds.

A third term, **misophonia**, is sometimes used to describe an extreme dislike of specific sounds (Jastreboff & Hazell, 2004; Jastreboff & Jastreboff, 2013). Patients with misophonia often describe with remarkably precision their displeasure with sounds such as lip-smacking

LEADERS AND LUMINARIES

David Baguley

David Baguley earned a master's degree in audiology at the University of Manchester, an MBA (Open University), and a PhD from the University of Cambridge in the United Kingdom. Dr. Baguley is the Head of Service, Audiology/Hearing Implants at Cambridge University Hospitals in the United Kingdom. He is also a fellow at Wolfson College, University of Cambridge, and Visiting Professor at Anglia Ruskin University, Cambridge, and at the University of Bristol. Dr. Baguley has over 120 peer-reviewed publications and has authored several books and many book chapters. He is a coauthor of a recent book entitled *Living with Tinnitus and Hyperacusis*.

Dr. Baguley is an internationally recognized expert and lecturer on tinnitus and hyperacusis. Through his writings and lectures, he has inspired innumerable audiologists to provide clinical services to patients with tinnitus and hyperacusis. Awards received by Dr. Baguley include the British Society of Audiology T. S. Littler Prize (1992), the American Academy of Audiology International Award in Hearing (2006), and the British Tinnitus Association Shapiro Prize (2005, 2008).

or chewing sounds produced by a family member. *Misophonia* is sometimes used instead of the term *phonophobia*.

Relation of Tinnitus and Hyperacusis

There are similarities between tinnitus and hyperacusis, but also a number of distinct differences. Involvement of the brain in the reaction to sound holds true for the two problems. Certain parts of the brain, such as the limbic system, play an important role in the reaction to sound for patients with tinnitus and hyperacusis. Cochlear function offers an example of a difference. Almost all patients with tinnitus have cochlear dysfunction and many have hearing loss, whereas most patients with hyperacusis have normal hearing sensitivity and normal cochlear function.

Up to one-half of persons with bothersome tinnitus describe the development of additional intolerance to environmental sounds (Baguley & Andersson, 2007; Hall, 1998; Hall & Haynes, 2000). However, audiologists regularly encounter children and adults with hyperacusis who have no complaints about tinnitus. Hyperacusis is the only concern for these patients.

Explanations for Hyperacusis

Hyperacusis has a physiological and a psychological basis (Baguley & Andersson, 2007; Marriage & Barnes, 1995). The brain explanations already described for hyperacusis are somewhat similar to those already reviewed for tinnitus (Baguley, 2003; Baguley & Andersson, 2007; Katzenell & Segal, 2001). Greater-than-normal excitation of the brain in response to sound is a common feature of both problems. In tinnitus patients and in hyperacusis patients the emotional response to sound involves activation of the limbic system and the fear of certain sounds reflects activation of the autonomic nervous system. However, the release of excitatory neurotransmitters in patients with hyperacusis is not due to cochlear dysfunction as it is in tinnitus. Instead, excitation and hyperactivity in the auditory regions of the brain is triggered by stress, anxiety, and/or fatigue.

Diagnosis of Hyperacusis

Patient History. We will now briefly review the steps in assessment of patients with the chief complaint of intolerance to loud sounds. You will notice clear similarities in the diagnostic processes for tinnitus and hyperacusis. Figure 15.7 summarizes major components of the patient history and the diagnostic test battery for hyperacusis patients. As with tinnitus, one of the first goals is to determine whether the patient has a disease that includes hyperacusis as a symptom. Patients with a history suggesting the possibility of a disease or disorder are generally referred to a medical specialist like an otolaryngologist or neurologist.

The patient history also includes questions about medications sometimes associated with hyperacusis. The patient is questioned about the kinds of sounds he or she finds annoying or uncomfortable and about sounds that are well tolerated. Finally, audiologists often attempt to quantify the impact of hyperacusis on quality of life. The Tinnitus Handicap Inventory described earlier can be adapted for patients with hyperacusis.

Diagnostic Hearing Test Battery. Hearing assessment for patients complaining of intolerance to sound includes the usual test procedures with slight modifications. Pure tone hearing thresholds are evaluated for conventional test frequencies but also for frequencies higher than 8000 Hz. Tympanometry is performed but acoustic reflex measurement is never performed. It is important to avoid the presentation of high-intensity and probably bothersome sounds to patients with hyperacusis.

Measurement of otoacoustic emissions is an important component of the test battery. Patients with hyperacusis typically express concern about possible damage to hearing with exposure to

FIGURE 15.7

Flowchart for assessment and management of hyperacusis.

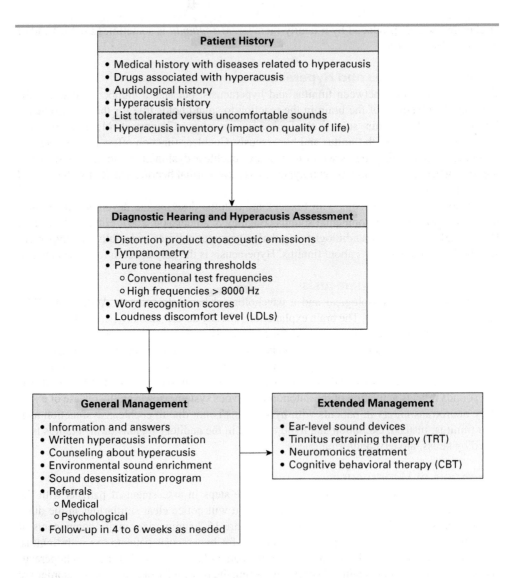

Patient History

- Medical history with diseases related to hyperacusis
- Drugs associated with hyperacusis
- Audiological history
- Hyperacusis history
- List tolerated versus uncomfortable sounds
- Hyperacusis inventory (impact on quality of life)

Diagnostic Hearing and Hyperacusis Assessment

- Distortion product otoacoustic emissions
- Tympanometry
- Pure tone hearing thresholds
  ○ Conventional test frequencies
  ○ High frequencies > 8000 Hz
- Word recognition scores
- Loudness discomfort level (LDLs)

General Management

- Information and answers
- Written hyperacusis information
- Counseling about hyperacusis
- Environmental sound enrichment
- Sound desensitization program
- Referrals
  ○ Medical
  ○ Psychological
- Follow-up in 4 to 6 weeks as needed

Extended Management

- Ear-level sound devices
- Tinnitus retraining therapy (TRT)
- Neuromonics treatment
- Cognitive behavioral therapy (CBT)

loud and annoying sounds. Some patients actually describe pain when they hear loud sounds. Documentation of normal otoacoustic emissions for test frequencies above 1000 Hz provides a patient with reassuring evidence that cochlear function is normal. Based on normal findings for otoacoustic emissions testing, an audiologist can explain to the patient that there is no reason for concern about damage to the ears or hearing from exposure to everyday sounds.

The measurement of loudness discomfort levels (LDLs) is the final step in the diagnostic process. You learned in Chapter 6 about the technique for estimating loudness discomfort level for tones and for speech. LDLs in dB HL provide quantification of a patient's intolerance to sound and means for evaluating the benefit of hyperacusis management.

Management of Hyperacusis

There are clear similarities in the management of patients with tinnitus and hyperacusis. The plan for management of hyperacusis, like tinnitus, is based on the patient's history and results of a comprehensive diagnostic assessment of auditory function. Also, counseling addressing the patient's specific concerns plays a critical role in the management of both types of auditory disorders. Figure 15.7 summarizes general and more extended or specialized management options for patients with hyperacusis.

General Management. Management begins with an in-depth counseling session about hyperacusis with the adult patient or with parents and sometimes other family members of pediatric patients. The audiologist explains that hyperacusis is a well-defined and not uncommon problem. Patients or parents of patients inevitably have questions about hyperacusis that must be clearly answered. Patients and family members typically do not understand hyperacusis. Patients with hyperacusis like those with tinnitus often have misconceptions that fuel excessive anxiety and fear. One of the most common is the misconception that loud and annoying sounds cause permanent damage to ears and hearing.

Environmental sound enrichment is very effective in the promotion of tolerance to loud sounds, just as it is for reducing the perception of bothersome tinnitus. Audiologists sometimes implement an informal program of "graded exposure" to reduce the patient's fearful response to certain sounds. Desensitization to sound is usually achieved with regular exposure to sounds the patient considers very annoying. During the desensitization sessions, parents of children with hyperacusis explain that the sounds might be scary but they aren't really dangerous.

Let's consider a patient who is particularly annoyed by sounds like a vacuum cleaner, an emergency vehicle siren, or a slamming door. The patient or a family member makes a recording of these sounds or downloads examples from the Internet. Then the patient listens to the sounds for 10 to 15 minutes several times each week beginning at very soft levels and then at progressively higher-intensity levels. Importantly, the patient controls the intensity level of the sounds during the listening sessions.

Treatment options for tinnitus are also effective in the management of hyperacusis (Baguley & Andersson, 2007; Jastreboff & Jastreboff, 2000). The common themes for these management strategies are reduction or elimination of fear and anxiety associated with sound and therapy to "retrain" the brain's excessive and negative response to sound. The most commonly applied treatment options are listed in Figure 15.7. Treatments for hyperacusis are explained in recent textbooks (Baguley & Andersson, 2007 McKenna, Baguley, & McFerran, 2010).

We will conclude the discussion of hyperacusis with a brief case report of an actual patient that illustrates the assessment and management process.

Case Report: Hyperacusis

History. The patient was an 18-year-old female freshman student at a major university who was majoring in music. An otolaryngologist in a nearby city referred the patient to an audiologist who specializes in hyperacusis. The patient's mother accompanied her to the audiology clinic. According to the history they gave, onset of hyperacusis occurred ten months earlier when the patient was exposed to a high-intensity squealing sound at a recording studio in the university music department.

Since then the patient had not been able to tolerate everyday environmental sounds. She was annoyed when her roommate and friends laughed and talked loudly. She was reluctant to enter public settings like restaurants and even classrooms at the university due to worry about loud sounds. As she related the history, the patient cried often and expressed serious concerns about the need to change her plans for a music career.

Before her visit to the hyperacusis specialist, the patient underwent hearing assessment at another audiology clinic and then at the office of the referring otolaryngologist. Following each previous hearing assessment the patient was told that the results showed a sensorineural hearing loss due to noise exposure. She was advised to protect herself from loud sound and

FIGURE 15.8

Distortion product otoacoustic emissions (DPOAEs) for a 18-year-old female with severe intolerance to loud sounds (hyperacusis).

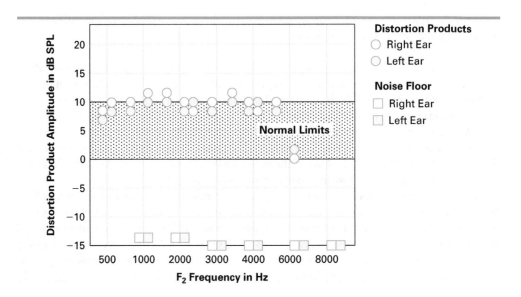

specifically instructed to avoid use of her iPod. The patient's physician prescribed the drug Xanax to treat her extreme anxiety.

Hyperacusis Assessment. The patient reported on the day of the hyperacusis evaluation that she was unable to tolerate loud sound during 100% of her waking hours. Her hyperacusis interfered with daily activities like social events and concerts and with her ability to concentrate while studying. Her sensitivity to sound also interfered with sleeping. On a scale of 0 (no problem) to 10 (life is ruined), the patient rated the impact of her hyperacusis at 8. The patient's score was 88 on the Tinnitus Handicap Inventory when she answered questions for hyperacusis rather than tinnitus. In combination, these findings confirmed that the patient's hyperacusis had a major negative impact on her quality of life.

Figure 15.8 depicts the patient's otoacoustic emission findings. Distortion product otoacoustic emission amplitudes were well within normal limits for test frequencies of 500 Hz up to 6000 Hz.

Tympanograms were normal for both ears. Word recognition was excellent (100%).

Pure tone audiometry was initially performed with insert earphones. Hearing thresholds were 10 dB HL or better for test frequencies of 250 Hz through 2000 Hz and also for 8000 Hz. There was for the right ear a notch-type deficit in the hearing threshold (25 dB nHL) at 4000 Hz when testing was done with insert earphones. However, for the right ear there was a notch-type deficit in the hearing threshold (30 dB nHL) at 3000 Hz when testing was done with supra-aural earphones. The patient's hearing threshold for a 6000-Hz tone decreased to 20 dB HL in the left ear for insert earphones but her threshold was −5 dB HL at the same frequency with a supra-aural earphone. A deficit in hearing thresholds was unexpected, given the previously recorded normal otoacoustic emissions. And, the apparent differences in hearing thresholds for insert versus supra-aural earphones was quite curious. The source of the discrepancy in findings was not clear. However, the audiologist questioned the validity of a hearing loss due to the inconsistencies between pure tone thresholds and normal otoacoustic emissions. Tympanograms were normal for both ears. Word recognition was excellent (100%).

Using special supra-aural earphones, high-frequency pure tone audiometry was conducted for test frequencies of 10,000 through 20,000 Hz. Hearing thresholds in each ear were consistently between 0 and 10 dB for all frequencies. Loudness discomfort levels (LDLs) were measured next. LDLs were in the range of 65 to 80 dB HL. The intensity levels producing discomfort were lower than normal and confirmed the patient's report of sensitivity to loud sounds.

Management. The patient and her mother were counseled immediately after testing was completed. The audiologist explained hyperacusis and gave the patient written information about hyperacusis. The patient and her mother were given an opportunity to ask questions. All test findings were explained, with an emphasis on the normal otoacoustic emissions findings and the evidence of normal hearing sensitivity for test frequencies from 500 Hz to 20,000 Hz. The patient was told that hearing testing confirmed reduced tolerance to sound. She was also told unequivocally that her hearing was normal and that test results showed no evidence of damage to her ears.

The following management plan was recommended. The patient was encouraged to resume regular daily use of her iPod at a low comfortable volume. The audiologist also recommended consistent use of a desktop environmental sound device in her dormitory room. Customized musician earplugs were made for the patient to wear during activities like sports events and concerts where there was the likelihood of loud sounds. The audiologist advised the patient to resume normal activities without worry about her hearing or the possibility of hearing loss. The patient was scheduled to return to the clinic in four weeks for a follow-up visit. The patient and her mother were visibly relieved at the end of the counseling session.

Follow-up. The patient returned to the clinic four weeks after the initial visit. She came alone, without her mother. The patient reported that she was following all recommendations. She now could tolerate everyday sounds, including her roommates' talking and laughing. The patient said she was no longer anxious and in her words "was happy for the first time in the past year." The audiologist advised the patient to continue with the same plan and to return to the clinic one year later.

At the follow-up visit one year after the beginning of treatment, quality of life was markedly improved based on the 0–10 scale and the Tinnitus Handicap Inventory. Repeat measurement of Loudness Discomfort Levels confirmed greater tolerance to loud sounds. The patient was encouraged to follow the plan as outlined a year earlier and to contact the audiologist if she had any concerns. Follow-up communication with the patient confirmed that she graduated from the university with a degree in music and moved to another city to pursue graduate studies in music composition and songwriting.

PULLING IT ALL TOGETHER

You now appreciate the importance of accurate diagnosis and effective management of four different and interesting patient populations: patients with false hearing loss, exaggerated hearing loss, tinnitus, and hyperacusis. Children and adults with these diverse auditory problems clearly differ from patients with more typical sensorineural hearing loss. The clinical principles you've read about throughout the book also guide audiologists in the assessment and management of these challenging patients. A thorough patient history is invaluable for prompt identification and diagnosis of the problems. Comprehensive hearing assessment with carefully selected tests, including objective measures, leads to accurate description of auditory status. Information from the history and hearing testing is applied in the development of a management plan.

READINGS

Baguley, D. M., & Andersson, G. (2007). *Hyperacusis: Mechanisms, diagnosis, and therapies.* San Diego: Plural Publishing.

Henry, J. A., Trune, D. R., Robb, M. J. A., & Jastreboff, P. J. (2007). *Tinnitus retraining therapy: Patient counseling guide.* San Diego: Plural Publishing.

Henry, J. A., Zaugg, T., Myers, P., & Kendall, C. (2010). *Progressive tinnitus management: Clinical handbook for audiologists.* San Diego: Plural Publishing.

Henry, J. L., & Wilson, P. H. (2002). *Tinnitus: A self-management guide for the ringing in your ears.* Boston: Allyn & Bacon.

Jastreboff, P. J. (2004). *Tinnitus retraining therapy: Implementing the neurophysiological model.* Cambridge UK: Cambridge University Press.

McKenna, L., Baguley, D. M., & McFerran, D. (2010). *Living with tinnitus and hyperacusis.* London: Sheldon Press.

Tyler, R. S. (2000). *Tinnitus handbook.* San Diego: Singular Publishing.

Tyler, R. S. (2005). *Tinnitus treatment: Clinical protocols.* New York: Thieme.

16

Management Strategies in Selected Patient Populations and Preparation of Patient Reports

LEARNING OBJECTIVES

In this chapter, you will learn:

- About diverse types of patients that audiologists assess and treat
- What is meant by "early intervention for hearing loss" in children
- How appropriate management of hearing loss in infants has a lifelong impact
- Responsibilities of audiologists and speech pathologists who manage hearing loss in school-age children
- How audiologists and speech pathologists in school systems help children with hearing impairment
- The main steps involved in programming a cochlear implant
- About challenges faced by audiologists when managing patients with neurofibromatosis II (NF II)
- How and why audiologists monitor auditory system and facial nerve function in the operating room when patients undergo some types of surgery
- The reason a multidisciplinary approach is important for management of auditory neuropathy spectrum disorder (ANSD)
- About different evidence-based techniques and strategies audiologists and speech pathologists use in the management of auditory processing disorders (APD) in children and adults
- How audiologists and speech pathologists contribute to identification and intervention for APD in a school system
- How audiologists can contribute to the effective management of a vestibular disorder called benign paroxysmal positional vertigo (BPPV)

KEY TERMS

Benign paroxysmal positional vertigo (BPPV)
Bottom-up or stimulus-driven approach
Canalith repositioning procedure
Collaborative consultation model
Comfortable level
Educational audiology
Epley maneuver
Expert model
Maximum stimulation level
Tertiary care hospital
Threshold (T) of stimulation
Top-down or strategy-driven approach
Upper stimulation level

CHAPTER FOCUS

The profession of audiology has changed dramatically since its beginnings over sixty years ago. The scope of audiology practice now includes a wide range of diagnostic and rehabilitation services provided to highly diverse patient populations. Audiologists are involved in the management of hearing loss in patients of all ages, from newborn infants to elderly adults. Some patients under the care of audiologists do not even have hearing loss. Audiologists contribute to the management of additional debilitating health problems, including tinnitus, facial nerve dysfunction, and vestibular disturbances.

Management often takes place far beyond the walls of the audiology clinic, in locations as different as an operating room in a hospital or a classroom in a school. Although management sometimes involves precise

CHAPTER FOCUS *Concluded*

programming of complex computer-based technology like cochlear implants, it may also consist of compassionate counseling or relatively simple physical maneuvers requiring no equipment.

In this final chapter you will be introduced to a sample of the remarkably different types of patients managed by audiologists today. The etiologies for hearing loss and related disorders discussed in this chapter have very serious and in some cases devastating effects on patient quality of life. The handicaps associated with the different types of hearing loss and related disorders severely disrupt daily activities, including communication, mobility, work, and social interactions, and sometimes even threaten life itself.

To be accurate, it is doubtful that any single audiologist or speech pathologist anywhere in the world is involved on a daily basis in the management of all of the patient populations described in the chapter. Recognizing the considerable knowledge and skills required for provision of standard of care to special patient populations, audiologists and speech pathologists tend to specialize in the management of subsets of the patient populations reviewed in this chapter. For example, one audiologist and one speech pathologist focusing on pediatric services might be involved in early intervention for hearing loss in preschool children, management of school-age children with auditory processing disorders, or perhaps the provision of audiology services to selected children in a local school system. In contrast, an audiologist with a primarily adult practice might divide clinical time between monitoring auditory and facial nerve function during surgical procedures, managing patients with tinnitus, and providing rehabilitation services to persons with vestibular dysfunction. Audiologists and speech pathologists employed in major university hospitals often represent multiple specialties. Together as a team they provide each of the management services covered in the chapter.

The overall goal of this chapter is to give you a glimpse into the role of audiologists and speech pathologists in habilitation and rehabilitation. Audiologists and speech pathologists are responsible for the diagnosis and management of patients with a wide range of etiologies for hearing loss and communication disorders. The types of patients discussed here represent only a small segment of the larger patient population. The information in this chapter supplements the review in the preceding chapter of diagnosis and management for three additional patient groups that audiologists encounter in clinical practice, namely, those with false or exaggerated hearing loss, tinnitus, and hyperacusis.

Early Intervention for Infant Hearing Loss

Definition and Benefits of Early Intervention

Early intervention for infant hearing loss is now defined as beginning within six months after birth. You learned in Chapter 10 about the "1-3-6 Principle" that guides the sequence of events leading to early intervention. Optimally, identification of hearing loss via hearing screening is completed within the first month after the child is born. Diagnosis of hearing loss is made by 3 months, and appropriate intervention for the hearing loss is implemented before the child is 6 months old.

The rationale for early intervention is quite straightforward. Early intervention leads to "significantly better outcomes in vocabulary development, receptive and expressive language, syntax, speech production, and social-emotional development. Children enrolled in early intervention within the first year of life have also been shown to have language development within the normal range of development at 5 years of age" (JCIH, 2007, p. 902).

The principle underlying the benefits of early intervention for infant hearing loss is *brain plasticity*. We discussed brain plasticity earlier in the book. Development of hearing regions of the infant brain and acquisition of speech and language is highly dependent on auditory stimulation and consistent exposure to all of the acoustic features of speech. Beginning at birth normal-hearing children benefit from consistent daily exposure to a rich auditory and language environment. Neural pathways and connections are shaped and developed by incoming sound during the ten or twelve months before the child utters a word. Without early intervention, children with hearing loss are deprived of acoustic and speech stimulation that is necessary for normal neural development of the auditory system.

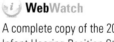 **Web**Watch

There are a number of websites with practical information about all aspects of the process of identification, diagnosis, and management of infant hearing loss, commonly referred to as early hearing detection and intervention (EHDI). You'll find interesting information on the websites for the American Academy of Audiology and the American Speech-Language-Hearing Association. Also, most states in the United States have website pages devoted to EDHI-related topics.

What Happens after Diagnosis of Infant Hearing Loss?

Management of infant hearing loss varies depending on the etiology and type of auditory dysfunction. You were introduced in Chapter 11 to causes of conductive hearing loss and medical and surgical treatments for middle ear disorders. Although audiologists invariably contribute to the diagnosis of middle ear disorders, management is often in the domain of medicine, and specifically otolaryngology. Later in this chapter we'll review the challenges associated with effective management of children with a specific group of neural hearing problems called auditory neuropathy spectrum disorders (ANSD). Here the focus is on management of the most commonly encountered type of permanent hearing impairment—sensory hearing loss due to cochlear dysfunction.

WebWatch

A complete copy of the 2007 Joint Committee on Infant Hearing Position Statement and follow-up clarification statements can be accessed online at the Pediatrics Journal on the website for the American Academy of Pediatrics (access content/120/4/898.full).

Case Scenario. Let us assume an infant was diagnosed with a sensory hearing loss. Here's how the hearing loss for this particular baby was confirmed and diagnosed. Within thirty-six hours after the child was born, hearing screening was performed in the well-baby nursery of a small birthing hospital. Hearing screening with an automatic otoacoustic emissions (OAEs) technique yielded a "refer" outcome for both ears. In compliance with hospital policy requiring a two-step hearing screening approach, a second hearing screening was soon completed using an automated auditory brain stem response (AABR) technique. AABR screening technique also produced a bilateral "refer" outcome.

Before the child was discharged from the hospital, a follow-up diagnostic hearing assessment was scheduled for two months later at a larger tertiary care hospital in a city about forty miles away. A **tertiary care hospital** is usually a major medical center that includes many different physician specialties, providing a wide range of services. Patients are often referred to the tertiary care center by primary care physicians and by physicians at smaller local or regional hospitals.

The infant's parents arrived with their child at the audiology clinic for an 8 a.m. appointment. Parents had closely followed clinic instructions for sleep deprivation of their child. That is, the child was not allowed to fall asleep until quite late the night before. Parents and their child awoke early the morning of the appointment to permit enough time for the one-hour drive to the audiology clinic. While father drove the car, mother remained in the back seat and consistently stimulated the child to prevent him from taking a nap.

As soon as the child arrived at the clinic front desk, an audiologist escorted the family back to the test area where the child was prepared for ABR measurement. Skin on the forehead and each earlobe was scrubbed vigorously with gritty liquid. The child cried lustily during the ABR preparation process. Acoustic immittance measurements were then performed. The child's tympanograms were normal in each ear, but there was no evidence of acoustic reflex activity even at the high intensity level of 100 dB HL. Otoacoustic emission testing was done next. No evidence of OAEs was detected bilaterally for test frequencies in the region of 2000 to 8000 Hz. The absence of acoustic reflexes and OAEs suggested the likelihood of hearing loss.

As final preparations were made for ABR measurement, including placement of electrodes and insert earphones, the audiologist explained the procedure to parents. Room lights were turned off and mother was encouraged to feed her child to increase the likelihood that the child would fall asleep. ABR recording was underway within five minutes as the child slept naturally.

Approximately thirty to forty minutes later, ABR measurement with click and tone burst stimulation was complete. The ABR waveforms recorded with tone burst stimuli permitted frequency-specific estimation of the child's auditory thresholds. Results confirmed a moderate-to-severe (50- to 65-dB HL) sensory hearing loss in both ears in the frequency region of 500 to 4000 Hz. The audiologist quietly and quickly examined the ears as the child slowly awoke from sleep. Before the child was fully awake, the audiologist inserted into each ear canal a small piece of specially shaped foam called an "oto-block." The audiologist then made ear mold impressions of each ear.

The audiological diagnosis was permanent moderate-to-severe hearing loss in each ear. What happened next? First, the audiologist and the family members relocated to another room in the clinic for an initial counseling session. The very important process of counseling family members about newly diagnosed childhood hearing loss was reviewed in Chapter 14. Following this "personal adjustment" counseling session and with the parents' full support and approval, the audiologist mailed the ear mold impressions off to a laboratory where custom ear molds were manufactured for the child. Forms were immediately completed for purchase of two digital hearing aids specifically selected to meet the child's hearing needs. Hearing aids were purchased with assistance from Medicaid and a designated fund in the state where the parents lived.

Consistent with 2007 Joint Committee on Infant Hearing (JCIH) guidelines for management of children with permanent sensory hearing loss, the audiologist communicated with the child's primary care physician about the need for consultation with other medical specialists. The audiologist specifically recommended referral of the child to an otolaryngologist, an ophthalmologist (eye specialist), and a genetics expert.

The 2007 JCIH report states "physicians including pediatricians" serve as an infant's "medical home," and they work with audiologists, educators, and others in the delivery of appropriate healthcare services following a coordinated family-centered approach. Although audiologists play a critical and major role in the management of infants with permanent hearing loss, appropriate and effective intervention requires a coordinated team approach.

Two weeks later and within three months after birth, the family returned to the audiology clinic in the tertiary hospital for additional counseling and also for hearing aid fitting. Electroacoustical measurements two days earlier when the hearing aids were delivered to the clinic showed that they were in good working order. You learned in Chapter 13 about how hearing aid performance is measured with special equipment. The hearing aids were coupled to the ear molds with properly sized tubing while the child rested comfortably in mother's arms. The next step was measurement of hearing aid performance with the child wearing the hearing aids.

Probe-microphone measurements of hearing aid performance were described in Chapter 13 and equipment was shown in Figure 13.11. A tiny probe tube was inserted into each ear canal sequentially. Real ear measurements of the hearing aids were performed to verify that amplification was appropriate and adequate for the child's hearing loss. Hearing aids were adjusted for the child's hearing loss using a computer-based prescriptive fitting program called Desired Sensation Level (DSL) (Seewald, 1992). The clinic visit with the child's family included detailed instruction on hearing aid operation and an explanation about battery insertion and proper disposal.

A follow-up visit was scheduled before the family departed from the clinic, including an appointment with a speech pathologist. The follow-up clinic visit was important for counseling and ongoing monitoring of hearing aid performance and "surveillance for auditory skills and language milestones" (JCIH, 2007, p. 891).

The initial hearing aid fitting as just described was the first step in the family's journey to effective communication. It was followed by close and regular documentation of the child's communication abilities, regular re-evaluation of hearing and hearing aid performance, and adjustments in management as necessary to optimize communicative outcome. Throughout the diagnostic and habilitation process, the audiologist and speech pathologist consistently updated the child's pediatrician with written reports and progress notes.

Concluding Comments

A plan for habilitation/rehabilitation of infant hearing loss is always customized to meet the needs of a child and the child's family. The scenario just described highlights principles guiding habilitation and rehabilitation efforts for all children with newly diagnosed permanent hearing loss. The "*1-3-6 Principle*" was followed in the case scenario. Hearing screening was completed by one month, diagnosis of hearing loss was made by three months, and intervention was initiated by six months after the child's birth. Also, the audiologist and speech pathologist took a family-centered approach to habilitation. The child's parents and family members were closely involved in each step of the decision-making process.

Finally, a multidisciplinary team contributed to the child's habilitation for hearing loss. The team included physicians as well as the audiologist and a speech pathologist. Importantly, there was at each step in the habilitation process close communication with child's primary care physician. The pediatrician has ultimate responsibility for management of the child's healthcare.

Management of Hearing Loss in Schools

What Is Educational Audiology?

Educational audiology is a specialty area in the profession. An educational audiologist is responsible for meeting the hearing needs of children in a school system, most often an elementary school. Educational audiologists work closely with speech pathologists in a school setting. Large public school systems in major metropolitan areas often employ a small number of full-time audiologists to provide comprehensive services to children enrolled in schools. The same school systems are likely to employ many more speech pathologists.

L E A D E R S   A N D   L U M I N A R I E S

Christine Yoshinago-Itano

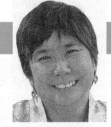

Dr. Christine Yoshinaga-Itano is Chair and Professor of Audiology in the Department of Speech, Language and Hearing Sciences and faculty in the Institute of Cognitive Science within the Center for Neurosciences at the University of Colorado in Boulder. She is also on the faculty in the Department of Otolaryngology and Audiology at the University of Colorado in Denver and the Marion Downs Hearing Center and a faculty associate in the Women and Gender Studies Program. Dr. Yoshinaga-Itano received her bachelor's degree from the University of Southern California in Psychology, her master's degree in Education of the Hearing Impaired, and her PhD in Audiology and Hearing Impairment from Northwestern University. Dr. Yoshinaga-Itano is both an audiologist and a teacher of the deaf and hard of hearing. She has conducted research in the areas of language, speech, and social-emotional development of deaf and hard-of-hearing infants and children for almost forty years. In 1996 she developed the Marion Downs National Center. Since 1996, Dr. Yoshinaga-Itano has assisted many state departments of education and public health agencies, schools for the deaf and blind, and early intervention programs throughout the United States and its territories. In addition, she has served as a consultant for many countries currently developing their early hearing detection and intervention programs, including the United Kingdom, Canada, Australia, New Zealand, Japan, China, Korea, Austria, Belgium, Poland, Spain, Austria, Denmark, Sweden, Norway, The Netherlands, Mexico, Chile, Argentina, Brazil, Thailand, Philippines, and South Africa.

Rationale for Educational Audiology

Audiology services are an important component of public education and essential for school system compliance with federal regulations. All children have a right to "a free and appropriate education in the least restrictive environment (LRE)." Table 16.1 summarizes federal legislation relevant to hearing services in the classroom. Appropriate education includes full and consistent access to an adequate acoustic and auditory learning environment in a school.

Learning during the early school years, from preschool through the third or fourth grade depends mostly on the auditory modality. Children will later acquire much information by reading books and other educational materials. Classroom instruction in elementary school until the age of 8 or 9 years is largely verbal. Consequently, hearing and listening abilities and the acoustic classroom environment are very important factors in a child's academic performance

TABLE 16.1

Federal legislation for public education that pertains to hearing and educational audiology.

IDEA (Individuals with Disabilities Education Act)
To be eligible for special education services (funded by the Federal government) children with hearing loss must show adverse educational effects as a result of the hearing loss. Special hearing services are described in an Individualized Educational Plan (IEP).
Rehabilitation Act of 1973 (Section 504)
A child with a physical impairment that substantially limits one or more life activities, including hearing impairment that affects speech perception and listening ability in the classroom, has a right to accommodation in a regular education setting. The need for accommodations and services must be documented, such as by an audiologist or speech pathologist.

TABLE 16.2

Responsibilities and duties of educational audiologists.

Audiology Services
• Comprehensive hearing assessments
• Management of students with hearing aids
• Management of students with assistive devices
• Coordinate school hearing screening programs
• Instruction in speech reading and listening skills
• Referral of students to physicians and other health professionals
• Counsel family members about hearing loss and its effects

Education
• Training of school staff on hearing and related topics
• Educate students about the dangers of high levels of noise and music
• Increase community awareness of hearing and related topics

Adapted from the Educational Audiology Association.

and success. This point is succinctly summarized with a common saying: "From kindergarten through the third grade children learn to read. After that, children read to learn." An educational audiologist working closely with a speech pathologist plays a critical role in assuring that school-age children reach their academic potential, particularly children with hearing problems.

Responsibilities of Educational Audiologists

Table 16.2 summarizes some of the duties of educational audiologists.

Audiologists conduct or coordinate annual hearing screenings throughout the school system, sometimes in collaboration with school nurses. Diagnostic hearing assessments in relatively large school systems are typically conducted in a self-sufficient clinical facility that includes sound-treated rooms and hearing test instrumentation.

Audiologists also travel from school to school to service hearing-impaired children with hearing aids, cochlear implants, and FM technology. Moderate-size and smaller cities or counties usually do not employ full-time or permanent audiologists. Instead, these school systems contract with local audiologists to provide some or all of the hearing services to children on either a regular or an "as-needed" basis. Figure 16.1 shows a Doctor of Audiology fourth-year student conducting hearing screening of a kindergarten student in a quiet classroom.

Educational Audiologists Are Experts and Advocates

Audiologists working in the school setting are advocates for the children they serve. Requisite knowledge of audiologists working in schools includes: (1) understanding how the education system functions, (2) awareness of federal and other legislation relating to hearing

FIGURE 16.1

Photograph of a fourth-year Doctor of Audiology student performing hearing screening of child in a kindergarten classroom in an elementary school using a portable diagnostic audiometer with insert earphones.

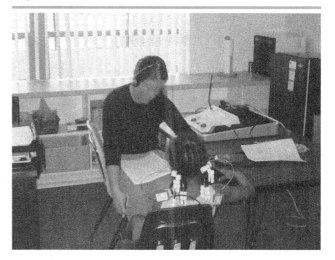

(i) Web Watch

The Educational Audiology Association (EAA) is an organization for audiologists who provide hearing services in educational settings. The website for the EAA is a good resource for information on the topic, including position statements on educational issues, publications on audiology services in the school setting, and availability of monetary grants and awards. Also on the website you can view a PowerPoint presentation entitled "School-Based Audiology Services At-A-Glance." You may be interested in knowing that the EAA is on Facebook.

and hearing services, (3) special learning needs of children with hearing impairment, (4) technologies available to improve speech perception and classroom listening, including hearing aids, classroom amplification systems, and personal FM devices, and (5) accommodations available to children with hearing impairment. In addition to providing direct services to children, audiologists inform and update other educational personnel on hearing, hearing impairment, and the operation and maintenance of hearing technology. Educational personnel include speech-language pathologists, classroom teachers, school psychologists, reading specialists, and special education teachers.

Models for Management of Hearing Loss in Schools

Two general models are used to meet the objective of improving access to verbal instruction and speech perception in the classroom. The **collaborative consultation model** generally involves provision of management services to the hearing-impaired child in the school environment, as just described. With the **expert model**, the school system consults with a professional, like an audiologist or speech pathologist, who has expertise that is not available in the school system. For example, a child may be referred by the school to an audiology clinic for reprogramming of a cochlear implant or for diagnostic assessment of auditory processing.

Classrooms Are Noisy

All children are at risk for listening difficulties in the classroom. Most classrooms are noisy and not ideal environments for listening and learning. Listening in a classroom is especially difficult for young children who have immature auditory systems and for children of any age with either a hearing loss or a central auditory processing disorder.

The signal-to-noise ratio (SNR) is quite adverse in a typical classroom. The difference between the intensity level of a teacher's voice and background noise in an elementary school classroom varies between +7 dB and −5 dB. The signal-to-noise ratio is even less favorable for children who are furthest from the teacher. Highly adverse listening conditions are also commonplace in classrooms where floors consist of hard surfaces and in older schools.

There are now American National Standards Institute (ANSI) standards for acoustical properties of learning environments (ANSI, 2002). You were introduced to ANSI standards earlier in the book in discussions about calibration and equipment used in hearing testing. The ANSI standards for classrooms call for a +15 dB SNR, with background noise less than 36 dBA. The classroom standard essentially defines an appropriate and least restrictive environment for learning in schools.

Management Strategies in the School Population

We will conclude this brief review of management of hearing loss in schools with specific examples of how an audiologist and a speech pathologist can help students. Children with some form of hearing impairment like a hearing loss or auditory processing disorder are most at risk for speech perception, listening, reading, and learning problems in noisy classrooms.

One important role of the audiologist is to contribute whenever possible to enhancement of the classroom listening environment for all children. Improvement in classroom acoustics is especially important for children with hearing impairment and other children who are struggling academically. Enhancement of the listening environment may involve use of classroom FM systems, acoustic modifications in the classroom, and/or recommendations for teaching adaptations, like seating a child near the teacher during classroom instruction.

L E A D E R S   A N D   L U M I N A R I E S

Cheryl deConde Johnson

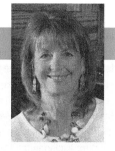

Cheryl deConde Johnson received her bachelor's degree from the University of California, Santa Barbara, her master's degree from the University of Northern Colorado, and her EdD in Special Education Administration: Audiology and Deaf Education, also at the University of Northern Colorado. Dr. Johnson currently provides consulting services regarding educational audiology and deaf education through her practice, The ADEvantage. She holds adjunct faculty appointments in audiology at the University of Colorado and the University of Northern Colorado and in deaf education at the University of Arizona. She was previously an audiology and deaf education consultant with the Colorado Department of Education. She's held positions as a school-based educational audiologist, an early intervention provider, and a coordinator in public school programs serving deaf and hard-of-hearing students. Dr. Johnson is co-author of the *Educational Audiology Handbook* as well as numerous articles and book chapters. As a parent of a grown daughter with rubella-based hearing loss, Dr. Johnson applies her personal and professional experience throughout her work and as co-founder and Board President of Hand & Voices.

Audiologists and speech pathologists serve hearing-impaired children who use hearing aids or cochlear implants in a school setting. The role of the audiologist varies, depending on the extent of services available in the school system. The audiologist may be involved in (1) identification of a child with hearing impairment through hearing screening, (2) diagnostic assessment of children with hearing loss, and (3) acquiring and fitting hearing aids or programming cochlear implants for students who need them.

An audiologist working in a school setting almost always collaborates with speech pathologists. Audiologists and speech pathologists work together on rehabilitation of the child, on instruction of classroom teachers on operation and care of hearing aids, and in assuring that the hearing aids or cochlear implants are functioning properly. Audiologists and speech pathologists also monitor a student's communication and academic progress to assure that hearing services are effective.

Finally, audiologists determine and document whether personal FM technology is needed for a child in the school setting. An audiologist advocates for the use of FM technology with or without amplification. The need for FM technology may be based on various factors, including the degree and nature of hearing loss or auditory processing disorder, the child's grades, or test results documenting speech perception abilities with and without FM technology in noisy listening conditions.

Patients with Cochlear Implants

Cochlear implants offer the opportunity for effective oral communication to persons with no usable hearing. You learned in Chapter 13 about cochlear implant technology. Following cochlear implantation and completion of an appropriate rehabilitation program with an audiologist and a speech pathologist, a person with profound hearing loss or deafness can typically go about daily activities like someone with normal hearing. Children with cochlear implants often develop normal speech and language and attend classes with hearing children. Cochlear implant users can listen to the radio, watch and hear television, and talk on the telephone.

WebWatch

Information on cochlear implants is available from a variety of sources, including textbooks and the Internet. You'll find some fascinating and rather dramatic YouTube videos of children hearing sound for the first time and adults rediscovering the wonder of sound. Websites for manufacturers of cochlear implants are a handy starting point for exploring the topic online. Here in alphabetical order are websites for the three manufacturers of cochlear implants: Advanced Bionics, Cochlear Americas, and Med-El.

A complete description of intervention for hearing impairment with cochlear implants is far beyond the scope of our review. Cochlear implant services are truly a specialty area within the profession of audiology. The American Board of Audiology (ABA) offers a specialty certification in cochlear implants. During their graduate education, Doctor of Audiology students take two or three courses on cochlear implant topics, supplemented by clinical observations and many hours of practicum experience. Here you'll be introduced to one of the critical components of management of cochlear implants, the programming process.

Programming Cochlear Implants

Hearing for the First Time or Once Again. The programming process for new cochlear implant patients was until recently quite complicated and time consuming. A high level of knowledge and skill in combination with considerable clinical experience is still needed to optimize patient performance with cochlear implants. However, each manufacturer now offers one or more streamlined signal coding strategies to be used as a starting point for converting critical properties of sound into an electrical signal that provides benefit to the patient.

Cochlear implant programming of the external speech processor begins on the day the device is first activated or "turned on." Activation is scheduled at an appropriate interval following the cochlear implantation surgery. The surgeon must first verify that the implantation site is sufficiently healed. In addition, before the audiology clinic visit, the surgeon usually reviews findings on radiological tests like X-rays to assure that the electrode array is properly inserted. The time required for initial mapping or programming of the external speech processor ranges from a few hours to an entire day.

ClinicalConnection

Audiologists and speech pathologists work together in the management of patients with cochlear implants. Management requires special clinical knowledge of technology that is not used with other patient populations. Cochlear implant components were reviewed in Chapter 13.

The clinic visit for cochlear implant activation is an exciting and emotional time for the patient, family members, and the audiologist. When a young, severely hearing-impaired child first responds to sound, tears of joy are a common sight in the clinic room. Emotions are also very strong when an elderly patient who has lost all sensation of sound hears a favorite song or hears his or her spouse utter the three words "I love you!"

The Programming Process. We will now discuss the main principles and goals of the programming process. Since the 1980s, a new and rather extensive vocabulary has evolved for describing and discussing cochlear implants. Estimation of the **threshold (T) of stimulation** is one of the essential goals in cochlear implant programming. What level of electrical stimulation is needed for the patient to just detect the presence of a signal? Threshold levels are measured separately for electrical stimulation delivered to individual electrodes. Threshold measurement in older children and adults is conducted much like pure tone hearing testing, with the patient responding verbally or manually whenever he or she hears a sound corresponding to the programmed electrical pulse signal. Other strategies for threshold assessment must often be used for young children, including non-behavioral test techniques involving electrophysiological measurements.

Another basic and routine cochlear implant measurement is the **maximum stimulation level** or **upper stimulation level** that is still a **comfortable level**. Manufacturers use different terminology in referring to this level for cochlear implant stimulation, including "most comfortable level," "maximum comfort level," and simply the "C" level. Accurate estimation of the upper stimulation level has an important influence on sound quality, speech recognition, and cochlear implant performance in general.

A number of other measurements and manipulations of stimulus parameters are also regularly included in cochlear implant programming, including determination of the dynamic range of electrical stimulation, features of the electrical pulses, the rate of stimulation, and at least a half-dozen other stimulus-related variables.

Ironically, even as research and development contribute to increasingly more complex and sophisticated cochlear implant technology, programming is becoming more efficient, quick, and simple. Manufacturers of the latest cochlear implants include user-friendly interface equipment and software with multiple pre-set programs to maximize programming success while minimizing programming time. Figure 16.2A shows an example of a simple "remote assistant" for programming the cochlear implant external speech processor shown in Figure 16.2B. Some cochlear implant systems include easily selected programs for different listening settings, such as one-on-one conversation, listening in noisy settings, or listening to music.

Another feature available with some cochlear implants automatically switches settings to optimize hearing when a patient begins using a telephone. Portable remote monitoring devices with easy to follow icons allow audiologists and even patients to quickly troubleshoot problems with cochlear implant operation.

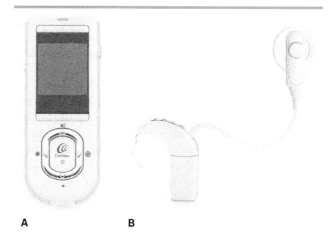

FIGURE 16.2

A remote device **(A)** for assisting an audiologist in programming a cochlear implant external speech processor **(B)**. Photos courtesy of Cochlear Americas.

A   B

Evaluating Performance of Cochlear Implants

Speech Perception. The overall objective in management of patients with cochlear implants is improved communication. A number of different measures are used to document performance of cochlear implants. Performance is documented in the clinic by assessing a patient's ability to recognize words and sentences. Speech recognition performance is usually evaluated with visual cues, like watching the speaker, and then without the cues, and also in quiet and noisy conditions.

Factors in Cochlear Implant Performance. Performance of cochlear implants is influenced by a variety of factors. As a rule, the sooner the patient is implanted after hearing loss onset the better the communication outcome. Cochlear implant performance is also affected by other subjective factors, such as motivation and cognitive functioning.

One of the most important determinants of cochlear implant success is not directly related to the patient but, rather, how accurately an audiologist programs the cochlear implant. As you've just learned, a cochlear implant program must result in audibility of soft sounds and minimize discomfort with loud sounds. There are many other components and dimensions to cochlear implant programming that affect performance and communication. The audiologist is responsible for selecting and modifying the program that controls cochlear implant operation for a specific patient.

Challenges of CI Programming in Children. An audiologist's skill in programming a cochlear implant is important for all patients. However, optimizing cochlear implant settings and processing is critical for young children who require consistent and complete access to sound for normal auditory, speech, and language development. Cochlear implant programming is particularly challenging in young children who cannot provide the audiologist with verbal impressions or descriptions of sound. Also, young children cannot be evaluated with the formal measures of speech perception that are used regularly with older children and adults.

We've focused here on the critical role of the audiologist in programming cochlear implants. Management of patients with cochlear implants, however, requires a team approach, also involving important contributions from speech pathologists, otolaryngologists, and sometimes other professionals, like psychologists. Team members work closely and communicate regularly during each step of the process, including evaluation for candidacy, surgical implantation, cochlear implant activation, and habilitation or rehabilitation.

Concluding Comments

There is no doubt that cochlear implants can dramatically improve communication. Children with profound hearing impairment who undergo cochlear implantation under the age of 2 years and receive appropriate habilitation services generally develop normal, age-appropriate speech and language. Pediatric cochlear implant users are usually enrolled in regular schools. Although children with cochlear implants may require additional special education services, most will be able to attend regular education classes with normal-hearing peers. Cochlear implants in children with post-lingual hearing loss typically have excellent ability to recognize speech and communicate effectively. The term *post-lingual* hearing loss indicates that the onset was after the child developed speech and language.

Retrocochlear Auditory Dysfunction in Adults

Vestibular Schwannoma (Acoustic Neuroma)

Recalling the discussion about vestibular schwannomas in Chapter 12, you may suspect that audiologists contribute only to early identification and diagnosis of retrocochlear auditory dysfunction and not to management. However, since the 1980s audiologists have performed an important service during surgical treatment for patients undergoing operations that put the auditory system and also the facial nerve at risk for damage. Intra-operative neurophysiological monitoring of the auditory system and facial nerve is within the scope of practice for audiology.

You learned in Chapters 9 and 12 about application of the ABR measurement technique in the diagnosis of retrocochlear auditory dysfunction. The wave I component of the ABR waveform arises from the cochlear end of the auditory nerve, whereas later components like wave III and wave V are generated from brain stem structures. Analysis of the inter-wave latencies from ABR wave I to wave III and wave V provides a sensitive index of auditory nerve and brain stem functioning.

Audiologists in the Operating Room. Some audiologists perform services in the operating room monitoring both auditory and facial nerve function during surgery to remove tumors. Figure 16.3 shows an audiologist in an operating room prior to intra-operative monitoring of auditory function in a child scheduled for surgery affecting the auditory system. You learned in Chapter 12 how tumors growing in the internal auditory canal press upon the auditory nerve and facial nerve. Intra-operative monitoring involves repeated ABR recordings during surgical procedures that put the auditory system at risk. An audiologist immediately reports changes in auditory or facial nerve responses during surgery to the surgeon. The surgeon modifies the surgery as necessary to

FIGURE 16.3

An audiologist prepared to monitor with the auditory brainstem response function of the ear, auditory nerve, and brainstem during surgery putting these structures at risk. A Doctor of Audiology student is on hand to observe the intra-operative monitoring process. The audiologist operating an auditory brainstem response system and the student observer are located in the left portion of the photograph.

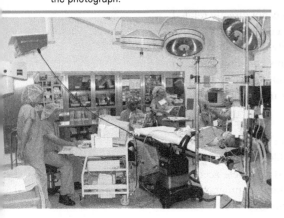

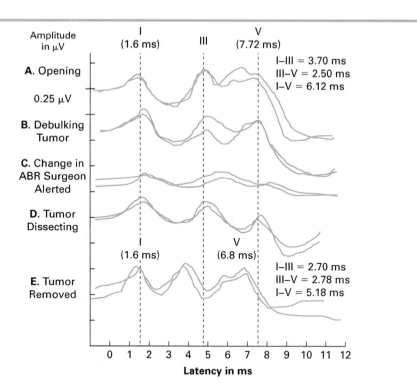

Amplitude in μV

I (1.6 ms) III V (7.72 ms)

A. Opening

I–III = 3.70 ms
III–V = 2.50 ms
I–V = 6.12 ms

0.25 μV

B. Debulking Tumor

C. Change in ABR Surgeon Alerted

D. Tumor Dissecting

I (1.6 ms) V (6.8 ms)

E. Tumor Removed

I–III = 2.70 ms
III–V = 2.78 ms
I–V = 5.18 ms

0 1 2 3 4 5 6 7 8 9 10 11 12

Latency in ms

FIGURE 16.4

A series of auditory brain stem response (ABR) waveforms were recorded continuously during surgical removal of a vestibular schwannoma. Major surgical events labeled in the figure are: **(A)** the beginning of surgery, **(B)** removal of portions of the tumor, **(C)** a change in the ABR requiring notification of the surgeon, **(D)** further removal of tumor, and **(E)** conclusion of surgery with tumor removed.

prevent damage to auditory structures or the facial nerve. The goal of the monitoring is preservation of hearing and facial nerve function.

Intraoperative Analysis of ABR Findings. Figure 16.4 shows a series of ABR waveforms recording continuously during surgical removal of an acoustic tumor. Major surgical events are labeled in the figure. Close analysis of the waveforms reveals an increase in the time interval between Wave I and Wave III and the overall latency from Wave I to Wave V that occurred during manipulation of the tumor during removal. You'll recall from Chapter 9 that the term *latency* refers to the time between the stimulus and the appearance of ABR waves. The change in the ABR was promptly reported to the otologist and neurosurgeon who were performing the surgery. After brief consultation with the audiologist, the surgeons decided to alter the surgical approach to the tumor. The ABR showed improvement at the end of surgery, confirming preservation of auditory functioning.

Concluding Comments. Modification of surgical technique based on intra-operative neurophysiological monitoring can lead to improved auditory, facial nerve, and neurological outcome. Audiologists who provide information that permits preservation of hearing and facial nerve function contribute importantly to effective management of patients with retrocochlear auditory dysfunction such as that caused by a vestibular schwannoma.

Neurofibromatosis II (NF II)

Special Challenges in Management of NF II. Patients with neurofibromatosis II (NF II) pose a rehabilitation challenge for audiologists. NF II was reviewed in Chapter 12. It is characterized by tumors involving the right and left auditory nerves. Patients with the diagnosis of NF II have bilateral neural hearing loss that progressively worsens as tumors grow. Hearing is usually better on one side than the other.

Patients with a vestibular schwannoma on one side usually rely on hearing in the non-tumor ear for effective communication. That is usually not an option for patients with NF II since the hearing loss is bilateral. Hearing aids provide limited or no benefit for patients with NF II because speech perception is characteristically poor for patients with neural auditory dysfunction.

As a patient's bilateral tumors continue to grow, they pose a serious health risk, and surgical management is almost always necessary. Enlarging tumors may press upon vital brain stem structures that are involved in controlling breathing and heart function. Unfortunately, surgical removal of a neurofibroma almost always results in total loss of hearing because auditory nerve fibers from the cochlea and the artery leading to the cochlea are embedded within the tumor.

For patients with profound cochlear hearing loss in both ears and intact auditory nerve function, a cochlear implant is usually a good management option. However, cochlear implants are not helpful to patients with NF II because damage to the auditory nerves caused during removal of the tumors eliminates the route for electrical stimulation traveling from the cochlear implant to the brain.

Management Options for NF II.   How can audiologists help patients who are diagnosed with NF II? Audiologists who participate in assessment and monitoring of auditory status of patients with NF II counsel the patient and family members regarding options for preserving effective communication. As hearing loss progresses, management with hearing aids can be considered. FM technology either alone or coupled with a hearing aid may greatly assist with communication, particularly in noisy listening settings. You learned about FM technology in Chapter 13.

The relatively slow and somewhat predictable progression of bilateral hearing loss also allows adequate time for instruction in speech reading and other strategies for "living with hearing loss." For younger adult patients, intervention may also include vocational counseling to assist the patient in selecting or changing to an occupation that can be successfully pursued by someone with severe hearing loss or deafness. Professional psychological counseling may be indicated for some patients with NF II.

Auditory Neuropathy Spectrum Disorder (ANSD)

Accurate Diagnosis Is Essential for Appropriate Management

Auditory neuropathy spectrum disorder (ANSD) was reviewed in Chapter 12. Our discussion there included a definition of the disorder, etiologies associated with it, and the test battery used for diagnosis of ANSD. You will recall that the main goal of the diagnostic process for ANSD is to determine as precisely as possible the location of dysfunction in the auditory system. In particular, differentiation among three sites of dysfunction is important for accurate diagnosis. The three sites are (1) inner hair cells, (2) the synapse between the inner hair cells and auditory nerve fibers, and (3) the auditory nerve.

 ClinicalConnection

Diagnosis of ANSD is extremely challenging. It requires a team approach. Audiologists involved in the diagnostic process must apply the latest techniques for objective hearing assessment, including auditory evoked responses like electrocochleography (ECochG). Objective clinical procedures used to diagnose ANSD were reviewed in Chapters 8 and 9.

Accurate diagnostic information on the site of auditory dysfunction in ANSD is critical for its appropriate and effective management. A multidisciplinary team approach is necessary for diagnosis and management of ANSD, with contributions from numerous medical specialists. Clinical experience has confirmed that management of ANSD is very challenging. *Evidence-based Guidelines for Identification and Management of Infants and Young Children with Auditory Neuropathy Spectrum Disorder* (Bill Daniels Center for Children's Hearing, 2008) provide valuable information for audiologists and other professionals with responsibility for helping patients with possible ANSD. We will briefly review here family-centered audiological management of the disorder.

Management Options

Audiologists use a diverse assortment of techniques and technologies for rehabilitation with ANSD including:

- Amplification (hearing aids)
- Personal FM devices
- Cochlear implants
- Sign language, including formal and informal methods (e.g., Babysigns.com)
- Visual cues and support, like lip reading and cued speech techniques

No single management strategy is appropriate for all patients with ANSD. A multidisciplinary team must carefully develop an individualized intervention plan based on a patient's specific diagnosis and communication status. The conventional emphasis on early intervention, prior to 6 months, and the rather straightforward step-by-step rehabilitation process followed in the management of patients with sensory hearing loss does not apply to ANSD.

Management of children and adults with ANSD proceeds relatively slowly and cautiously. Management decisions such as the implementation of hearing aid use may need to be reconsidered or even abandoned depending on the patient's communication status. Audiologists and families alike are sometimes frustrated by the inability to confidently settle on a long-term predictable plan for effective management and the possibility of little or no progress in communication status. The importance of family-centered counseling in the management of ANSD cannot be overstated.

 WebWatch

A panel of experts on ANSD developed the 2008 Guidelines for Identification and Management of Infants and Young Children with Auditory Neuropathy Spectrum Disorder. The experts combined their extensive clinical experiences with ANSD with published information from the scientific literature in preparing the document. You will find a link to download the document from the Children's Hospital Colorado website. A search for ANSD Guidelines should provide a link to the PDF.

Auditory Processing Disorders (APD)

Evidence-Based Management

You were first introduced to auditory processing disorders in Chapter 12. Our review there included a definition of APD, its etiologies in children and adults, and discussion of a test battery used for diagnostic assessment of peripheral and central auditory processing disorders.

Management plans for patients with APD are based largely on history and diagnostic test findings, just as they are for patients with other hearing problems. Management must also take into account non-auditory disorders that often coexist with APD, such as speech-language impairment, attention deficits, and reading disorders. A multidisciplinary approach to management is necessary for patients with APD. Audiologists and speech pathologists play key roles in management. Other team members may include psychologists, educators, medical specialists, occupational therapists, and sometimes others.

WebWatch

A recent and comprehensive document on auditory processing disorders is readily available via the Internet. At the website of the American Academy of Audiology you can download the Clinical Practice Guidelines on the Diagnosis, Treatment and Management of Children and Adults with Central Auditory Processing Disorder.

Refinement of Terminology. In this chapter and elsewhere in the book we have used the term *management* in discussion of habilitation and rehabilitation of patients with hearing loss and related disorders. The American Academy of Audiology Clinical Practice Guidelines document on APD, however, makes a clear distinction among three terms used in discussions of rehabilitation.

To quote the document, "Management, intervention, and treatment are commonly used terms associated with the habilitation or rehabilitation of persons affected by (C)APD and other disorders. The terms are defined as follows for purposes of this document. Intervention is an encompassing term referring to one or more actions taken in order to produce an effect and alter the course of a disease, disorder, or pathological condition. Treatment is any specific procedure used to prevent, remediate (i.e., cure), or ameliorate a disease, disorder, or pathological condition. Management refers to compensatory approaches (e.g., strategies, technologies) used to reduce the impact of deficits that are resistant to remediation" (American Academy of Audiology, 2010, p. 6).

Early Identification Is Best

Exploiting Brain Plasticity. Management for APD takes advantage of the principle of brain plasticity that you've read about elsewhere this chapter and earlier in Chapter 12. As stated in the American Academy of Audiology Clinical Practice Guidelines, "Early identification followed by intensive intervention exploits the brain's inherent plasticity. Successful treatment outcomes are dependent on stimulation and practice that induce cortical reorganization (and possibly reorganization of the brain stem), which is reflected in behavioral change" (American Academy of Audiology, 2010, p. 23)

Early Diagnosis. Diagnosis of APD should occur as soon as possible after onset in children or adults. And, diagnosis should be followed by intensive management efforts to achieve maximum benefits. Parents of children diagnosed with APD and also adults with APD often ask: "Is this a permanent problem? Will my child (or will I) always need to use a device or undergo therapy for my hearing problem?" In years past, audiologists and speech pathologists were hard pressed to provide a definite answer to these two reasonable questions. Now, research evidence clearly shows that auditory processing can almost always be improved with intervention, and auditory processing disorders can often be remediated. The change in outlook for management of APD is directly due to recognition of the important role of neural plasticity in rehabilitation (Hornickel, Zecker, Bradlow, & Kraus, 2012; Johnston et al., 2009).

Early Intervention. Optimally, the diagnostic and rehabilitative process for a child with APD begins soon after someone raises concerns about hearing or listening. APD in children is most often first suspected in the elementary school years. However, younger children with older siblings who have already been diagnosed with APD may benefit from earlier identification because parents and teachers have heightened awareness of APD characteristics. Optimal outcome of management efforts for APD is reflected in more effective and efficient communication. For children, optimal outcome is also reflected in improved academic performance.

Risk Factors for APD. Recognition of risk factors contributes to earlier identification of APD. As noted in Chapter 12, screening for APD using risk factors, paper-and-pencil inventories, or a formal screening test like a dichotic listening procedure are all options for early detection of APD in children.

Early identification and diagnosis of APD in adults is also dependent on an awareness of APD in audiologists, speech pathologists, and other healthcare professionals like physicians and psychologists. Traumatic brain injury (TBI), for example, is a clear risk factor for APD. Various healthcare professionals are in a position to refer for diagnostic assessment an adult patient who has suffered TBI, perhaps from a motor vehicle accident or a military combat incident. It is not uncommon for adults with possible APD to be self-referred. That is, the patient realizes a problem with hearing or listening and arranges to see an audiologist.

A Multidisciplinary Approach to Management

Bottom Up versus Top Down. Management decisions are made mostly from information gathered in the patient history and from the pattern of findings emerging from diagnostic hearing assessment. Effective management of APD combines coordination of bottom-up and top-down strategies by a multidisciplinary team.

Audiologists most often implement **bottom-up or "stimulus-driven"** management programs. The goal with this approach is to improve auditory perception skills for non-speech and speech stimuli. We will consider two bottom-up strategies. One strategy is implementation of a combination auditory and visual training program to develop or strengthen specific auditory skills and to permanently "reorganize" the auditory nervous system. The Earobics™ program reviewed earlier in Chapter 14 is a good example of a multisensory program for training auditory and visual perception. Another example of the bottom-up approach includes techniques to enhance the acoustic environment and signal-to-noise ratio, such as classroom and personal FM systems and other classroom modifications (Johnston et al., 2009).

Speech pathologists and other educational personnel like teachers, special educators, and psychologists are more likely to offer **top-down or "strategy-driven"** forms of intervention for children and adults diagnosed with APD. The goal of top-down remediation for APD is to enhance and optimize the brain's effective and efficient utilization of auditory information. Examples of top-down management include (1) strategies that involve language and cognitive skills like memory and attention, (2) strategies for learning and instructional modifications, and (3) accommodations and compensatory methods in the home and school settings.

Case Scenario. We'll take a moment here to review a clinical pathway to illustrate the link between APD diagnostic test results and management decisions. Figure 16.5 is a flowchart of one common pathway for management of APD. The patient is an 8-year-old boy who is in the clinic for a full diagnostic assessment of auditory processing. His mother and second-grade classroom teacher are very concerned about the child's poor academic progress. A psychoeducational evaluation conducted in the school system that included an intelligence or "IQ" test showed normal cognition. However, the boy was retained at the end of the first grade due to poor grades and classroom performance.

Let us begin with a brief summary of the patient history at the top of Figure 16.5. Mother reported a long history of recurring ear infections during preschool and early school years. Since the child was in kindergarten, classroom teachers had often commented to mother that he didn't seem to hear well. He confused classroom instructions. Much of the school day he was inattentive and "tuned out" what the teacher was saying. Mom emphasized that her child had low self-esteem. The boy recently made remarks like "I'm stupid." Five audiograms conducted within the past three years were all described as "within normal limits."

Figure 16.5 also summarizes test findings for the patient. A comprehensive hearing assessment showed evidence of auditory dysfunction. Hearing thresholds were in the 15 to 20 dB HL range for all test frequencies from 250 to 8000 Hz. Distortion product otoacoustic emissions were either absent or far below the normal amplitude region for test frequencies of 500 to 8000 Hz. The child's performance on most tests of auditory processing was within age-referenced normal limits for an 8-year-old child. However, his performance was markedly abnormal on three different measures of speech perception in noise.

Speech perception scores were less than 50% even for relatively favorable signal-to-noise ratios of +5 to +7 dB. Word recognition in quiet, however, was excellent (100%). Noting periods of inattentiveness during the hearing assessment, the audiologist performed a test to evaluate the child's ability to sustain attention during an auditory task. The boy's scores were below normal expectations for an 8-year-old on the Auditory Continuous Performance Test.

FIGURE 16.5

A flowchart showing the
relationship between
patient history, auditory
findings, and manage-
ment strategy for an
8-year-old boy with a
profile consistent with
auditory processing
disorder.

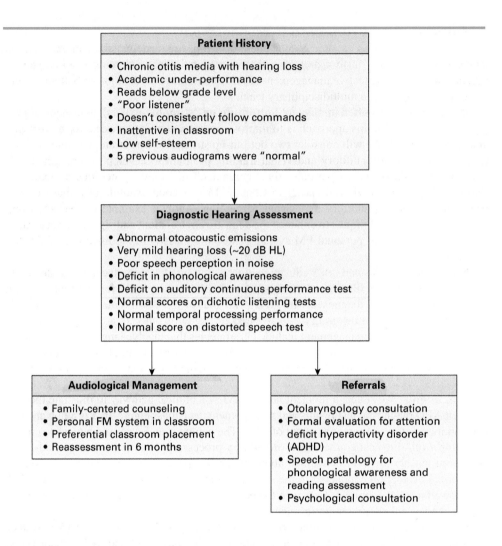

Patient History

- Chronic otitis media with hearing loss
- Academic under-performance
- Reads below grade level
- "Poor listener"
- Doesn't consistently follow commands
- Inattentive in classroom
- Low self-esteem
- 5 previous audiograms were "normal"

Diagnostic Hearing Assessment

- Abnormal otoacoustic emissions
- Very mild hearing loss (~20 dB HL)
- Poor speech perception in noise
- Deficit in phonological awareness
- Deficit on auditory continuous performance test
- Normal scores on dichotic listening tests
- Normal temporal processing performance
- Normal score on distorted speech test

Audiological Management

- Family-centered counseling
- Personal FM system in classroom
- Preferential classroom placement
- Reassessment in 6 months

Referrals

- Otolaryngology consultation
- Formal evaluation for attention deficit hyperactivity disorder (ADHD)
- Speech pathology for phonological awareness and reading assessment
- Psychological consultation

Based on these diagnostic test findings, the audiologist made the recommendations for management summarized in Figure 16.5. Considerable time was devoted to counseling the mother, father, and child about the test findings and how the child's hearing impairment interfered with communication and probably classroom performance. Counseling efforts were also directed to helping the child understand that his problem with hearing was causing difficulties in school and that there was help for the problem.

A personal FM system was strongly recommended. Steps were taken to order the device immediately. The teacher was asked to remain close to the child during classroom instruction to enhance the child's listening performance and attention. In addition, the audiologist referred the child to an otologist for evaluation of the mild hearing loss.

The patient was also referred to a neuropsychologist who specialized in evaluation and management of attention deficit hyperactivity disorder (ADHD), including the inattentive type. The neuropsychologist was also asked to provide counseling services for the documented psychosocial problems the child was experiencing. At the end of the visit to the audiology clinic, an appointment was made for a reassessment of auditory function. The follow-up visit in six months focused particularly on the assessment of speech perception in noise.

Management of APD in children often yields, in a relatively short period of time, remarkable improvement in auditory function, psychosocial status, reading, and academic performance (Hornickel et al., 2012; Johnston et al., 2009). The most effective intervention for APD begins as early as possible. Effective intervention is almost always intensive and focused on auditory deficits demonstrated in diagnostic testing, whether the patient is a child or an adult.

Finally, it bears repeating that an audiologist and a speech pathologist are the two key team members in management of APD. Indeed, close professional collaboration between audiology and speech pathology is essential for thorough assessment and effective management of children and adults with APD.

Rehabilitation of Balance and Vestibular Disorders

Dizziness, disequilibrium, imbalance, and vertigo are symptoms of a wide array of diseases and disorders affecting many bodily systems. Audiologists work closely with physicians and particularly otolaryngologists in the diagnosis of the diseases and disorders producing these symptoms. For some patients, the diagnostic process reveals a vestibular abnormality involving the inner ear. Medical or surgical management by physicians is sometimes effective in minimizing or resolving disturbances of vestibular function. However, not all vestibular abnormalities can be successfully managed with medicine or surgery.

Effective nonmedical management is very important because vestibular disorders are often debilitating and even devastating. Patients may experience severe dizziness or vertigo with changes in position, such as sitting up in bed or turning the head to one side. Secondary physical problems may also develop from the lack of normal movement. The dizziness or vertigo often interferes with daily activities, including walking, driving, and working. For patients with such abnormalities, nonmedical management is often a viable and remarkably effective option.

Vestibular rehabilitation is most often carried out by physical therapists specializing in providing services to patients with balance disorders. However, rehabilitation of vestibular and balance disorders is also within the audiology scope of practice. Audiologists provide vestibular rehabilitation to patients with certain vestibular disturbances.

Benign Paroxysmal Positional Vertigo (BPPV)

The following discussion highlights nonmedical evidence-based management by audiologists of a vestibular disorder known as **benign paroxysmal positional vertigo (BPPV)**. The term will be more easily understood with a brief explanation of each word. *Benign* means the disorder is not malignant or life threatening. The term *paroxysmal* refers to strengthening and weakening changes in intensity of the symptoms that are characteristic of the disorder. *Positional* changes of the head or body provoke the abnormal response. The head or body changes occur during daily activities such as rolling over in bed or getting out of bed. *Vertigo*, a sensation of spinning, is the primary symptom of BPPV. The vertigo in BPPV is associated with nystagmus (eye movements) that usually last for less than one minute.

Diagnosis of BPPV. Benign paroxysmal positional vertigo accounts for about 20% of all persons with dizziness and up to one-half of older persons who have dizziness. An audiologist or otolaryngologist can make the diagnosis of BPPV in an office with a proper history and the Dix-Hallpike maneuver. The Dix-Hallpike procedure was depicted in Figure 10.6, in Chapter 10. A patient sitting on an examination table is helped into the supine position with the head hanging downward and 45° to the right or the left. The final movement of the head produces rapid eye movements called nystagmus. The cause of BPPV is abnormal relocation of tiny particles called otoconia from the utricle into the posterior semicircular canal in the vestibular

FIGURE 16.6

The four photographs show a patient undergoing sequentially the four steps (**A, B, C, D**) in a canalith repositioning maneuver for treatment of benign paroxysmal positional vertigo (BPPV). Photos courtesy of Devin McCaslin.

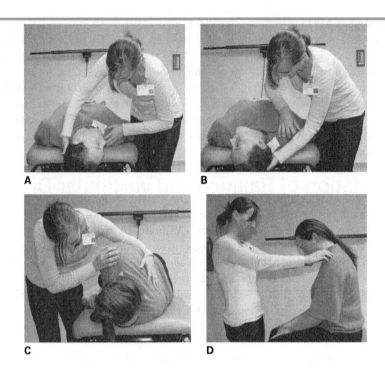

organ. Vestibular system anatomy was reviewed toward the end of Chapter 3 and vestibular assessment was covered at the end of Chapter 10.

Intervention for BPPV. BPPV may resolve without treatment within about two months of onset. However, due to the debilitating impact of the disorder on quality of life, treatment is generally requested by patients and recommended by audiologists and physicians. The **canalith repositioning procedure** is a commonly applied technique for treatment of BPPV. The term *canalith* refers to the tiny otoconia in the vestibular organ. The procedure is also called the **Epley maneuver**, named after John Epley, who first described a similar procedure.

 WebWatch

On the Internet you'll find a number of different YouTube videos and other websites showing various steps in the canalith repositioning procedure or the Epley maneuver.

The canalith repositioning or Epley maneuver requires only about fifteen minutes and is usually carried out in a clinic examination room. The photographs in Figure 16.6 illustrate the procedure. The patient's head is moved sequentially through four different positions, remaining in each position for about 30 seconds. The goal of the maneuver is to move the otoconia particles from the posterior semicircular canal back into the utricle.

The canalith repositioning procedure successfully treats BPPV in about 80% of patients. However, BPPV recurs in approximately one of three patients undergoing the procedure. In such cases, the same treatment is repeated.

Writing Patient Reports

The last section of the final chapter of the book is devoted to a brief discussion of patient report writing. It is a logical place for a review of this important topic. A patient report is a description of the analysis of test findings. It also includes an interpretation of the test findings in the context of the patient's history and sometimes other diagnostic test results. A patient report usually concludes with recommendations for management or referral to other specialists.

You've been introduced elsewhere in the book to all of the information that goes into a patient report. In Chapter 4 and again in Chapter 10 you learned about the importance of a patient history. We reviewed in Chapters 5 through 9 test procedures and test batteries that audiologists use in the diagnosis of hearing loss in children and adults. Then, in Chapters 11 and 12 you studied a variety of disorders and diseases that cause hearing loss or result in auditory dysfunction affecting the ear and the brain. Later chapters were devoted to technology and techniques that are applied in the habilitation and rehabilitation of children and adults with hearing loss. All of this information is brought to bear in preparing a patient report.

Components of a Patient Report

A patient report is the official written documentation of clinical services provided. Patient reports may vary considerably in format, length, and content. However, four essential components of a patient report are almost always included: (1) identifying information about the patient, such as full name, birth date, and medical record or social security number, (2) a listing of the hearing tests performed, (3) a summary of test findings, and (4) recommendations for further assessment or management based on the test findings.

Responsibility for a Patient Report

The person who is responsible for information in a written report signs it. The audiologist or speech pathologist that evaluated or provided services to the patient typically signs the patient report. The signing audiologist or speech pathologist must hold appropriate credentials, such as licensure by a state and/or clinical privileges at a hospital. Other persons often assist with service delivery and participate in preparation of a patient report. Assistants include graduate students in clinical training, technicians, or clerical support staff. However, the audiologist or speech pathologist has full responsibility for the accuracy of every component of the report.

Patient Reports Are Legal Documents

A patient report is a legal document. A brief explanation of this statement may be helpful. The patient report is a factual summary of information that is known about the patient and a description of all services provided to the patient. In the event of legal proceedings involving the patient, the person signing the report is held accountable for all statements included the report. From a legal perspective, it is very important for an audiologist or speech pathologist to document in the report all clinical observations, test findings, and/or services provided. The description of all clinical observations, test findings, and services provided in the patient report is proof that they actually occurred. There is no evidence that clinical services were provided unless they are documented in a written report.

Patient Privacy and Security

The very important principles of patient confidentiality, privacy, and security, reviewed in Chapter 4, apply directly to patient reports. Indeed, a patient report consists almost entirely of protected health information that must remain confidential. Patient reports in any format, whether hardcopy or electronic, must be stored in a secure location. Printed hardcopies of reports in medical or clinical charts must be stored in a locked cabinet or room. Electronic versions of the reports must be stored in password-protected files on encrypted computers or share drives and transmitted only via secure email systems or as password-protected documents.

Patient Report Scenario

A simple and real-world example of the importance of written documentation in a patient report will help you appreciate the concept. The patient is a 45-year-old male who comes to the clinic with the chief complaint of decreased hearing in the right ear. An audiologist performs an otoscopic inspection before beginning a hearing assessment. Clinical policy dictates routine otoscopic inspection for every patient.

Let us assume that otoscopic inspection for this particularly patient reveals a clear perforation of the right tympanic membranes. Unfortunately, on an especially hectic day in the clinic, the audiologist does not mention the otoscopic inspection in the patient report. As a consequence, there is no documentation of the abnormal findings.

Now let's fast forward to the end of same day. While relaxing at home, the patient is bothered by itching ear canals. In an attempt to relieve the itching sensation, the patient repeatedly wiggles a cotton swab tip deeper and deeper into his right ear canal. The patient experiences a sudden sharp pain and then notices blood on the cotton swab tip. An immediate late night trip to the emergency department of the local hospital confirms a perforation of the right tympanic membrane.

Inappropriately associating the tympanic membrane perforation with a complication of his hearing assessment earlier in the day, the patient secures legal representation to seek compensation for pain suffered as a result of the perforation and medical costs incurred for its diagnosis and treatment. Within a few days the audiologist receives a court order to submit the patient report and other documents from the clinic visit. Legal proceedings are pending. Legal defense hinges on proof that the audiologist was not responsible for the tympanic membrane perforation. Unfortunately, the audiologist's case is complicated by the lack of documentation in the patient report and chart notes. There is no proof that the tympanic membrane was perforated when the patient entered the audiology clinic and first underwent otoscopic inspection of the ear.

Common Features of Effective Patient Reports

More than fifty years ago, James Jerger published a short paper with the interesting title "Scientific Writing Can Be Readable" (Jerger, 1962). You may recall Jerger's name from the review of the development of audiology as a profession in Chapter 1. Jerger remains a major figure in clinical audiology. Although the paper offers advice to persons preparing manuscripts for publication in professional journals, it is also remarkably appropriate for writing patient reports. As Jerger notes, "In scientific reporting the object is to convey to the reader what you did, why you did it, and what you found" (Jerger, 1962, p. 101). At the conclusion of the paper, he summarizes four steps to improve professional writing (Jerger, 1962, p. 104).

To help you appreciate the contribution of writing style to the clarity and understandability of a patient report, each step is followed here by "before and after" examples from patient reports. That is, passages from patient reports are shown first in the original form and then with revisions according to a specific recommendation.

- "Write short sentences. Use a new sentence for each new thought."

  Before: *Ms. Susan Johnson was scheduled for a hearing assessment at the University Speech and Hearing Center on August 1, 2010, where she reported that she had a hearing loss and also experienced some ringing tinnitus that was greater in the right ear than in the left ear, beginning in approximately July of 2010 and attributed to attendance at a Deaf Lion concert in the football stadium.*

  After: *Ms. Susan Johnson underwent a hearing assessment at the University Speech and Hearing Center on August 1, 2010. Her chief complaints were bilateral hearing loss and also tinnitus, greater for the left ear. Ms. Johnson first noticed her tinnitus in July 2010 after attending an outdoor rock concert.*

- "Avoid artificiality and pompous embellishment. Write it the way you would say it."

  Before: *Considering her complaint of hearing loss, it was decided to conduct hearing testing of Ms. Johnson by means of the Hughson-Westlake technique using a two-channel diagnostic audiometer with TDH-59 earphones in a double-walled sound-treated test room. Hearing thresholds were obtained with good test reliability and indicated that hearing sensitivity was better than 20 dB hearing level (HL) for pure tone frequencies of 250 Hz, 500 Hz, 1000 Hz, 2000 Hz, 3000 Hz, 4000 Hz, and 8000 Hz.*

After: *Pure tone audiometry showed hearing sensitivity within normal limits bilaterally. An audiogram accompanies this report.*

[Note: The audiogram includes details about the audiometer, earphones, test reliability, and other pertinent information.]

- "Use active verb construction whenever possible. Avoid the passive voice."

Before: *It was found that Ms. Johnson had very good word recognition when words were presented at a comfortable level of 40 dB HL in quiet, including scores of 100% when words were presented to the right ear and 96% when words were presented to the left ear.*

After: Ms. Johnson's word recognition scores in quiet were excellent for the right ear (96%) and the left ear (100%) at an intensity level of 40 dB HL.

[Note: The audiogram includes a table or graph showing speech audiometry findings.]

- "Use personal pronouns when it is natural to do so."

Before: *It was recommended that Ms. Johnson consider the use of hearing aids and it was suggested that she consider making an appointment for an evaluation of the possible use of hearing aids.*

After: *We recommend a hearing aid consultation to explore the possible use of amplification.*

Effective reports are simple, clear, accurate, and supported by clinical and test findings. Importantly, a well-written report contributes to patient management and outcome. A patient report has no value if it is not read or not understood by the recipient. Adhering to the four simple steps just described will make reports more readable and understandable.

Preparation of Reports

Reports for new patients in a clinic may be prepared "from scratch" with all information dictated for transcription by someone else, or from a template that includes much of the generic information found in most reports. Students in an audiology or a speech pathology graduate-level educational program are often assigned the duty of preparing a draft of the patient report as part of their clinical training. A preceptor or supervisor then reviews and edits the report before printing and signing a final version.

In the interest of efficiency, practicing audiologists and speech pathologists are more likely to dictate reports that are then typed and printed, making use of templates or other strategies for quick yet accurate report preparation. The template consists of the skeleton or framework for a typical report, including phrases and statements that appear in most reports. Details for a specific patient, such as his or her identifying information and details of test findings, are written and inserted by the person preparing the report.

Some audiologists and clinics prepare patient reports utilizing special software programs that permit the selection from pull-down menus of commonly used "buzz words," phrases, and statements. The statements are then inserted into the text of the report. For example, if test results are normal, the audiologist might select from a pull-down menu labeled "Pure Tone Audiometry" the statement "Pure tone audiometry revealed normal hearing sensitivity in both ears for test frequencies from 250 to 8000 Hz." The statement is automatically inserted into the patient's clinical report.

Report Formats

Different patient report formats are used in audiology, depending on the test setting, the types of patients undergoing clinical services, the purpose of the report, and who will be reading the report.

Chart Note. A *chart note* format is quite common for reporting findings of patients who are tested in a hospital setting. A chart note is a brief "bottom line" type of report, usually hand-written in the appropriate section of the medical chart of the patient staying in the hospital.

An example of a chart note is shown in Figure 16.7. The chart note summarizes findings for hearing assessment of a young woman who was an inpatient in the hospital where she was being treated with chemotherapy for a brain tumor. The chemotherapy included carboplatin, a potentially ototoxic medication. The patient was transported to the audiology clinic in a wheelchair. The note was written by a Doctor of Audiology student immediately after completion of testing, signed by the student's preceptor in clinic, and then inserted in the patient's hospital record.

Similar chart notes are often written in the medical charts of patients admitted for a day or less to a clinic or laboratory facility for tests or to an operating room for diagnostic or treatment procedures. Patients who receive services in a facility within a day and then leave for home are called *outpatients,* whereas those who spend one or more nights in a medical facility like a hospital are referred to as *inpatients.* The chart note might be supplemented with a printout of test results, such as an audiogram, tympanograms, or auditory brain stem response waveforms.

SOAP Format. Some audiologists follow a medical format commonly known as *SOAP* when preparing chart notes or brief reports of test findings or updating a patient's status. SOAP is a handy acronym for each of the headings in the report: *S*ubjective, *O*bjective, *A*ssessment, and *P*lan.

The *Subjective* section of the report usually consists of the patient's history, chief complaints, other symptoms, and information given by the patient, caregiver, or family members. The *Objective* section consists of clinical observations, measurements, and test findings. A physician

FIGURE 16.7

An example of an audiology chart note handwritten by a Doctor of Audiology (AuD) student into the medical record or chart of an inpatient who underwent hearing test procedures following chemotherapy as treatment for a brain tumor. Chemotherapy included carboplatin, a potentially ototoxic medication. A clinical preceptor (licensed audiologist) who supervised the student signed the chart note.

History / Physical Examination / Progress Notes

June 2, 2012 (10am)

    The patient underwent a hearing assessment in the audiology clinic. Hearing thresholds were well within normal limits for both ears. Word recognition scores were excellent (100%) bilaterally. Otoacoustic emission amplitudes were also within normal limits in each ear for test frequencies up to 8000 Hz. An audiogram is included with this note.

Impressions: Test results are consistent with normal peripheral auditory function. A full report to follow.

James W Hall PhD
Pager 352-000-0007

would include findings from the physical examination and laboratory test findings in the Objective section. This information is comparable to that found in the Results section of a report.

The *Assessment* section includes the diagnosis or diagnoses and the same information as an Impressions section. Finally, treatment and management plans and recommendations are listed in the *Plan* section of the SOAP format report. The SOAP format may also be followed with a progress report or an update on patient management.

Summary Report. A variation of the chart note is sometimes written on an audiogram form. The brief summary of the analysis of test findings is supplemented with detailed information displayed numerically or graphically on the audiogram form. The written portion of the report at the top of the form consists only of a "bottom line" explanation of the outcome of testing, and sometimes a listing of recommendations.

The audiogram summary report format is often employed in an audiology or otolaryngology clinic setting where many patients are tested in a relatively short period of time. The brief summary report is common in settings where the recipient or recipients of the report typically have access to other patient findings like the history and the results of physical examination. In these settings, like an otolaryngology clinic, the recipients of the report are very familiar with hearing test procedures and terminology.

Narrative Letter Report. An audiologist generally prepares in letter format a more formal narrative report of the findings for other recipients, such the patient, parents of the patient, or a patient's family doctor. A *narrative letter report* is a common format for documenting and disseminating a patient's hearing test findings. The report is in the form of a letter addressed to the healthcare professional or some other person who referred the patient to audiology.

In its simplest form, each paragraph in a letter report focuses on a category of information regarding the patient. For example, the first paragraph identifies the patient, when and where he or she was evaluated, and perhaps includes a highlights of the patient's history in a sentence or two. Paragraph two summarizes test results. The final two paragraphs provide an interpretation of the test results followed by a listing of recommendations for further assessment or management.

A variation of the narrative report format includes headings for categories of information. The report may begin with a display of demographic and identifying information, such as patient name, birth date, medical record number, and date of assessment, followed by a description of the purpose of the evaluation and, perhaps, a brief patient history.

Subsequent categories of information are clearly defined by headings that are in bold font and/or capitalized, such as: *Results, Impressions, and Recommendations.* The headings provide a guide to the reader to facilitate quick access to patient information that is most relevant to the recipient of the report. The narrative report format with these headings is also suitable for a progress report, that is, an updated description of the patient's status and ongoing management based on findings during a clinic visit occurring some time after the initial assessment.

Example of a Narrative Report. Figure 16.8 shows an example of a one-page narrative report prepared within a few hours after diagnostic hearing assessment of a young child in an outpatient audiology clinic. The report begins with a statement about the purpose of the assessment. The Results section provides details about which procedures were used in the hearing assessment. This information will probably be meaningful to the otolaryngologist who will receive the report and certainly to any audiologist who is involved in follow-up hearing assessments.

Although the child's primary care physician may not understand all of the terminology in the report, the outcome of testing and the management plan are clearly and simply explained

FIGURE 16.8   An example of letter-type report for a patient referred from a primary care physician and who underwent hearing test procedures in an audiology clinic. As illustrated by this example, the report is typically printed on letterhead for the clinic.

NOVA SOUTHEASTERN UNIVERSITY
Health Professions Division
Department of Audiology
3200 South University Drive
Fort Lauderdale, Florida 33328
(954) 262-7745 Fax: (954) 262-2908
www.nova.edu/aud

Audiology Report: Objective Assessment of Auditory Function

RE:	Bambina, Isabella
MR#:	00000001
DOB:	7/27/2009
DOS:	12/20/2009
DX:	389.90

Isabella underwent hearing assessment at the Speech and Hearing Center on the above date. Parents report that Isabella did not pass newborn hearing screening at another hospital. Review of medical records showed no risk factors for progressive or delayed-onset hearing loss. The purpose of the assessment today was to estimate ear-specific auditory thresholds within the speech frequency region.

RESULTS: Otoscopy revealed clear external auditory canals and normal appearing tympanic membranes bilaterally. Acoustic immittance measurement yielded normal (type A) tympanograms. An acoustic reflex was observed in the uncrossed (ipsilateral) condition with right and left ear broadband noise (BBN) stimulation at 70 dB HL. Distortion product otoacoustic emissions (DPOAEs) were recorded bilaterally over a test frequency region of 1000 to 8000 Hz. DPOAE amplitudes were within the normal region for each ear. An ABR was recorded using a conventional clinical protocol in both ears. A reliable ABR was recorded bilaterally for click and tone burst stimulation (500, 1000, and 4000 Hz) at intensity levels down to 20 to 30 dB nHL. Estimated thresholds are plotted on an attached graph.

IMPRESSIONS: Today's auditory findings are consistent with hearing sensitivity within normal limits throughout the speech frequency region in both ears. Hearing sensitivity is adequate for normal speech and language acquisition.

RECOMMENDATIONS:

- Findings were explained to Isabella's parents. They acknowledged understanding the information.
- Isabella will be re-evaluated in 6 to 9 months with behavioral hearing test procedures. An assessment can be scheduled earlier if there are parental or physician concerns about hearing or speech/language acquisition.

Marlene Malleus

Marlene Malleus, Au.D., CCC-A, FAAA
Clinical Audiologist (Provider # 0000)

CC: Medical Records	*O. Titus, M.D.*	*Emily Petite, M.D.*
	Otolaryngology	*Pediatrics*

in the Impressions and Recommendations sections of the report. The most important message to be delivered following the comprehensive hearing assessment, and the information that is of most interest to the pediatrician who referred the child, is simply and unequivocally stated: "Hearing sensitivity is within normal limits and adequate for normal speech and language acquisition."

Brevity and simplicity are very important attributes for a report of audiological findings, particularly in a report sent to a physician. Most physicians are most interested in the answers to two simple, related questions: Does the patient have a hearing problem? If so, what should be done about it? This is particularly relevant for very busy primary care providers lacking extensive academic background and training in hearing, hearing disorders, and audiology.

Lengthier multipage narrative reports are often required for patients undergoing more extensive audiological assessment, including those requiring long-term intervention with more than one management approach. For example, reports prepared for children or adults evaluated for auditory processing disorders (APD) may be two or more pages. The report typically includes adequate description of findings for the multiple tests administered, a list of recommendations for further assessment, and a comprehensive plan for intervention.

Patient Ambulatory Summary Record. Audiologists working in a medical setting are now sometimes required to complete and maintain an ambulatory summary record for each patient who receives services in the clinic. The dual purposes for the record are (1) to document information that would be needed to medically manage the patient in an emergency situation, and (2) to improve the patient's healthcare. Information included in the patient ambulatory summary record is not directly related to the patient's audiology history, hearing test results, or plans for rehabilitation.

The ambulatory summary record consists of a listing of medications, including prescription and over-the-counter drugs and herbal preparations. The report is usually prepared following a brief interview with the patient at each audiology clinic visit. The summary record also lists allergies or reactions to drugs, foods, or latex. Medical diagnoses and conditions and operations and other invasive procedures are entered on the report form.

Finally, the summary report notes other patient appointments for healthcare services, including physicians, rehabilitation specialists, and medical diagnostic tests. In the unfortunate and unlikely event that the patient has a medical emergency in the audiology clinic, information on the ambulatory summary record is essential for prompt and appropriate medical treatment. The information is also useful in the diagnosis and management of hearing and related disorders, such as vestibular disturbances and tinnitus.

Patient Reports and Referral Sources
Referrals to and from Audiologists. Other professionals sometimes refer patients to audiologists for hearing assessment and management. Or, conversely, audiologists may refer patients to other healthcare professions for medical or other specialized diagnostic evaluation and management. Audiologists and speech pathologists commonly interact with various healthcare professionals. Physicians who refer patients to audiologists and speech pathologists include primary care physicians, like pediatricians, and medical specialists, such as otolaryngologists, neurologists, ophthalmologists, and developmental pediatricians. Audiologists and speech pathologists refer patients to each these types of physicians.

Patient-related communications and reports also involve other healthcare professionals, among them psychologists, occupational therapists, nurses, and geneticists. Audiologists often prepare patient reports exclusively for one of these healthcare professionals. In such cases, the content, terminology, and level of detail of the report take into account the recipient's professional specialty and knowledge of audiology.

PULLING IT ALL TOGETHER

A review of current strategies applied in management of hearing loss and related disorders in challenging patient populations is a fitting way to conclude a book about audiology today. Management of patient groups included in this chapter requires considerable audiology knowledge and skill. Much of the information we have covered earlier in the book was applied in addressing the hearing and balance problems represented in this sample of patients. Diagnosis of and intervention for severe-to-profound hearing loss in young children is perhaps the most challenging responsibility facing audiologists. It requires a high level of technical skill with diagnostic tools like auditory evoked responses as well as rehabilitation technology such as hearing aids and cochlear implants.

Considerable knowledge and skill is also necessary to improve communicative function and outcome in adults and children with complex problems such as auditory processing disorders, auditory neuropathy spectrum disorders, and other disorders affecting the retrocochlear pathways and central auditory nervous system. And, knowledge of different anatomy and an entire new skill set are required for effective management of balance disorders.

Audiologists have the education and training to provide the high-level clinical services described in this chapter. No other health profession is prepared to take on the responsibility. Audiologists who provide services like those included in this chapter contribute importantly to patient quality of life and overall health.

Finally, you were introduced in this chapter to report writing. You learned about different report formats and the importance of communicating hearing test results simply, clearly, and accurately.

READINGS

American Academy of Audiology. (2010). *Auditory processing disorders clinical guidelines.* audiology.org

Baguley, D. M. (2002). Mechanisms of tinnitus. *British Medical Bulletin, 63,* 195–212.

Baguley, D. M., & Andersson, G. (2007). *Hyperacusis: Mechanisms, diagnosis, and therapies.* San Diego: Plural Publishing.

Boothroyd, A., & Gatty, J. (2012). *The deaf child in a hearing family: Nurturing development.* San Diego: Plural Publishing.

Eggermont, J. J., & Roberts, L, E. (2004). The neuroscience of tinnitus. *TRENDS in Neuroscience 27,* 676–682.

Hornickel, J., Zecker, S. G., Bradlow, A. R., & Kraus, N. (2012). Assistive listening devices drive neuroplasticity in children with dyslexia. PNAS pnas.org/cgi/doi/10.1073/pnas.1206628109

Guidelines for Identification and Management of Infants and Young Children with Auditory Neuropathy Spectrum Disorder. Guidelines Development Conference at NHS 2008, Como, Italy.

Jerger, J. (1962). Scientific writing can be readable. *Asha, 4,* 101–104.

Johnston, K. N., John, A. B., Kreisman, N. V., Hall, J. W. III, & Crandell, C. C. (2009). Multiple benefits of personal FM system use by children with auditory processing disorder. *International Journal of Audiology, 48*(6), 371–383.

Joint Committee on Infant Hearing. (2007). Year 2007 position statement: Principles and guidelines for early detection and intervention programs. *Pediatrics, 120,* 898–921.

Richburg, C. M., & Smily, D. F. (2012). *School-based audiology.* San Diego: Plural Publishing.

Seewald, R. (1992). The desired sensation level method for fitting children: version 3.0. *Hearing Journal, 45,* 36–41.

Shaywitz, S. E., Morris, R., & Shaywitz, B. A. (2008). The education of dyslexic children from childhood to young adulthood. *Annual Review of Psychology, 59,* 451–475.

Glossary

ABR See Auditory brain stem response.

ABG See Air-bone gap.

ABLB See Alternate binaural loudness balance.

Acoustic immittance A term coined to refer to either acoustic *im*pedance or acoustic ad*mittance*.

Acoustic neuroma A usually benign tumor affecting the auditory nerve (8th cranial nerve). The proper term is a vestibular schwannoma.

Acoustic ohms and mhos Units used to report acoustic immittance measurements. Acoustic impedance is described in **acoustic ohms,** whereas the reciprocal entity, acoustic admittance, is described in **acoustic mhos**.

Acoustic reflex Contraction of one or both middle-ear muscles in response to an intense sound. Contraction of the stapedius muscle is typically measured in clinical audiology.

ADA See Americans with Disabilities Act.

AER See Auditory evoked responses.

Admittance Ease of energy flow through the middle ear system.

Air-bone gap (ABG) The difference in decibels (dB) between air conduction and bone hearing thresholds of 10 dB or more. Air conduction thresholds are poorer than bone conduction thresholds at the same frequency in the same ear.

Air conduction The route taken by sounds that are presented to the ear with earphones or a loudspeaker. Sounds reach the inner ear by traveling from the outer ear and through the middle ear.

ALDs See Assistive listening devices.

Alternate binaural loudness balance (ABLB) A test procedure for assessing recruitment in a patient with unilateral hearing loss. A sensory hearing loss shows abnormal growth of loudness in comparison to a normal ear.

Alzheimer's dementia A disease characterized by diminished cognitive function and especially memory abilities in selected elderly persons. It accounts for up to 70% of dementias found in the aging population.

Ambient noise Background acoustic noise in an environment such as room where hearing testing takes place.

American Sign Language (ASL) A manual communication method that involves signs representing words or meanings. ASL is a popular signing method in the United States.

Americans with Disabilities Act (ADA) A U.S. public law (P.L. 101-336) enacted in 1990 to give equal opportunity for individuals with disabilities.

Amplitude The amount of vibration movement of a mass from the position of rest to the farthest point from the position of rest. Also, a measure of the size or magnitude of an auditory evoked response wave usually made from either a peak to a preceding or following trough or from the peak of a wave to some index of baseline. Amplitude of an evoked response is expressed in microvolts.

Anomalies: Abnormalities or malformations in structures such as the outer ear or the inner ear.

APD See Auditory processing disorder.

Apex The low-frequency region of the cochlea at the opposite end from the base near the stapes.

Articulation index A measure of speech perception that quantifies the audibility of speech.

Artificial ear A device for calibrating the sound produced by earphones used in air conduction hearing testing. It consists of a 6 cm^3 coupler to connect an earphone to a microphone.

Artificial mastoid A device for calibrating bone-conduction vibrators that is connected to a sound level meter that documents the intensity level in either decibels or units of force.

Ascending technique A technique for estimation of pure tone hearing thresholds that begins at a level below a person's likely hearing threshold with presentation of stimulus sounds at progressively higher levels.

ASL   See American Sign Language.

Assistive listening devices (ALDs)   Electrical devices consisting of a microphone worn by a talker and earphones on or loudspeakers near a listener. An assistive listening device improves the signal-to-noise ratio of speech versus background noise and therefore speech perception. Also known as hearing assistance technologies (HAT).

Attenuate   To reduce the intensity level of a sound. Ear plugs attenuate noise levels that reach the inner ear.

Audiogram of familiar sounds   An audiogram form showing the level and the general frequency region of speech sounds and also common sounds like a whisper, a lawnmower, and jet airplane.

Audiological rehabilitation   Treatment of those with hearing loss after birth (acquired hearing loss) to improve communication using hearing aids and other devices, therapy, speechreading, and counseling. Formerly referred to as aural rehabilitation.

Audiology   The profession of specialists in hearing assessment and non-medical management of persons with hearing loss.

Audiometer   *(pronounced aw dee AH muhter)* A device for measuring hearing. The operator of an audiometer can change the frequency and the intensity level of sounds in hearing testing.

Audiometric frequencies   The frequencies typically included in hearing testing including 250 Hz, 500 Hz, 1000 Hz, 2000 Hz, 4000 Hz, and 8000 Hz.

Audiometric zero   A term used to describe 0 dB HL (hearing level) on an audiogram. Average hearing threshold for persons with entirely normal hearing sensitivity.

Auditory brain stem response (ABR)   Electrical activity evoked (stimulated) by very brief sounds that originates from the 8th nerve or auditory portions of the brain stem. The ABR consists of five waves and is usually recorded from the surface of the scalp and external ear. The ABR is used in hearing testing of infants and young children and in detection of auditory abnormalities affecting the auditory nerve and brain.

Auditory evoked potential(s)   See auditory evoked response(s).

Auditory evoked responses (AERs)   Electrical activity evoked (stimulated) by sounds arising from auditory portions of the peripheral or central nervous system and recorded with electrodes. AERs include but are not limited to the electrocochleography (ECochG),

auditory brainstem response, auditory middle-latency response, auditory late response, and P300 response.

Auditory Neuropathy Spectrum Disorder (ANSD)   A complex collection of auditory disorders that interfere with hearing and especially speech perception in quiet and noise. Possible sites of dysfunction in ANSD include the inner hair cells, the auditory nerve, and the synapse between the inner hair cells and the nerve fibers. Formerly known as auditory neuropathy and auditory dys-synchrony.

Auditory-oral approach   An educational strategy for children with profound hearing loss that emphasizes the development of amplified residual hearing and spoken language utilizing speech-reading cues as a supplement to the auditory signal.

Auditory processing disorder (APD)   Disorder in the efficient and effective processing of auditory information anywhere in the auditory system from the ear to the highest levels of the brain. Audiologists and speech pathologists assess and manage APD in patients ranging from children who experienced difficulties in school to adults with traumatic brain injury,

Auditory training   Therapy to develop and enhance auditory skills to maximize use of hearing abilities in persons with hearing loss or auditory processing disorders.

Auditory-verbal approach   An educational strategy for children with profound hearing impairment that emphasizes the child's residual hearing through the use of amplification with the goal of developing listening skills through natural communication. With this approach, a child is placed in mainstream education beginning in preschool years.

Aural atresia   Malformation of the outer and often middle ear. In some cases there is no pinna.

Aural rehabilitation   Treatment of those with hearing loss after birth (acquired hearing loss) to improve communication using hearing aids and other devices, therapy, speechreading, and counseling.

Auricle   Outer ear consisting of cartilage.

Automated audiometry   Hearing testing under computer control.

Baha   See Bone-anchored hearing aid.

Behavioral audiometry   Hearing testing that requires a behavioral response from a patient like raising a hand, pressing a button, or repeating a word. Behavioral audiometry is influenced by a number of listener variables like motivation, attention, alertness, and understanding of the task.

Behind-the-ear (BTE) A hearing aid style consisting of a C-shaped hearing aid located on and behind the outer ear with a tube leading into the external ear canal.

Benign paroxysmal positional vertigo (BPPV) A vestibular disorder characterized by vertigo associated with changes in head position. BPPV can be successfully treated by audiologists and physicians in a clinic office with special maneuvers.

Best practices The adherence to standard of care in clinical practice; following evidence-based clinical practices.

Binaural integration The ability to integrate or effectively listen to different sounds presented simultaneously to each ear in a dichotic task.

Binaural separation The ability to effectively listen to sounds presented to one ear while different sounds are presented simultaneously to the other ear in a dichotic task.

Bing test A test to measure the occlusion effect that can be performed with a tuning fork or audiometer. The Bing test is useful in trying to determine whether a hearing loss is conductive.

Board certification In audiology the highest credential for clinical practice offered by the American Board of Audiology (ABA).

Bone-air gap A statistically predictable test finding in which hearing thresholds with bone conduction stimulation are slightly greater (poorer) than hearing thresholds with air conduction stimulation.

Bone-anchored hearing aid (Baha) A surgically implantable device for stimulating the cochlea via bone conduction. Baha devices are suitable for patients with unilateral hearing loss and some patients with conductive hearing loss.

Bone conduction Transmission of sound (mechanical vibrations) from the surface of the skull at the mastoid or forehead to the fluids of the cochlea. Sounds are then perceived in the usual way.

Bone vibrator A small device (usually black plastic on the exterior with electronic components within, about an inch square) that is used to present sounds (vibrations) to the skull in bone conduction auditory assessment. A Radioear B-71 oscillator (vibrator) is recommended for AER stimulation. Sometimes called a bone **oscillator**.

Bottom up or stimulus-driven approach Auditory training that focuses on improving the quality of auditory signals and developing auditory perception skills.

BPPV See Benign paroxysmal positional vertigo.

Brain plasticity The ability of the central nervous system, especially the brain, to change and reorganize with stimulation.

Brain stem Part of the central nervous system above the spinal cord that contains important auditory centers as well as centers that control vital life functions like breathing and heart activity.

BTE See Behind-the-ear.

C See Comfortable level.

Calibration Electronic or psychoacoustic determination that an electrical device (such as an amplifier) or an acoustic transducer (an earphone) is functioning according to defined characteristics. The term usually also implies correction of the device if necessary.

Caloric tests Vestibular tests conducted with irrigation of the external ear canal using cool or warm water or air to stimulate the vestibular portion of the inner ear. Caloric stimulation produces rapid eye movements called nystagmus. Caloric testing is part of elecronystagmography or videonystagmography.

Canalith repositioning procedure Maneuvers of the head that are used in treating the a disorder known as benign paroxymal positional vertigo (BPPV).

Candidacy (for hearing aid) When a person meets criteria for the use of a hearing aid.

CANS See Central auditory nervous system.

Carrier phrase A phrase such as "say the word" or "you will say" that precedes every presentation of an item in a word recognition test in speech audiometry. A carrier phrase is not always used in word recognition testing.

CC See Chief complaint.

Central auditory nervous system (CANS) The auditory system beginning with the cochlear nucleus in the brainstem and including also pathways and auditory regions in the thalamus and the cerebrum.

Central masking A change in hearing threshold in one ear associated with the presentation of masking noise to the opposite ear at a relatively low level that is not adequate to crossover to mask the test ear.

Cerebral cortex   The thin outermost layer of the cerebrum. The auditory cortex is located on the superior surface of the temporal lobe in the cerebrum.

Cerebrovascular accident (CVA)   A stroke; brain damage resulting from interruption of blood supply to the brain.

Cerumen   Ear wax, a sticky acidic substance normally secreted from ceruminous glands within the walls of the external auditory canal. Ceremen plays a role in protecting the ear.

Chief complaint (CC)   Main problem that brings a person to a healthcare professional. For patients seeking care from an audiologist, chief complaints often include hearing loss, dizziness, and tinnitus.

Cholesteatoma   Pronounced *koh less teeah TOH mah*. Skin-like material that grows inward from the tympanic membrane and into the middle ear space. A cholesteatoma is a serious ear disease that requires medical attention.

CIC   See Completely-in-the-canal.

Clinical scholar   A professional who has expertise in providing patient services combined with research education and experience.

Closed-set response test   A type of speech audiometry procedure that includes a relatively small and fixed number of items like words or sentences that the patient responds to.

Cochlea   Pronounced *KOH kleeah*. The inner ear located within the temporal bone of the skull. The cochlea consists of important structures for hearing, including the inner and outer hair cells, the basilar membrane, the stria vascularis, and many other structures

Cochlear implants   Complex electrical devices that are used in the management of persons with severe or profound hearing loss consisting of external components for picking up sound and converting the sound to electrical signals and internal components for delivering the electrical signals to the auditory nerve.

Cocktail party (noise) effect   The phenomenon of hearing multiple voices at the same time and with concentration perceiving the speech of a single speaker

Code of ethics   A document developed by a professional organization for guiding the professional behavior of its members. Audiologists and speech pathologists are expected to abide by their respective Codes of Ethics.

Cognitive variables   Cognitive factors that can affect performance on hearing tests.

Collaborative consultation model   Provision of management services to the hearing impaired or speech-language impaired children within a school environment.

Comfortable (C) level   In programming a cochlear implant the level of electrical stimulation producing sound that is perceived as comfortable to the patient.

Competing message   A form of background sound during speech testing consisting of an ongoing meaningful story as opposed to noise or unintelligible multi-talker babble.

Completely-in-the-canal (CIC)   A hearing aid that fits entirely within the external ear canal.

Compression   See condensation. In amplification, limiting amplification of higher-intensity (louder) sounds in comparison to amplification of lower intensity (fainter) sounds.

Concha   The bowl-shaped region of the outer ear that helps to collect sound before it passes into the external auditory canal.

Condensation   Region of a sound wave characterized by increased density of molecules. Opposite of rarefaction. Acoustic stimulus produced by a positive electrical pulse activating a transducer like an earphone to produce condensation stimulus polarity.

Conditioned play audiometry (CPA)   A technique for hearing testing in young children that trains the patient to perform a game-type activity like dropping blocks into a bucket or putting pegs into holes in a board every time a sound is heard.

Configuration of hearing loss   The shape of an audiogram determined by how the degree of hearing loss changes as a function of the test frequency. Common configurations are flat, rising, and sloping hearing losses

Content counseling   A form of counseling that involves explaining test results and answering questions about hearing and test findings. Also called informational counseling.

Contralateral pathways   In acoustic reflex measurement the pathways involved in activation of the acoustic reflex when the stimulus sound is presented to one ear and changes in acoustic immittance due to contraction of the stapedius muscle are measured in the opposite ear.

Cortilymph   The thick fluid located within the organ of Corti in the cochlea.

Coupler   A specially designed device for connecting an earphone with a microphone of a sound-level meter. Also used to describe a small device that connects the acoustic tube of an insert earphones with a foam or rubber tip.

CPA   See Conditioned play audiometry.

Craniofacial abnormalities   Abnormalities from birth involving the head and face including the ear. Examples are deformations in the external ear and tags or pits in front of the ear.

Critical band   The part of a band of noise in a region above and below the frequency of a pure tone. A tone is barely detectable when the level of the critical band is the same as the level of the tone. Further increases in the frequency width beyond the critical band do not result in more effective interference with detection of the pure tone.

Cross hearing   Stimulus sound presented to the test ear at a level exceeding the inter-aural attention (insulation) provided by the head for air or bone conduction crosses over to and is detected in the non-test ear

Cross masking   Masking noise presented to the non-test ear at a sufficiently high level to crossover to interfere with hearing in the test ear. Also called over-masking.

Cued speech   A communication strategy for improving speech reading where sounds that are not visible as movements of the lips or tongue are identified with additional visual cues in the form of hand-shapes located near the mouth.

CVA   See Cerebrovascular accident.

Cycle   A complete 360-degree course of a single sine wave from beginning to end.

Cytomegalovirus (CMV)   A virus in the herpes family that is a serious cause of hearing loss in children. Hearing loss in CMV is progressive. It may initially only involve one ear.

Damping   Decrease in the amplitude of a vibrating body over time.

daPa   See decaPascal.

dB   See Decibel.

Deaf community   A group of people who communicate with sign language and who usually share the belief that deafness is a difference in human experience and not a disability.

Deaf Culture   A term used to describe the Deaf community. See Deaf community.

decaPascal (daPa)   A unit of pressure used in acoustic immittance measurements, such as tympanometry.

Decibel (dB)   A unit of sound intensity level. A dB is the logarithm of the sound pressure of a sound to a reference sound pressure (usually 0.0002 dynes/cm^2). For adult patients, hearing threshold levels of 0 to 20 dB are considered to be within the normal range. Units for describing decibels include dB hearing level (HL), sound pressure level (SPL), sensation level (SL) and, for auditory evoked responses, dB normal hearing level (dB nHL).

Degree of hearing loss   The extent or severity of a deficit in hearing thresholds. Degree of hearing loss on an audiogram is often described with terms like mild, moderate, and severe.

Dehiscence   A thinning of bone or a small opening in bone as in superior semicircular canal dehiscence in the vestibular apparatus.

Dementia   An impairment in cognitive and intellectual function that is generally related to advancing age. Features of dementia often include disorientation and deficits in memory and judgment.

Demyelinating disease   Neurological disorder resulting from abnormalities in the myelin surrounding neurons. Multiple sclerosis is an example of a demyelinating disease.

Descending-ascending method   A procedure for estimating hearing threshold that involves repeating the process of decreasing sound levels in 10 dB steps until the patient doesn't hear the stimulus and then increasing the level in 5 dB level steps until the patient responds again.

Dichotic listening task   A test that involves simultaneous presentation of a different sound like two different words or sentences to each ear. The patient usually responds by repeating the speech stimulus.

Differential diagnosis   The process of systematically reducing the number of explanations for the cause of a health problem like a hearing loss based on a review of the patient history and the analysis of findings for diagnostic tests.

Digitally programmable hearing aid   An analog hearing aid that digitally controls some circuits.

Displacement   When an object is displaced from one point to another point. Displacement is constantly changing over time, Displacement in a waveform is referred to as amplitude.

Distorted speech tests   Special tests of auditory processing that consist of alterations in the frequency or timing features to make the tests more sensitive to detecting deficits in auditory function.

Distortion product otoacoustic emissions (DPOAEs)   Sounds recorded in the external ear canal associated with activation and movements of the outer hair cells in the cochlea in response to stimulation with two closely spaced pure tones. Distortion products are evidence of outer hair cell functioning.

Distortional bone conduction   One of the three forms of bone conduction stimulation in which vibrations of the bones surrounding the cochlea are transmitted through cochlear fluids to hair cells.

Doctor of Audiology (AuD) degree   A degree awarded after completion of a three- or four-year graduate program in audiology; it is necessary for the practice of audiology.

DPgram   A graph showing the amplitude of distortion product otoacoustic emissions plotted as a function of the stimulus frequency (usually the f2 stimulus). See Distortion product otoacoustic emissions.

DPOAEs   See Distortion product otoacoustic emissions.

Early hearing detection and intervention (EHDI)   A term used to describe formal programs within the United States for newborn hearing screening, the diagnosis of infant hearing loss, and early intervention for infant hearing loss.

Ear mold   A device that connects a hearing aid to the patient's external ear canal. Ear molds are often custom-made for a particular patient.

Ear mold impression   Soft pliable material with the consistency of thick toothpaste that is injected into the ear canal prior to manufacture of a custom ear mold. Ear mold impression material becomes firm within a few minutes. It is removed from the external ear canal and usually shipped to a special laboratory where it is made into an ear mold.

Earobics   A computer-based auditory training program for developing auditory processing and pre-reading skills.

Ear specific   A term used to describe test results that result from stimulation of only the right or the left ear without involvement of the non-test ear.

Educational audiology (audiologist)   An audiologist working usually in a school setting who has responsibility for hearing care of students there.

Effective masking (EM)   The level of noise that is necessary to eliminate perception of or to mask any stimulus sound that reaches the non-test ear. Stimulus sound reaching the non-test ear at 20 dB HL is masked out with effective masking of at least 40 dB.

Efferent auditory system   The descending auditory pathways in the central nervous system that serve an inhibitory function. The efferent system ends with efferent fibers that connect with the hair cells in the inner ear.

EHDI   See Early Hearing Detection and Intervention.

Elasticity   The capacity of an object that has been deformed to return to its natural shape

Electroacoustical measurement/Electroacoustic procedures   Auditory tests involving the presentation of a sound stimulus and detection of an auditory response by the measurement of sound in the ear canal. Acoustic immittance measurements and otoacoustic emissions are examples of electroacoustic procedures.

Electrodes   Devices that make contact with the body and conduct bioelectrical activity from the body via a wire lead to recording equipment. The electrode may consist of different materials including metal in the shape of a small cup or an adhesive material integrated with conducting gel. Electrodes in auditory evoked response measurement detect activity in the ear and the brain. An electrode may also be used to deliver electrical stimulation to the body in a test of facial nerve function called electroneuronography (ENoG).

Electronystamography (ENG)   A group of vestibular tests that involve measurement of eyeball movements (nystagmus) that are spontaneous or that follow different types of stimulation of the vestibular system.

EM   See Effective masking.

Endolymph   A thick fluid in the auditory and vestibular portions of inner ear and specifically within the scala media.

Epley maneuver   A clinical repositioning maneuver performed in an office and used to treat a disorder known as benign paroxymal positional vertigo (BPPV) in which floating particles in a semicircular canal are relocated. Named after Dr. John Epley.

Erroneous hearing loss   See Pseudohypacusis, False hearing loss, and Exaggerated hearing loss.

Eustachian tube   A passageway that permits communication between the middle ear space on each side and the posterior region of the mouth (the nasopharynx).

It's lined with mucous membrane and normally closed toward the end near the mouth.

Exaggerated hearing loss An apparent hearing loss that is greater than actual hearing loss due to dysfunction within the auditory system. Also known as pseudohypacusis.

Expert model An approach for delivery of services when a school system consults with a professional, like an audiologist or speech pathologist, who has expertise that is not available in the school system.

External ear canal The passageway or channel in the outer ear leading from the concha to the tympanic membrane.

False hearing loss An apparent hearing loss that is not due to dysfunction of the auditory system and is not real. Also known as pseudohypacusis or erroneous hearing loss.

FastForWord A computer-based auditory training program that is specifically designed to develop the ability to rapidly process auditory information.

Feedback A whistling sound produced when sound from the receiver in a hearing aid is escapes from the ear canal and enters the microphone of the hearing aid where it is amplified again.

Filtered word test A test of auditory processing consisting of words with high frequency information removed to reduce redundancy.

Flat hearing loss configuration Hearing thresholds on an audiogram that are similar at different test frequencies.

fMRI See Functional magnetic resonance imaging.

Forced vibration Vibration of an object that is maintained by the application of ongoing external energy.

Foreign body (foreign objects) Term used to describe anything out of the ordinary in the external ear canal such as raisins, pebbles, insects, and other assorted small objects.

Foreign objects Term used to describe anything out of the ordinary in the external ear canal such as raisins, pebbles, insects, and other assorted small objects.

Frenzel goggles Special goggles that magnify the appearance of the eyes used in testing vestibular functions.

Frequency A property of sound defined as the number of complete cycles or oscillations of a vibrating body in a specified unit of time (e.g., 1000 cycles/second). Frequency is usually indicated with the abbreviation Hz (for Hertz).

Functional hearing loss See Pseudohypacusis, False hearing loss, and Exaggerated hearing loss.

Functional magnetic resonance imaging (fMRI) A dynamic brain imaging technique that displays metabolic activity in the brain during some type of stimulation, such as listening to words or other sound.

Gain (hearing aid) Increase in the amplitude or energy of an electrical signal with amplification. Gain is the difference between the input signal and the output signal.

Gaze test A test within the ENG test battery that measures eye movements (nystagmus) while the eyes are in different horizontal positions.

Gestation (Gestational age) The time in weeks after conception. A full-term birth is 40 weeks. Premature infants with a gestational age of as little as 26 to 27 weeks can now survive with intensive care.

Hearing aids Electrical devices that amplify sound to improve hearing and communication.

Hearing aid selection The process of determining the hearing aid style and characteristics most likely to provide maximum benefit for hearing and communication.

Hearing assistance technology (HAT) See Assistive listening devices.

Hearing Handicap Inventory for the Elderly-Screening Version (HHIE-S) A popular and brief inventory or tool for determining the impact of hearing loss on daily activities and communication.

Hearing in Noise Test (HINT) A test of speech perception that involves repeating sentences in the presence of speech spectrum noise. Testing is conducted at different speech-to-noise ratios.

Hearing science The area of science that focuses on the ear and hearing. Hearing scientists often have specific interests such as psychoacoustics, the anatomy or physiology of a particular region of the auditory system, or neurophysiological measures of auditory function.

Hermetic seal In audiology, an airtight seal or connection between a rubber probe tip and the walls of the external ear canal.

Hyperacusis Abnormally decreased tolerance to everyday loud sounds.

Impedance (Z) A measure of total opposition to energy (current) flow in an electrical, mechanical, or acoustical system. Inter-electrode impedance in evoked response measurement is the opposition to current flow between a pair of electrodes, reported as electrical resistance in ohms.

Incus Second ossicle within the middle ear space that is connected laterally to the malleus and medially to the stapes.

Industrial audiology The area of audiology that focuses on prevention and documentation of noise-related hearing loss in work settings.

Inertia The resistance of any object to change its shape or its state of motion.

Inertial bone conduction Bone conduction stimulation that is produced by the lag in movement between the vibrations of the bone surrounding the ear and the movement of the stapes in and out of the oval window.

Information counseling See Content counseling.

Informed consent A document signed by a patient or research subject indicating agreement to participate in clinical testing or treatments, or a well-defined research study

Initial masking (IM) The lowest level of noise presented to the non-test ear during masking. The level of initial masking is equivalent to the hearing threshold in the non-test ear.

Inner hair cells Very small cells arranged in a single row in the cochlea with stereocilia ("hairs") on the top that communicate with auditory nerve fibers at the bottom. There are about 3500 inner hair cells in a human cochlea.

Insert earphones A type of earphone consisting of a transducer built into a small box and an acoustic tube for delivery of the sound stimulus to the ear. The tube is coupled to the ear by means of a small foam or rubber probe tip.

Instantaneous displacement Displacement of a point on a waveform at a specific time.

Intensity The magnitude of sound energy per unit area. The term is commonly used in describing sound levels used in hearing testing.

Interaural attenuation The isolation or attenuation produced by the head when sound is presented to one ear before it crosses over to the other (non-test ear). Inter-aural attenuation is greater for insert earphones (at least 60 dB) than for supra-aural earphones (at least 40 dB).

There is no inter-aural attenuation for bone conduction (0 dB).

In-the-canal (ITC) A small hearing aid style that fits entirely within the external auditory canal.

In-the-ear (ITE) A hearing aid style that fits entirely within the concha of the outer ear and extends into the external auditory canal.

Inverse square law The principle of physics that defines the decrease in sound intensity as a function of the square of the distance from the source of the sound.

Ipsilateral pathways In acoustic reflex measurement the pathways involved in activation of the acoustic reflex when the stimulus sound is presented to one ear and changes in acoustic immittance due to contraction of the stapedius muscle are measured in the same ear.

ITC See In-the-canal.

ITE See In-the-ear.

Labyrinth The complex fluid-filled passageways within the auditory and vestibular portions of the ear that are enclosed within the temporal bone including the bony labyrinth and the membranous labyrinth.

LACE See Listening and Communication Enhancement.

LDL See Loudness discomfort level.

Licensure Credential required by states in the United States in the regulation of audiologists, speech pathologists, and other professionals.

Linear amplification Increase in sound output from a hearing aid that is proportional to the sound input.

Listening and Communication Enhancement (LACE) A computer-based or online auditory training program for development of different skills important in communication including speech perception in noise and cognitive factors involved in hearing. The LACE program is designed for adults with hearing loss to improve listening skills.

Listening check Daily verification of the output of audiometers and earphones conducted with a known normal-hearing person. Sometimes called biological calibration.

Localization to sound Determining the specific location of a source of a sound in space in horizontal and vertical directions.

Loudness The psychological correlate to sound intensity. Increases in sound intensity are perceived as increased loudness. The relationship between intensity and loudness is not one-to-one but, rather, logarithmic.

Loudness discomfort level (LDL) The level of sound perceived as unpleasant or uncomfortably loud. Also known as uncomfortable loudness level (UCL).

Loudness recruitment Abnormal growth in the perception of loudness. A feature of sensory hearing loss due to abnormal function of the outer hair cells.

Malignant The tendency of a pathology like a tumor to progressively worsen and potentially cause death. In describing tumors, the term *malignant* often refers to cancer.

Malingerer See Pseudohypacusis.

Malingering Consciously and willfully faking or exaggerating a hearing loss motivated by personal gain like financial compensation or to avoid an obligation. See False and Exaggerated hearing loss.

Malleus The first of the three tiny bones (ossicles) connecting the tympanic membrane to the inner ear. The umbo of the malleus rests against the inner surface of the tympanic membrane and can usually be seen with otoscopic examination of the ear. The malleus connects the tympanic membrane to the incus.

Manometer A meter for measuring air pressure. Acoustic immittance devices include a manometer to measure air pressure in the ear canal during tympanometry.

Manual approaches Manual education of children with profound hearing loss emphasizes the development and reliance on sign language for communication with little or no use of residual hearing abilities.

Masking (masker) Noise presented to the non-test ear in a hearing test procedure. Common masking noises are either broadband or narrowband noise. Masking is used in an attempt to prevent a response from the non-test ear due to possible stimulus crossover from the test ear.

Masking dilemma Briefly, when the level of masking noise that is adequate to mask the non-test ear crosses over to the mask the test ear (cross masking occurs)

Maximum masking The highest intensity level of masking noise that can be presented to the non-test ear before the noise level exceeds inter-aural attention for the earphone and cross masking occurs and the test ear is affected by over-masking.

Maximum stimulation level The highest level of electrical stimulation for a cochlear implant before a patient experiences discomfort.

MCL See Most comfortable level.

Medical home A patient-centered model for health delivery involving a team led by a physician for comprehensive and continuous provision of healthcare.

Ménière's disease Pathology affecting the cochlea and resulting in sensory (sensorineural) hearing impairment. Characteristic signs and symptoms are tinnitus, vertigo, sensation of ear fullness, and a fluctuating, often low frequency, sensorineural hearing loss.

Meningiomas Tumors that arise from the meninges surrounding the brain in the region of the auditory nerve that can cause hearing loss.

Meningitis An inflammation of the meninges, the tissue that is a protective covering of the brain and the spinal cord.

Microtia Pronounced *my CRO shia*. Abnormally small and/or deformed outer ear.

Minimum masking The lowest level of noise presented to the non-test ear that masks hearing and prevents detection of stimulus sound crossing over from the test to the non-test ear.

Misophonia Decreased tolerance to sound characterized by a severe dislike or aversion to specific sounds, usually sounds produced by bodily activities like chewing and lip smacking.

MLV See Monitored live voice.

mmH$_2$O A unit of pressure expressed as millimeters (mm) of water (H$_2$O) pressure.

Monaural frequency distorted speech tests Tests involving speech like words with some frequencies removed that are presented to one ear at a time.

Monitored live voice (MLV) Presentation mode for speech audiometry using speech spoken into a microphone with visual monitoring of the voice level on a meter or digital display.

Most comfortable level (MCL) Hearing level judged by a listener to be comfortable (not too loud and not to soft). The level at which most people prefer to listen to sound.

Multi-talker babble Recording of ongoing speech of two or more speakers that is unintelligible.

Myringotomy Pronounced *meer ing GAH toh mee*. A surgical procedure that involves making a small incision or cut in the tympanic membrane usually to drain fluid from the middle ear space. A myringotomy is performed before insertion of tympanostomy tubes into the tympanic membrane.

Natural auditory-oral approach A family-centered variation of the auditory-oral strategy that maximizes normal daily parent-child interaction to promote development of effective communication.

Neoplasm *Gr. neos,* new, *plasma,* thing. A tumor within the body, literally, a new growth. An anti-neoplastic drug is given to stop, or reduce, the growth of a tumor.

Neurodegenerative disease A neurologic disease that leads to a deterioration of function including auditory abnormalities.

Neurofibroma Tumor arising from the skin and/or from peripheral nerves.

Neuroradiology Imaging of the central nervous system including computerized tomography (CT) and magnetic resonance imaging (MRI).

Nonorganic hearing loss See False hearing loss, Exaggerated hearing loss, or Pseudohypacusis.

Nystagmus Horizontal or less commonly vertical movements of the eyeballs. Nystagmus may result from stimulation of the vestibular (balance) system. Recording nystagmus with electrodes placed around the eyes during stimulation of the vestibular system is a technique called electronystagmography (ENG).

OAEs See Otoacoustic emissions.

Objective auditory procedures Auditory tests that do not require a behavioral response from a patient. Otoacoustic emissions, acoustic immittance measures, and auditory evoked responses are examples of objective auditory tests.

Occlusion effect Perception of increased loudness of a bone conducted tone stimulus when an ear is covered with an earphone or when the external auditory canal is occluded with an insert ear tip. The occlusion effect also occurs for patients with middle ear disorder and conductive hearing loss.

Open fit-BTE hearing aid A behind-the-ear hearing aid design that consists of a tube that leads to but does not block the external auditory canal opening.

Open-set response test A speech recognition test that includes many different items like words. With an open-set response test patients have no advanced notice about which word they are about to hear.

Organ of Corti The sensory organ of hearing is located on the basilar membrane of the cochlea (inner ear). It contains inner and outer hair cells as well as supporting cells. Mechanical energy is transduced to bioelectrical energy at the organ of Corti.

Oscillate To vibrate and move back and forth.

Osseotympanic bone conduction One of the three mechanisms of bone conduction hearing. With osseotympanic bone conduction, sound energy from vibrations of the skull produced in the external ear canal reaches the tympanic membrane and then activates the cochlea.

Otitis externa Infection involving the external ear canal walls.

Otitis media A general term for various forms of middle ear disease, such as serous otitis media, otitis media with effusion, purulent otitis media, and chronic otitis media. Otitis media is one of the most common childhood diseases and usually produces a conductive hearing loss.

Otoacoustic emissions (OAEs) Acoustic energy measured within the ear canal that is produced by the cochlea, specifically movement or motility of outer hair cells. Evoked OAEs, including transient (TEOAEs), and distortion-product (DPOAE) otoacoustic emissions are generated by acoustic stimulation of the ear.

Otolaryngology Medical specialty dealing with medical and surgical treatment of diseases and disorders affecting the ears, nose, and throat (ENT).

Otologist A physician who specializes in medical and surgical treatment of ear diseases. An otologist is an otolaryngologist, commonly called an ear, noise, and throat (ENT) physician.

Otology Specialty within otolaryngology specializing in diagnosis and treatment of ear and related problems like vestibular or balance disorders.

Otosclerosis A bony degenerative disease process that can involve the stapes footplate and/or the cochlea; also called otospongiosus.

Otoscope A device for illuminating the external auditory canal and examining the ear consisting of a light and cone-shaped speculum that fits into the opening of the ear canal.

Otoscopy Examination or inspection of the external ear canal and tympanic membrane with an illuminating device (see Otoscope).

Ototoxic   Pronounced *oh toh TAHX ick.* Drugs or medications that potentially damage the cochlea and cause hearing loss. Most ototoxic drugs interfere with metabolism of the hair cells in the cochlea.

Outer hair cells   Very small and highly metabolic cells arranged in three to four rows in the cochlea with more than 100 stereocilia ("hairs") on the top. Outer hair cells are capability of motility or changes in shape with activation by sound. There are about 12,000 outer hair cells in a human cochlea.

Oval window   One of two openings into the inner ear (cochlea) from the middle ear space. Vibrations transmitted through the middle ear are send via the stapes footplate through the oval window into the inner ear. See *Round window.*

Over-masking   When the level of masking noise presented to the non-test ear is sufficient to crossover to the test ear and interfere with detection of the stimulus sound.

Paralysis   Pronounced *pah RAH luh sus.* Loss of muscle function.

Paresis   Pronounced *pah REE sus.* Weakness of muscle function.

Patient history   A patient's description of health status including complaints, symptoms, and prior tests and treatments.

PB   See Phonemically balanced.

PBmax   Maximum score in word recognition performance for a list of phonetically (phonemically) balanced words.

PBmin   The minimum score in word recognition performance for a list of phonetically (phonemically) balanced words at an intensity level higher than the level producing the maximum score (PBmax). Used in the description of rollover in word recognition.

PB word lists   A list of twenty-five or fifty monosyllabic words that that contains the distribution of speech sounds (phonemes) as they are distributed in connected English speech.

Pediatric audiology   Evaluation of hearing and management of hearing loss in children.

Perforation   Pronounced *purr for AY shon.* A hole in the ear drum. A perforation may result from infection and rupture of the tympanic membrane due to buildup of infected fluid or traumatic damage to the tympanic membrane.

Performance intensity (PI) function   See Performance intensity function for PB words.

Performance intensity function for PB words (PI-PB function)   A graph displaying word recognition performance in percent correct on the y-axis as a function of the intensity level of the words on the x-axis.

Perilymph   Thick fluid within the scala vestibuli and the scala tympani in the cochlea and also within the vestibular portion of the ear.

Period   Duration in seconds of one complete cycle of a vibration or a pure tone. The period is the reciprocal of frequency. For example, the period of a 1000 Hz tone is 1/1000 second.

Peripheral auditory system   The portion of the auditory system that includes the outer ear, the middle ear, the inner ear, and the auditory nerve.

Phase   The zero voltage point at the beginning of the waveform of a stimulus or of a frequency component of a response waveform expressed in degrees or radians, such as 0 or 90 degrees. Phase of a response is related to latency.

Phonemically balanced (PB)   Also phonetically balanced. Characteristic of single-syllable words in which speech sounds (phonemes) are represented with the occurrence expected in conversational or written speech.

Phonophobia   Fear of certain sounds. See Hyperacusis and Misophonia.

PI-PB function   See Performance intensity function for PB words.

Pinna   The most visible outer portion of the ear consisting of a cartilage framework. The auricle. Parts of the pinna are the helix, the lobe, and the concha. The word *pinna* is derived from the Latin word for feather or wing.

Pitch   The psychological sensation related to the frequency of sound. High pitches correspond to high-frequency sounds and low pitches to low-frequency sounds.

Preauricular pits   Small indentations or holes in the skin in front of the ear.

Preauricular tag   A small outgrowth of skin in front of the ear.

Preferred method   A long-standing approach for conducting pure tone hearing testing in which sounds are decreased in intensity by 10 dB and then increased in intensity by 5 dB.

Presbycusis   Pronounced *press bee COO sis.* Decrease in hearing sensitivity associated with aging. Although hearing may first begin to show aging effects at 20 years, presbycusis usually does not cause speech perception difficulty and serious hearing impairment until age 60 or older.

Prescriptive hearing aid fitting   A method for determining the most appropriate amplification with a hearing aid for a specific patient based on description of the degree of hearing loss at different frequencies and other factors.

Prevalence   The proportion of a population or number of persons that has a specific condition or disorder like a hearing loss.

Probe tone   A tone presented to the ear via a probe in the external ear canal that is used in acoustic immittance measurements.

Pseudohypacusis   False or exaggerated hearing loss.

Psychoacoustics   Field focuses on study of the relation between the physical properties of sound (e.g., intensity and frequency) and the psychological or perceptual aspects of hearing (e.g., loudness and pitch).

Psychogenic hearing loss   A false hearing loss associated with psychological factors sometimes at the unconscious level.

Psychosocial (status or problems)   In audiology a patient's emotional or social status or response to hearing loss or related disorders including responses such as frustration, irritation, sense of isolation, anger, sadness.

PTA   See Pure tone average.

Pure tones   A single-frequency tonal sound, e.g.. 1000 Hz; a sinusoid. See related term Simple harmonic motion.

Pure tone average (PTA)   The average of hearing threshold levels in dB HL. The pure tone average is usually at test frequencies of 500, 1000, and 2000 Hz. These frequencies are in the speech frequency region.

Quality of life   A index of general well-being and health status.

Rarefaction   Region of a sound wave characterized by less dense molecules. Opposite of condensation. Acoustic stimulus produced by a negative electrical pulse activating a transducer like an earphone.

REA   See Right ear advantage.

Receiver   In a hearing aid, the component that receives an amplified electrical signal and converts it to sound that is delivered to a patient's ear.

Receiver-in-the-canal (RIC)   A relatively recent hearing aid design with the receiver producing sound located within the external auditory canal.

Reference equivalent threshold sound pressure levels (RETSPLs)   Sound level values that are determined from calibrating sounds with a sound level meter connected to a specific type of coupler.

Resonance frequency   The natural frequency for vibration of an object where vibrations occur with the least external force.

Retrocochlear   Referring to the eighth cranial nerve or central auditory nervous system pathways. Retrocochlear auditory dysfunction often refers only to dysfunction involving the eighth (auditory) nerve.

Retrocochlear disorder   Abnormality in the auditory system that involves the eighth cranial nerve, or other structures toward the central nervous system from the inner ear. An "acoustic tumor" (really a vestibular schwannoma) is an example of retrocochlear pathology.

RETSPLs   See Reference equivalent threshold sound pressure levels.

RIC   See Receiver-in-the-canal.

Right ear advantage (REA)   Better (higher) scores on dichotic listening tests when stimuli (e.g., words) are presented to the right versus left ears.

Rising hearing loss configuration   An audiogram configuration or shape with poorer hearing in the low frequencies improving to better hearing in the high frequency region.   Often reflects a conductive hearing impairment when bone conduction hearing is normal.

R/O   See Rule out.

Rollover   A somewhat paradoxical decrease in performance (percent correct) scores for a speech audiometry procedure at highest stimulus intensity level versus maximum scores at a lower intensity level. Rollover of greater than 20% is often considered a sign of retrocochlear auditory dysfunction.

Rollover index   A number describing the amount of rollover in word recognition scores in comparison to the maximum word recognition score.

Round window   One of two openings in the bony wall of the inner ear connecting the inner ear to the middle ear. The round window, which is covered with a thin membrane, acts as a pressure release valve permitting movement of inner ear fluids with movement of the stapes footplate. See Oval window.

Rule out (R/O) In audiology, to eliminate as a possibility a disease or disorder as an explanation of a patient's auditory problem. For example, age-related hearing loss was ruled out by the patient's age of 8 years.

Saccade test A vestibular test that records eye movements as a person looks at a visual stimulus that repeatedly moves in a horizontal direction.

SAL See Sensorineural acuity level technique.

SAT See Speech awareness threshold.

Scope of practice A document describing the clinical activities that are appropriate and "within the scope" of practice for a profession like audiology or speech pathology.

SDT See Speech detection threshold.

SEE See Signing Exact English.

Sensorineural Hearing loss due to cochlear (sensory) or eighth nerve (neural) auditory dysfunction. Most hearing impairments described as sensorineural are actually just sensory. The term "nerve deafness" is often used inappropriately to describe sensory hearing loss due to common etiologies, such as exposure to high intensity noise and aging. Also sometimes referred to as neurosensory.

Sensorineural acuity level (SAL) technique A test for estimating bone conduction hearing levels based on a comparison of pure tone air conduction hearing thresholds in quiet versus with at least 50 dB of narrowband noise presented via bone conduction. Bone conduction hearing is calculated with an analysis of the shift or increase in hearing thresholds with noise.

Signal-to-noise ratio (SNR) The ratio of an acoustical or electrical signal to background (non-response) acoustical or electrical activity (noise).

Signing Exact English (SEE) A manual communication system that utilizes much of the same vocabulary as American Sign Language (ASL) plus grammatical features and English syntax

Simple harmonic motion Movement of an object back and forth to produce multiple vibrations.

Site-of-lesion The location of dysfunction, pathology, or abnormality within the auditory system.

SLM See Sound level meter.

Sloping hearing loss configuration A term used in describing the configuration of a pure tone audiogram, that is, how hearing loss varies as a function of test frequency. A sloping configuration shows progressively greater hearing loss for higher test frequencies. A common audiogram pattern, a sloping hearing loss is often associated with age related cochlear dysfunction.

SNR See Signal-to-noise ratio.

SOAEs See Spontaneous otoacoustic emissions.

Sound field In audiology sound from a loudspeaker in an enclosed area like a sound-treated test room.

Sound-field testing Hearing testing with sounds presented to a patient with a loudspeaker in a sound-treated test room. The patient does not wear earphones in sound-field testing.

Sound level meter (SLM) A device for measuring and quantifying sound intensity level in decibels (dB) sound pressure level (SPL).

Sound pressure level (SPL) The amount or intensity of a sound, such as an acoustic stimulus for evoked responses, expressed in decibels (dB); an intensity level of 0 dB SPL is the smallest amount of displacement of air molecules caused by a sound that can be just be detected by the human ear at a given frequency; a physical scale for intensity level. The normal hearing SPL decibel (dB) reference is 20 micropascals, i.e., dB SPL = 20 log (Po/Pref), where Po is observed instantaneous pressure and Pref = 20 pascals.

Special speech audiometry Speech audiometry tests in addition to word recognition in quiet that are used in the assessment of auditory processing including speech-in-noise tests, frequency- or time-disordered speech tests, and dichotic listening procedures. Also called diagnostic speech audiometry.

Speech awareness threshold (SAT) Hearing level at which a patient can just detect the presence of a speech signal. Also called speech detection threshold (SDT).

Speech detection threshold (SDT) See Speech awareness threshold (SAT).

Speech discrimination Distinguishing between two speech items that differ in only one speech sound like "cat" versus "bat." Sometimes inaccurately used to describe speech recognition.

Speech frequency region Frequencies within the 500 to 2000 or 3000 Hz region that are important for the perception of speech.

Speech materials Consonant-vowel combinations, words, sentences, and other forms of speech used in speech audiometry.

Speech-in-noise test A common type of test of auditory processing that requires recognition of a speech signal like a word or sentence in the presence of some type of background noise or speech.

Speech noise Noise with energy within the spectrum or frequency region of speech.

Speech reception threshold (SRT) The lowest speech level at which a listener can correctly repeat or recognize approximately 50% of a small series of words. See Speech recognition threshold.

SPL See Sound pressure level.

Spondee threshold (ST) Lowest level at which approximately 50% of two-syllable spondee words can be correctly repeated.

Spondee words Two-syllable words with equal stress on each syllable such as *toothbrush, airplane, sidewalk*. Also called spondaic words.

Spontaneous otoacoustic emissions (SOAEs) Energy produced by outer hair cells and detected in the external ear canal in the absence of any outside acoustic stimulus.

Standard of care The level of healthcare and degree of prudence and caution required of a qualified individual.

Stapedius muscle The smallest muscle in the human body, attached to the posterior portion of the neck of the stapes and innervated by a branch of the seventh (facial) cranial nerve. The stapedius muscle contracts in response to high-intensity sounds. See Acoustic stapedial reflex.

Stapes Pronounced *STAY pees*. A tiny, stirrup-shaped bone (ossicle) within the medial portion of the middle ear space connecting another ossicle (the incus) to the oval window of the cochlea.

Stenger test A clinical test based on the Stenger principle that is used in diagnosis of unilateral false or exaggerated hearing loss.

Stenosis Pronounced *stih NO sis*. In audiology, a restriction or even total occlusion of the external auditory canal.

Supra-aural earphones Earphones that rest on the pinna with a diaphragm aligned with the opening of the external auditory canal.

Supra-threshold level A level above a person's hearing threshold. For example, word recognition testing is conducted at a supra-threshold level.

Syndromes Collections of signs and symptoms associated with specific diseases or conditions.

Talk Back An electronic connection for communication between an audiologist outside of a sound room and the patient inside the sound room. A TalkBack system consists of a microphone and earphones or a loudspeaker for the tester and for the patient.

Temporal bone A very hard skull bone enclosing the external ear canal, the middle and inner ear, and within the internal auditory canal, the eighth (auditory) cranial nerve.

Temporal integration A measure of processing of brief durations of sound. Hearing thresholds are progressively elevated for sounds as duration decreases below 200 ms.

Temporal lobe One of the four major lobes of the brain. Auditory regions are located in the temporal lobe.

Tensor tympani muscle Connected to the malleus in the middle ear the tensor tympani muscle contracts with bodily activities like chewing and also in a startle-type response to very high intensity sounds. The tensor tympani muscle is innervated by the trigeminal (5th cranial) nerve. The other smaller muscle in the middle ear is the stapedius muscle.

TEOAEs See Transient evoked otoacoustic emissions.

Tertiary care hospital A large hospital offering high level of comprehensive care by specialists to persons with a variety of health problems. Many tertiary care hospitals are located in medical centers in urban areas or on a university campus.

Test battery A collection of auditory tests that are applied in the diagnosis of auditory dysfunction. Usually each test in the battery contributes different information on auditory function.

Test reliability See Test-retest reliability.

Test-retest reliability The agreement between results from one test to the next for the same patient under the same test conditions. Also called test repeatability.

Test validity The degree to which a test finding accurately reflects a disorder that is tested.

Thalamus A sub-cortical oval shaped structure on each side of the central nervous system that serves as a major relay station for sensory pathways (auditory, visual, somatosensory) between the brainstem and cortex. The medial geniculate body, an important auditory structure, is located on the posterior portion of thalamus.

Threshold In audiology the level of sound that is just barely detected. Typically, threshold is defined as the level of sound in dB HL that can be detected about 50% of the times it is presented.

Tinnitus The perception of a noise in the ear like ringing, cricket sound, or roaring even when there is no external sound; a phantom sound. Tinnitus is not a disease but, rather, a symptom associated with many disorders of the auditory system.

TM Tympanic membrane.

Tone bursts Very brief (less than 1 second) tone stimuli. Tone burst stimuli are effective in eliciting an auditory brainstem response.

Top-down or strategy-driven approach Treatment strategies that focus on high-level cognitive and linguistic functions rather than perception of sounds and the listening environment.

Total communication A combination education approach for persons with severe or profound hearing loss that includes both oral methods for hearing speech and also manual or sign language methods.

Transcranial hearing Hearing sounds that travel across or around the head from one ear to the other. Most transcranial hearing occurs via bone conduction from one ear to the cochlea on the other side.

Transcranial transmission loss The reduction in the intensity of a sound stimulus as it travels from the test ear to the nontest ear. See Interaural attenuation.

Transducer An electroacoustic device for converting energy from one form to another. An earphone is a transducer that converts electrical energy to acoustic energy (sound).

Transient evoked otoacoustic emissions (TEOAEs) Energy associated with stimulation of outer hair cells in the cochlea in response to very brief sounds like clicks.

Traveling waves Systematic movements of the basilar membrane progressing from the base near the stapes footplate toward the apex. Deformations of the basilar membrane activate the outer and inner hair cells in the cochlea.

TTS See Temporary threshold shift.

Tuning fork A metal device with a stem and two tines that produces a specific frequency like 500 Hz with vibration after it is struck on the hand.

Tympanic membrane Three-layer membrane that vibrates in response to even very small levels of sound. The outer layer consists of skin, the middle layer connective tissue, and the inner layer is mucous membrane. Commonly called the eardrum.

Tympanogram A graph showing measurement of tympanic membrane mobility as a function of air pressure changes within the ear canal. Tympanograms are classified into types, e.g., type A, type B, and type C.

Tympanometry Measurement of tympanic membrane mobility as a function of air pressure changes within the ear canal.

Under-masking When the level of masking noise presented to the non-test ear is not adequate to prevent the test stimulus from being heard in the non-test ear.

UNHS Universal newborn hearing screening.

Universal newborn hearing screening (UNHS) Hearing screening of all babies in a defined area (e.g., state, province, country).

Upper stimulation level The highest level of electrical stimulation producing sound that is comfortable.

Validation In hearing aid fitting, the process of determining that a patient is getting as much benefit as possible from amplification in daily communication.

VEMP See Vestibular evoked myogenic potential.

Verification In hearing aid fitting, verification is the process for making sure that a hearing aid is properly amplifying sound for a specific patient.

Vertigo A symptom of balance and specifically vestibular disorder. The patient experiences a spinning sensation, or senses that the environment is spinning around him or her.

Vestibular evoked myogenic potential (VEMP) Momentary reduction in contraction of the sternocleidomastoid muscle in response to high intensity low frequency stimulation of an ear and activation of the saccule within the vestibular apparatus.

Vestibular schwannoma A tumor arising from the schwann cells of the superior or inferior vestibular nerve. With growth, the tumor can press upon the auditory portion of the auditory nerve. Also known as an acoustic neuroma or acoustic tumor.

Vestibular system Portion of the nervous system that is responsible for maintaining a person's equilibrium and position in space. The vestibular system consists of structures in the ear, vestibular nerves, and collections of vestibular nerves in the brainstem with connections also to eye muscles and large muscle groups in the trunk of the body.

Vibration Back and forth movements of an object that give rise to sound energy.

Vibrotactile response A sensation of feeling with the presentation of high-intensity and low-frequency bone conduction sounds.

Video-nystagmography (VNG) Measurement of nystagmus (eye movements) with special magnifying goggles during various vestibular tests.

Video otoscopy Visualization of the external ear canal and tympanic membrane with a computer or video monitor during inspection of the ear.

Visual reinforcement Use of light, picture, or mechanical play activity to maintain a child's attention during behavioral hearing testing and to reinforce responses to sound.

VNG See Video-nystagmography.

Warble tones Slight and rapid change or modulation the frequency of pure tones used in hearing testing with loudspeakers in a sound-treated room to minimize the likelihood of constructive or destructive interference.

Wavelength Distance between the same point on two successive cycles of a pure tone.

Weber test A test performed with a tuning fork or an audiometer to measure the lateralization of forehead presented bone conducted sound to the right ear, the left ear, or the middle of the head. The Weber test is usually performed with low-frequency pure tones like 250 and 500 Hz.

Word recognition Repetition or identification of words presented in a list during hearing testing.

Z See Impedance.

References

Agrawal, S. K., Blevins, N. H., & Jackler, R. K. (2009). Vestibular schwannomas and other skull base neoplasms. In J. B. Snow Jr. & P. A. Wackym (Eds.), *Ballenger's otorhinolaryngology—head and neck surgery* (17th ed., pp. 413–433). Shelton CT: BC Decker.

Agrawal, Y., Platz, E. A., Niparko, J. K. (2008). Prevalence of hearing loss and differences by demographic characteristics among US adults: Data from the National Health and Nutrition Examination Survey, 1999–2004. *Archives of Internal Medicine, 168,* 1522–1530.

American Academy of Audiology. (1997). Identification of hearing loss and middle ear dysfunction in preschool and school aged children. Position Statement. *Audiology Today, 9,* 21–23.

American Academy of Audiology. (2003). Pediatric amplification guidelines. Retrieved October 21, 2012, from www.audiology.org/resources/documentlibrary/documents/pedamp.pdf

American Academy of Audiology. (2004). Scope of Practice. www.audiology.org Retrieved February 18, 2013.

American Academy of Audiology. (2010). *Clinical practice guidelines: Diagnosis, treatment and management of children and adults with central auditory processing disorder.* Accessed November 16, 2010 from www.audiology.org/resources/documentlibrary/Documents/CAPD%20Guidelines%208-2010.pdf

American Academy of Audiology. (2010). Position statement: Audiology assistants. www.audiology.org/resources/documentlibrary/Documents/2010_AudiologyAssistant_Pos_Stat.pdf

American Academy of Pediatrics, Task Force on Newborn and Infant Hearing. (1999). Newborn and infant hearing loss: Detection and intervention. *Pediatrics, 103,* 527–530.

American Academy of Pediatrics & American Academy of Family Physicians, Subcommittee on Management of Acute Otitis Media. (2004, March). *Clinical practice guideline: Diagnosis and management of acute otitis media.* Retrieved July 10, 2012, from www.aap.org

American Medical Association (AMA). (2008). *Guides to permanent hearing impairment* (6th ed.). www.ama-assn.org/go/amaguidessixthedition-errata

American National Standards Institute. (1987). American National Standards specifications for instruments to measure aural acoustic impedance and admittance (aural acoustic immittance). ANSI S3.39-1987. New York: Author.

American National Standards Institute. (1999). *Maximum permissible ambient noise levels for audiometric test rooms.* ANSI S3.1-1999. New York: Author.

American National Standards Institute. (2002). *Acoustical performance criteria, design requirements, and guidelines for schools.* ANSI S12.60-2002. New York: Author.

American National Standards Institute. (2003). *American national standard for specification of hearing aid characteristics.* ANSI S3.22-2003. New York: Author.

American National Standards Institute. (2004). *American national specification for audiometers.* ANSI S3.6-2004. New York: Author.

American National Standards Institute. (2004a). Methods for manual pure-tone threshold audiometry. ANSI S3.21-2004. New York: Author.

American National Standards Institute. (2010). Specifications for audiometers. ANSI S3.6-2010. New York: Author.

American Speech-Language-Hearing Association Subcommittee on Speech Audiometry. (1979). Guidelines for determining the threshold level for speech. *Asha, 21,* 353–355.

American Speech-Language-Hearing Association Subcommittee on Speech Audiometry. (1988). Guidelines for determining the threshold level for speech. *Asha, 30,* 85–89.

American Speech-Language-Hearing Association (ASHA). (1990). *Guidelines for audiometric symbols.* Rockville, MD: Author. Available from www.asha.org/policy

American Speech-Language-Hearing Association. (1997). Guidelines for audiological screening. Rockville, MD: Author. www.asha.org

American Speech-Language-Hearing Association. (2004). *Scope of practice in audiology.* Retrieved February 18, 2013, from www.asha.org/policy/SP2004-00192.htm

American Speech-Language-Hearing Association (ASHA). (2005a). *Guidelines for manual pure-tone threshold audiometry.* Rockville, MD: Author. Available from www.asha.org/policy

American Speech-Language-Hearing Association. (2005b). *(Central) auditory processing disorders [Technical Report].* Retrieved July 10, 2011, from www.asha.org/docs/html/TR2005-00043.html

Amiani, A. M. (2001). Efficacy of directional microphone hearing aids: A meta-analytic perspective. *Journal of the American Academy of Audiology, 12,* 202–214.

Andéol, G., Guillaume, A., Micheyl, C., Savel, S., Pellieux, L., & Moulin, A. (2011). Auditory efferents facilitate sound localization in noise in humans. *The Journal of Neuroscience, 31,* 6759–6763.

Anderson, H., Barr, V., & Wedenberg, E. (1970). Early diagnosis of VIIIth nerve tumours by acoustic reflex tests. *Acta Otolaryngologica, 263,* 232–237.

Arts, H. A., & Neely, J. G. (2001). Intratemporal and intracranial complications of otitis media. In B. J. Bailey, K. H. Calhoun, G. B. Healy, H. C. Pillsbury, J. T. Johnson, R. T. Jackler, & M. E. Tardy (Eds.), *Head and neck surgery—otolarynoglogy. Volume II* (3rd ed., pp. 1759–1772). Philadelphia: Lippincott Williams & Wilkins.

Ashmore, J. (2008). Cochlear outer hair cell motility. *Physiological Reviews, 88,* 173–210.

Attias, J., Bresloff, I., & Furman, V. (1996). The influence of the efferent auditory system on otoacoustic emissions in noise induced tinnitus. *Acta Otolaryngologica, 116,* 534–539.

Bagatto, M., & Scollie, S. (2011). Current approaches to the fitting of amplification to infants and young children. In R. Seewald & A. M. Tharpe (Eds.), *Comprehensive handbook of pediatric audiology* (pp. 527–552). San Diego: Plural Publishing.

Baguley, D. M. (2002). Mechanisms of tinnitus. *British Medical Bulletin, 63,* 195–212.

Baguley, D. M. (2003). Hyperacusis. *Journal of the Royal Society of Medicine, 96,* 582–585.

Baguley, D. M., & Andersson, G. (2007). *Hyperacusis: Mechanisms, diagnosis, and therapies.* San Diego: Plural Publishing.

Baguley, D. M., Bartnik, G., Kleinjung, T., Savastano, M., & Hough, E. A. (2013). Troublesome tinnitus in childhood and adolescence: Data from expert centres. *International Journal of Pediatric Otorhinolaryngology 77,* 248–251.

Balatsouras, D.G., Kaberos, A., Korres, S., Kandiloros, D., Ferekidis, E., & Economou, C. (2003). Detection of pseudohypacusis: A prospective randomized study of the use of otoacoustic emissions. *Ear & Hearing, 24,* 518–527.

Bandura, A. (1969). Social learning theory of identificatory processes. In D. A. Goslin (Ed.), *Handbook of socialization theory and research* (pp. 213–262). Chicago: Rand McNally.

Baran, J. A., & Musiek, F. E. (1999). Behavioral assessment of the central auditory nervous system. In F. E. Musiek & W. F. Rintelmann (Eds.), *Contemporary perspectives in hearing assessment* (pp. 375–413). Boston: Allyn & Bacon.

Barry, S. J. (1994). Can bone conduction thresholds really be better than air? *American Journal of Audiology, 3,* 21–22.

Beasley, D. S., Schwimmer, S., & Rintelmann, W. F. (1972). Intelligibility of time-compressed CNC monosyllables. *Journal of Speech and Hearing Research, 15,* 340–350.

Békésy, G. von. (1947). A new audiometer. *Acta Otolarynoglogica, 35,* 411–422.

Bentler, R., & Chiou, L. K. (2006). Digital noise reduction: an overview. *Trends in Amplification, 10,* 67–82.

Berlin, C. I. (1999). *The efferent auditory system.* San Diego: Singular Publishing.

Bentler, R., & Kramer, S. E. (2000). Guidelines for choosing a self-report outcome measure. *Ear and Hearing, 21,* 37S–49S.

Berger, K. W. (1984). *The hearing aid, its operation and development* (3rd ed.). Livonia, MI: National Hearing Aid Society.

Berger, K. W .(1988). History and development of hearing aids. In M. C. Pollack (Ed.), *Amplification for the hearing impaired* (3rd ed., pp. 1–20). Orlando, FL: Grune & Stratton.

Berk, R. L., & Feldman, A. S. (1958). Functional hearing loss in children. *New England Journal of Medicine, 259,* 214–216.

Berlin, C. I., Lowe-Bell, S. S., Jannetta, P. J., & Kline, D. G. (1972). Central auditory deficits after temporal lobectomy. *Archives of Otolaryngology, 96,* 4–10.

Bess, F. H., & Tharpe, A. M. (1986). An introduction to unilateral sensorineural hearing loss in children. *Ear and Hearing, 7,* 3–13.

Bill Daniels Center for Children's Hearing. (2002). *Guidelines for identification and management of infants and young children with auditory neuropathy spectrum disorder.* Denver: Children's Hospital Colorado.

Bocca, E., Calearo, C., Cassinari, V., & Migliavacca, F. (1954). Testing "cortical" hearing in temporal lobe tumours. *Acta Otolaryngologica, 44,* 289–304.

Boothroyd, A. (1968). Developments in speech audiometry. *Sound, 2,* 3–10.

Boothroyd, A. (2007). Adult aural rehabilitation: What is it and does it work? *Trends in Amplification, 11,* 63–71.

Brackmann, D. E., & Green, J. D. (2001). Cerebellopontine angle tumors. In B. J. Bailey, K. H. Calhoun, G. B. Healy, H. C. Pillsbury, J. T. Johnson, R. T. Jackler, & M. E. Tardy (Eds.), *Head and neck surgery—otolarynoglogy. Volume II* (3rd ed., pp. 1899–1917). Philadelphia: Lippincott Williams & Wilkins.

Branch, W., Kern, D., Haidet, P., Weissmann, P., Gracey, C. F., Mitchell, G., & Inui, T. (2001). The patient-physician relationship: Teaching the human dimension of care in clinical settings. *Journal of the American Medical Association, 286,* 1067–1074.

Bratt, G. W., Rosenfeld, M. A. L., & Williams, D. W. (2007). NICD/VA hearing aid clinical trial and follow up: Background. *Journal of the American Academy of Audiology, 18,* 274–281.

Brigande, J. V., & Heller, S. (2009). Quo vadis, hair cell regeneration? *National Neuroscience, 12,* 679–685.

Briggs, R. J. S., Eder, H. C., Seligman, P. M., Cowan, R. S. C., Plant, K. L., Dalton, J., Money, D. K., & Patrick, J. F. (2008). Initial clinical experience with a totally implantable cochlear implant research device. *Otology & Neurotology, 29,* 114–119.

Brinkley, D. (2011). *Supporting deaf children and young people: Strategies for intervention, inclusion and improvement.* New York: Continuum Press.

British Association of Otorhinolaryngologists – Head & Neck Surgeons Clinical Practice Advisory Group. (2002, Spring). *Clinical effectiveness guidelines acoustic neuroma (vestibular schwannoma).* BAO-HNS Document 5. London: The Royal College of Surgeons of England.

Broadbent, D. E. (1954). The role of auditory localization in attention and memory span. *Journal of Experimental Psychology, 47*(3), 191–196.

Brockenbrough, J. M., Rybak, L. P., & Matz, G. J. (2001). Ototoxicity. In B. J. Bailey, K. H. Calhoun, G. B. Healy, H. C. Pillsbury, J. T. Johnson, R. T. Jackler, & M. E. Tardy (Eds.), *Head and neck surgery—otolarynoglogy. Volume II* (3rd ed., pp. 1893–1898). Philadelphia: Lippincott Williams & Wilkins.

Brownell, W. E., Bader, C. R., Bertrand, D., & Ribaupierre, Y. (1985). Evoked mechanical responses of isolated outer hair cells. *Science, 227,* 194–196.

Bunch, C. C. (1929). Age variations in auditory acuity. *Archives of Otolaryngology, 9,* 625–636.

Bunch, C. C. (1943). *Clinical audiometry.* St. Louis: Mosby.

Cameron, S., & Dillon, H. (2007). Development of the Listening in Spatialized Noise-Sentences Test (LISN-S). *Ear and Hearing, 28,* 196–211.

Cameron, S., Dillon, H., & Newall, P. (2006). The Listening in Spatialized Noise test: Normative data for children. *International Journal of Audiology, 4,* 99–108.

Campbell, K. C. M. (2006). *Pharmacology and ototoxicity for audiologists.* Clifton Park, NY: Delmar Cengage Learning.

Canlon, B., Illing, R. B., Walton, J. (2010). Cell biology and physiology of the aging central auditory pathway. In S. Gordon-Salant, R. D. Frisina, A. N. Popper, & R. R. Fay (Eds.), *The aging auditory system* (pp. 39–74). New York: Springer.

Carhart, R. (1946). Speech reception in relation to pattern of pure tone loss. *Journal of Speech and Hearing Disorders, 11,* 97–108.

Carhart, R. (1946). Tests for selection of hearing aids. *Laryngoscope, 56,* 780–794.

Carhart, R. (1950). Clinical application of bone conduction audiometry. *Archives of Otolaryngology, 51,* 798–808.

Carhart, R. (1957). Clinical determination of abnormal auditory adaptation. *Archives of Otolaryngology, 65,* 32–39.

Carhart, R. (1961). Tests for malingering. *Transactions of the American Academy of Ophthalmology and Otolaryngology, 65,* 437.

Carhart, R., & Jerger, J. F. (1959). Preferred method for clinical determination of pure-tone threshold. *Journal of Speech & Hearing Disorders, 24,* 330–345.

Causse, J. R., & Causse, J. B. (1984). Otospongiosis as a genetic disease. Early detection, medical management, and prevention. *American Journal of Otology, 5,* 211–223.

Chaiklin, J. H. (1959). The relation among three selected auditory speech thresholds. *Journal of Speech and Hearing Research, 2,* 237–243.

Chaiklin, J. B. (1967). Interaural attenuation and cross-hearing in air conduction audiometry. *Journal of Auditory Research, 7,* 413–424.

Chermak, C. D., & Musiek, F. E. (2011). Neurological substrate of central auditory processing deficits in children. *Current Pediatric Reviews, 7,* 241–251.

Children's Hospital of Colorado. (2008). *Guidelines for identification and management of infants and young children with auditory neuropathy spectrum disorders.* Denver: Author.

Chole, R. A., & Nason, R. (2009). Chronic otitis media and cholesteatoma. In J. B. Snow Jr. & P. A. Wackym (Eds.), *Ballenger's otorhinolaryngology—head and neck surgery* (17th ed., pp. 217–227). Shelton, CT: BC Decker.

Chung, K. (2004a). Challenges and recent developments in hearing aids. Part I. Speech understanding in noise, microphone technologies and noise reduction algorithms. *Trends in Amplification, 8,* 83–124.

Chung, K. (2004b). Challenges and recent developments in hearing aids. Part II. Feedback and occlusion effect reduction strategies, laser shell manufacturing processes, and other signal processing technologies. *Trends in Amplification, 8,* 125–154.

Clark, J. G. (1981). Uses and abuses of hearing loss classification. *Asha, 23,* 493–500.

Clark, J. G. (2007). Patient-centered practice: Aligning professional ethics with patient goals. *Seminars in Hearing, 38,* 163–170.

Clark, M. (2007). *A practical guide to quality interaction with children who have a hearing loss.* San Diego: Plural Publishing.

Clemis, J. D., & McGee, T. (1979). Brainstem electric response audiometry in the differential diagnosis of acoustic tumors. *Laryngoscope, 89,* 31–42.

Cohen, M., & Phillips, J. A. III. (2012). Genetic approach to evaluation of hearing loss. *Otolaryngology Clinics of North America, 45,* 25–39.

Coles, R. R. A., & Priede, V. M. (1970). On the misdiagnosis resulting from incorrect use of masking. *Journal of Laryngology and Otology, 84,* 41–64.

Colquitt, J. L., Jones, J., Harris, P., Loveman, E., Bird, A., Clegg, A. J., Baguley, D. M., Proops, D. W., Mitchell, T. E., Sheehan, P. Z., & Welch, K. (2011). Bone-anchored hearing aids (BAHAs) for people who are bilaterally deaf: A systematic review and economic evaluation. *Health Technology Assessment, 15,* 1–200.

Conn, M., Dancer, J., & Ventry I. M. (1975). A spondee list for determining speech recognition threshold without prior familiarization. *Journal of Speech and Hearing Disorders, 40,* 388–396.

Cord, M. T., Walden, B. E., & Atack, R. M. (1992). *Speech recognition in noise test (SPRINT) for H-3 profile.* Unpublished manuscript. Bethesda, MD: Walter Reed Army Medical Center.

Cornelisse, L., Seewald, R., & Jamieson, D. (1995). The input/output formula: A theoretical approach to the fitting of personal amplification devices. *Journal of the Acoustical Society of America, 97,* 1854–1864.

Cotanche, D. A. (1987). Regeneration of hair cell stereo-cilliary bundles in the chick cochlea following severe acoustic trauma. *Hearing Research, 30* (2–3), 181–195.

Cox, R. M., & Alexander, G. C. (1995). The abbreviated profile of hearing aid benefit. *Ear & Hearing, 16,* 176–186.

Cox, R. M., & Alexander, G. C. (1999). Measuring satisfaction with amplification in daily life: The SADL. *Ear and Hearing, 20,* 306–320.

Cox, R. M., Alexander, G. C., Taylor, I. M., & Gray, G. A. (1997). The contour test of loudness perception. *Ear and Hearing, 18,* 388–400.

Crandell, C. C., Smaldino, J. J., & Flexer, C. (1992). *Sound-field FM applications: Theory and practical applications.* San Diego: Singular Publishing.

Crawford, J. V. (2012, June 27). Cochlear function. Retrieved from http://emedicine.medscape.com/article/874533-overview

Cruickshanks, K. J., Wiley, T. L., Tweed, T. S., Klein, B. E., Klein, R., Mares-Perlman, J. A. & Nondahl, D. M. (1998). Prevalence of hearing loss in older adults in Beaver Dam, Wisconsin. The epidemiology of hearing loss study. *American Journal of Epidemiology, 148,* 879–886.

Cullington, H. E., & Zeng, F-G. (2011). Comparison of bimodal and bilateral cochlear implant users on speech recognition with competing talker, music perception, affective prosody discrimination, and talker identification. *Ear and Hearing, 32,* 16–20.

Curry, E. T., & Cox, B. P. (1966). The relative intelligibility of spondees. *Journal of Auditory Research, 6,* 419–424.

Dahle, A. J., Fowler, K. B,. Wright, J. R., Boppana, S. B., Britt, W. J., & Pass, R. F. (2000). Longitudinal investigation of hearing disorders in children with congenital cytomegalovirus. *Journal of the American Academy of Audiology, 11,* 283–290.

Dallos, P. (2008). Cochlear amplification, outer hair cells and prestin. *Current Opinions in Neurobiology, 18,* 370–376.

Darrow, D. H., Dash, N., & Derkay, C. S. (2003). Otitis media: Concepts and controversies. *Current Opinions in Otolaryngology Head and Neck Surgery, 11,* 416–423.

Davis, H. (1948). The articulation area and the social adequacy index for hearing. *Laryngoscope, 58,* 761–778.

Davis, H. (1983). An active process in cochlear mechanics. *Hearing Research, 9,* 79–90.

Davis, H., Davis, P. A., Loomis, A. L., Harvey, E. N., & Hobart, G. (1939). Electrical reactions of the human brain to auditory stimulation during sleep. *Journal of Neurophysiology, 2,* 500–514.

de Boer, J., & Thornton, A. R. (2008). Neural correlates of perceptual learning in the auditory brainstem: Efferent activity predicts and reflects improvement at a speech-in-noise discrimination task. *The Journal of Neuroscience, 28,* 4929–4937.

DeBonis, D. A., & Donohue, C. L. (2004). *Survey of audiology: Fundamentals for audiologists and health professionals.* Boston: Allyn & Bacon.

de Jong, M. A., Adelman, C., Rubin, M., & Sohmer, H. (2012). Combined effects of salicylic acid and furosemide and noise on hearing. *Journal of Occupational Medicine and Toxicology, 7,* 1.

Delage, D., & Tuller, L. (2007). Language development with mild-moderate hearing loss: Does language normalize with age? *Journal of Speech, Language, and Hearing Research, 50,* 1300–1313.

Del Bo, L., & Ambrosetti, U. (2007). Hearing aids for treatment of tinnitus. In B. Langguth, G. Hajak, T. Kleinjung, A. Cacace, & A. R. Moller (Eds.), *Progress in Brain Research, 166,* 341–345.

Denes, P., & Naunton, P. F. (1952). Masking in pure tone audiometry. *Proceedings of the Royal Society of Medicine, 45,* 790–794.

DePalma, R. G., Burris, D. G., Champion, H. R., & Hodgson, M. J. (2005). Blast injuries. *New England Journal of Medicine, 352,* 1335–1342.

Dhar, S., & Hall, J. W. III. (2012). *Otoacoustic emissions: Principles, procedures, and protocols.* San Diego: Plural Publishing.

Diaz, R. C. (2009). Inner ear protection and regeneration: A "historical" perspective. *Current Opinion on Otolaryngology Head & Neck Surgery, 17,* 363–372.

Dillon, H., James, A. M., & Ginis, I. (1997). Client Oriented Scale of Improvement (COSI) and its relationship to several other measures of benefit and satisfaction provided by hearing aids. *Journal of the American Academy of Audiology, 8,* 27–43.

Dirks, D. D., Kamm, C., Bower, D., & Betsworth, A. (1977). Use of performance-intensity functions for diagnosis. *Journal of Speech and Hearing Disorders, 42,* 408–415.

Dirks, D., & Malmquist, C. (1964). Changes in bone conduction thresholds produced by masking in the nontest ear. *Journal of Speech and Hearing Research, 7,* 271–278.

DiSogra, R. (2008). *Adverse drug reactions and audiology practice.* Retrieved January 10, 2013, from www.audiology.org

Dix, M., Hallpike, C., & Hood, J. (1948). Observations upon the loudness recruitment phenomenon with especial reference to the differential diagnosis of disorders of the internal ear and VIIIth nerve. *Journal of Laryngology and Otology, 62,* 671–686.

Dixon, R. F., & Newby, H. A. (1959). Children with nonorganic hearing problems. *Archives of Otolaryngology, 70,* 619–623.

Djupesland, G. (1975). Advanced reflex considerations. In J. Jerger (Ed.), *Handbook of clinical impedance audiometry* (pp. 85–126). Dobbs Ferry, NY: American Electromedics Corporation.

Dobie, R. A. (2001). Noise-induced hearing loss. In B. J. Bailey, K. H. Calhoun, G. B. Healy, H. C. Pillsbury, J. T. Johnson, R. T. Jackler, & M. E. Tardy (Eds.), *Head and neck surgery—otolaryngology. Volume II* (3rd ed., pp. 1883–1891). Philadelphia: Lippincott Williams & Wilkins.

Dobie, R. A. (2008). The burdens of age-related and occupational noise-induced hearing loss in the United States. *Ear & Hearing, 29,* 565–577.

Dobie, R. A., & Doyle, K. J. (2009). Idiopathic sudden onset hearing loss. In J. B. Snow Jr. & P. A. Wackym (Eds.), *Ballenger's otorhinolaryngology—head and neck surgery* (17th ed., pp. 279–282). Shelton, CT: BC Decker.

Doerfler, L., & Stewart, K. (1946). Malingering and psychogenic deafness. *Journal of Speech Disorders, 11,* 181–186.

Doshi, J., Sheehan, P., & McDermott, A. L. (2012). Bone anchored hearing aids in children: An update.

International Journal of Pediatric Otorhinolaryngology, 76, 618–622.

Downs, M. P., & Sterritt, G. M. (1967). A guide to newborn and infant hearing screening programs. *Archives of Otolaryngology, 85,* 38–44.

Drake, A. F., Makielski, K., McDonald-Bell, C., & Atcheson, B. (1995). Two new otolaryngologic findings in child abuse. *Archives of Otolaryngology Head and Neck Surgery, 121,* 1417–1420.

Dror, A. A., & Avraham, K. B. (2009). Hearing loss: Mechanisms revealed by genetics and cell biology. *Annual Review of Genetics, 43,* 411–437.

Dubno, J., Lee. F-S., Klein, A. J., & Matthews, L. J. (1995). Confidence limits for maximum-word recognition scores. *Journal of Speech and Hearing Research, 38,* 490–502.

Dun, C. A., Faber, H. T., de Wolf, M. J., Cremers, C. W., & Hol, M. K. (2011). An overview of different systems: The bone-anchored hearing aid. *Advances in Otorhinolaryngology, 71,* 22–31.

Durrant, J. D., & Feth, L. L. (2013). *Hearing sciences: A foundational approach.* Boston: Pearson Education.

Edge, A. S. B., & Chen, Z. Y. (2008). Hair cell regeneration. *Current Opinions in Neurobiology, 18,* 377–382.

Egan, J. P. (1948). Articulation testing methods. *Laryngoscope, 58,* 955–991.

Egan, J. P., & Hake, H. W. (1950). On the masking pattern of a simple auditory stimulus. *Journal of the American Acoustical Society, 22,* 622–630.

Eggermont, J. J., & Roberts, L. E. (2004). The neuroscience of tinnitus. *Trends in Neuroscience, 27,* 676–682.

Elliott, L. L., & Katz, D. (1980). *Development of a new children's test of speech discrimination* (Technical Manual). St. Louis, MO: Auditec.

Elpern, B. S., & Naunton. R. F. (1963). The stability of the occlusion effect. *Archives of Otolaryngology, 77,* 376–382.

Engel, G. L. (1977). The need for a new medical model: A challenge for biomedicine. *Science, 196,* 129–136.

Fagelson, M. A. (2007). The association between tinnitus and post traumatic stress disorder. *American Journal of Audiology, 16,* 107–117.

Feeney, P. M., Grant, I. L., & Marryott, L. P. (2003). Wideband energy reflectance measurements in adults with middle-ear disorders. *Journal of Speech, Language, and Hearing Research, 46,* 901–911.

Feldmann, H. (1970). *A history of audiology: A comprehensive report and bibliography from the earliest beginnings to the present.* Chicago: Beltone Institute for Hearing Research.

Fletcher, H. (1921). *An empirical theory of telephone quality.* AT&T Internal Memorandum 101 (unpublished).

Fletcher, H. (1950). A method of calculating hearing for speech from an audiogram. *Acta Otolaryngologica (Supplement 90),* 26–37.

Fletcher, H., & Munson, W.A. (1933). Loudness, its definition, measurement, and calculation. *Journal of the Acoustical Society of America, 5,* 82–105.

Fletcher, H., & Munson, W. A. (1937). Relation between loudness and masking. *Journal of the American Acoustical Society, 9,* 1–10.

Fletcher, H., & Steinberg, J. C. (1929). Articulation testing methods. *Bell System Technical Journal, 8,* 806–854.

Formby, C., & Musiek, F. E. (2011). The legacies of Ira Hirsh and Robert Jirsa. *The Hearing Journal, 64,* 20–24.

Fortnum, H. M. (1992). Hearing impairment after bacterial meningitis: A review. *Archives of Diseases in Children, 67,* 1128–1133.

Fortnum, H. M., Summerfield, A. Q., Marshall, D. H., Davis, A. C., & Bamford, J. M. (2001). Prevalence of permanent childhood hearing impairment in the United Kingdom and implications for universal neonatal hearing screening: Questionnaire based ascertainment study. *British Medical Journal, 323,* 1–6.

Fowler, E. P. (1936). Differences in loudness response of the normal and hard-of-hearing ear at intensity levels slightly above threshold. *Annals of Otology, Rhinology & Laryngology, 45,* 1029–1039.

Fraser, F. C., Sproule, J. R., & Halal, F. (1980). Frequency of brancho-oto-renal (BOR) syndrome in children with profound hearing loss. *American Journal of Medical Genetics, 7,* 341–349.

French, N. R., & Steinberg, J. C. (1947). Factors governing intelligibility of speech sounds. *Journal of the Acoustical Society of America, 19,* 90–119.

Friderichs, N., Swanepoel, D. W., & Hall, J. W. III. (2012). Efficacy of a community based infant hearing screening programme utilising existing clinical personnel in Western Cape, South Africa. *International Journal of Pediatric Otorhinolaryngology, 76,* 552–559.

Friedland, D. R., & Minor, L. B. (2009). Meniere disease, vestibular neuritis, benign paroxysmal positional vertigo, superior semicircular canal dehiscence, and vestibular migraine. In J. B. Snow Jr. & P. A. Wackym (Eds.), *Ballenger's otorhinolaryngology—head and neck surgery* (17th ed., pp. 313–331). Shelton CT: BC Decker.

Friedland, D. R., Pensak, M. L., & Kveton, J. F. (2009). Cranial and intracranial complications of acute and chronic otitis media. In J. B. Snow Jr. & P. A. Wackym (Eds.), *Ballenger's otorhinolaryngology—head and neck surgery* (17th ed., pp. 229–238). Shelton, CT: BC Decker.

Fuchs, P. A., Glowatzki, E., & Moser, T. (2003). The afferent synapse of cochlear hair cells. *Current Opinions in Neurobiology, 13,* 452–458.

Gantz, B. J., Dunn, C. C., Walker, E. A., Kenworthy, M., Van Voorst, T., Tomblin, B. & Turner, C. (2010). Bilateral cochlear implants in infants: A new approach—Nucleus Hybrid S12 project. *Otology and Neurotology, 31,* 1300–1309.

Gates, G. A., et al. (2008). Central auditory dysfunction in older persons with memory impairment or Alzheimer's dementia. *Archives of Otolaryngology—Head & Neck Surgery, 134,* 771–777.

Gates, G. A., Couropmitree, N. N., & Myers, R. H. (1999). Genetic associations in age-related hearing thresholds. *Archives of Otolaryngology—Head & Neck Surgery, 125,* 654–659.

Gates, G. A., & Mills, J. H. (2005). Presbycusis. *Lancet, 366,* 1111–1120.

Gelfand, S. A., Schwander, T., & Silman, S. (1990). Acoustic reflex thresholds in normal and cochlear-impaired ears: Effects of no response rates on 90th percentiles in a large sample. *Journal of Speech and Hearing Disorders, 55,* 198–205.

Gelfand, S. A., & Silman, S. (1993). Functional components and resolved thresholds in patients with unilateral nonorganic hearing loss. *British Journal of Audiology, 27,* 29–34.

Gerard, J. M., Thill, M. P., Chantrain, G., Gersdorff, M., & Deggouj, N. (2012). Esteem 2 Middle Ear Implant: Our experience. *Audiology Neurotology, 22,* 267–274.

Gertner, J. (2012). *The idea factory: Bell Labs and the great age of American innovation.* New York: The Penguin Press.

Ghorayeb, B. Y., Yeakley, J. W., Hall, J. W. III, & Jones, E. B. (1987). Unusual complications of temporal bone fractures. *Archives of Otolaryngology—Head and Neck Surgery, 113,* 749–753.

Girgia, A., & Sanson-Fisher, R. W. (1995). Breaking bad news: Consensus guidelines for medical practitioners. *Journal of Clinical Oncology, 13,* 2449–2456

Gold, T. (1948). Hearing II. The physical basis of the action of the cochlea. *Proceedings of the Royal Society of London Series B. Biological Sciences, 135,* 492–498.

Goldstein, R. (1966). Pseudohypacusis. *Journal of Speech and Hearing Disorders, 31,* 341–352.

Gordon, K. A., & Papsin, B. C. (2009). Benefits of short inter-implant delays in children receiving bilateral cochlear implants. *Otology and Neurotology, 30,* 319–331.

Gordon-Salant, S. (2005). Hearing loss and aging: New research findings. *Journal of Rehabilitation Research & Development, 42,* 9–24.

Gradenigo, G. (1893). On the clinical signs of the affections of the auditory nerve. *Archives of Otology, 22,* 213–215.

Grantham, D. W., Ashmead, D. H., Haynes, D. S., Hornsby, B. W., Labadie, R. F., & Ricketts, T. A. (2012). Horizontal plane localization in single-sided deaf adults fitted with a bone-anchored hearing aid (Baha). *Ear and Hearing, 33,* 595–603.

Green, D. M., & Watson, C. S. (1992). Acoustical Society of America Gold Medal Award: Ira Hirsh. asa. aip.org/encomia/gold/hirsh.html

Grothe, B., Pecka, M., & McAlpine, D. (2010). Mechanisms of sound localization in mammals. *Physiological Review, 90,* 983–1012.

Grove, A. K. (2010). The challenge of hair cell regeneration. *Experimental Biology and Medicine, 4,* 434–446.

Gulya, A. J. (2001). Infections of the labyrinth. In B. J. Bailey, K. H. Calhoun, G. B. Healy, H. C. Pillsbury, J. T. Johnson, R. T. Jackler, & M. E. Tardy (Eds.), *Head and neck surgery—otolaryngology. Volume II* (3rd ed., pp. 1869–1881). Philadelphia: Lippincott Williams & Wilkins.

Guthrie, L. A., & Mackersie, C. L. (2009). A comparison of presentation levels to maximum word recognition scores. *Journal of the American Academy of Audiology, 20,* 381–390.

Hall, J. L. (1972). Auditory distortion products f2-f1 and 2f1-f2. *Journal of the Acoustical Society of America, 51,* 1863–1871.

Hall, J. W. III. (1982). Quantification of the relationship between crossed and uncrossed acoustic reflex amplitude. *Ear and Hearing, 3,* 296–300.

Hall, J. W. III. (1983). Diagnostic applications of speech audiometry. *Seminars in Hearing, 4,* 179–204.

Hall, J. W. III. (1985). The acoustic reflex in central auditory dysfunction. In M. L. Pinheiro & F. E. Musiek (Eds.), *Assessment of central auditory dysfunction: Foundations and clinical correlates* (pp. 103–130). Baltimore: Williams & Wilkins.

Hall, J. W. III. (1987). Contemporary tympanometry. *Seminars in Hearing, 8,* 319–327.

Hall, J. W. III.. (1991). The classic site-of-lesion test battery: Foundation of diagnostic audiology. In W. Rintelmann (Ed.), *Hearing assessment* (2nd ed., pp. 653–677). Austin TX: Pro-Ed.

Hall, J. W. III. (1992). *Handbook of auditory evoked responses.* Boston: Allyn & Bacon.

Hall, J. W. III. (1998). Hyperacusis . . . It's real and it hurts! *The Hearing Journal, 51,* 10–14.

Hall, J. W. III. (2000). *Handbook of otoacoustic emissions.* San Diego: Singular Publishing.

Hall, J. W. III. (2004). An ounce of prevention is worth a pound of cure. *Tinnitus Today, 29,* 14–16.

Hall, J. W. III. (2007a). Auditory processing disorders (APD): Evidence in support of assessment and management. *The Hearing Journal, 61,* 10–15.

Hall, J. W. III. (2007b). *New handbook of auditory evoked responses.* Boston: Allyn & Bacon.

Hall, J. W. III, & Bellis, T. J. (2008). Assessment and management of auditory processing disorders: It's real, it's here, and it's mainstream audiology. *Audiology Today, 20,* 42–44.

Hall, J. W. III, Berry, G. A., & Olson, K. (1982). Identification of serious hearing loss with acoustic reflex data: Clinical experience with some new guidelines. *Scandinavian Audiology, 11,* 251–255.

Hall, J. W. III, Bratt, G. W., Schwaber, M. K., & Baer, J. E. (1993). Dynamic sensorineural hearing loss (SNHL): Implications for audiologists. *Journal of American Academy of Audiology, 4,* 399–411.

Hall, J. W. III, & Chandler, D. (1994). Tympanometry in clinical audiology. In J. Katz (Ed.), *Handbook of clinical audiology* (4th ed., pp. 283–299). Baltimore: Williams & Wilkins.

Hall, J. W. III, Freeman, B., & Bratt, G. (1994). The role of audiology in health care reform models and perspectives. *Audiology Today, 6,* 16–18.

Hall, J. W. III, & Ghorayeb, B. Y. (1991). Diagnosis of middle ear pathology and evaluation of conductive hearing loss. In J. T. Jacobson & J. L. Northern (Eds.), *Diagnostic audiology* (pp. 161–198). Austin, TX: Pro-Ed.

Hall, J. W. III, & Haynes, D. S. (2000). Audiologic assessment and consultation of the tinnitus patient. *Seminars in Hearing, 22,* 37–49.

Hall, J. W. III, Huangfu, M., Gennarelli, T. A., Dolinskas, C. A., Olson, K., & Berry, G. A. (1983). Auditory evoked response, impedance measures and diagnostic speech audiometry in severe head injury. *Otolaryngology Head and Neck Surgery, 91,* 50–60.

Hall, J. W. III, & Mueller, H. G. III. (1997). *Audiologists' desk reference. Volume I. Diagnostic audiology: Principles, procedures, and practices.* San Diego: Singular Publishing Group.

Hall, J. W. III, & Swanepoel, D. (2010). *Objective assessment of hearing.* San Diego: Plural Publishing.

Hall, J. W. III, Winkler, J. B., Herndon, D. N., & Gary, L. B. (1988). Auditory brainstem response in young burn wound patients treated with ototoxic drugs. *International Journal of Pediatric Otorhinolaryngology, 12,* 187–203.

Halloran, D. R., Wall, T. C., Evans, H. H., Hardin, J. M., & Woolley, A. L. (2005). Hearing screening at well-child visits. *Archives of Pediatric and Adolescent Medicine, 159,* 949–955.

Harris, D. A. (1958). A rapid and simple technique for the detection of nonorganic hearing loss. *Archives of Otolaryngology, 68,* 758–760.

Harris, J. P. (1983). Immunology of the inner ear. Response of the inner ear to antigen challenge. *Otolaryngology Head & Neck Surgery, 91,* 18–32.

Harris, J. P. (2001). Autoimmune inner ear disease. In B. J. Bailey, K. H. Calhoun, G. B. Healy, H. C. Pillsbury, J. T. Johnson, R. T. Jackler, & M. E. Tardy (Eds.), *Head and neck surgery—otorhinoglogy. Volume II* (3rd ed., pp. 1933–1940). Philadelphia: Lippincott Williams & Wilkins.

Harris, J. P., Gopen, G., & Keithley, E. (2009). Autoimmune inner ear disease and other autoimmune diseases with inner ear involvement. In J. B. Snow Jr. & P. A. Wackym (Eds.), *Ballenger's otorhinolaryngology—head and neck surgery* (17th ed., pp. 305–312). Shelton, CT: BC Decker.

Harris, L. K., Van Zandt, C. E., & Rees, T. H. (1997). Counseling needs of children who are deaf and hard of hearing. *The School Counselor, 44,* 271–279.

Hawkins, J. E., & Stevens, S. S. (1950). Masking of pure tones and of speech by white noise. *Journal of the American Acoustical Society, 22,* 6–13.

Haynes, D. S., Young, J. A., & Wanna, G. B. (2010). Middle ear devices from past to present. *ENT & Audiology News, 19,* 82–84.

Hecox, K., & Galambos, R. (1974). Brain stem auditory evoked responses in human infants and adults. *Archives of Otolaryngology, 99,* 30–33.

Heller, M. F., & Berman, M. (1953). Tinnitus aurium in normally hearing persons. *Annals of Otology, 62,* 73–83.

Henry, J. A., Dennis, K. C., & Schechter, M. A. (2005). General review of tinnitus: Prevalence, mechanisms, and management. *Journal of Speech, Language, and Hearing Research, 48,* 1204–1235.

Henry, J. A., Trune, D. R., Robb, M. J. A., & Jastreboff, P. J. (2007). *Tinnitus retraining therapy: Patient counseling guide.* San Diego: Plural Publishing.

Henry, J. A., Zaugg, T., Myers, P., & Kendall, C. (2010). *Progressive tinnitus management: Clinical handbook for audiologists.* San Diego: Plural Publishing.

Hirsh, I. J., & Bowman, W. D. (1953). Masking of speech by bands of noise. *Journal of the American Acoustical Society, 25,* 1175–1180.

Hirsh, I. J., Davis, H., Silverman, S. R., Reynolds, E. G., Eldert, E., & Bensen, R. W. (1952). Development of materials for speech audiometry. *Journal of Speech and Hearing Disorders, 17,* 321–337.

Hodgetts, B. (2011). Other implantable devices: Bone-anchored hearing aids. In R. Seewald & A. M. Tharpe (Eds.), *Comprehensive handbook of pediatric audiology* (pp. 585–598). San Diego: Plural Publishing.

Holenweg, A., & Kompis, M. (2010). Non-organic hearing loss: New and confirmed findings. *European Archives of Otorhinolaryngology, 267,* 1213–1219.

Holmes, A., Kileny, P. R., & Hall, J. W. III. (2011). The legacies of Margo Skinner and Roger Ruth. *The Hearing Journal, 64,* 10–14.

Holstad, B. A. (2011). FM systems. In J. R. Madell & C. Flexer (Eds.), *Pediatric audiology casebook* (pp. 235–243). New York: Thieme Medical Publishers.

Holt, L. A., Margolis, R. H., & Cavanaugh, R. M. (1991). Developmental changes in multifrequency tympanograms. *Audiology, 30,* 1–24.

Holte, L. A., & Margolis, R. H. (1987). Screening tympanometry. *Seminars in Hearing, 8,* 329–338.

Hood, J. D. (1955). Auditory fatigue and adaptation in the differential diagnosis of end-organ disease. *Annals of Otology, Rhinology & Laryngology, 64,* 507–518.

Hood, J. D. (1960). The principles and practice of bone-conduction audiometry. *Laryngoscope, 70,* 1211–1228.

Hornickel, J., Zecker, S. G., Bradlow, A. R., & Kraus, N. (2012). Assistive listening devices drive neuroplasticity in children with dyslexia. *Proceedings of National Academy of Sciences, 109,* 16731–16736.

Hudgins, C. V., Hawkins, J. E., Karlin, J. E., & Stevens, S. S. (1947). The development of recorded auditory tests for measuring hearing loss for speech. *Laryngoscope, 40,* 57–89.

Hudspeth, A. J. (1989). How the ear works. *Nature, 341,* 397–404.

Hugdahl, K. (1988). *Handbook of dichotic listening: Theory, methods, and research.* Chichester, England: John Wiley & Sons.

Hughson, W., & Westlake, H. (1944). Manual for program outline for rehabilitation of aural casualties both military and civilian. *Transactions of the American Academy of Ophthalmology and Otolaryngology, Supplement 48,* 1–15.

Humes, L. E. (1996). Evolution of prescriptive fitting approaches. *American Journal of Audiology, 5,* 19–23.

Hunter, L. L., Feeney, M. P., Lapsley Miller, J. A., Jeng, P. S., & Bohning, S. (2010). Wideband reflectance in newborns: normative regions and relationship to hearing screening results. *Ear & Hearing, 31,* 599–610.

Hunter, L. L., & Margolis, R. H. (1992). Multifrequency tympanometry: Current clinical application. *American Journal of Audiology, 1,* 33–43.

Hunter, L. L., & Shahnaz, N. (2013). *Acoustic immittance measures: Basic and advanced principles.* San Diego: Plural Publishing.

Hurley, R. M., & Sells, J. P. (2003). An abbreviated word recognition protocol based on item difficulty. *Ear and Hearing, 24,* 111–118.

Jacobson, G. P., & Shepard, N. T. (2007). *Balance function assessment and management.* San Diego: Plural Publishing.

Jahrsdoerfer, R. A., & Hall, J. W. III. (1986). Congenital malformations of the ear. *American Journal of Otology, 7,* 267–269.

Jahrsdoerfer, R. A., Yeakley, J. W., Hall, J. W. III, Robbins, K. T., & Gray, L. C. (1985). High resolution CT scanning and ABR in congenital aural atresia—patient selection and surgical correlation. *Otolaryngology—Head and Neck Surgery, 93,* 292–298.

Jastreboff, P. J., Gray, W. C., & Gold, S. L. (1996). Neurophysiological approach to tinnitus patients. *The American Journal of Otology, 17,* 236–240.

Jastreboff, P. J., & Hazell, J. W. P. (2004). *Tinnitus retraining therapy: Implementing the neurophysiological model.* Cambridge, UK: Cambridge University Press.

Jastreboff, P. J., & Jastreboff, M. M. (2000). Tinnitus retraining therapy (TRT) as a method for treatment of tinnitus and hyperacusis patients. *Journal of the American Academy of Audiology, 11,* 162–177.

Jastreboff, P. J., & Jastreboff, M. M. (2013). Using TRT to treat hyperacusis, misophonia and phonophobia. *ENT & Audiology News, 21,* 88–90.

Jenkins, H. A., & McKenna, M. J. (2009). Otosclerosis. In J. B. Snow Jr. & P. A. Wackym (Eds.), *Ballenger's oto-rhinolaryngology—head and neck surgery* (17th ed., pp. 247–251). Shelton, CT: BC Decker.

Jerger, J. (1952). A difference limen test and its diagnostic significance. *Laryngoscope, 62,* 1316–1322.

Jerger, J. (1960a). Békésy audiometry in the analysis of auditory disorders. *Journal of Speech and Hearing Research, 3,* 275–287.

Jerger, J. (1960). Observations on auditory behavior in lesions of the central auditory pathways. *Archives of Otolarygology, 71,* 797–806.

Jerger, J. (1970). Clinical experience with impedance audiometry. *Archives of Otolaryngology, 92,* 311–324.

Jerger, J. (Ed.). (1975). *Handbook of clinical impedance audiometry.* Dobbs Ferry, NY: American Electromedics.

Jerger, J. (1976). Proposed audiometric symbol system for scholarly publications. *Archives of Otolaryngology, 102,* 33–36.

Jerger, J. (1980). Research priorities in auditory science . . . The audiologist's view. *Annals of Otology, Rhinology, and Laryngology, 89* (Supplement 74), 134–135.

Jerger, J. (2009). *Audiology in the USA.* San Diego: Plural Publishing.

Jerger, J. (2013). Why the audiogram is upside down. *International Journal of Audiology, 52,* 146–150.

Jerger, J., Anthony, L., Jerger, S., & Mauldin, L. (1974a). Studies in impedance audiometry. III. Middle ear disorders. *Archives of Otolaryngology, 99,* 165–171.

Jerger, J., Burney, P., Mauldin, L., & Crump, B. (1974b). Predicting hearing loss from the acoustic reflex. *Journal of Speech and Hearing Disorders, 39,* 11–22.

Jerger, J., Harford, E., Clemis, J. & Alford, B. (1974). The acoustic reflex in eighth nerve disorders. *Archives of Otolaryngology, 99,* 409–413.

Jerger, J., & Hayes, D. (1977). Diagnostic speech audiometry. *Archives of Otolaryngology, 103,* 216–222.

Jerger, J., & Jerger, S. (1965). Clinical evaluation of SAL audiometry. *Journal of Speech and Hearing Research, 8,* 103–128.

Jerger, J., & Jerger, S. (1967). Psychoacoustic comparison of cochlear and VIIIth nerve disorders. *Journal of Speech and Hearing Research, 10,* 659–688.

Jerger, J., & Jerger, S. (1971). Diagnostic significance of PB word functions. *Archives of Otolaryngology, 93,* 573–580.

Jerger, J., & Jerger, S. (1974). Diagnostic value of Békésy comfortable loudness tracings. *Archives of Otolaryngology, 99,* 351–360.

Jerger, J., & Jerger, S. (1975). Clinical validity of central auditory tests. *Scandinavian Audiology, 4,* 147–163.

Jerger, J., & Jerger, S. (1975a). A simplified tone decay test. *Archives of Otolaryngology, 101,* 403–407.

Jerger, J., Jerger, S., & Mauldin, L. (1972a). The forward-backward discrepancy in Békésy audiometry. *Archives of Otolaryngology, 96,* 400–406.

Jerger, J., Jerger, S., & Mauldin, L. (1972). Studies in impedance audiometry. I. Normal and sensorineural ears. *Archives of Otolaryngology, 96,* 513–523.

Jerger, J., & Musiek, F. E. (2000). Report of the consensus conference on the diagnosis of auditory processing disorders in school-aged children. *Journal of the American Academy of Audiology, 11,* 467–474.

Jerger, J., Oliver, T., & Pirozzolo, F. (1989). Speech understanding in the elderly. *Ear and Hearing, 10,* 79–89.

Jerger, J., Shedd, J., & Harford, E. (1959). On the detection of extremely small changes in sound intensity. *Archives of Otolaryngology, 69,* 200–211.

Jerger, J., Speaks, C., & Trammell, J. (1968). A new approach to speech audiometry. *Journal of Speech and Hearing Disorders, 33,* 318–328.

Jerger, J., & Tillman, T. (1960). A new method for clinical determination of sensorineural acuity level (SAL). *Archives of Otolaryngology, 71,* 948–953.

Jerger, J. F., Tillman, T.W., & Peterson, J. L. (1960). Masking by octave bands of noise in normal and impaired ears. *Journal of the American Acoustical Society, 32,* 385–390.

Jerger, S. (1984). Speech audiometry. In J. Jerger (Ed.), *Pediatric audiology* (pp. 71–93). San Diego: College-Hill Press.

Jerger, S., & Jerger, J. (1974). Audiological comparison of cochlear and eighth nerve disorders. *Annals of Otology, Rhinology & Laryngology, 83,* 275–286.

Jerger, S., & Jerger, J. (1977). Diagnostic value of crossed versus uncrossed acoustic reflexes: Eighth nerve and brainstem disorders. *Archives of Otolaryngology, 103,* 445–453.

Jerger, S., Lewis, S., Hawkins, J., & Jerger, J. (1980). Pediatric speech intelligibility test. I. Generation of the test materials. *International Journal of Pediatric Otorhinolaryngology, 2,* 217–230.

Jewett, D. L., Romano, M. N., & Williston, J. S. (1970). Human auditory evoked potentials: Possible brainstem components detected on the scalp. *Science, 167,* 1517–1518.

Jewett, D. L., & Williston, J. S. (1971). Auditory evoked far fields averaged from the scalp of humans. *Brain, 4,* 681–696.

Jodar, L., Feavers, I. M., Salisbury, D., & Granoff, D. M. (2002). Development of vaccines against meningococcal disease. *Lancet, 359,* 1499–1508.

Johnston, K. N., John, A. B., Kreisman, N. V., Hall, J. W. III, & Crandell, C. C. (2009). Multiple benefits of personal FM system use by children with auditory processing disorder. *International Journal of Audiology, 48,* 371–383.

Joint Committee on Infant Hearing. (1994). Position Statement. *Asha, 36,* 38–41.

Joint Committee on Infant Hearing. (2007). Year 2007 Position Statement. Principles and guidelines for early hearing detection and intervention programs. *Pediatrics, 120,* 898–921.

Kaltenbach, J. A. (2007). The dorsal cochlear nucleus as a contributor to tinnitus: Mechanisms underlying the induction of hyperactivity. In B. Langguth, G. Hajak, T. Kleinjung, A. Cacace, & A. R. Moller. *Progress in brain research, 166,* 89–106.

Kaltenbach, J. A. (2011). Tinnitus: Models and mechanisms. *Hearing Research, 276,* 52–60.

Kamm, C. A., Dirks, D. D., & Mickey, M. R. (1978). Effect of sensorineural hearing loss on loudness discomfort level and most comfortable loudness judgments. *Journal of Speech and Hearing Research, 21,* 668–681.

Kamm, C. A., Morgan, D. E., & Dirks, D. D. (1983). Accuracy of adaptive procedure estimates of PB-max level. *Journal of Speech and Hearing Disorders, 48,* 202–209.

Kaplan, H., Garretson, C., & Baily, S. (1985). *Speech reading: A way to improve understanding.* Washington DC: Gallaudet University Press.

Kates, J. M. (2005). Principles of digital dynamic-range compression. *Trends in Amplification, 9,* 45–76.

Katz, J. (1962). The use of staggered spondaic words for assessing the integrity of the central auditory nervous system. *Journal of Auditory Research, 2,* 327–337.

Katzenell, U., & Segal, S. (2001). Hyperacusis: Review and clinical guidelines. *Otology & Neurotology, 22,* 321–326.

Kei, J., Mazlan, R., Hickson, L., Gavranich, J., & Linning. R. (2007). Measuring middle ear admittance in newborns using 1000 Hz tympanometry: A comparison of methodologies. *Journal of the Academy of Audiology, 18,* 739–748.

Keith, R. (Ed.). (1977). *Central auditory dysfunction.* New York: Grune & Stratton.

Keith, R. (1994). *SCAN - A: A Test for Auditory Processing Disorders in Adolescence and Adults.* San Antonio, TX: Psychological Corporation.

Keith, R. W. (2000). Development and standardization of SCAN-C test for auditory processing disorders in children. *Journal of the American Academy of Audiology, 11,* 438–445.

Keith, R., & Anderson, J. (2007). Dichotic listening tests. In F. E. Musiek & G. D. Chermak (Eds.), *Handbook of (central) auditory processing disorders. Volume I. Auditory neuroscience and diagnosis* (pp. 207–230). San Diego: Plural Publishing.

Kemp, D. T. (1978). Simulated acoustic emissions from within the human auditory system. *Journal of Acoustical Society of America, 64,* 1386–1391.

Kemp, D. T. (1980). Towards a model for the origin of cochlear echoes. *Hearing Research, 2,* 533–548.

Kileny, P. R., & Seewald, R. (2011). The legacies of Robert Galambos and Judith Gravel. *The Hearing Journal, 64,* 12, 14, 16

Killion, M. C., & Mueller, H. G. (2010). Twenty years later: A NEW count-the-dots method. *The Hearing Journal, 63,* 10–15.

Killion, M. C., Niquette, P. A., Gudmundsen, G. I., Revit, L. J., & Banerjee, S. (2004). Development of a quick speech-in-noise test for measuring signal-to-noise ratio loss in normal hearing and hearing impaired listeners. *Journal of the Acoustical Society of America, 116*(4), 2395–2405.

Killion, M. C., Wilbur, L. A., & Gudmundsen, G. I. (1985). Insert earphones for more interaural attenuation. *Hearing Instruments, 36,* 34.

Kimura, D. (1961). Some effects of temporal-lobe damage on auditory perception. *Canadian Journal of Psychology, 15,* 157–165.

Kleihues, P., Burger, P. C., & Scheithauer, B. W. (1993). The new WHO system classification of brain tumors. *Brain Pathology, 3,* 255–268.

Klockhoff, I. (1961). Middle ear muscle reflexes in man: A clinical and experimental study with special reference to diagnostic problems in hearing impairment. *Acta Otolaryngologica,* Supplement 164, 1–92.

Kochkin, S. (2007). MarkeTrak VII: Obstacles to adult non-user adoption of hearing aids. *The Hearing Journal, 51,* 30–41.

Kochkin, S. (2010). MarkeTrak VIII: Consumer satisfaction with hearing aids is slowly increasing. *The Hearing Journal, 63,* 19–32.

Kochkin, S. (2009). MarkeTrak VIII: 25-year trends in the hearing health market. *Hearing Review, 16,* 12–31.

Kochkin, S. (2011). MarkeTrak VIII: Reducing patient visits through verification and validation. *Hearing Review, 18,* 10–12.

Kochkin, S. (2012). MarkeTrak VIII: The key influencing factors in hearing aid purchase. *Hearing Review, 19,* 12–25.

Kochkin, S., & Kuk, F. (1997). The binaural advantage: Evidence from subjective benefit and customer satisfaction data. *The Hearing Review, 4,* 29ff.

Konkle, D. F., & Rintelmann, W. F. (Eds.). (1983). *Principles of speech audiometry.* Baltimore: University Park Press.

Kreisman, N. V., John, A. B., Kreisman, B. M., Hall, J. W. III, & Crandell, C. C. (2012). Psychosocial status of children with auditory processing disorder. *Journal of the American Academy of Audiology, 22,* 222–233.

Kricos, P. B. (2000a). Family counseling for children with hearing loss. In J. Alpiner & P. McCarthy (Eds.), *Rehabilitative audiology: Children and adults* (3rd ed., pp. 399–433). Philadelphia: Lippincott, Williams & Wilkins.

Kricos, P. B. (2000b). The influence of nonaudiological variables on audiological rehabilitation outcomes. *Ear & Hearing, 21,* 7S–14S.

Kricos, P. B. (2007). Hearing assistive technology considerations for older individuals with dual sensory loss. *Trends in Amplification, 11,* 273–280.

Kricos, P. B. (2009). Providing hearing rehabilitation to people with dementia presents unique challenges. *The Hearing Journal, 62,* 39–40, 42–43.

Kricos, P. B., & Holmes, A. E. (1996). Efficacy of audiologic rehabilitation for older adults. *Journal of the American Academy of Audiology, 7,* 219–229.

Kricos, P. B., & McCarthy, P. (2007). From ear to there: A historical perspective on auditory training. *Seminars in Hearing, 28,* 89–98.

Kruel, E. J., Nixon, J. C., Kryter, K. D., Bell, D. W., Lang, J. S., & Schubert, E. D. (1968). A proposed clinical test of speech discrimination. *Journal of Speech and Hearing Research, 11,* 536–552.

Kryter, K. D. (1962). Methods for the calculation and use of the Articulation Index. *Journal of the Acoustical Society of America, 34,* 1689–1697.

Kujawa, S. G. (2009). Noise-induced hearing loss. In J. B. Snow Jr. & P. A. Wackym (Eds.), *Ballenger's otorhinolaryngology—head and neck surgery* (17th ed., pp. 265–272). Shelton, CT: BC Decker.

Lalaki, P., Hatzopoulous, S., Lorito, G., Kochanek, K., Silwa, L., & Skarzynski, H. (2011). *Medical Science Monitor, 17,* MT 65–62.

Lambert, P. R. (2001). Congenital aural atresia. In B. J. Bailey, K. H. Calhoun, G. B. Healy, H. C. Pillsbury, J. T. Johnson, R. T. Jackler, & M. E. Tardy (Eds.), *Head and neck surgery—otolaryngology. Volume II* (3rd ed., pp. 1745–1757). Philadelphia: Lippincott Williams & Wilkins.

Lawson, G. D., & Peterson, M. E. (2011). *Speech audiometry.* San Diego: Plural Publishing.

Lebo, C. P., Smith, M. F. W., Mosher, E. R., Jelonek, S. J., Schwind, D. R., Decker, K. E., Krusemark, H. J., & Kurz, P. L. (1994). Restaurant noise, hearing loss, and hearing aids. *Western Journal of Medicine, 161,* 45–49.

Lehrer, N. D., Hirschenfang, S., Miller, M. H., & Radpour, S. (1964). Nonorganic hearing problems in adolescents. *Laryngoscope, 74,* 64–69.

Le Prell, C. G., Gagnon, P. M., Bennett, D. C., & Ohlemiller, K. K. (2011). Nutrient-enhanced diet reduces noise-induced damage to the inner ear and hearing loss. *Translational Research, 158,* 38–53.

LePrell, C., Hensley, B. N., Campbell, K. C. M., Hall, J. W. III, & Guire, K. (2011). Evidence of hearing loss in a "normally-hearing" college-student population. *International Journal of Audiology, 50 Supplement 1,* S21–23.

Le Prell, C. G., & Spankovich, C. J. (2012). Noise-induced hearing loss: Detection, prevention, and management. In M. Sanna, A. Devaiah, & C. de Souza (Eds.), *Otology-neurotology.* Stuttgart, Germany: Thieme.

Lesperance, M. M., Hall, J. W. III, Bess, F. H., Jain, P., Ploplis, B., San Agustin, T. B., Skarka, H., Smith, R. J. H., Wills, M., & Wilcox, E. R. (1995). A gene for autosomal dominant nonsyndromic hereditary hearing impairment maps to 4p16.3. *Human Molecular Genetics, 4,* 1967–1972.

Levitt, H. (1987). Digital hearing aids: A tutorial review. *Journal of Rehabilitation Research and Development, 24,* 7–20.

Lewis, D., & Eiten, L. (2011). FM systems and communication access for children. In R. Seewald & A. M. Tharpe (Eds.), *Comprehensive handbook of pediatric audiology* (pp. 553–564). San Diego: Plural Publishing.

Lewkowicz, D. J., & Hansen-Tift, A. (2012). Infants deploy selective attention to the mouth of a talking face when learning speech. *Proceedings of the National Academy of Sciences (PNAS), Early Edition,* 2–6.

Liberman, M. C. (1982). Single neuron labeling in the cat auditory nerve. *Science, 216,* 1239–1241.

Liden, G., Nilsson, G., & Anderson, H. (1959a). Masking in clinical audiometry. *Acta Otolaryngologica, 50,* 125–136.

Liden, G., Nilsson, G., & Anderson, H. (1959b). Narrow-band masking with white noise. *Acta Otolaryngologica, 50,* 116–124.

Lieu, J. E. (2004). Language and educational consequences of unilateral hearing loss in children. *Archives of Otolaryngology Head & Neck Surgery, 130,* 524–530.

Lieu, J. E., Tye-Murray, N., Karzon, R. K., & Piccirillo, J. F. (2004). Unilateral hearing loss is associated with worse speech-language scores in children. *Pediatrics, 125,* 1348–1355.

Lin, H. W., Furman, A. C., Kujawa, S. G., & Liberman, M. C. (2011). Primary neural degeneration in the guinea pig cochlea after reversible noise-induced threshold shift. *Journal of the Association for Research in Otolaryngology, 12,* 605–616.

Lin, L. M., Bowditch, S., Anderson, M. J., May, B., Cox, K. M., & Niparko, K. (2006). Amplification in the rehabilitation of unilateral deafness: Speech in noise and directional hearing effects with bone-anchored hearing and contralateral routing of signal amplification. *Otology and Neurology, 27,* 172–182.

Lockwood, A., Salvi, R. J., & Burkard, R. (2003). Tinnitus. *New England Journal of Medicine, 347,* 904–910.

Lockwood, A. H., Salvi, R. J., Coad, M. L., Towlsey, J. L., Wack, D. S., & Murphy, B. W. (1998). The functional neuroanatomy of tinnitus: Evidence for limbic system links and neural plasticity. *Neurology, 50,* 114–120.

Lovett, B. J., & Johnson, T. L. (2010). Review of SCAN-3 for Adolescents and Adults: Tests for Auditory Processing Disorders. *Journal of Psychoeducational Assessment, 28,* 603–607.

Lucente, F. E., & Hanson, M. (2009). Diseases of the external ear. In J. B. Snow Jr. & P. A. Wackym (Eds.), *Ballenger's otorhinolaryngology—head and neck surgery* (17th ed., pp. 191–199). Shelton, CT: BC Decker.

Lunner, T., Hellgren, J., Arlinger, S., & Elberling, C. (1998). Non-linear signal processing in digital hearing aids. *Scandinavian Audiology, 27,* Supplement 49, 40–49.

Lüscher, E., & Zwislocki, J. J. (1951). The difference limen of intensity variations of pure tones and its diagnostic significance. *Journal of Laryngology & Otology, 65,* 486–510.

Luterman, D. (2008). *Counseling persons with communication disorders and their families* (5th ed). Austin, TX: ProEd.

Lynn, G. E., & Gilroy, J. (1972). Neuro-audiological abnormalities in patients with temporal lobe tumors. *Journal of Neurological Science, 17,* 167–184.

Lyons, A., Kei, J., & Driscoll, C. (2004). Distortion product otoacoustic emissions in children at school entry: A comparison with pure-tone screening and tympanometry results. *Journal of the American Academy of Audiology, 15,* 702–715.

MacIennan-Smith, F., Swanepoel, D., & Hall, J. W. III. (2013). Validity of diagnostic pure tone audiometry without a sound-treated environment in adults. *International Journal of Audiology, 52,* 66–73.

Margolis, R. H. (2004). In one ear and out the other—what patients remember. *The Hearing Journal, 57,* 10–17.

Margolis, R. H. (2010). A few secrets about bone-conduction testing. *The Hearing Journal, 63*(10), 12, 14, 16–17.

Margolis, R. H., & Hunter, L. L. (1999). Tympanometry: Basic principles and clinical applications. In F. E. Musiek & W. F. Rintelmann (Eds.), *Contemporary perspectives in hearing assessment* (pp. 89–130). Boston: Allyn & Bacon.

Margolis, R. H., & Popelka, G. R. (1977). Interaction among tympanometric variables. *Journal of Speech and Hearing Research, 20,* 447–462.

Margolis, R. H., & Saly, G. L. (2008). Distribution of hearing loss characteristics in a clinical population. *Ear and Hearing, 29,* 524–532.

Marriage, J., & Barnes, N. M. (1995). Is central hyperacusis a symptom of 5-hydroxytryptamine (5-HT) dysfunction? *Journal of Laryngology & Otology, 109,* 915–921.

Marschark, M., Lang, H. G., & Albertini, J. A. (2006). *Educating deaf students: From research to practice.* London: Oxford University Press.

Martin, F. N. (1966). Speech audiometry and clinical masking. *Journal of Auditory Research, 6,* 199–203.

Martin, F. N. (1974). Minimum effective masking levels in threshold audiometry. *Journal of Speech and Hearing Disorders, 39,* 280–285.

Martin, F. N., Armstrong, T. W., & Champlin, C. A. (1994). A survey of audiological practices in the United States in 1992. *American Journal of Audiology, 3,* 20–26.

Martin, F. N., & Blythe, M. E. (1977). On the cross hearing of spondaic words. *Journal of Auditory Research, 17,* 221–224.

Martin, F. N., Champlin, C. A., & Chambers, J. A. (1998). Seventh survey of audiometric practices in the United States. *Journal of the American Academy of Audiology, 9,* 95–104.

Martin, F. N., & Clark, J. G. (2012). *Introduction to audiology* (11th ed.). Boston: Pearson/Allyn & Bacon.

Martin, F. N., & DiGiovanni, D. (1979). Central masking effects on spondee thresholds as a function of masker sensation level and masker sound pressure level. *Journal of the American Auditory Society, 4,* 141–146.

Martin, F. N., Hawkins, R. R., & Bailey, H. A. T. (1962). The non-essentiality of the carrier phrase in phonetically balanced (PB) word testing. *Journal of Auditory Research, 2,* 319–322.

Martin, F. N., Krueger, J. S., & Bernstein, M. (1999). Diagnostic information transfer to hearing impaired adults. *Tejas, 16,* 29–32.

Martin, F. N., Severance, G. K., & Thibodeau, L. (1991). Insert earphones for speech recognition testing. *Journal of the American Academy of Audiology, 2,* 55–58.

Martin, N. A. (1946). Psychogenic deafness. *Annals of Otology, Rhinology & Laryngology, 55,* 81–89.

Matzker, J. (1959). Two new methods for the assessment of central auditory functions in cases of brain disease. *Annals of Otology, Rhinology & Laryngology, 68,* 1155–1197.

McKay, S., Gravel, J., & Tharpe, A. M. (2008). Amplification considerations for children with minimal or mild bilateral hearing loss and unilateral hearing loss. *Trends in Amplification, 12,* 43–54.

McKenna, L., Baguley, D. M., & McFerran, D. (2010). *Living with tinnitus and hyperacusis.* London: Sheldon Press.

McPherson, B. (2010). Innovative technology in hearing instruments: Matching needs in the developing world. *Trends in Amplification, 16,* 209–214.

Merzenich, M. M., Jenkins, W. M., Johnston, P., Schreiner, C., Miller, S. L., & Tallal, P. (1996). Temporal processing deficits of language-learning impaired children ameliorated by training. *Science, 271,* 77–81.

Metz, O. (1946). The acoustic impedance measured on normal and pathologic ears. *Acta Otolaryngologica* (Stockholm), Supplement 63, 3–254.

Metz, O. (1952). Threshold of reflex contraction of muscles of middle ear and recruitment of loudness. *Archives of Otolaryngology, 55,* 536–543.

Meyer, A. C., & Moser, T. (2010). Structure and function of cochlear afferent innervation. *Trends in Amplification, 14,* 170–191.

Meyer, C., & Hickson, L. (2012). What factors influence help-seeking for hearing impairment and hearing aid adoption in older adults? *International Journal of Audiology, 51,* 66–74.

Miller, E. (1989). Language impairment in Alzheimer's type dementia. *Clinical Psychology Review, 9,* 181–195.

Mills, J. H., Megerian, C. A., & Lambert, P. R. (2009). Presbyacusis and presbyastasis. In J. B. Snow Jr. & P. A. Wackym (Eds.), *Ballenger's otorhinolaryngology—head and neck surgery* (17th ed., pp. 333–342). Shelton, CT: BC Decker.

Milner, B., Taylor, S., & Sperry, R. (1968). Lateralized suppression of dichotically presented digits after commissural section in man. *Science, 161,* 184–185.

Miyamoto, R. T., & Kirk, K. I. (2001). Cochlear implants and other implantable auditory prostheses. In B. J. Bailey, K. H. Calhoun, G. B. Healy, H. C. Pillsbury, J. T. Johnson, R. T. Jackler, M. E. Tardy (Eds.), *Otolaryngology—head and neck surgery. Volume II* (3rd ed., pp. 1949–1959). Philadelphia: Lippincott Williams & Wilkins.

Mueller, G., & Killion, M. (1990). An easy method for calculating the Articulation Index. *The Hearing Journal, 45,* 14–17.

Mueller, H. G. III, & Hall, J.W. III. (1998). *Audiologists' desk reference. Volume II: Audiologic management, rehabilitation, and terminology* (pp. 230–239). San Diego: Singular Publishing Group.

Mueller, H. G., Hawkins, D. B., & Northern, J. L. (1992). *Probe microphone measurements: Hearing aid selection and assessment.* San Diego: Singular Publishing Group.

Mukerji, S., Windsor, A. M., & Lee, D. J. (2010). Auditory brainstem circuits that mediate the middle ear reflex. *Trends in Amplification, 14,* 170–191.

Mullin, W. J., Gerace, W. J., Mestre, J. P., & Velleman, S. L. (2003). *Fundamentals of sound with applications to speech and hearing.* Boston: Allyn & Bacon.

Munro, K. J., & Agnew, N. (1999). A comparison of interaural attenuation with the Etymotic ER-3A insert earphone and the Telephonies TDH-39 supra-aural earphone. *British Journal of Audiology, 33,* 259–262.

Murray, D. J., & Hanson, J. V. (1992). Application of digital signal processing to hearing aids: A critical survey. *Journal of the American Academy of Audiology, 3,* 145–152.

Murray, M., Miller, R., Hujoel, P., & Popelka, G. R. (2011). Long-term safety and benefit of a new intraoral device for single-sided deafness. *Otology Neurotology, 32,* 1262–1269.

Musiek, F. E. (1983). Assessment of central auditory dysfunction: The dichotic digits test revisited. *Ear & Hearing, 4,* 79–83.

Musiek, F. E. (1986). Neuroanatomy, neurophysiology, and central auditory assessment. Part III. Corpus callosum and efferent pathways. *Ear and Hearing, 7,* 349–358.

Musiek, F. E., & Baran, J. A. (2007). *The auditory system: Anatomy, physiology, and clinical correlates.* Boston: Allyn & Bacon.

Musiek, F. E., Bornstein, S. P., & Rintelmann, W. F. (1995). Transient evoked otoacoustic emissions and pseudohypacusis. *Journal of the American Academy of Audiology, 6,* 293–301.

Musiek, F. E., & Chermak, G. D. (2007). *Handbook of (central) auditory processing disorder: Volume 1: Auditory neuroscience and diagnosis.* San Diego: Plural Publishing.

Musiek, F. E., Wilson, D. H., & Pinheiro, M. L. (1979). Audiological manifestations in "split-brain" patients. *Journal of the American Auditory Society, 5,* 25–29.

Myklebust, H. R. (1954). *Auditory disorders in children: A manual for the differential diagnosis.* New York: Grune and Stratton.

National Institute on Deafness and Other Communication Disorders (NIDCD). (2010). www.nidcd.nih.gov/health/ statistics/quick.htm

National Institutes of Health. (1993). *NIH Consensus Statement. Early identification of hearing impairment in infants and young children.* Online 1993, March 1-3, *11,*1–24.

National Institutes of Health Consensus Panel. (1991, December 11–13). Acoustic neuroma. *NIH Consensus Statement Online, 9* (40), 1–24.

National Institute of Neurological Disorders and Stroke, NINDS (www.ninds.nih.gov).

Nelson, D. I., Nelson, R. Y., Concha-Barrientos, C., & Fingerhut, M. (2005). The global burden of occupational noise-induced hearing loss. *American Journal of Industrial Medicine, 48,* 446–458.

Nelson, E. G., & Hinojosa, R. (2006). Presbycusis: A human temporal bone study of individuals with downward sloping audiometric patterns of hearing loss and review of the literature. *Laryngoscope, 116, Supplement 112,* 1–12.

Newby, H. A. (1979). *Audiology* (4th ed). Englewood Cliffs, NJ: Prentice-Hall.

Newman, C. W., Jacobson, G. P., & Spitzer, J. B. (1996). Development of the Tinnitus Handicap Inventory. *Archives of Otolarynoglogy-Head & Neck Surgery, 122,* 143–148.

Newman, L. (2005, October 5). Communication of clinical report of data from Speech-Language Pathology, Army Audiology and Speech Center, Walter Reed Army Medical Center.

Niemeyer, W., & Sesterhenn, G. (1974). Calculating the hearing threshold from the stapedial reflex threshold for different sound stimuli. *Audiology, 13,* 421–427.

NIH Consensus Panel. (1991, December 11–13). Acoustic neuroma. NIH Consensus Statement Online, *9* (40), 1–24.

Nilsson, M., Soli, S., & Sullivan, J. (1994). Development of the Hearing in Noise Test for the measurement of speech reception thresholds in quiet and in noise. *Journal of the Acoustical Society of America, 95,* 1085–1099.

Nitchie, E. B. (2007). *Lip-reading principles and practice.* Melbourne Australia: Book Jungle.

Nober, E. H. (1970). Cutile air and bone conduction thresholds of the deaf. *Exceptional Children, 36,* 571–579.

Norena, A. J., & Farley, B. J. (2013). Tinnitus-related neural activity: Theories of generation, propagation, and centralization. *Hearing Research, 295,* 161–171.

Oestreicher, E., Wolfgang, A., & Felix, D. (2002). Neurotransmission of the cochlear inner hair cell synapse: Implications for inner ear therapy. *Advances in Otorhinolaryngology, 59,* 131–193.

Ohlemiller, K. K. (2004). Age-related hearing loss: The status of Schuknecht's typology. *Current Opinions in Otolaryngology Head and Neck Surgery, 12,* 439–443.

Olsen, W., & Matkin, N. (1979). Speech audiometry. In W. F. Rintelmann (Ed.), *Hearing assessment* (pp. 133–206), Baltimore: University Park Press.

Olsen, W., & Noffsinger, D. (1974). Comparison of one new and two old tests of auditory adaptation. *Archives of Otolaryngology, 99,* 94–99.

Pacala, J. T., & Yueh, B. (2012). Hearing deficits in the older patient: "I didn't notice anything." *Journal of the American Medical Association, 307,* 1185–1194.

Pai, I., Kelleher, C., Nunn, T., Pathak, N., Jindal, M., O'Connor, A. F., & Jiang, D. (2012). Outcome of bone-anchored hearing aids for single-sided deafness: A prospective study. *Acta Otolaryngologica, 132,* 751–755.

Paradise, J. L., Dollaghan, C. A., Campbell, T. F., Feldman, H. M., Bernard, B. S., Colborn, K., Rockette, H. E., Janoski J. E., Pitcairn, D. L., Sabo, D. L., Kurs-Lasky, M., & Smith, C. G. (2010). Language, speech sound production, and cognition in three-year-old children in the relation to otitis media in their first three years of life. *Pediatrics, 105,* 1119–1130.

Peck, J. E. (2011). *Pseudohypacusis: False and exaggerated hearing loss.* San Diego: Plural Publishing.

Pederson, O. T., & Studebaker, G. A. (1972). A new minimal contrasts closed-response-set speech test. *Journal of Auditory Research, 12,* 187–195.

Perez, R., de Almeida, J., Nedzelski, J. M., & Chen, J. M. (2009). Variations in the "Carhart notch" and overclosure after laser-assisted stapedotomy in otosclerosis. *Otology Neurotology, 30,* 1033–1036.

Perlman, H. B. (1938). Hyperacusis. *Annals of Otology, Rhinology & Laryngology, 47,* 947–953.

Pichora-Fuller, M. K., & Singh, G. (2006). Effects of age on auditory and cognitive processing: Implications for hearing aid fitting and audiologic rehabilitation. *Trends in Amplification, 10,* 29–59.

Pinheiro, M. L., & Tobin, H. (1969). Interaural intensity difference for intracranial lateralization. *Journal of the Acoustical Society of America, 46,* 1482–1487.

Pisoni, D. B., & Remez, R. (Eds.). (2005). *The handbook of speech perception.* Oxford: Blackwell.

Poe, D. S., & Gopen, Q. (2009). Eustachian tube dysfunction. In J. B. Snow Jr., & P. A. Wackym (Eds.), *Ballenger's otorhinolaryngology—head and neck surgery* (17th ed., pp. 201–208). Shelton, CT: BC Decker.

Pokorni, J. L., Worthington, C. K., & Jamison, P. J. (2004). Phonological awareness intervention: Comparison of FastForWord, Earobics, and LiPS. *The Journal of Educational Research, 3,* 147–158.

Popelka, G. R. (2010). SoundBite hearing system by Sonitus Medical: A new approach to single-sided deafness. *Seminars in Hearing, 31,* 393–409.

Popelka, G. R., Derebery, J., Blevins, N. H., Murray, M., Moore, B. C., Sweetow, R. W., Wu, B., & Katsis, M. (2010). Preliminary evaluation of a novel bone-conduction device for single sided deafness. *Otology Neurotology, 31,* 492–497.

Post, J. C., & Kerschner, J. E. (2009). Otitis media and middle-ear effusions. In J. B. Snow Jr. & P. A. Wackym (Eds.), *Ballenger's otorhinolaryngology—head and neck surgery* (17th ed., pp. 209–227). Shelton, CT: BC Decker.

Pratt, S. R., Kuller, L., Talbott, E. O., McHugh-Pemu, K., Buhari, A. M., & Xu, X. (2009). Hearing loss in black and white elders: Results of the cardiovascular study. *Journal of Speech & Hearing Research, 52,* 973–989.

Psarommatis, I., Kontorinis, G., Kontrogiannis, A., Douniadakis, D., & Tsakanikos, M. (2009). Pseudohypacusis: The most frequent etiology of sudden hearing loss in children. *European Archives of Oto-Rhino-Laryngology, 266,* 1857–1861.

Ramesh, A.V., Panwar, S.S., Nilkanthan, A., Nair, S. & Mehra, P.R. (2012). Auditory neuropathy spectrum disorder: Its prevalence and audiological characteristics in an Indian tertiary hospital. *International Journal of Pediatric Otorhinolaryngology, 76,* 1351–1354.

Raphael, L. J., Borden, G. J., & Harris, K. S. (2006). *Speech science primer: Physiology, acoustics, and perception of speech* (5th ed.). Baltimore: Lippincott, Williams & Wilkins.

Rasmussen, J., Olsen, S. O., & Nielsen, L. H. (2012). Evaluation of long-term patient satisfaction and experience with the Baha^R bone conduction implant. *International Journal of Audiology, 51,* 194–199.

Reger, S. (1935). Loudness level contours and intensity discrimination of ears with raised auditory threshold. *Journal of the Acoustical Society of America, 7,* 73.

Reger, S. N., & Kos, C. M. (1952). Clinical measurements and implications of recruitment. *Annals of Otology, Rhinology & Laryngology, 61,* 810–823.

Ricci, G., Volpe, A. D., Faralli, M., Longari, F., Lancione, C., Varricchio, A. M., & Frenguelli, A. (2011). Bone-anchored hearing aids (Baha) in congenital aural atresia: Personal experience. *International Journal of Pediatric Otorhinolaryngology, 75,* 342–346.

Ricketts, T. A. (2000). Impact of noise source configuration on directional hearing aid benefit and performance. *Ear and Hearing, 21,* 194–205.

Ricketts, T. A., De Chicchis, A., & Bess, F. H. (2001). Hearing aids and assistive listening devices. In B. J. Bailey, K. H. Calhoun, G. B. Healy, H. C. Pillsbury, J. T. Johnson, R. T. Jackler, & M. E. Tardy (Eds.), *Otolaryngology—head and neck surgery. Volume II* (3rd ed., pp. 1961–1972). Philadelphia: Lippincott Williams & Wilkins.

Ricketts, T. A., & Mueller, H. G. (1999). Making sense of directional microphone hearing aids. *American Journal of Audiology, 8,* 117–127.

Riedner, E. D., & Efros, P. L. (1995). Nonorganic hearing loss and child abuse: Beyond the sound booth. *British Journal of Audiology, 29,* 195–197.

Rintelmann, W. F., & Harford, E. R. (1963). The detection and assessment of pseudohypacusis among school-age children. *Journal of Speech and Hearing Disorders, 28,* 141–152.

Ritenour, A. E., Wickley, A., Ritenour, J. S., Kriete, B. R., Blackbourne, L. H., Holcomb, J. B., & Wade, C. E. (2009). Tympanic membrane perforation and hearing loss from blast overpressure in Operation Enduring Freedom and Operation Iraqi Freedom wounded. *Journal of Trauma, 64,* S174–S178.

Roberts, J., Hunter, L., Gravel, J., Rosenfeld, R., Berman, S., Haggard, M., Hall, J., Lannon, C., Moore, D., Vernon-Feagans, L., & Wallace, I. (2004). Otitis media, hearing loss, and language learning: Controversies and current research. *Journal of Developmental & Behavioral Pediatrics, 25,* 110–122.

Robertson, D. (1984). Horseradish peroxidase injection of physiologically characterized afferent and efferent neurones in the guinea pig spiral ganglion. *Hearing Research, 13,* 113–121.

Roland, P. S., Easton, D., & Meyerhoff, W. L. (2001). Aging in the auditory and vestibular system. In B. J. Bailey, K. H. Calhoun, G. B. Healy, H. C. Pillsbury, J. T. Johnson, R. T. Jackler, & M. E. Tardy (Eds.), *Head and neck surgery—otolaryngology. Volume II* (3rd ed., pp. 1941–1947). Philadelphia: Lippincott Williams & Wilkins.

Roland, P. S., & Meyerhoff, W. L. (2001). Otosclerosis. In B. J. Bailey, K. H. Calhoun, G. B. Healy, H. C. Pillsbury, J. T. Johnson, R. T. Jackler, & M. E. Tardy (Eds.), *Head and neck surgery—otolaryngology. Volume II* (3rd ed., pp. 1829–1841). Philadelphia: Lippincott Williams & Wilkins.

Roland, P. S., & Pawlowski, K. S. (2009). Ototoxicity. In J. B. Snow Jr. & P. A. Wackym (Eds.), *Ballenger's otorhinolaryngology—head and neck surgery* (17th ed., pp. 273–278). Shelton, CT: BC Decker.

Roseberry-McKibbin, C. (1997). Working with linguistically and culturally diverse clients. In K. Shipley (Ed.), *Interviewing and counseling in communicative disorders* (pp. 151–173). Baltimore: Williams & Wilkins.

Rosenfeld, R. M., Brown, L., Cannon, C. R., et al. (2006). Clinical practice guideline: Acute otitis externa. *Otolaryngology—Head & Neck Surgery, 134,* S5–S23.

Ross, M., & Lerman, J. (1970). Picture identification test for hearing-impaired children. *Journal of Speech and Hearing Research, 13,* 44–53.

Russo, N. M., Hornickel, J., Nicol, T., Zeckler, S., & Kraus, N. (2010). Biological changes in auditory function following training in children with autism spectrum disorders. *Behavioral and Brain Functions, 6,* 60.

Russo, N. M., Nicol, T. G., Zecker, S. G., Hayes, E. A., & Kraus, N. (2005). Auditory training improves neural timing in the human brain. *Behavioural Brain Research, 156,* 95–103.

Ryals, B. M., & Rubel, E. W. (1988). Hair cell regeneration after acoustic trauma in adult coturnix quail. *Science, 240,* 1774–1776.

Ryan, A., & Dallos, P. (1975). Effect of absence of cochlear outer hair cells on behavioral auditory threshold. *Nature, 253,* 44–46.

Sanchez-Longo, L. P., Forster, F. M., & Auth, T. L. (1957). A clinical test for sound localization and its application. *Neurology, 7,* 653–655.

Sanders, J.W. (1972). Masking. In J. Katz (Ed.), *Handbook of clinical audiology.* Baltimore: Williams & Wilkins.

Sanders, J. W., & Hall, J. W. III. (1999). Clinical masking. In F. E. Musiek & W. F. Rintelmann (Eds.), *Contemporary perspectives in hearing assessment* (pp. 67–87). Boston: Allyn & Bacon.

Saunders, G., & Echt, K. (2007). An overview of dual sensory impairment in older adults: Perspectives for rehabilitation. *Trends in Amplification, 11,* 243–258.

Savage, J., & Waddell, A. (2012, February 3). *Tinnitus.* Clinical evidence (Online). Retrieved February 3, 2012, from www.ncbi.nlm.nih.gov/pubmed/22331367

Schaub, A. (2008). *Digital hearing aids.* New York: Thieme Medical Publishers.

Schuknecht, H., & Woellner, R. (1955). An experimental and clinical study of deafness from lesions of the cochlear nerve. *Journal of Laryngology, 69,* 75–97.

Schuknecht, H. F. (1964). Further observations on the pathology of presbycusis. *Archives of Otolaryngology, 80,* 369–382.

Schuknecht, H. F. (1993). *Pathology of the ear* (2nd ed). Philadelphia: Lea & Febiger.

Schultz, M. S., & Schubert, E. D. (1969). A multiple choice discrimination test (MCDT). Laryngoscope, 79, 382–399.

Schum, D. J. (2010, March/April). Wireless connectivity for hearing aids. *Advance for Audiologists,* 24–26. Retrieved September 15, 2012, from www.advance-web.com/aud

Schwaber, M. K., & Hall, J . W. III. (1992). Cochleo-vestibular nerve compression syndrome: I. Clinical features and audiovestibular findings. *Laryngoscope, 102,* 1020–1029.

Schwander, M., Kachar, B., & Muller, U. (2010). Review series: The cell biology of hearing. *Journal of Cell Biology, 190, 9*–20.

Schweitzer, C. (1997). Development of digital hearing aids. *Trends in Amplification, 2,* 41–77.

Seewald, R. (1992). The desired sensation level method for fitting children: version 3.0. *Hearing Journal, 45,* 36–41.

Selters, W. A., & Brackmann, D. E. (1977). Acoustic tumor detection with brain stem electric response audiometry. *Archives of Otolaryngology, 103,* 181–187.

Shambaugh, F. E., Jr., & Scott, A. (1964). Sodium fluoride for arrest of otosclerosis. *Archives of Otolaryngology, 80,* 263.

Shargorodsky, J., Curhan, S. G., Curhan, G. C., & Eavey, R. (2010). Change in prevalence of hearing loss in US adolescents. *Journal of the American Medical Association, 304,* 772–778.

Shockley, W. W., & Stucker, F. J. (1987). Squamous cell carcinoma of the external ear: A review of 75 cases. *Otolarynoglogy—Head & Neck Surgery, 97,* 308–312.

Sinha, S. (1959). *The role of the temporal lobe in hearing.* Master's thesis. McGill University.

Sivian, L. J., & White, S. D. (1933). Minimal audible sound fields. *Journal of the Acoustical Society of America, 4,* 288–321.

Sklare, D. A., & Denenberg, L. J. (1987). Interaural attenuation for tubephone insert earphones. *Ear and Hearing, 8,* 298–300.

Smith, R. J. H., Kochhar, A., & Friedman, R. A. (2009). Hereditary hearing impairment. In J. B. Snow Jr. & P. A. Wackym (Eds.), *Ballenger's otorhinolaryngology—head and neck surgery* (17th ed., pp. 289–303). Shelton, CT: BC Decker.

Snik, A., Verhaegen, V., Mulder, J., & Cremers, C. (2010). Cost-effectiveness of implantable middle ear hearing devices. *Advances in Otorhinolaryngology, 69,* 14–19.

Snyder, J. M. (1973). Interaural attenuation characteristics in audiometry. *Laryngoscope, 73,* 1847–1855.

Soli, S. (2008). Some thoughts on communication handicap and hearing impairment. *International Journal of Audiology, 47* (6), 285–286.

Speaks, C., & Jerger, J. (1965). Method for measurement of speech identification. *Journal of Speech & Hearing Research, 8,* 185–194.

Sprinzl, G. M., & Riechelmann, H. (2010). Current trends in treating hearing loss in elderly people: A review of the technology and treatment options—a mini-review. *Gerontology, 56,* 351–358.

Staab, W. J., & Lybarger, S. F. (1994). Characteristics and use of hearing aids. In J. Katz (Ed.), *Handbook of clinical audiology* (4th ed., pp. 657–722). Baltimore: Williams & Wilkins.

Stapells, D. R. (2000). Threshold estimation by tone-evoked auditory brainstem response: A literature meta-analysis. *Journal of Speech-Language Pathology and Audiology, 24,* 74–83.

Starr, A., & Achor, L. J. (1975). Auditory brainstem responses in neurological diseases. *Archives of Neurology, 32,* 761–768.

Starr, A., Picton, T. W., Sininger, Y. S., Hood, L. J., & Berlin, C. I. (1996). Auditory neuropathy. *Brain, 119,* 741–753.

Steiger, J. R. (2005). Audiologic referral criteria: sample clinic guidelines. *The Hearing Journal, 58,* 38–42.

Stevens, S. S. (1935). The relation of pitch to intensity. *Journal of the Acoustical Society of America, 6,* 150–154.

Stevens, S. S., Volkman, J., & Newman, E. (1937). A scale for the measurement of the psychological magnitude pitch. *Journal of the Acoustical Society of America, 8,* 185–190.

Stewart, C. M., Clark, J. H., & Niparko, J. K. (2011). Bone-anchored devices in single-sided deafness. *Advances in Otorhinolaryngology, 71,* 92–102.

Stewart, D., Mehl, A., Hall, J. W. III, Carroll, M., & Bramlett, J. (2000). Newborn hearing screening with automated auditory brainstem response (AABR): A multisite study. *Journal of Perinatology, 20,* s128–s131.

Stockard, J. J., & Rossiter, V. S. (1977). Clinical and pathologic correlates of brain stem auditory response abnormalities. *Neurology, 27,* 316–325.

Strasnick, B., Glasscock, M. E., Haynes, D. S., McMenomey, S. O., & Minor, L. B. (1994). The natural history of untreated acoustic neuromas. *Laryngoscope, 104,* 1115–1119.

Strouse, A,. Hall, J. W. III, & Berger, M. (1995). Central auditory processing in Alzheimer's disease. *Ear & Hearing, 16,* 230–238.

Strunk, C. L., & Lambert, P. R. (2001). Intratemporal and intracranial complications of otitis media. In B. J. Bailey, K. H. Calhoun, G. B. Healy, H. C. Pillsbury, J. T. Johnson, R. T. Jackler, M. E. Tardy (Eds.), *Head and neck surgery—otolarynoglogy. Volume II* (3rd ed., pp. 1787–1797). Philadelphia: Lippincott Williams & Wilkins.

Studebaker, G. A. (1962). On masking in bone-conduction testing. *Journal of Speech and Hearing Research, 5,* 215–227.

Studebaker , G. A. (1967). Clinical masking of the non-test ear. *Journal of Speech and Hearing Disorders, 32,* 360–371.

Studebaker, G. A. (1967). Intertest variability and the air bone gap. *Journal of Speech and Hearing Disorders, 32,* 82–86.

Surr, R. K., Montgomery, A. A., & Mueller, H. G. (1985). Effect of amplification on tinnitus among new hearing aid users. *Ear and Hearing,* 6, 71–75.

Swanepoel, D., Clark, J. L., Koekemoer, D., Hall, J. W. III, Krumm, M., Ferrari, D. V., McPherson, B., Olusanya, B. O., Mars, M., Russo, I., & Barajas, J. J. (2010). Tele-health in audiology: The need and potential to reach underserved populations. *International Journal of Audiology,* 49, 195–202.

Swanepoel, D., Clark, J. L., Koekemoer, D., Hall, J. W., III, Krumm, M., Ferrari, D. V., McPherson, B., Olusanya, B. O., Mars, M., Russo, I., & Barajas, J. J. (2010). Tele-health in audiology: The need and potential to reach underserved populations. *International Journal of Audiology, 49,* 195–202.

Swanepoel, D., & Hall, J. W. III. (2010). A systematic review of telehealth applications in audiology. *Telemedicine and e-Health, 16,* 181–200.

Swanepoel, D., & Louw, B. (Eds.). (2010). *HIV/AIDS related communication, hearing, and swallowing disorders.* San Diego: Plural Publishing.

Swanepoel, D., Storbeck, C., & Friedland, P. (2009). Early hearing detection and intervention in South Africa. *International Journal of Pediatric Otolaryngology, 73,* 783–786.

Sweetow, R. W., & Palmer, C. V. (2005). Efficacy of individual auditory training in adults: A systematic review. *Journal of the American Academy of Audiology, 16,* 494–504.

Sweetow, R. W., & Sabes, J. H. (2006). The need for and development of an adaptive listening and communication enhancement (LACE™) program. *Journal of the American Academy of Audiology, 17,* 538–558.

Tarazi, F. I., & Schetz, J. A. (Eds.). (2011). *Neurological and psychiatric disorders.* New York: Humana Press.

Terkildsen, K., Huis in't Veld, F., & Osterhammel, P. (1977). Auditory brainstem responses in the diagnosis of cerebellopontine angle tumors. *Scandinavian Audiology, 6,* 43–47.

Terkildsen, K., & Nielson, S. (1960). An electroacoustic impedance measuring bridge for clinical use. *Archives of Otolaryngology, 72,* 339–346.

Terkildsen, K., & Thomsen, K. A. (1959). The influence of pressure variations on the impedance of the human eardrum. *Journal of Laryngology & Otology, 73,* 409–418.

Tharpe, A. M. (2007). Unilateral hearing loss in children: A mountain or molehill? *The Hearing Journal, 7,* 10, 14–16.

Thomsen, J., Terkildsen, K., & Osterhammel, P. (1978). Auditory brain stem responses in patients with acoustic neuromas. *Scandinavian Audiology, 7,* 179–183.

Thornton, A. R., & Raffin, M. J. M. (1978). Speech discrimination scores modeled as a binomial variable. *Journal of Speech and Hearing Research, 21,* 507–518.

Tillman, T., & Carhart, R. (1966). *An expanded test for speech discrimination utilizing CNC monosyllabic words: Northwestern University Test No. 6.* Brooks Air Force Base, TX: USAF School of Aerospace Medicine Technical Report.

Tillman, T. W. R., Carhart, R., & Wilber, L. (1963). *A test for speech discrimination composed on CNC monosyllabic words. Northwestern University Auditory Test No. 4. Technical Documentary Report No. SAM-TDR-62-135.* Brooks Air Force Base, TX: USAF School of Aerospace Medicine.

Tonndorf, J. (1964). Animal experiments on bone conduction: Clinical conclusions. *Annals of Otology, Rhinology & Laryngology, 73,* 659–678.

Trotter, M. I., & Donaldson, I. (2008). Hearing aids and tinnitus therapy: A 25-year experience. *The Journal of Laryngology & Otology, 128,* 1052–1056.

Tye-Murray, N. (2008). *Foundations of aural rehabilitation: Children, adults, and their family members* (3rd ed.). Clifton Park, NY: Delmar Cengage Publishing.

Ullrich, K., & Grimm, D. (1976). Most comfortable listening level presentation versus maximum discrimination for word discrimination material. *Audiology, 15,* 338–347.

Valente, M. (Ed.). (2002). *Strategies for selecting hearing aids and verifying hearing aid fittings.* New York: Thieme Medical Publishers.

Valente, M., Abrams, H., Benson, D., Chisolm, T., Citron, D., Hampton, D., Loavenbruck, A., Ricketts, T., Solodar, H., & Sweetow, R. (2006). Guidelines for the audiologic management of adult hearing impairment. *Audiology Today, 18,* 32–36.

Van Camp, K. J., Margolis, R. H., Wilson, R. H., Creten, W. L., & Shanks, J. E. (1986). Principles of tympanometry. *ASHA Monograph, 24.*

Van Hecke, H. I. (1994). Emotional responses to hearing loss. In J. G. Clark & F. N. Martin (Eds.), *Effective counseling in audiology: Perspectives and practice* (pp. 93–115). Englewood Cliffs NJ: Prentice Hall.

Ventry, I. M., Chaiklin, J. B., & Dixon, R. F. (Eds.). (1971). *Hearing measurement: A book of readings.* New York: Appleton-Century-Crofts.

Ventry, I. M., & Weinstein, B. E. (1982). The Hearing Handicap Inventory for the Elderly: A new tool. *Ear and Hearing, 3,* 128–134.

Verhagen, C. V. M., Hol, M. K. S., Coppens-Schellekens, W., Snik, A. F. M., & Cremers, C. W. R. (2008). The Baha softband: A new treatment for young children with bilateral congenital aural atresia. *International Journal of Pediatric Otorhinolaryngology, 72,* 1455–1459.

Verhaegen, V. J., Mulder, J. J., Cremers, C. W., & Snik, A. F. (2012). Application of active middle ear implants in patients with severe mixed hearing loss. *Otology Neurotology, 33,* 297–301.

Verhaert, N., Fuchsmann, C., Tringali, S., Lina-Granade, G., & Truy, E. (2011). Strategies of active middle ear implants for hearing rehabilitation in congenital aural atresia. *Otology Neurotology, 32,* 639–645.

Vrabec, J. T. (2001). Surgical management of vestibular disorders. In B. J. Bailey, K. H. Calhoun, G. B. Healy, H. C. Pillsbury, J. T. Johnson, R. T. Jackler, & M. E. Tardy (Eds.), *Head and neck surgery—otolaryngology. Volume II* (3rd ed., pp. 2011–2019). Philadelphia: Lippincott Williams & Wilkins.

Wackym, P. A., Balaban, C. D., & Schumacher, T. S. (2001). Medical management of vestibular disorders and vestibular rehabilitation. In B. J. Bailey, K. H. Calhoun, G. B. Healy, H. C. Pillsbury, J. T. Johnson, R. T. Jackler, & M. E. Tardy (Eds.), *Head and neck surgery—otolaryngology. Volume II* (3rd ed., pp. 1993–2010). Philadelphia: Lippincott Williams & Wilkins.

Wackym, P. A., & Runge-Samuelson, C. (2009). Cochlear and auditory brainstem implantation. In J. B. Snow Jr. & P. A. Wackym (Eds.), *Ballenger's otorhinolaryngology—head and neck surgery* (17th ed., pp. 363–388). Shelton CT: BC Decker.

Walsh, F. (1996). The concept of family resilience: Crisis and challenge. *Family Process, 35,* 261–281.

Waltzman, S. B., & Roland, J. T. Jr. (2009). *Cochlear implants.* New York: Thieme Medical Publishers.

Wazen, J. J., Spitzer, J. B., Ghossaini, S. N., Fayad, J. N., Niparko, J. K., Cox, K., Brackmann, D. E., & Soli, S. D. (2003). Transcranial contralateral cochlear stimulation in unilateral deafness. *Otolaryngology-Head & Neck Surgery, 129,* 248–254.

Weaver, E. G., & Bray, C. W. (1930). Auditory nerve impulses. *Science, 71,* 215.

Wegel, R. L. (1931). A study of tinnitus. *Archives of Otolaryngology, 14,* 158–165.

Wegel, R. L., & Lane, G. I. (1924). The auditory masking of one pure tone by another and its probable relation to the dynamics of the inner ear. *Physiological Review, 23,* 266–285.

Weinstein, B., Spritzer, J., & Ventry, I. (1986). Test-retest reliability of the Hearing Handicap for the Elderly. *Ear & Hearing, 7,* 295–299.

Welling, D. B., & Packer, M. D. (2009). Trauma to the middle ear, inner ear, and temporal bone. In J. B. Snow Jr. & P. A. Wackym (Eds.), *Ballenger's otorhinolaryngology—head and neck surgery* (17th ed., pp. 253–263). Shelton, CT: BC Decker.

Wiley, T. L., Chappell, R., Carmichael, L., Nondahl, D. M., & Cruickshanks, K. J. (2008). Changes in hearing thresholds over 10 years in older adults. *Journal of the American Academy of Audiology, 19,* 281–292.

Wilson, R. H. (2003). Development of a speech in multitalker babble paradigm to assess word-recognition performance. *Journal of the American Academy of Audiology. 14,* 453–470.

Wilson, R. H., & Burks, C. A. (2005). Use of 35 words for evaluation of hearing loss in signal-to-babble ratio: A clinical protocol. *Journal of Rehabilitation Research & Development, 42,* 839–852.

Wilson, R. H., & Cates, W. B. (2008). A comparison of two word-recognition tasks in multitalker babble: Speech recognition in noise test (SPRINT) and

Words-in-Noise Test (WIN). *Journal of the American Academy of Audiology, 19,* 548–556.

Wilson, R. H., & Margolis, R. H. (1983). Measurements of auditory thresholds for speech stimuli. In D. F. Konkle & W. F. Rintelmann (Eds.), *Principles of speech audiometry* (pp. 79–126). Baltimore: University Park Press.

Wilson, R. H., McArdle, R. A., & Smith, S. L. (2007). An evaluation of the BKB-SIN, HINT, Quick SIN, and WIN materials on listeners with normal hearing and listeners with hearing loss. *Journal of Speech, Language, and Hearing Research, 50,* 844–856.

Wilson, R. H., & Strouse, A. L. (1999). Auditory measures with speech signals. In F. E. Musiek & W. F. Rintelmann (Eds.), *Contemporary perspectives in hearing assessment* (pp. 21–66). Boston: Allyn & Bacon.

Wolfe, J., & Schafer, E. C. (2010). *Programming cochlear implants* (pp. 115–127). San Diego: Plural Publishing.

Wolframm, M. D., Giarbini, N., & Streitberger, C. (2012). Speech-in-noise and subjective benefit with active middle ear implant omni-directional microphones: A within-subjects comparison. *Otology Neurotology, 33,* 618–622.

Woodson, E. A., Reiss, L. A., Turner, C. W., Gfeller, K., & Gantz, B. J. (2010). The Hybrid cochlear implant: A review. *Advances in Otorhinolaryngology, 67,* 125–134.

World Health Organization (WHO). (2011). *Burden of disease from environmental noise—Quantification of healthy life years lost in Europe.* Bonn: The WHO European Centre for Environment and Health.

Yacullo, W. S. (1999). Clinical masking in speech audiometry: A simplified approach. *American Journal of Audiology, 8,* 106–116.

Yogev, R., & Tan, T. (2011). Meningococcal disease: The advances and challenges of meningococcal disease prevention. *Human Vaccines, 8,* 828–837.

Yoshinaga-Itano, C. (2003). From screening to early identification and intervention: Discovering predictors to successful outcomes for children with significant hearing loss. *Journal of Deaf Students and Deaf Education, 8,* 11– 30.

Yoshinaga-Itano, C., Sedley, A. L., Coulter, D. K., & Mehl, A. L. (1998). Language of early- and later-identified children with hearing loss. *Pediatrics, 102,* 1161–1171.

Zapala, D. A., Stamper, G. C., Shelfer, J. S., Walker, D. A., Karatayli-Ozgursoy, S., Ozgursoy, O. B., & Hawkins, D. B. (2010). Safety of audiology direct access for Medicare patients complaining of hearing impairment. *Journal of the American Academy of Audiology, 21,* 365–379.

Zheng, X. Y., Shen, W., He, D. Z., Long, K. B., Madison, I. D., & Dallos, P. (2000). Prestin is the motor protein of cochlear outer hair cells. *Nature, 405,* 149–155.

Zwicker, E., & Harris, F. P. (1990). Psychoacoustical and ear canal cancellation of (2f1-f2)-distortion products. *Journal of the Acoustical Society of America, 87,* 2583–2591.

Zwislocki, J. (1953). Acoustic attenuation between ears. *Journal of the Acoustical Society of America, 25,* 752–759.

Zwislocki, J. (1963). An acoustic method for clinical examination of the ear. *Journal of Speech and Hearing Research, 6,* 303–314.

Author Index

Subject Index